THE UNIQUE HERBAL

NEW INSIGHTS INTO ANCIENT MEDICINES

VOLUME FOUR (M-R)

ROBERT DALE ROGERS (RH) AHG

CONTENTS

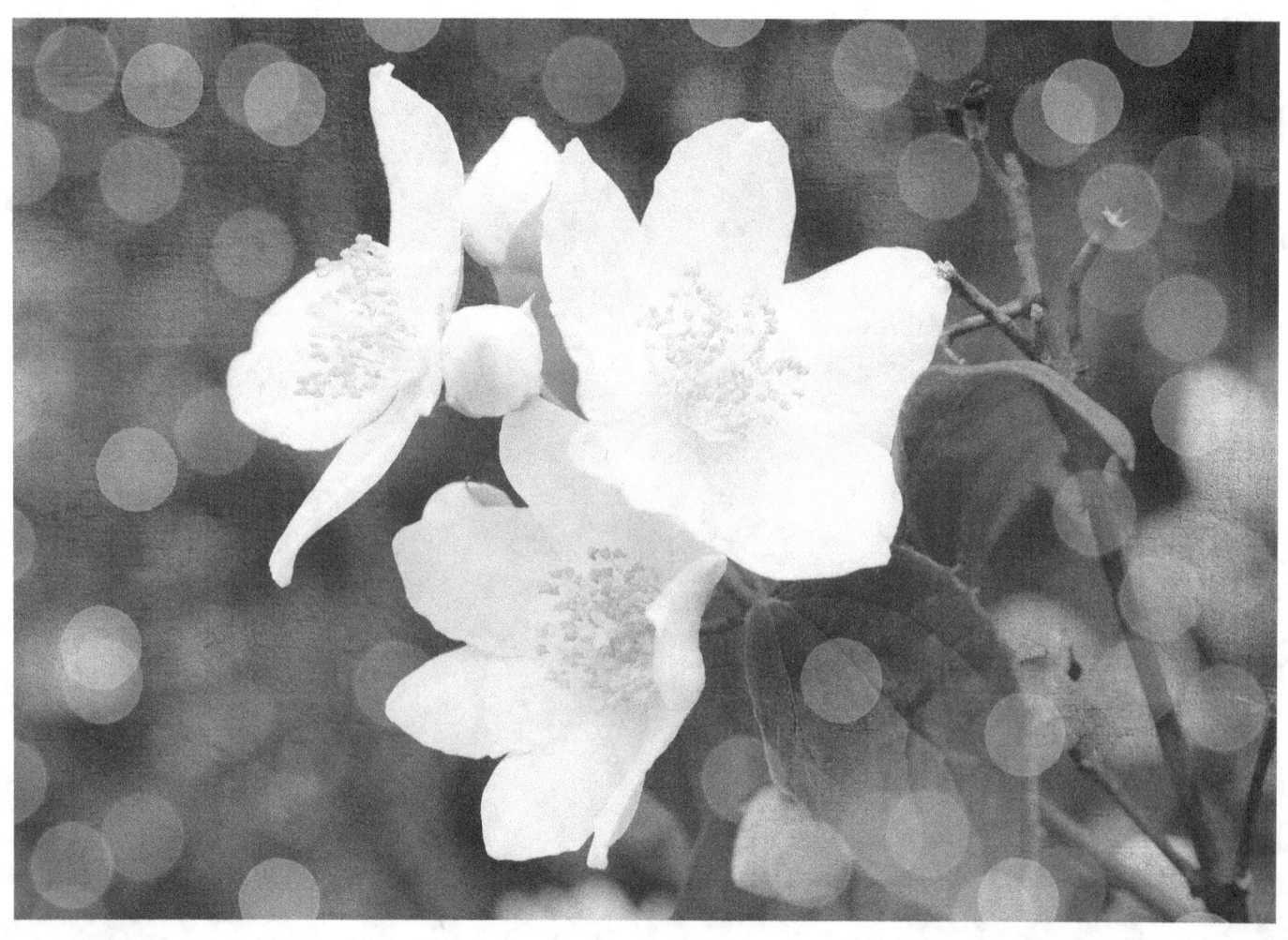

INTRODUCTION

Over the years, I have accumulated some information, a bit of knowledge and even a little wisdom about medicinal plants.

Many of the healing herbs in this volume set are relatively unknown; and some are little used in day-to-day clinical practice. Some are well known, but not utilized to their full extent of possibilities.

It is my hope that these pages may lead to a new and expanded materia medica, and a wider appreciation of many, often neglected, overlooked, and useful medicinal plants.

North American herbals tend to repeat, with increasingly useful additions, the same hundred or so plant medicines. The purpose of this book is to expand that awareness and hope that other herbalists will begin to look at the plants in their backyard and explore, observe and experience for themselves.

In turn, we could reconnect and continue the work begun in past centuries by the Eclectics and other plant people.

Like some of my previous publications, this book records indigenous use of medicinal herbs, garnered respectfully from the oral tradition, as well as work by various cultures around the world, the Eclectic physicians, modern herbalists, and recent scientific findings on various plant constituents.

It also includes homeopathic usage, essential oils, hydrosols, gemmotherapy, flower essences, personality traits, spiritual properties and astrological correspondences.

Please contact me if you wish to contribute; I am always learning.

Some Other Books by Robert Dale Rogers - www.amazon.com/author/robertdalerogers

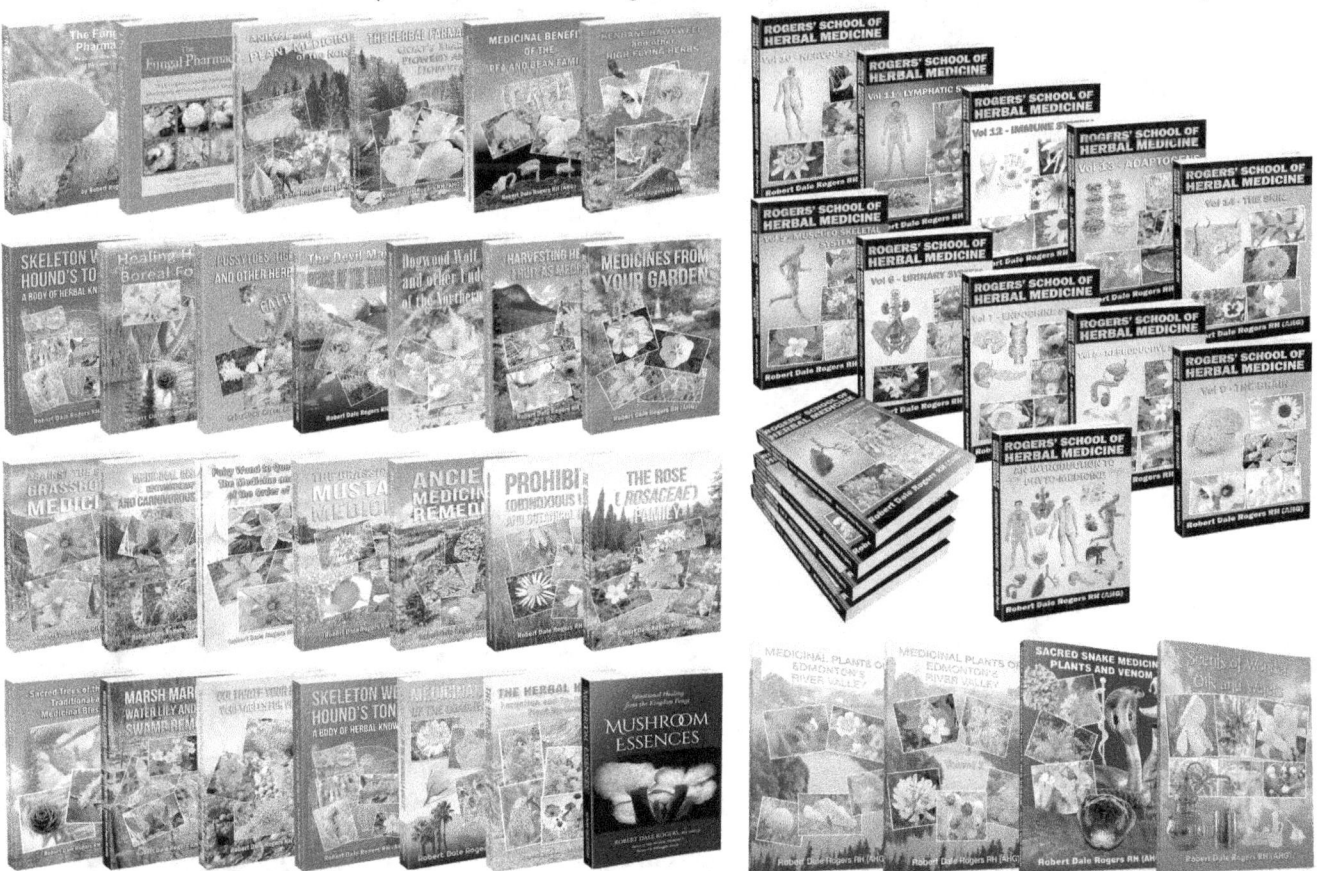

www.selfhealdistributing.com or www.scentsofwonder.ca - email: scents@telusplanet.net - Fax: 1 780-439-9540

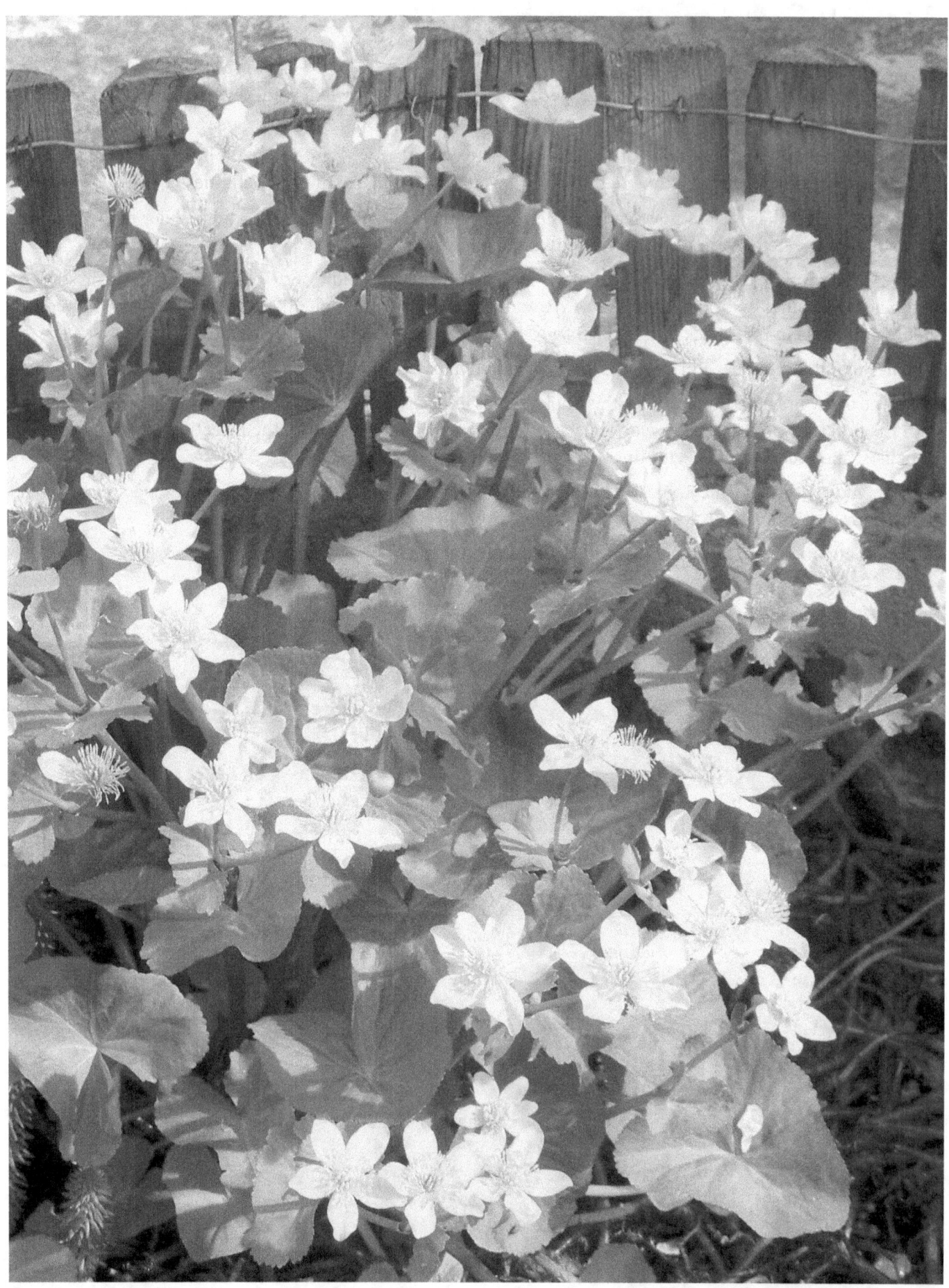

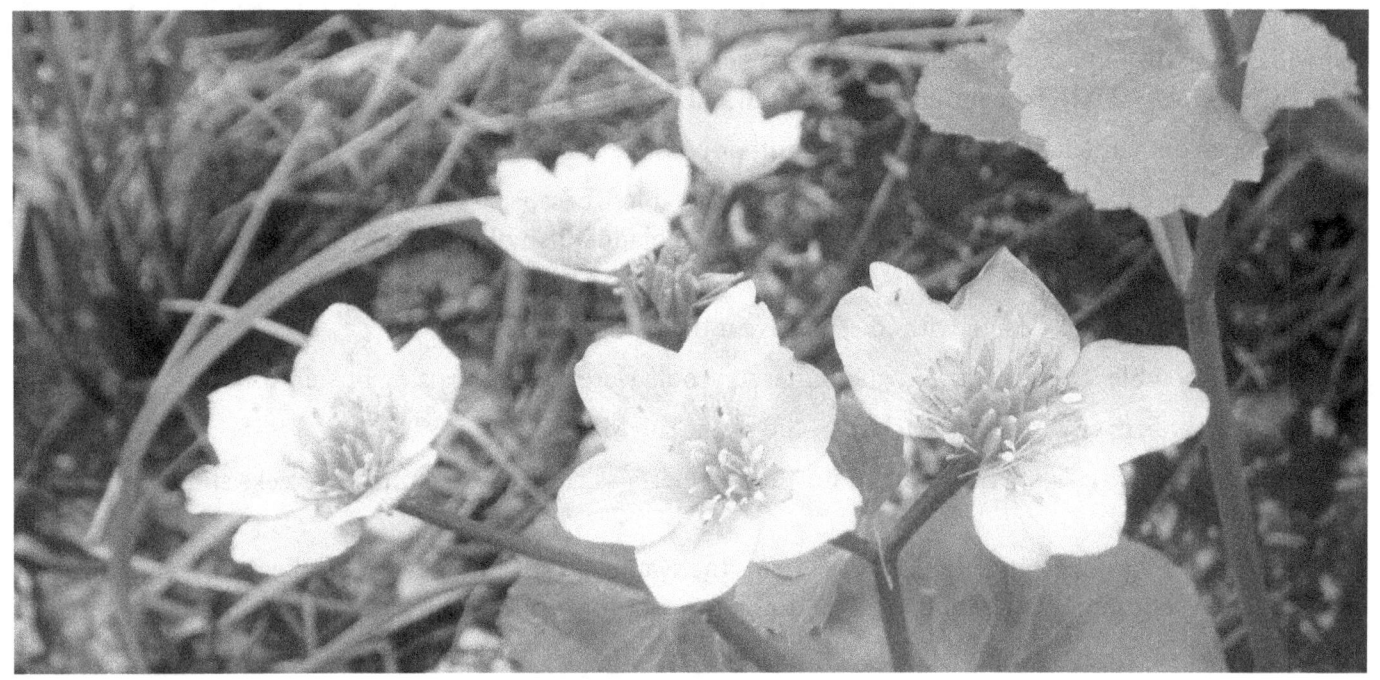

MARSH MARIGOLD

MARSH MARIGOLD
KING CUPS
(*Caltha palustris* L.)
(*C. arctica* R. Brown) not accepted
(*C. palustris ssp.arctica* [R. Br.] Hult.) not accepted
WHITE MARSH MARIGOLD
MOUNTAIN MARIGOLD
(*C. leptosepala* DC.)
(*C. biflora* DC.) not accepted
(*C. howellii* Huth.) not accepted
FLOATING MARSH MARIGOLD
(*C. natans* Pall.)
(*Thacla natans* [Pall. ex Georgi] Deyl & Sojak) not accepted
PARTS USED- flowers, leaves

O velvet bee! You're a dusty fellow!
You've powdered your legs with gold.
O brave marsh marybuds, rich and yellow.
Give me your money to hold.   **JEAN INGELOW**

"And the Wild Marsh-Marigold shines like fire
in swamps and hollows gray".   **TENNYSON**

"King cups by the river, so shiny you'd think the bees
Could see their faces in them".   **JOHN MOORE**

Caltha is from the Greek **KALATHOS**, meaning goblet. Or from **CALATHUS**, a small round twig basket made 2000 years ago. Persephone was collecting wild flowers in a Calathus when carried off by Pluto. Palustris means, "of the marsh or wet place".

1

Marsh Marigold and Marybuds date back to the Middles Ages, when the plant was dedicated to the Virgin Mary, and widely used in Church celebrations. It may be derived from the Anglo Saxon **MERSC**, a marsh; along with **MEARGEALLA**, **MEARH** meaning horse, and **GEALLA**, meaning a gall or blister.

The Anglo Saxon name for marsh, **MERE**, is another possible derivation.

It was at one time called Meargealla, a horse blob, or Mare-Blob, because the tight round buds suggested a round swelling. This derives from **MERE** a marsh, and **BLOB** a bladder. An older name **VERRUCARIA** is related to its use of burning off warts.

The habit of opening and closing with the sun gave it the name **SOLSEQUIA**.

The flowers resemble large buttercups, and buttercup roots were used for raising blisters as a counter-irritant.

The plant symbolizes "I wish I were rich", and the birth date March 9th.

I have found Marsh Marigold flowering in northern Alberta as early as mid April, in creeks still rimmed with ice and snow.

To some native tribes, the name translates as "opens the swamps." The Chippewa used the root decoction as an emetic, diaphoretic and expectorant. Women drank the root in combination with other herbs during times of separation from the other tribe members during menstruation.

The root tea was combined with wild currant stems to treat colds.

The Ojibwa mixed the plant tea with maple syrup as a cough syrup that was popular amongst early European settlers.

Poultices of the boiled and mashed roots were applied to wounds and sores. In Russia, the plant was used for dressing and cleansing skin lesions and sores.

The Iroquois infused the smashed roots and drank it to vomit and antidote a love charm. Infusions of the leaves and stalk were added to combinations when a diuretic was required. The Onondaga called the plant **GANAWAHA'KS** meaning, "makes a hole in the swamp."

Eskimos of Alaska used (dry) leaf infusions to relieve constipation.

In Europe, farmers would hang the flowers over their houses and barns on May Day to protect them from fairies and witches. Garlands were woven to wear on this celebration of fertility and growth.

In Ireland and the Isle of Man, the flower garlands are still used in May Day celebrations.

The leaves make an acceptable potherb if picked early, and BOILED several times, discarding the water with each cooking. The plant contains protoanemonin, like the buttercups. The toxin is only removed by boiling, or thoroughly drying the plant.

In Ireland, the flowers were boiled into a posset or soup for heart ailments, and the stewed leaves applied to boils. In Scotland, a tincture of the whole plant in flower was used for anemia.

Robert Cooper was a close friend of Clarke and Compton Burnett, and a low potency prescriber in a fashion similar to Dr. Edward Bach of flower essence fame a few decades later. The Three C's (The Cooper Club) met regularly and exchanged cases and accounts of their findings.

Clarke wrote. "Cooper has used *Caltha palustris* with excellent effect in a case of uterine cancer, giving single doses of the mother tincture at long intervals."

The waxy, yellow flowers are a symbol of spring in the north.

They look exotic enough to be in the Amazon basin, and yet can survive the most extreme winters. Louis Lewin, in his 1924 publication, *Phantastica*, mentioned the indigenous people of southern Brazil smoked the leaves of *Caltha palustris*.

The herb is used in Asian medicine to treat arthritis and rheumatism.

The blossoms have been used as an ingredient in hair rinses and dry skin lotions. The flowers are infused and combined with fresh cream, for improving facial complexion.

The young buds are picked before opening, and preserved in vinegar, are used as a caper substitute.

The roots can be dug and boiled as an emergency food, suggested by some people to be similar in taste to sauerkraut.

The Mountain Marsh Marigold, or Elkslip can be used identically for food. They differ in that they have beautiful, white blossoms that sometimes poke up through the snow. Even more beautiful are the small, blue buds that precede the flowers. As the name suggests, it is only found in the mountains.

The root was chewed or crushed by various native tribes and used as a poultice to reduce inflammation and pain.

Floating Marsh Marigold can be found in the same areas as *C. palustris*, but has small white or pink sepals.

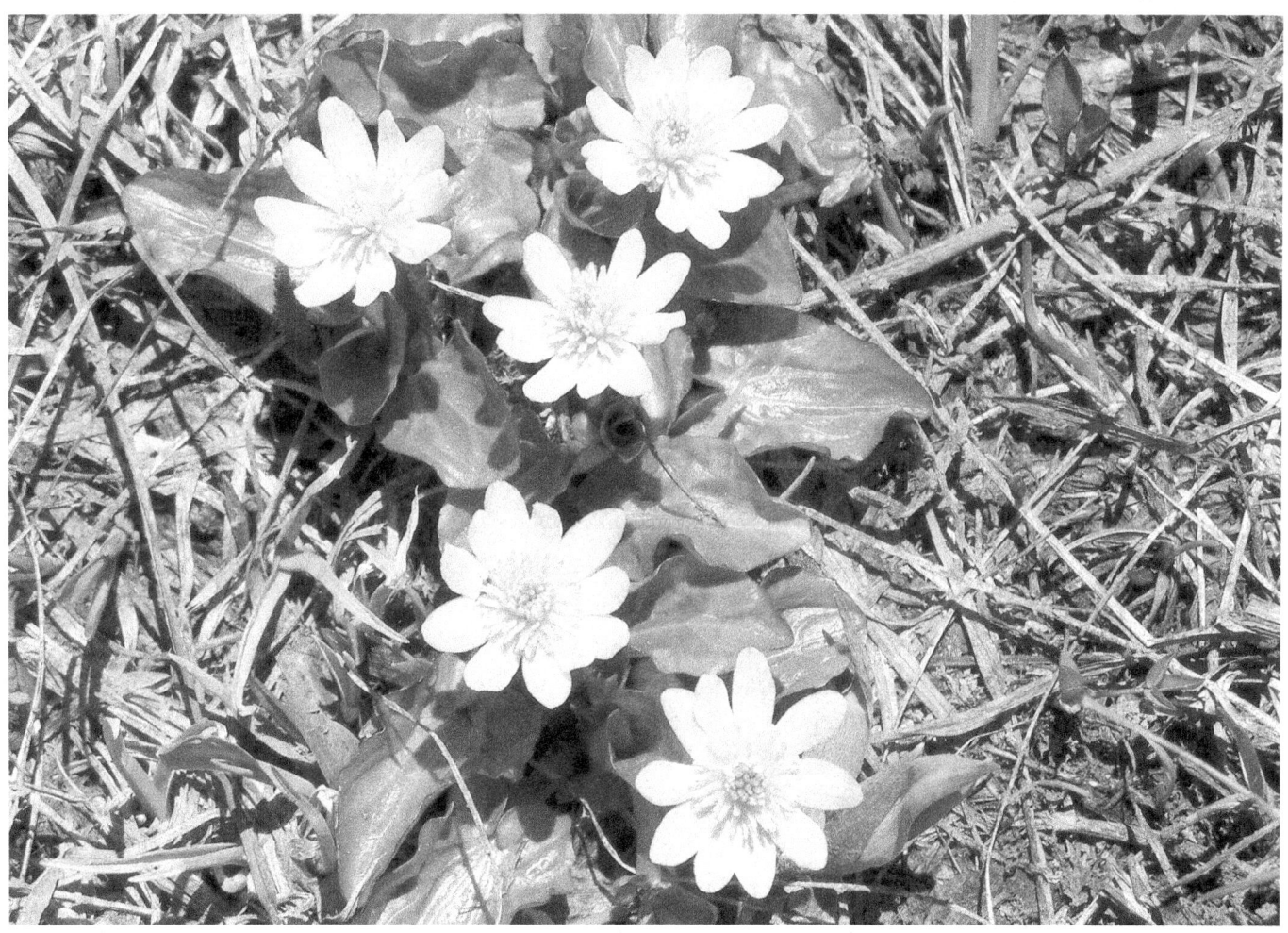

MOUNTAIN MARSH MARIGOLD

MEDICINAL

CONSTITUENTS- protoanemonin (0.3 mg/kg fresh weight), anemonin, caltholide, epi-caltholide, hederagenin and its acid, palustroside, saponins, choline, flavones, including sitosterol and its glucoside, and 16,17-dihydroxykauran-19-oic acid. Triterpene saponins, and lactones including calthoid and palustrolid; isoquinoline alkaloids (aphorine type) including corytuberin, mangoflorine and protopine; as well as scopoletin, helleborine, isorhamnetin and xanthophyllepoxyl.
roots- five triterpene glycosides.

Early use of the plant was recorded by a Dr. Withing. "It would appear that medicinal properties may be evolved in the gaseous exhalations of the flowers...being put into the bedroom of a girl who had been subject to fits, the fits ceased." Afterwards, infusions of the flowers became a successful way to treat epilepsy in both children and adults.

Marsh Marigold is an irritant, rubefacient, and secretory stimulant. It helps stimulate the flow of mucous in the lungs, digestive tract and uterus; as well as loosening dry mucous in the bronchials and sinuses. It is used medicinally in the treatment of whooping cough, bronchial catarrh and dysmenorrhea.

Work by Golenera et al, in 1979 found Marsh Marigold possesses both anti-inflammatory and hypocholesterinic activity.

It combines well with gum weed, as an energetic expectorant after a sinus or bronchial infection. Michael Moore, noted herbalist, suggests that it is useful in relieving sinus infections caused by tooth infections of the upper jaw.

There is some mild anti-spasmodic activity that make hot poultices useful in lower back pain, and colonic spasms. Facial paralysis is relieved by an application of hot leaf poultices, combing well with cow parsnip seed or root for this purpose.

The fresh juice from the leaves has been used to remove warts.

The tincture, in small, well-diluted doses appears to be effective in anemia.

The dried aerial plant lowers cholesterol levels, and raises blood sugar levels in rats in oral dosage, according to some Russian studies.

Formaldehyde induced inflammation has been reduced with the topical use of plant preparations in unspecified manner.

Saponins from the whole plant have shown spermicidal activity in human semen. Human relevance is unknown, probably none.

Extracts of *C. palustris* were investigated for immuno-stimulatory and anti-tumor properties. Powdered plant material was extracted in methanol, and the methanol extract was discarded. The residue was extracted successively with water (fraction A), 0.1 M NaOH (fraction B), 5% CH_3COOH (fraction C), and 1 M NaOH (fraction D). Fractions C and D (100 mcg/ml) enhanced lymphocyte recruitment to the generation cycle, and increased PHA-stimulated human lymphocyte proliferation by about 25%.

Fraction B (100 mcg/ml) reduced the rate of mitosis by ca. 15%, and fraction A had no proliferative effect. Fractions A and C stimulated granulocyte activation in the absence of PMA; in the presence of PMA, neither fraction influenced granulocyte activation. Fractions B and D inhibited granulocyte activation in the presence and absence of PMA. The proliferation rates of human Raji leukaemic cells were increased in the presence of fraction C, and decreased by 55% in the presence of fraction B.

Polysaccharide B has been found to exert significant effect on progression of collagen induced arthritis in lab studies, comparable to methotrexate as control. Suszko A et al, *J Ethnopharm* 2013 145(1): 109-17.

For medicinal herbal usage, only the dried aerial parts are used.

Magnoflorine is found in many medicinal plants, including black cohosh, gold thread, amur bark, and of course, magnolia blossoms and bark. The compound possesses anti-inflammatory and sedative activity.

Both corytuberine and magnoflorine, also found in Oregon grape root (*Mahonia aquifolium*), appear to be antagonists of alpha 1-adrenoceptors, suggestive of relaxing properties. Sotnikova R et al, *Methods Find Exp Clin Pharmacol* 1997 19(9): 589-97.

Protopine shows moderate anti-seizure activity in one study. Prokopenko Y et al, *Sci Pharm* 2015 84(3): 547-554. This suggests the early observations of Dr. Withing may be worthy of further consideration. Protopine is a major alkaloid found in California poppy (*Eschscholzia californica*), and Greater Celandine (*Chelidonium majus*).

Protopine affects the microtubule structures in living cells, without affecting tubulin polymerization *in vitro*, which led to cancer cell arrest in the G2/M phase. Wang X et al, *Molecules* 2016 21(7).

Alcohol extracts from the root of *C. palustris var. alba* possess activity against gastrointestinal nematodies, anti-oxidant and cytotoxic activity against human leukemia, lung, colon, cervix and prostate cell lines. Mubashir S et al, *Chin J Nat Med* 2014 12(8): 567-72. Native to Pakistan and western Himalayas, this is a widely cultivated nursery plant in North America.

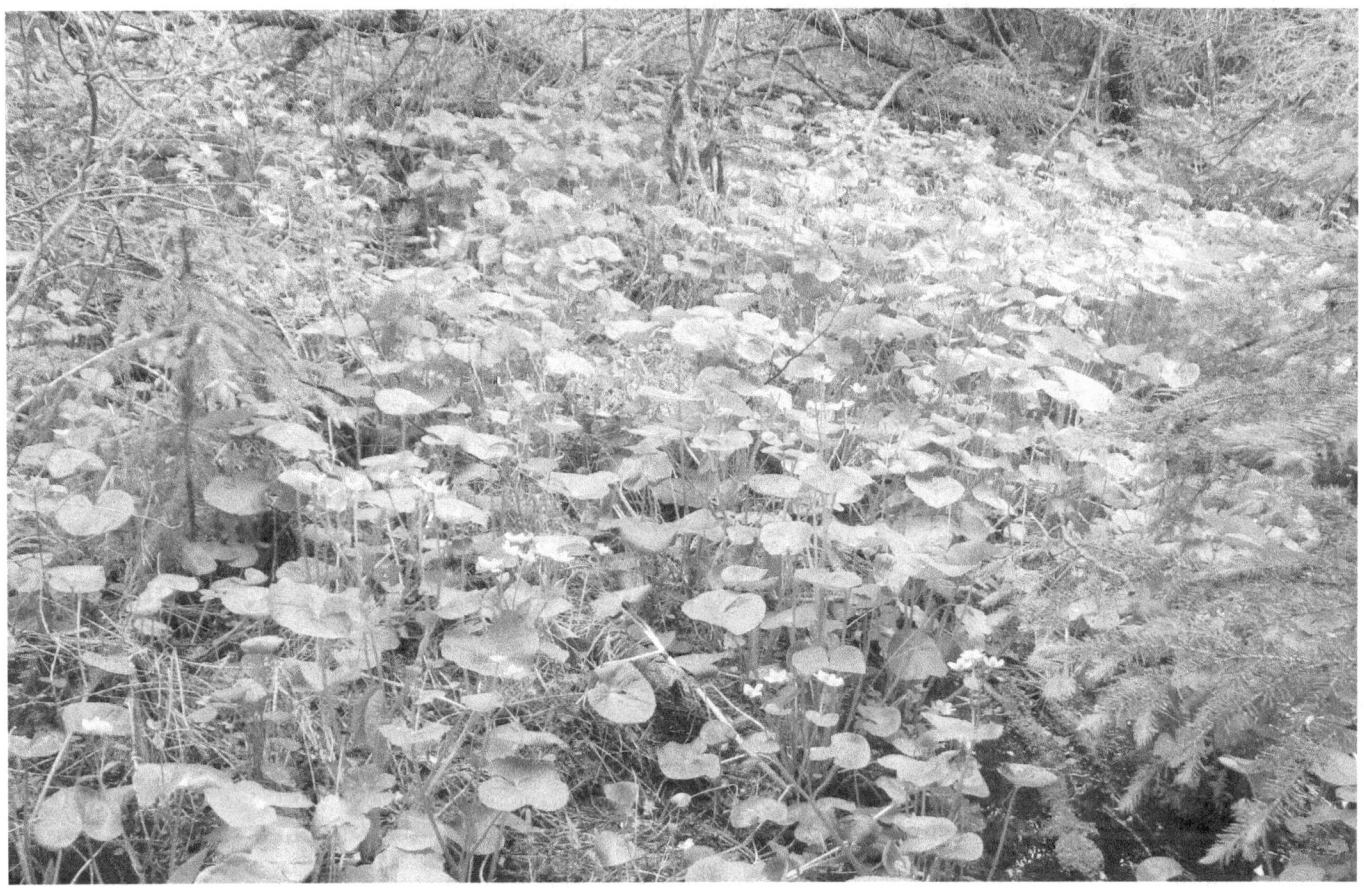

MARSH MARIGOLD SWAMP

Mountain Marigold (*C. leptosepala*) can be used in small amounts, dried, to stimulate the flow of mucous in the lungs, digestive tract and uterus, as well as loosen dried mucous from the bronchials and sinuses.

According to Michael Moore, Elkslip is an energetic expectorant without causing nausea, combining well with Grindelia for bronchial or sinus infection.

It is one of the better remedies for sinus troubles caused by tooth infections of the upper jaw. For this a cup of tea every three hours followed by hot and cold showers can quickly lessen the pain. Steep one tsp. of dried plant per pint of boiling water.

The herb is also anti-spasmodic, and a hot poultice of the dried leaves can be used in facial paralysis, combining well with cow parsnip seed tea internally. Hot tea of dried leaves induces sweating.

For lower back pain and intestinal cramping, a hot poultice can be used for temporary relief.

Freeman & Mongeau suggest it "helps us receive sunlight and absorb Vitamin D in winter." Not sure how.

This species lacks some of the pyrrolizidine and aporphine alkaloids found in Marsh Marigold, but again, dry carefully before use.

HOMEOPATHY

Marsh Marigold has done good work in gastric symptoms with abdominal pain, vomiting and diarrhea, especially when headache and singing in the ears are present. A feeling of the frequent urge to urinate may also be present.

It may also have favourable action in cellulitis, and watery skin blisters surrounded by a ring with much itching.

Caltha palustris, in mother tincture or low potency, may also be tried in great swelling of the face, especially around the eyes, and in itching eruptions on the thighs with pustules.

Good action is said observed in uterine cancer.

DOSE- Tincture to low potencies. The mother tincture is prepared from the fresh flowering plant. First a juice is made and then added to equal amount of 95% alcohol. Let sit for a week or so, and then filter.

This is based on the eating of the plant by a family of five persons living near Solingen, Germany, in 1817. They were compelled to eat the food due to bad circumstance and within half an hour exhibited above symptoms. On the third day an eruption of pemphigous vesicles as large as almonds appeared and these dried up in 48 hours. They all recovered.

SEED OIL

The seed oil of *C. palustris* yields two unusual polyunsaturated components, all cis-5, 11, 14-eicosatrienoic acid (23%) and all-cis-5,11, 14, 17-eicosatetraenoic acid (1%). The C18 monoene fraction (26%) is a 2:1 mixture of cis-5 and cis-9 octadecenoic acids.an

FLOWER ESSENCES

Marsh Marigold "shines" a light" on dark situations and helps shift-workers improve their sleep patterns.
OLIVE

Marsh Marigold brings the light of divine understanding to heal the deepest wounds of our personal and shared history.
LIGHT HEART

Marsh Marigold essence helps ensure that the thread of life's cycle will be found and pursued.   **MIRIANA**

Marsh Marigold (*C. leptosepala*) enables us to protect ourselves while giving to others. Opens our hearts to the postive. A remedy for depression associated with Seasonal Affective Disorder (SAD), keeping metabolism in balance. Use with St. John's Wort essence for strengthening the light of the aura to impact and invigorate the physical body. Useful for mid-life crises.
NETTLES AND MORE

PERSONALITY TRAITS

Water comes to this dark place out of sorrow. In the pool under broken alders, a chieftain of the Old North was killed in battle and his head carried on a stick away from where Tern meets Severn to high ground in the west. 'Usual is the wind from the east,' usual for a proud man and a thrush among thorns and the outcry against oppression, 'usual for crows to find flesh in a nook.' Unusual is gold fallen in mud to rise into the air and, through the river fog, sing for our eyes.
PAUL EVANS

ASTROLOGY

In the marsh marigold a further characteristic of the buttercups becomes evident. The green flower bud rises above the leaves, swells up, and finally unfolds in a radiant yellow. The corolla is five-petaled; it lacks, however, the calyx, as do most buttercup species. The calyx expresses blossom development becoming independent of vegetative life. Where there is no calyx, the development of leaves and blossoms is closely connected. With the marsh marigold, the flowering stage only gradually grows beyond the mere vegetative processes…The petals are…rather thick and substantial. Most importantly, they vary in their form from one another. The first petal to emerge still appears somewhat unshapely. Only towards the development of the last one does the complete form become apparent…It is dominated, generally speaking, by vegetative processes in the part of the plant influenced by Mercury. **KRANICH**

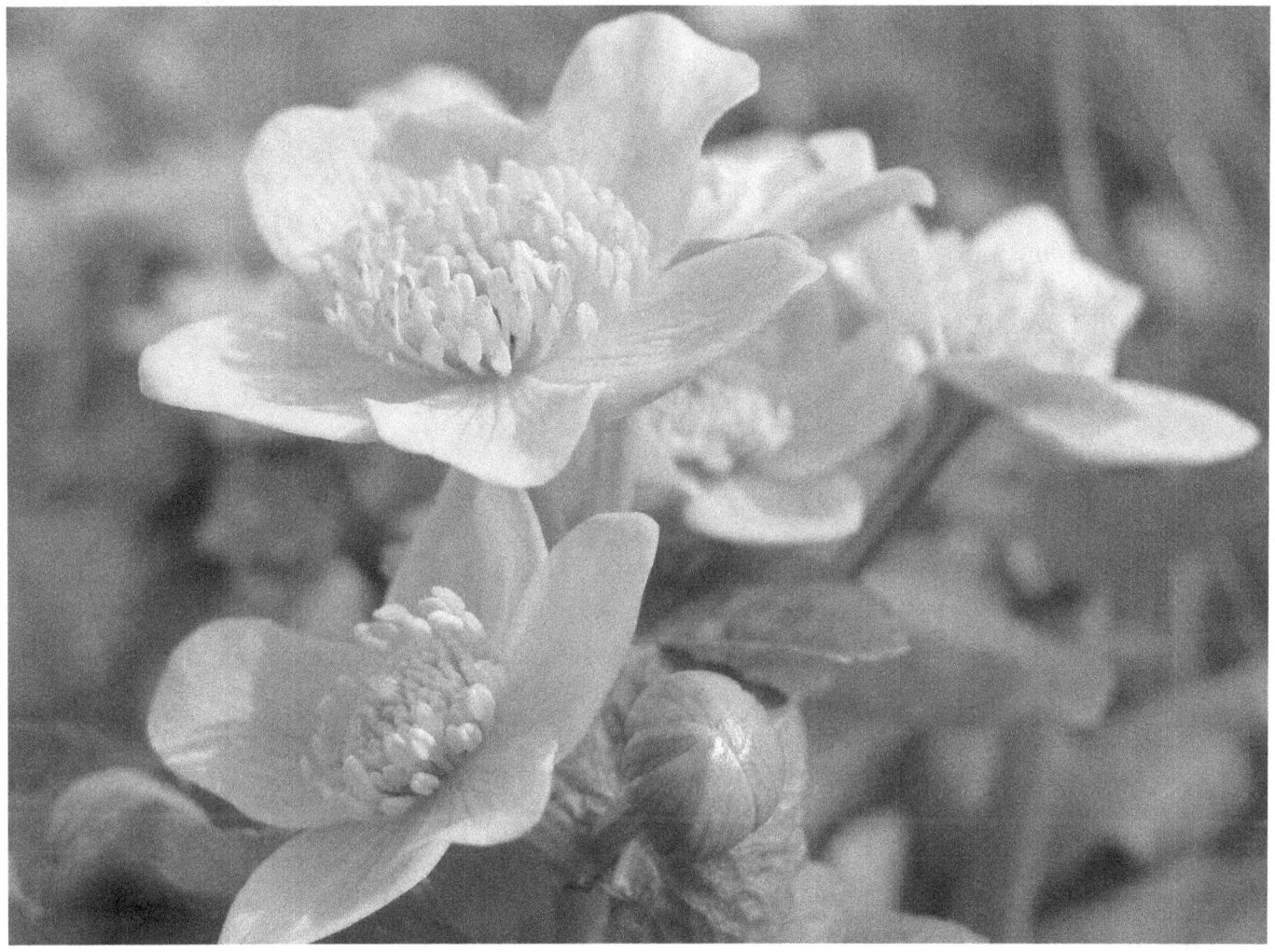

MARSH MARIGOLD

MYTHS AND LEGENDS

Catha was a German maiden who fell deeply in love with the Sun God. She would spend day and night in the fields, so that she could see him as much as possible. She eventually wasted away, and on the spot where she stood, the first marsh marigold appeared, in a form and colour that represented the sun. And on its petals was a drop that might have been dew or a tear of happiness at the maid's translation. **CHARLES SKINNER**

RECIPES

INFUSION- One tsp of dried leaf to one cup of water. Should not be taken for more than four days due to possibility of liver and kidney inflammation in sensitive individuals.

POULTICE- One ounce of dried leaves added to boiling water. Wring out and apply directly to affected area. Cover.

MEADOW PARSNIP
HEART LEAVED ALEXANDERS
(*Zizia aptera* [A. Gray] Fern.)
(*Z. cordata* W.D.J. Koch ex DC) not accepted
(*Z. aptera* var. *occidentalis* Fernald) not accepted
PURPLE MEADOW PARSNIP
(*Thaspium aureum* [L.] Nutt.) not accepted
(*T. trifoliatum* var. *aureum* [L.] Britton)
GOLDEN ALEXANDERS
MEADOW PARSNIP
(*Z. aurea* [L.] W.D.G Koch)
(*Thaspium aurea*) not accepted
(*Smyrnium aureum* L.) not accepted
HAIRY JOINT MEADOW PARSNIP
HAIRY SPINE THASPIUM
(*T. barbinode* [Michx.] Nutt.)
PARTS USED- aerial parts, root

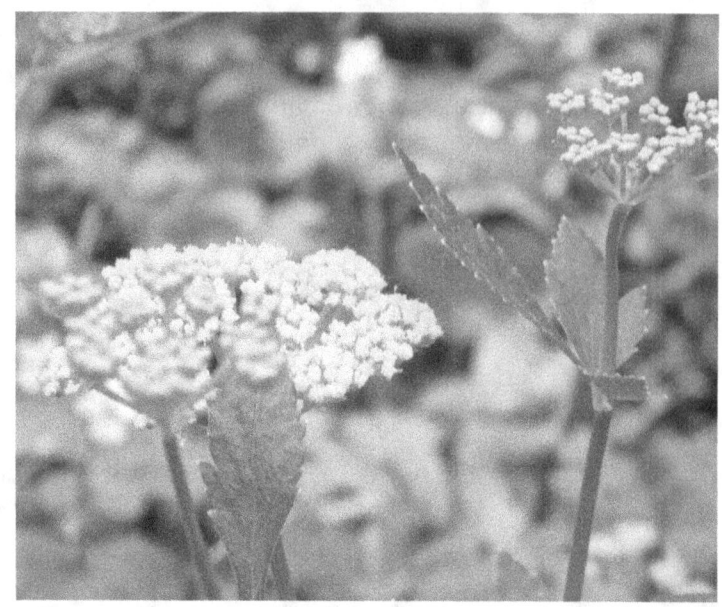

MEADOW PARSNIP

Zizia is named after the German botanist Johann Baptist Ziz. Aptera is from the Greek **A**, meaning without, and **PTERYX**, a wing, referring to the wingless fruit on the plant. Aurea or aureum means gold or golden. Thaspium is named after the island of Thapsus.

The plant is common to moist locations of my region, found near streams in open meadows. The closely related, and smaller Golden Alexanders is used in Homeopathy (see below), and is found further east into Manitoba.

Today, the genus Thaspium is considered distinct from Zizia, and identified by its winged, ribbed fruit. The flowers are somewhat paler yellow, but otherwise very similar looking.

Golden Alexanders root (*Z. aurea*) was used by Fox, and other indigenous healers for fevers. They used the flower stalks as part of compound, which included *Monarda* and Philadelphia Fleabane leaves, then powdered as snuff, to relieve sick headaches.

Meadow Parsnip (*T. barbinode*) root, **BUSIDJI'BIKUGUK**, meaning Plump root, was decocted by the Chippewa to aid children's colic. On the prairies, it is confined to the southeastern corner of Manitoba.

MEDICINAL

CONSTITUENTS- *A. aptera*- aerial part- rutin (quercetin-3-O-rhamnoglucoside), various coumarins, apertin, edultin, pteryxin, isosamidin (sesquiterpenoid), 9-senecioyloxy-columbianetin acetate, 9-(2&3- methylbutyryloxy)-columbia-netin acetates; apterin (benzopyran).
Root- isosamidin, pteryxin

Constance Rafinesque in *Medical Flora of the United States* 1830 suggested Zizia is "vulnerary, anti-syphilitic and sudorific."

Millspaugh reported the proving of Dr. E. E. Marcy on Meadow Parsnip as those of a nerve irritant.

"The tincture leaves a numb, fuzzy sensation on the tongue, followed by a feeling as if the tongue had been scalded with hot tea; my eyes began to water and smart; I ceased writing, and threw myself upon my lounge; my face then began to feel suffused with blood and soon became hot, especially the cheeks and forehead; drowsiness followed, and I fell into a distressingly dreamy sleep, lasting an hour. When I awoke, all symptoms had passed except the scalded sensation of the tongue, which lasted fully an hour longer."

Marcy wrote in the *North American Journal of Homeopathy*, 1855. "The odour of the root has been known to produce such an effect upon the system as to confine the subjects of its influence to bed for days. In these instances, nausea, faintness and lassitude, were the symptoms produced."

The seed tincture has been used for epilepsy.

Isosamidin is present in both the roots and aerial parts of Meadow Parsnip and exhibits both spasmolytic and coronary vaso-dilating activity.

Edultin inhibits *Pseudomonas aeruginosa* and *Staphylococcus aureus*. Ng TB et al, *Gen Pharmacol* 1996 27(7):1237-40.

Pteryxin is a dihydropyranocoumarin found in several members of the *Apiaceae* family.

Pteryxin is present in the aerial parts and roots, and is antispasmodic, with vaso-dilating properties. In rabbit studies, it relaxed the smooth muscle of trachea and pulmonary arteries. Zhao NC et al, *Biol Pharm Bull* 1999 22(9):984-7.

Pteryxin plays a key role in regulating lipid metabolism and improving energy production. It may be useful new natural compound for the anti-obesity market. Nugara RN et al, *Nutrition* 2014 30(10): 1177-84.

It shows strong anti-platelet aggregation activity, *in vitro*. Chen IS et al, *Phytochemistry* 1996 41(2): 525-30.

The compound is a strong butyrylcholinesterase inhibitor, suggesting benefit in the treatment of Alzheimer's disease. It is a more potent inhibitor than galanthamine. Orhan IE et al, *Food Chem Toxicol* 2017 17:30109-6.

The seed head, stem and leaves of *Z. aurea* show significant activity against *Staphylococcus aureus*. Borchardt et al, *J Med Plants Res* 20008 2:5.

HOMEOPATHY

Meadow Parsnip (*Z. aurea*) is used in conditions of excessive excitement, as in the hysteria present during or preceding menstruation. Intermittent neuralgia of the left ovary, with acrid and profuse leucorrhea, and delayed menses are other indications.

It is also indicated in cases of Sydenham's chorea, a disorder of the nervous system characterized by irregular, jerky movements caused by involuntary muscular contractions. Even fidgety legs, with lameness in arms and spasmodic twitching with unusual tired feeling may call for this remedy.

There may be depression, with alternating laughing and weeping moods. A pressure on top of the head and in the right temple, is associated with backache. **DOSE-** Tincture to third potency. The mother tincture is made from the whole fresh plant. Original proving by Marcy, and four others in 1855.

TALL MEADOW RUE
PURPLE MEADOW RUE
(*Thalictrum dasycarpum* Fisch. & Avé-Lall.)
WESTERN MEADOW RUE
(*T. occidentale* A. Gray)
FLAT-FRUITED MEADOW RUE
FEW FLOWERED MEADOW RUE
(*T. sparsiflorum* Turcz. ex Fisch. & C. A. Mey.)
VEINY MEADOW RUE
(*T. venulosum* Trel.)
(*T. confine* Fern.)
(*T. turneri* B. Boivin) not accepted
(*T. occidentale* **var. columbianum**) not accepted

COLUMBINE MEADOW RUE
(*T. aquilegiifolium* L.)
DUSTY MEADOW RUE
GLAUCOUS-LEAVED YELLOW MEADOW RUE
(*T. speciosissimum* L.)
(*T. flavum* **ssp. glaucum** [Desf.] Battan)
LOW MEADOW RUE
(*T. minus* L.)
YUNNAN MEADOW RUE
(*T. delavayi* Franch.)
(*T. dipterocarpum*)
PARTS USED- above ground

Thalictrum is from the Greek **THALIA**, meaning abundance, and good cheer. This is related to **THALLOS** from the Greek meaning green shoot, young sprout and **THALLEIN**, to thrive, bloom and grow luxuriantly; as well as Thalia, the blooming one, and the Muse of pastoral comedy and poetry. Some authors suggest Thalictrum means, plant with divided leaves, but I'm unsure of this explanation.

Rue is derived from the Latin **RUTA**, meaning bitter. Or it may derive from the Greek **REUO** "to set free", in reference to setting the body free from disease.

Rue may derive, according to some authors, from the Old English **HREOWAN** meaning sorrow, regret and sadness. I doubt it.

Dasycarpum means hairy-fruited. Sparsiflorum means few-flowered. Delavayi is named in honor of Pere Jean Marie Delavay, the 19th century botanist and explorer. Flavum means "pure yellow".

Meadow Rue, the *Thalictrum* genus, is not European Meadow Rue (*Ruta graveolens*). That being said, they do superficially look similar, and have some minor similarities of usage.

Pliny wrote *Thalictrum* "prevents hair falling out, or if it has already done so, restores it".

Dioscorides recommended *T. minus* leaves to heal old skin ulcers.

In England, the related *T. flavus* and *T. majus*, were known as Poor Man's Rhubarb, due to laxative effect of the roots. The former herb tops were boiled in ale for the same effect.

The related Early Meadow Rue (*T. dioicum*) grows further east and south of my region.

It was said that the roots of this plant were purgative and diuretic; and used for sciatica, snake bite and making spruce beer.

The leaves were added to spruce beer to act as a digestive tonic.

Low Meadow Rue (*T. minus*) was used in the Scottish Highlands as a purgative and vermifuge. A decoction was used by the women of Skye, for obstructed menses (abortifacient), while at Colonsay, the herb was used for rheumatism. The Gaelic name **RU BEG** means, "to flow".

Gilmore (1914) wrote of Tall Meadow Rue (*T. dasycarpum*) that, among the Teton Dakota, "the fruits on approaching maturity in August are broken off and stored away for their pleasant odor, for this purpose they are rubbed and scattered over the clothing. The Indians say the effect is enhanced by dampness. This, like all other odors used by Indians, is of slight, evansescent fragrance. They use no heavy scents; all are delicate and give a suggestion of wholesomeness and of the freedom of the uncontaminated outdoors."

The Pawnee mixed the root of Tall Meadow Rue with white clay, and rubbed it onto the nostrils of horses to increase their racing stamina. The Omaha used it as a horse snuff as well.

The Blackfoot used the partially ripened fruits of Western Meadow Rue, or **ATSIINAMIO** for their pleasant smell as well. The green seeds need to be picked when full, around the time that Saskatoon berries are red, because a week later, the seeds are dried and contain no scent.

In some indigenous tribes, like the Fox, it was used as a love potion. The seeds were put into the food of a quarreling couple, believing it would help them mend their differences. The Forest Potawatomi used seeds and leaves along with other plants to cure cramps. The seeds were put on the surface of poultices to make them more effective.

Various tribes, including the Ojibwa used a root decoction to relieve fevers, and heart palpitations.

The Gitksan of British Columbia chewed and swallowed the juice of Western Meadow Rue (*T. occidentale*) root for headache, eye trouble, and to loosen phlegm. It was also used to improve circulation, and relieve the pain of sore legs. Leaves and seeds were also placed on the aching muscles and cramps. A traditional name for the plant was Frog Parsnip, or **HAMOK GANAO**. Smith reported a small piece of the root was chewed and juice swallowed to cleanse the throat and improve circulation of blood.

In Montana, the Flathead decocted the dried seed heads as a hot tea for chills and colds, sometimes combining it with Sweet grass to make it more potent. The Nez Perce infused the seeds for colds, sore throats and fevers.

The Blood tribe, as told to French explorers, called it "Gros Ventre Scent", or the big stomach scent. They smudged the plant to keep away insects. They dried and chewed the seeds to make their hair fragrant, and grow long.

An infusion was given to relieve hiccups and aching chest.

The young furled plant can be steamed as a potherb, with a flavor like snow peas.

The Blackfoot call it **AT-SINA-MO**. Both this species and the flat-fruited Meadow Rue (*T. sparsifolium*) foliage was dried, ground to a fine powder, and administered by mouth to make a horse long-winded, spirited, and enduring.

The stems were used for straws, with more than one tribe naming it "hollow stem".

Flat-fruited, or Few-flowered Meadow Rue has separate male and female flowers on the same plant. The Cheyenne of Montana know it as "elk domesticated or horse medicine". The flowers were picked green and mixed with Anise Hyssop for personal and horse perfume. It was rubbed in the mane and tail to give an animal long-winded endurance.

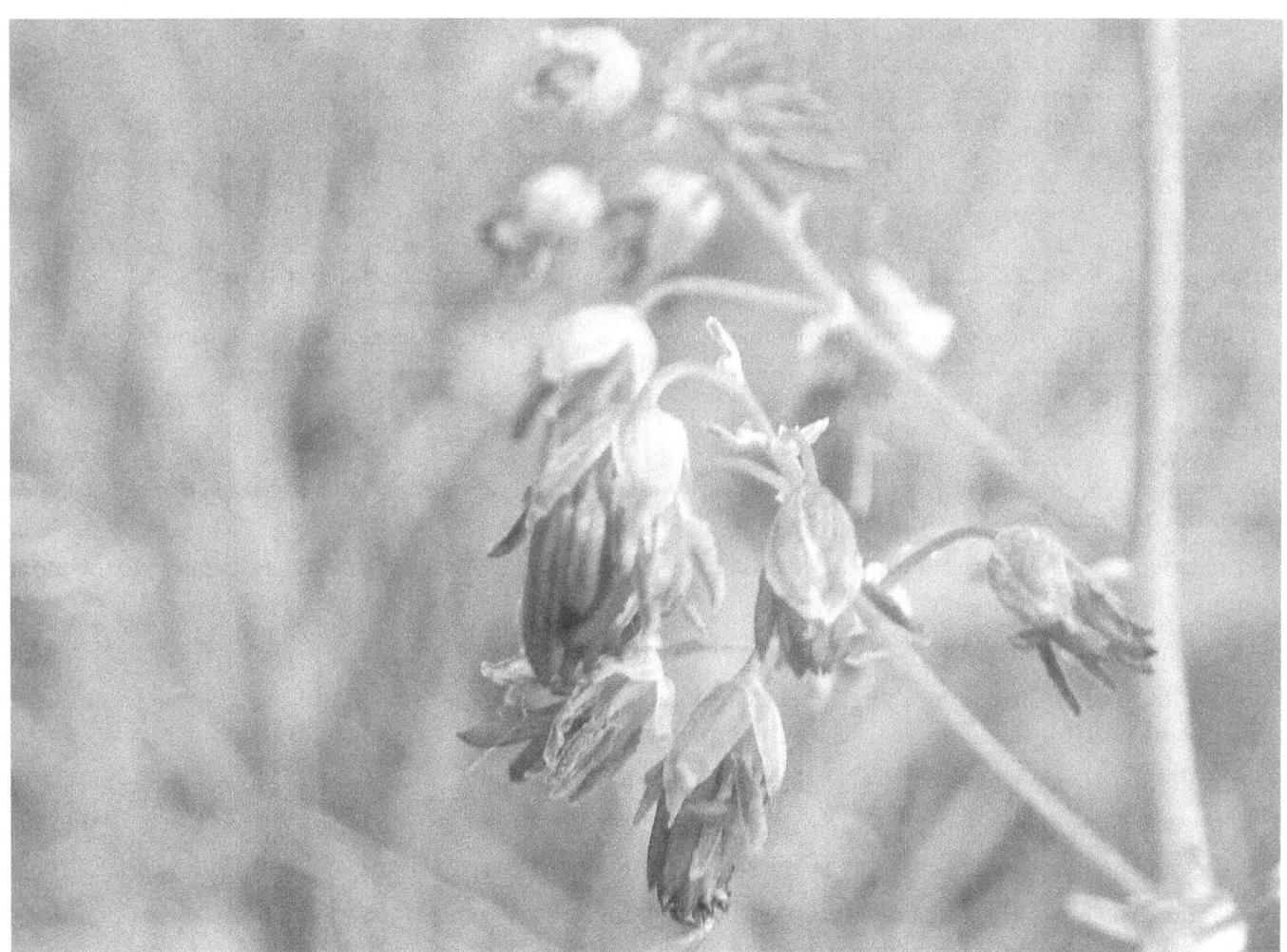

VEINY MEADOW RUE

In Traditional Chinese Medicine, the species *T. foliolosum*, or **TANG SONG CAO**, from the Cantonese is used.

Yunnan Meadow Rue (*T. delavayi*) is fully hardy to the prairies, and grows to one meter. I have seen it at the Botanic Garden of Calgary, and in the yard of my good friends on south side of Edmonton, Alberta.

Columbine, Dusty and Low Meadow Rue are all perennials that grow well on the prairies in backyards of full or partial sun. They can be easily propagated from root division.

The herb produces beautiful cut dried flowers, or wreaths can be woven from the plant while fresh, and flexible.

Low Meadow Rue, for example, has a growing period of 140 days; flowering lasting 14 days and fruiting another forty.

Thalicoside A (see below) content is always present, but highest (1.7-2.0%) between bud formation and the beginning of fruit ripening. Leaves contain on average 2.1% and flowers 1.5%.

Yellow Meadow Rue (*T. flavum*) can be recognized by its distinct semen-like odor.

MEDICINAL

CONSTITUENTS *T. dasycarpum* root- dehydrothalicarpine, thaliblastine, thalicarpine, magnoflorine (thalictrine), thalidasine, thalisopavine, norargemonine, dasycarponin, bis-norarge-monine, L-laudanidine, and corypalline.
stem and leaves- thalicarpine.
T. minus- thalicosides A-D, triterpene glycosides; various alkaloids including thalivarmine, thalsivasine, isothalisopavine, thalicberine, thalmelatine, thalipine, thalicarpine, glacucine, ocoteine, and berberine. Also contains methylthanmethine, alpha-allocryptopine, methylcanadine, thalictrimine, argemonine, aromoline, corunnine, dehydrothalicime, glaucine, jatrorrhizine, magnoflorine, N-methylargemonine, beta-N-methyl-canadine, thalmidine, palmitine, precoteine N-oxide, thalbadensine, thalicmidine, thalicmine, thalicminine, and thalicsimidine. Berberine content in the callus is 5.7 mg/gram of dry weight.
root- thaliadine, thaliadanine, adiantifoline; thalirabine, thaliracebine, thalphenine, benzylisoquinoline alkaloids, including 5'Hydroxythalidasine, Thalrugosaminine and)-Methylthalicberine.
T. sparsiflorum- O-methyltransferases
T. podocarpum root- various alkaloids, hernandezine, thalidezine, N-desmethylthalidezine, isothalidezine, thalistyline, thalistyline methodiiodide, N-desemethylthalistyline, berberine, columbamine, jatrorrhizine, palmatine, thalifendine,magnoflorine, oxyberberine, thaliglucinone and methothalistyline.
T. longistylum root- 12 alkaloids, berberine, columbamine, jatrorrhizine, magnoflorine, methothalistyline, N-desmethyl thalistyline, oxyberberine, palmatine, thalibrine, thalifendine, thaliglucinone, and thalistyline.
T. rugosum- thalrugosine, protothalipine (a protopine alkaloid), thaliglucinone, aporphine, columbamine, thalifendine, obaberine, homoaromoline, O-methylthalicberine and deoxy-thalidastine.
T. aquilegifolium- thalictoside and aquilegifolin.
T. flavum- root- berberine, pseudoberberine, thalfoetidine, northalfoetidine, northalidasine, northalrugosidine, thaligosidine, thalicberine, thaliglucinone, preocoteine, O-methylcassythine, armepavine.

Our native Meadow Rue has none of the effects on the nervous and reproductive systems attributed to the more famous, European Rue, *Ruta graveolens*.

As a tea, however, it does relieve some dizziness and ear problems.

A tea of the fresh or dried root can give relief to sinus headaches, while a tincture of the fresh root is a useful mild expectorant for the lungs, best when combined with mullein leaf.

The fresh leaves can be infused in hot water and then well strained and cooled; and used in an eyecup to relieve tired, sore eyes.

Meadow rue contains berberine, a bitter digestive tonic found in Oregon Grape root and Gold Thread.

Part of the problem for herbalists, has been the lack of study of our native plants. All of the saponins of meadow rue have anti-tumor activity, the most powerful being foetoside C, cyclofoetoside B, and thalicoside.

Thalictrum glycosides interfere with the formation of endometrium; increase FSH (follicle stimulating hormone) in the bloodstream and decrease LH (luteinizing hormone).

Thalidasine, a novel bis-benzyl-isoquinoline alkaloid has been found in our Tall Meadow Rue (*T. dasycarpum*). This alkaloid is a potent tumor inhibitor. Kupchan et al, *Journal of Organic Chemistry* 1969 34(12): 3884-8.

Thalicarpine, derived from Tall Meadow Rue, shows significant inhibitory activity against Walker intramuscular carcinosarcoma 256 over a wide dosage range; and is a potent anti-leukemic agent, with hypotensive activity. Kupchan SM et al, *J Pharm Sci* 1963 52:985-8. It also possesses anti-platelet aggregation, *in vitro*.

Thaliblastine is a cytotoxic alkaloid present in Purple/Tall Meadowrue.

The leaves and stems of latter species show activity against *S. aureus*. Borchardt et al, *J Med Plants Res* 2008 2:5.

In Russia, *T. minus* ssp. *elatum* has been studied for its alkaloid thaliblastine; and found to inhibit lung metastases.

Thaslisyline is another alkaloid isolated from various Thalictrum species. It is about one quarter as potent as d-tubocurarine in blocking neuromuscular transmissions in laboratory studies, with a pharmacological mechanism of action similar to the drug.

Obamegine, another alkaloid, does not exhibit this curare-like activity. It antagonizes the effects of phenylephrine on the aorta, and lowers blood pressure in normal hypertensive dogs for a short, transient time. The rhizomes mildly stimulate blood circulation and a tincture combined with hawthorn is a general good cardiac tonic.

For mild angina pain, a tincture of the seeds may be helpful.

It appears that both alkaloids exhibited alpha-adrenergic blockade, but the mechanism for the benefit on high blood pressure is still uncertain.

Alkaloids from *T. podocarpum* (see above) have been found to possess anti-microbial activity at concentrations of 100 micrograms/ml or less. Wu WN et al, *Lloydia* 1977 40(4):384-94.

Several alkaloids in *T. longistylum* (see above) possess hypotensive effects. Methothalistyline, N-desmethyl thalistyline, thalistyline and thalibrine have been found active against *Staphylococcus aureus* and *Mycobacterium smegmatis*. Thalistyline is the most active compound.

In studies by Ong et al, thaldicine was found as a novel alkaloid in *Thalictrum dioicum*. *Ann Pharm France* 1976 34(5-6):223-30.

Magnoflorine (thalictrine) has been found in five species of *Thalictrum* in Poland, in studies by Sobiczewska and Borkowski. Thalictrine is a very active cardiac poison that depresses heartbeat, but in large doses leads to convulsions and death.

Studies by Wu et al 1976 found several of the alkaloids from *T. rugosum* were anti-microbial.

Low meadow rue (*T. minus*) roots contain benzyl isoquinoline alkaloids that show activity against bovine mastitis. Mushtaq S et al, *J Ethnopharm* 2016 193:221-6.

The triterpene glycoside, talicoside, reduced levels of luteinizing hormone and increased serum follicle-stimulating hormone in rabbit studies. Korkhov VV et al, *Eksp Klin Farmakol* 1995 58(1):43-4. Human implications are uncertain.

Meadow Rue leaves can be dried, rolled and smoked as cigarettes for headache.

Tall Meadow Rue extracts, particularly isolated alkaloids, have been patented in Romania since 1986, as anti-tussive, anti-microbial, anti-inflammatory, anti-arrhythmia and cholagogue drugs.

Yellow meadow rue roots contain compounds with anti-parasitic activity. Ropivia J et al, *Molecules* 2010 15(9):6476-84.

Other species, such as *T. squarrosum*, have been used traditionally in Siberia for treating hypertension. This is not surprising considering the wealth of alkaloids from the roots of this genus with hypotensive activity.

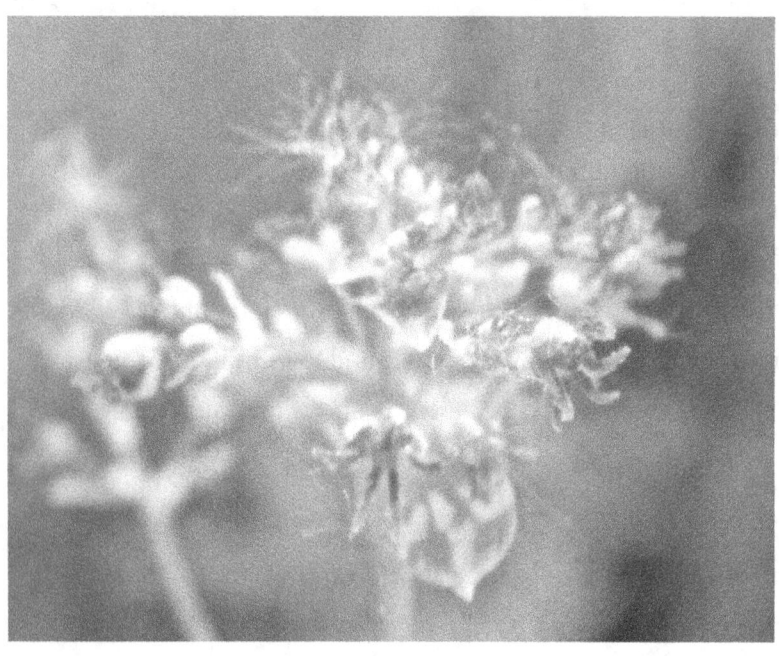

VEINY MEADOWRUE

Thaliadine, thaliadanine, adiantifoline, thalilrabine, thaliracebine, and thalphenine from *T. minus* roots all exhibit hypotensive action. Thalicoside A possesses anti-tumor activity.

Early work by the Eclectic physician Dr. King, found the root of the eastern North American Anemone Rue (*T. anemonoides*) useful in treating both internal and external hemorrhoids. Meadow rue was described in the 1916 *US Dispensatory* as a bitter and tonic, for vaginal infection.

Methothalistyline, from *T. podocarpum* is hypotensive as are several alkaloids from *T. rugosum* including thali-glucinone, obaberine, thalrugosine, homoaromoline, and O-methyl-thalicberine.

Yunnan Meadow Rue contains nine isoquinoline alkaloids, and berberine derivatives. Pseudoprotopine showed competitive inhibition activity in DA receptor binding assay, *in vitro*. Li et al, *Planta Medica* 2001 67:2.

ESSENTIAL OILS

The whole plant of *T. minus* has been steam distilled and found to possess 12 compounds comprising 100% of volatiles. These include thymol 66%, para-cymene 13%, gamma terpinene 7.3%, carvacrol 3.7% and 1.8 cineole 2%. Taherpour et al, *Nat Prod Res* 2008 22:2.

SEED OIL

From the seeds of Veiny Meadow Rue has been pressed an oil containing trans-5-hexadecenoic and trans-5, cis-9-octadecadienoic acids.

The seeds have attracted attention in Bulgaria, for their use as semi-drying oils.

Low Meadow Rue (*T. minus*) seed oil yields from 13.9-19.9%, with from 2-2.9% unsaponifiables. It has an iodine value of 163-173.

Both Veiny and Low Meadow Rue contain about 60% of acids with double bonds in the trans-5 position. Columbinic acid is found in some Meadow Rue species.

Its structure (trans-5, cis-9, cis-12 18:3 is remarkably similar to cis-6, cis-9, cis-12 18-3 of gamma linolenic acid, or GLA.

FLOWER ESSENCES

Meadow Rue is the flower essence that opens us to feel worthy of God's freely given love and favour.
GREEN HOPE

Western Meadow Rue essence is for dealing with people who repeat themselves even if you say you've already heard.
ROCKY MOUNTAIN

SPIRITUAL PROPERTIES

Much of the interesting lore of this old Indian herb is hinted at by its name. When translated, its Yuki moniker, **HOL-GA-SHEN**, and that of the Yokia, **E-WE BUCH-O-A**, both mean Coyote Angelica.

By the California Indians, for whom true Angelica was doubtless the most respected medicinal herb, of all the plants they knew, the coyote was considered the most cunning of all creatures.

Since this was true, it follows that a plant had to be considered very special in order to earn the label, "Coyote Angelica". The meadow rue qualified, it was so special that its virtues, like those of its namesakes, smacked of the world of magic and the realm of spirit. It was also as aromatic as Angelica; that in itself was like an omen. And yet, unlike Angelica, which was as gentle talisman, it was dangerously poisonous.

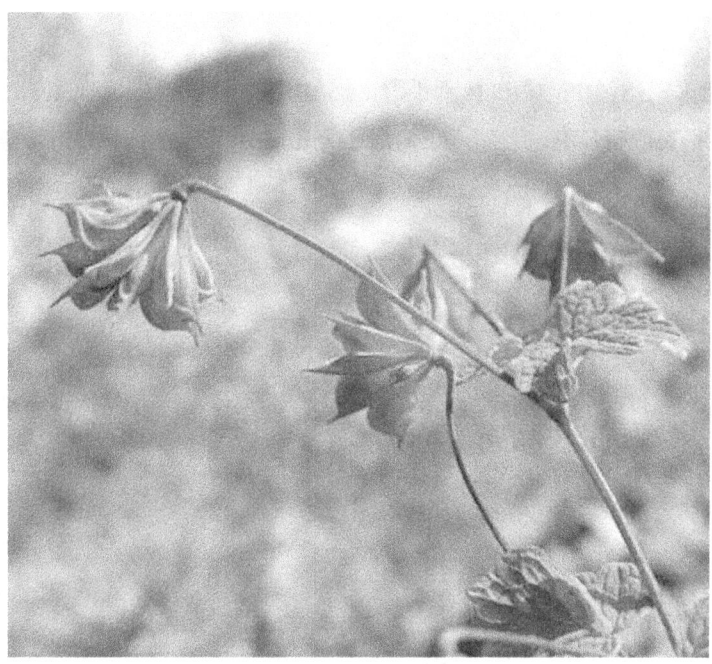

FLAT-FRUITED MEADOW RUE

Wasn't this a known fact? Hadn't a little white child once died from mistaking the stem of one for the stem of the other?

But wasn't it also true that the coyote was so cunning he could consume that poisonous plant and not be fazed by his folly? Couldn't he lope away unscathed after he'd gnawed at its lethal stems? And wasn't there a sense in which the immunity of the coyote only served to render the plant all the more dangerous to anyone else- like those who were already dead and buried, whose hard-won rest would be interrupted by terrible nightmares if the Coyote Angelica plant was allowed to grow on their graves?

Didn't the living Wailakis know this full well and thereby acted upon their knowledge? Wasn't it true that when the deceased would suddenly and inexplicably cross their minds they would hasten to the burial ground and uproot the Meadow Rue, which, according to their calculations, they were almost sure to find growing over the graves?

They'd dig it up at once and wash their heads in the juice from the crushed stems and crumbled leaves, as a kind of propitiation rite, to make certain that the deceased could rest well once more.

But the juice of the Meadow Rue was more than a cure for the bad dreams of the dead. Oddly enough, the same application that could quell those native nightmares could soothe the common headaches of the living, just as surely as if it were some beneficent decoction from an ordinary herb, wholly unadulterated by the coyote's cunning.

WESTRICH

ASTROLGY

The meadow rue …leaves are similarly pinnate. The division of the blade into numerous small leaflets goes farther, however. The leaves look like a continuously dividing system of stems whose ends have tiny pinnate leaves. They are divided to such a degree that their blades seem to dissolve into the atmosphere. The loose inflorescences expand beyond this centrifugal leaf development in a striking manner. The individual corollas are tiny and drop off prematurely. The blossoms form no interior. On the contrary, the numerous stamens radiate directly into space. The filaments are partially colored and so create the image of radiant flowering…In our entire vegetation, there is no other plant in which the Mars character of the development of the filaments determines the entire form in this manner. In the lesser meadow-rue, this process of dissolving even reaches a stage where the plant becomes wind-pollinated.

KRANICH

RECIPES

INFUSION- One tsp of dried leaf to one pint of hot water. Steep. Take one-half cup up to three times daily.

TINCTURE- The fresh root is tinctured at 1:2 and 50% alcohol.

SWAMP MILKWEED
(*Asclepias incarnata* L.)
SILKY MILKWEED
COMMON MILKWEED
INMORTAL ROOT
(*A. syriaca* L.)
(*A. cornuti* DC.) not accepted
SHOWY MILKWEED
(*A. speciosa* Torr.)
(*A. giffordii* Eastw.) not accepted
GREEN MILKWEED
(*A. viridiflora* Raf.)
(*Acerates viridiflora* [Raf.] Pursh ex Eaton) not accepted
LOW MILKWEED
DWARF MILKWEED
(*A. ovalifolia* Decne.)

EASTERN WHORLED MILKWEED
(*A. verticillata* L.)
BLOODFLOWER MILKWEED
SCARLET SILKWEED
WILD IPECACUANHA
(*A. curassavica* L.)
DESERT MILKWEED
(*A. subulata* Decne.)
BUTTERFLY WEED
PLEURISY ROOT
ORANGE MILKWEED
(*A. tuberosa* L.)
PARTS USED- leaf, flower, latex, root

As soft as silk, as white as milk,
As bitter as gall, I'm rather tall,
And a green coat covers me all!

In dusky pods the Milkweed
Its hidden silk has spun.

Asclepias cornuti pods…if you examine both inside and out, it a fairy-like casket shape, somewhat like a canoe. As they dry, they turn upward, crack and open by the seam along the convex or outer side—-revealing the brown seeds with thin, silvery parachutes like the finest unsoiled silk…some children call these manes of seed and silk fishes, and as they lie they somewhat resemble a plump, round, silvery fish with a brown head.
THOREAU

Asclepias is from the Greek ***ASKLEPIOS***, the God of Healing. In Latin, this became ***AESCULAPIUS***. In Greek and Roman art, this god carries the caduceus, a winged hazel rod encircled by a snake or two.

Among the ancient Greeks, Asklepios was revered as the founder of medicine. On one side was Hygieia, the goddess of wise living, and on the other Kanakeia, the goddess of cure alls. These became, of course, hygiene and panaceas (wonder drugs).

According to Robert Graves, this means, "unceasingly gentle". Other scholars suggest that **ASKO** and **ASKEO**, have two very different meanings. The latter meant "to form by art, decorate or adorn, to work out with skill". The former meant "to practice, train or exercise."

Shrines were devoted to his worship, where the sick or relatives came and made offerings. This was in hope that a specific cure would be revealed in dreams. He became very good at the art of healing, so good that he could bring the dead back to life. This incurred jealousy from the Gods, and Zeus incinerated him with a lightning bolt.

Incarnata means flesh-colored, at least the flesh color of pink northern Europeans. Syriaca is of Syria, because Linnaeus thought the plant came from there. In fact, it is native to North America. Speciosa means showy.

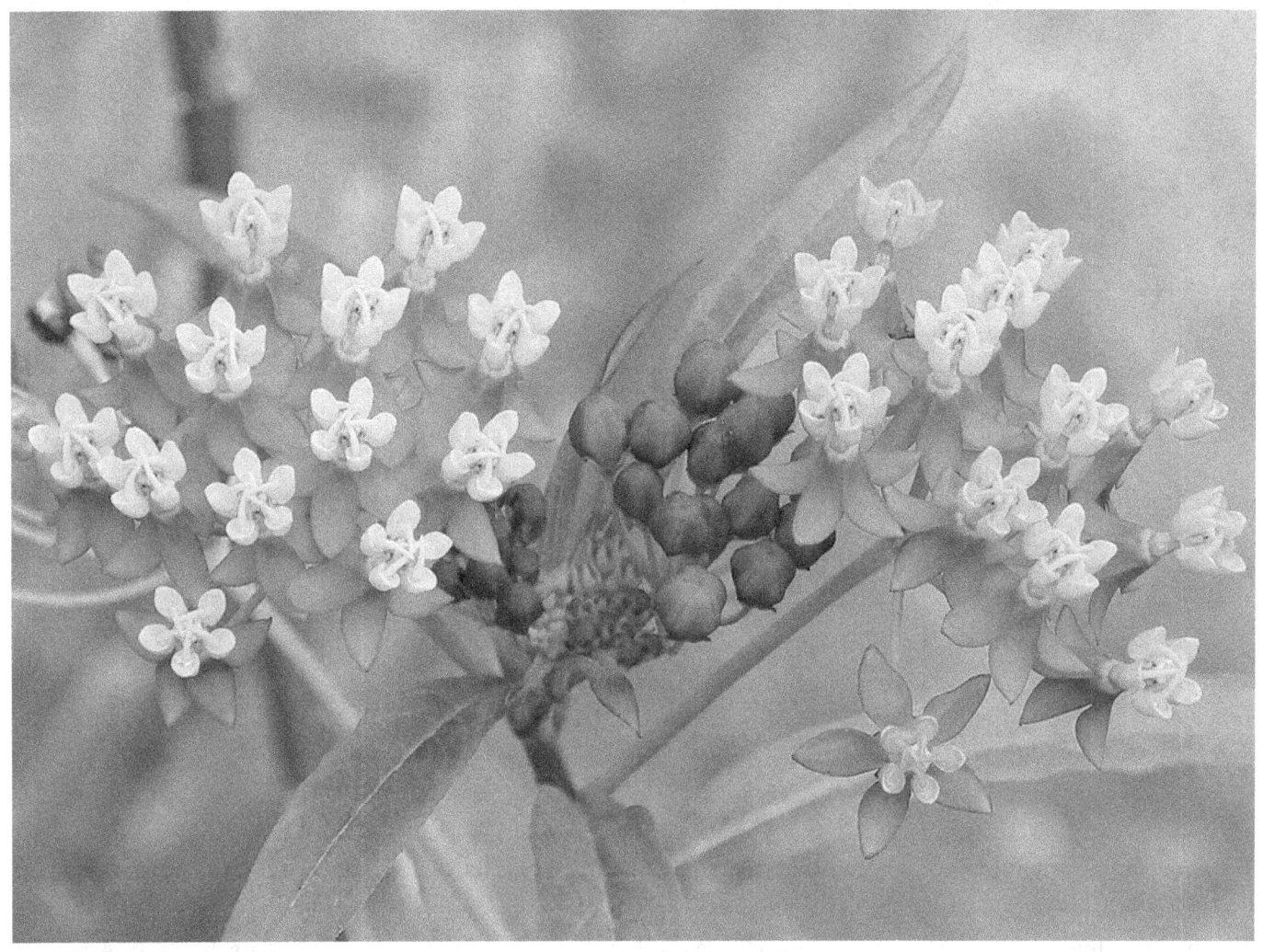

BLOOD FLOWER MILKWEED

Cornuti means horn-shaped, referring to the pods. Tuberosa means "full of swellings or knobs" referring to the root. Ovalifolia means oval-leaved, viridiflora is green-flowered.

Curassavicus is named for the Dutch Antilles island of Curacao; where the plant is native and common.

Milkweed is one of my favourite native plants. It amuses me with its manner of forming and releasing seedpods; and by its bold, primitive appearance.

Annora Brown wrote. "With its dark red turned-back petals, its high crown with exquisitely modeled hoods, its incurved horns, and the ingenious arrangement for compelling insects to work for it, it is not only a triumph in executive ability but in decorative design also".

Even amateur botanists can readily identify them for their strange appearance when seedpods are mature. These pods form the plant signature, looking like inflated lungs dispersing energy in all directions, according to Matthew Wood.

They can also be recognized by their heavy, narcotic smell, when in bloom.

The seeds are blessed with parachutes that distribute them far and away with the least zephyr of wind.

All the Milkweeds mentioned here are hardy perennials of the prairie, with the exception of Bloodflower, a widely cultivated annual from the tropics. Pleurisy root and Swamp Milkweed are from the eastern prairies, but hardy for transplant to the western regions.

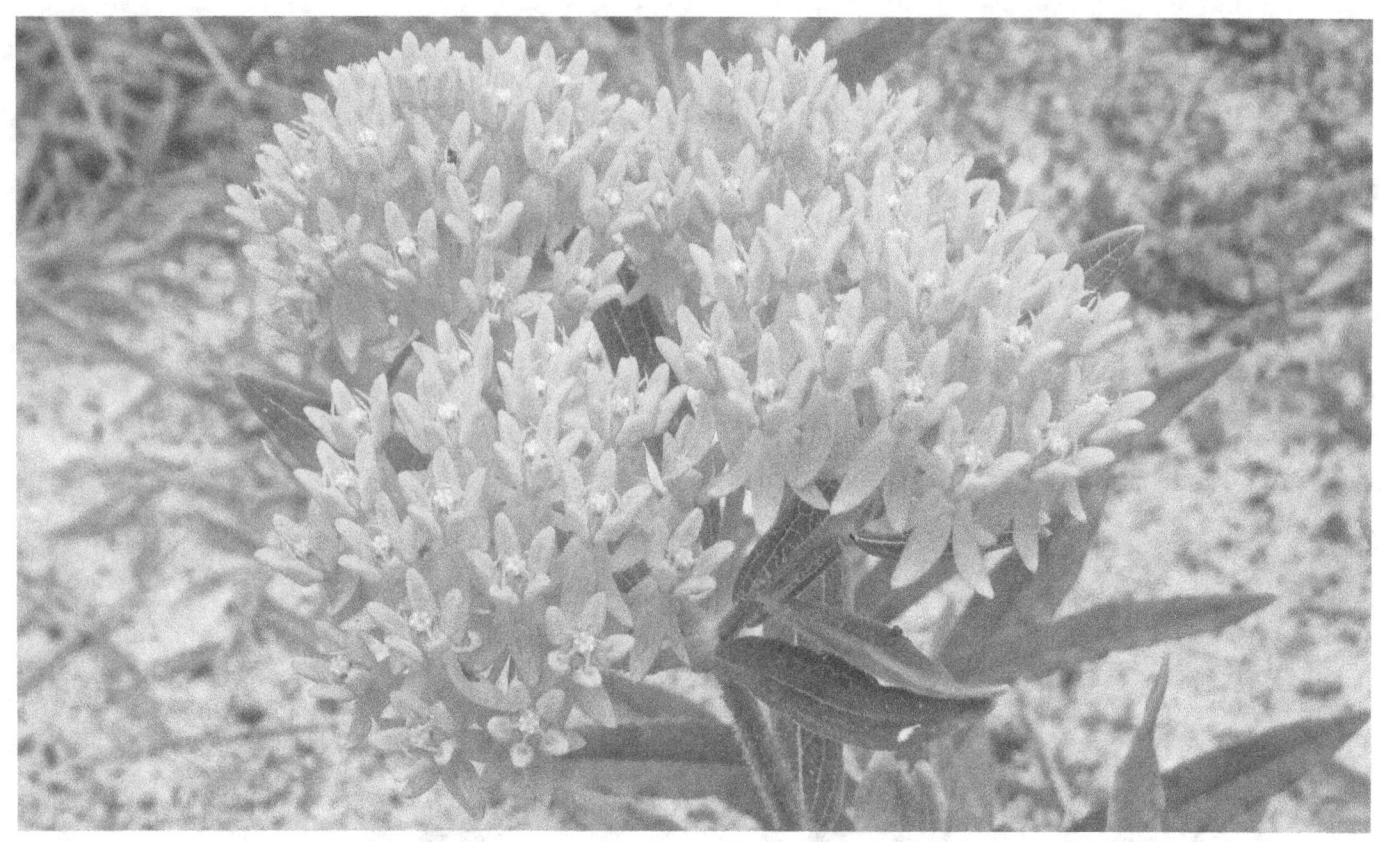

PLEURISY ROOT

The most famous member of the genus, Pleurisy root (*A. tuberosa*) is hardy to Zone 3, and is the most important herb commercially.

Like other milkweeds, the interesting seedpods are used in wreaths and flower arrangements. In South America, some tribes used the fiber from related Milkweed stems to make bowstrings.

Various indigenous people used milkweed tufts to make their buffalo hide robes warmer.

The fibers are hollow, and wick moisture away from the skin faster than pure down. The flowers are a crude sweetener; with a crystallized type of brown sugar made from the blossom nectar.

Numerous tribes prized pleurisy root for its main actions on the lungs and rheumatism. The Omaha even had a special ceremony surrounding the obtaining and distribution of this prized root. The called it **MAKAN SAKA**, meaning raw medicine; while to the neighboring Ponca it was **KIU MAKAN**, meaning wound medicine.

Both tribes ate the raw root for bronchial and lung troubles.

The Fox or Mesquakie name **ATISTE'I**, means knob on roots, very similar to the specific Latin name.

The Menomini call it the "deceiver", and consider it one of their most important medicines. The root was crushed for cuts, wounds and bruises.

One of their most important compounds was pleurisy root, ginseng root, Wild Cucumber (man in the ground) and sweet flag root. This represented four Indians in power.

The Cherokee called it wind root "for its ability to carry a message to the Great One", writes J.T. Garrett.

The beautiful orange and yellow flowers turn a deeper red as they mature, making them an eye striking addition to perennial flower beds, especially rock gardens and wilder gardens. It was named *Perennial Plant of the Year* for 2017, by the Perennial Plant Association. Long overdue I believe. In a poll of naturalists and scientists, it was chosen the fourth showiest wildflower of America.

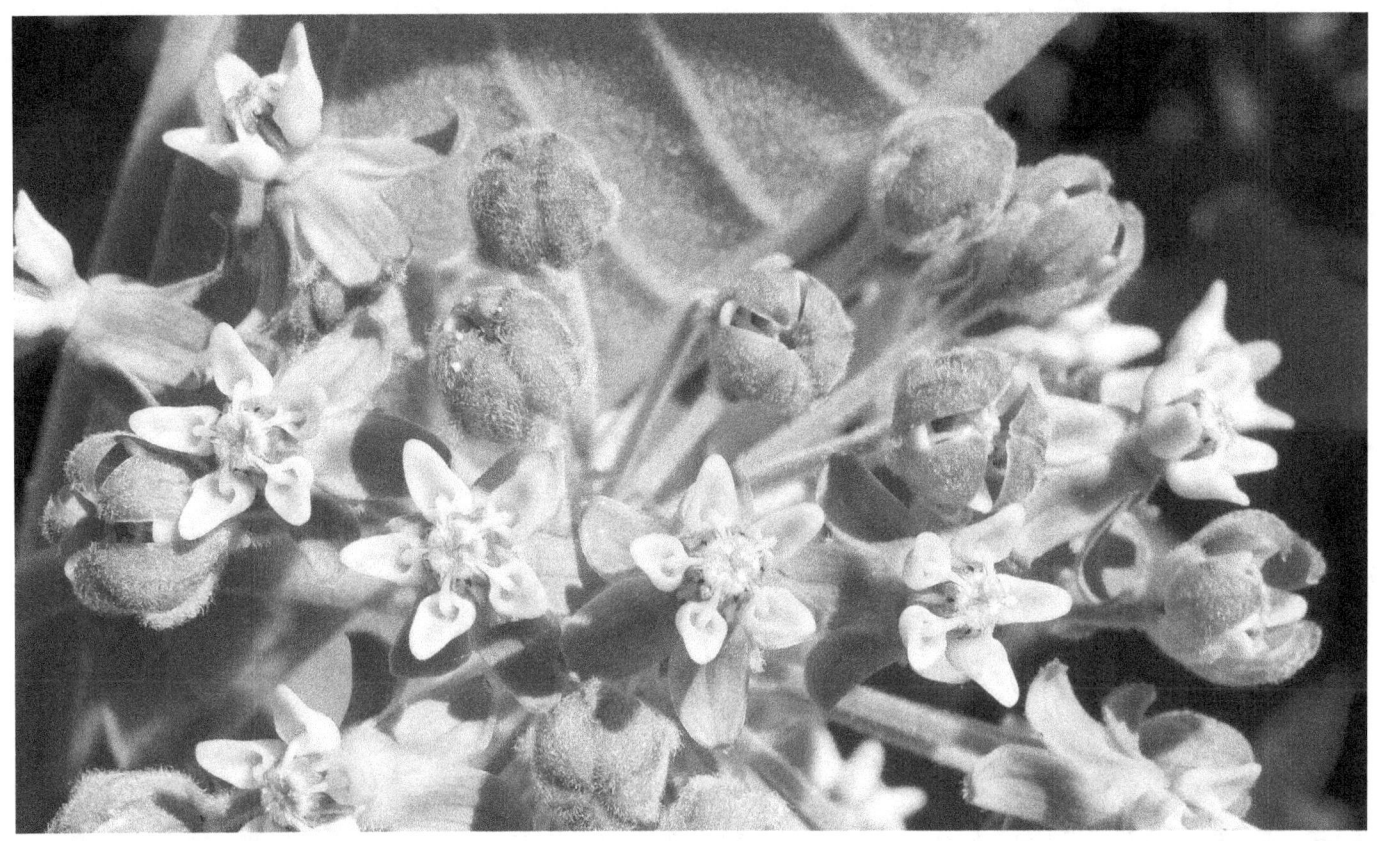

ASCLEPIAS SYRIACA

Unlike the other species, which have a white sap, Pleurisy root, unlike its cousins, has a clear or green juice. And unlike other Milkweed species, it has alternate leaves.

The root is up to 8 inches long, and white inside of an orange-red bark.

Pleurisy root fiber was used for clothing, rope and string, about five stalks to produce one foot of cord.

Textiles dating back to 700 BCE, found in Ohio, contain *Asclepias* fibers.

Both Showy and Silky Milkweed (*A. speciosa and A. syriaca*) are similar in appearance, and exude a sweet, narcotic smell from the flowers. The latter is known as Man Weed by the Forest Potawatomi.

Showy Milkweed is known as **CETIZBAXUPE**, by the Crow of southern Montana. The milky sap was mixed in water and taken internally, about a half cup four times daily, for swollen joints, according to Alma Hogan Snell.

The Omaha call it **MAKAN SAKA**, and the Lakota **CES'LOS'L PEJU'TA** according to Kahlee Keane, a local herbalist also known as Root Woman.

They are listed on the noxious weed list in Manitoba, meaning they can be destroyed where found. This has proven to impact the health of Monarch (*Anosia plexippus*) butterfly populations. A recent revision that allows for eradication on a complaint only basis may help the plants recover.

It is interesting to note that the green and yellow caterpillars feed on the leaves without any milk flowing, and yet a cut or tear will immediately result in a copious flow of white resin.

Flies, bees, butterflies and moths all enjoy the sweet nectar, but the plant has engineered a pollen trap that ensures heavy loads will be carried in exchange. If the insect is weak or too small, the tightening tenacious threads may be its death. Even bees can become so loaded with pollen sacs that they can fall to the ground and perish.

Swamp Milkweed (*A. incarnata*) was traditionally used as a root infusion by the Chippewa, for strengthening baths of children and adults. That may explain, in part, the name **BU'GISO'WIN** meaning, swimming.

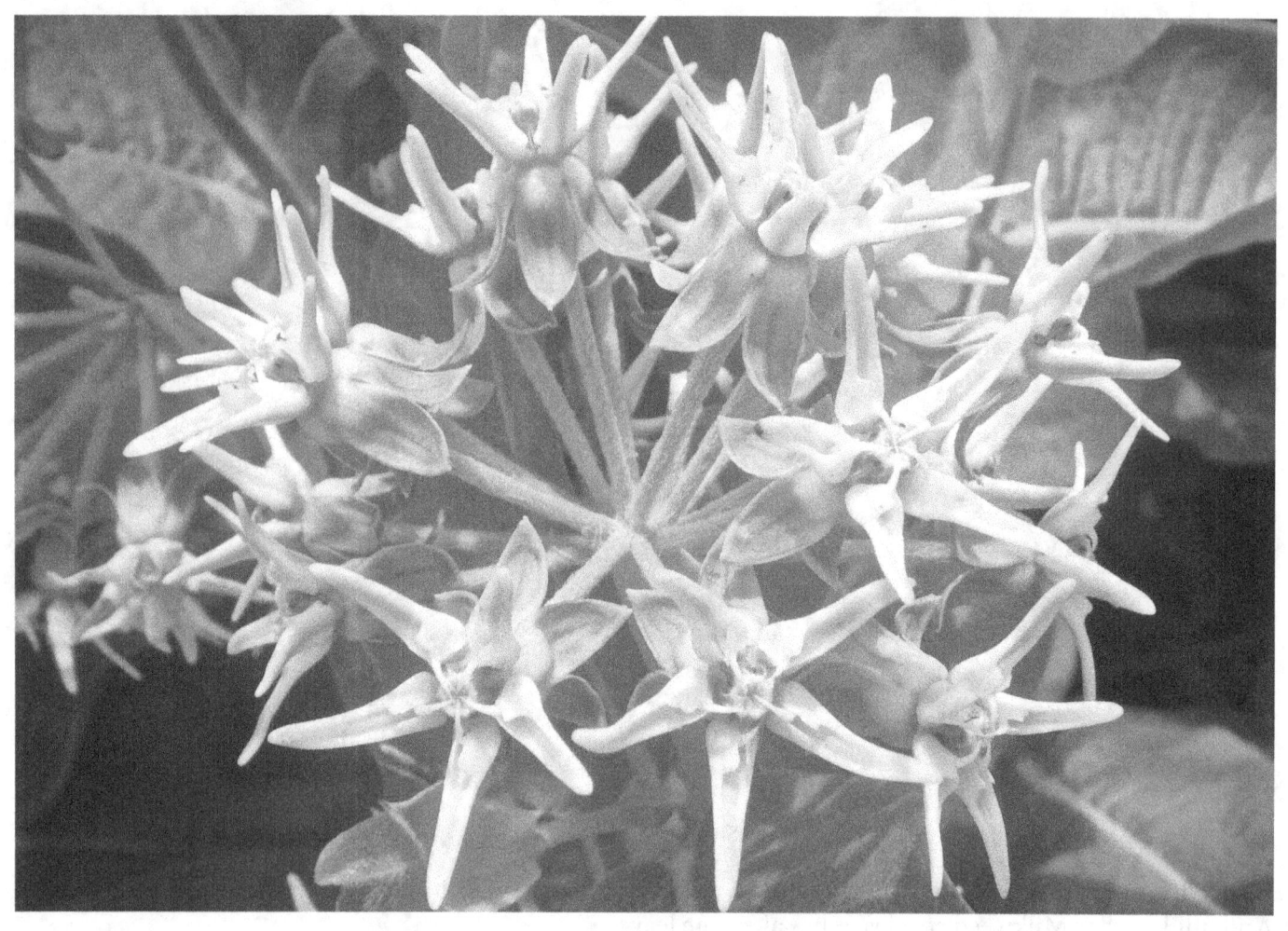

SHOWY MILKWEED FLOWERS

The Fox tribe used infusions internally as a powerful anthelmintic for tapeworms. Smith wrote that the root tea is said to drive worms from a person in an hour's time.

In smaller amounts, it was considered diuretic and carminative, and in larger doses, cathartic and emetic.

The Iroquois added cold infusions of the root to heal baby's navels. Internally it was used for too much or too little urine, with accompanying lower back pain.

The Lakota name is **WAHINHEYA IPI' YE** meaning, "medicine used to doctor gopher," in reference to swollen glands. The root was pulverized, and made into a fat-based salve for enlarged glands.

The stem bark of Swamp Milkweed was used by the Omaha tribe to make lariats, said to be stronger than those made of rawhide. The Pueblo cut it down when ripe, and rub it to separate the fibers. These threads are made into fishing lines and fine sewing thread. The Iroquois used the fiber to pull out diseased teeth.

The United States Department of Agriculture is investigating the nematode fighting properties of ground milkweed seeds.

Showy Milkweed (*A. speciosa*) plant tops were decocted by the Cheyenne as an eyewash for blindness and snow-blindness. The young, unopened flower buds were boiled in water with meat, and grease as a soup, thickened with seed flours, and in early days flavored with the layer underneath the hair of buffalo or deer hides. The green, immature fruit were peeled, and the inner layer under skin, eaten raw.

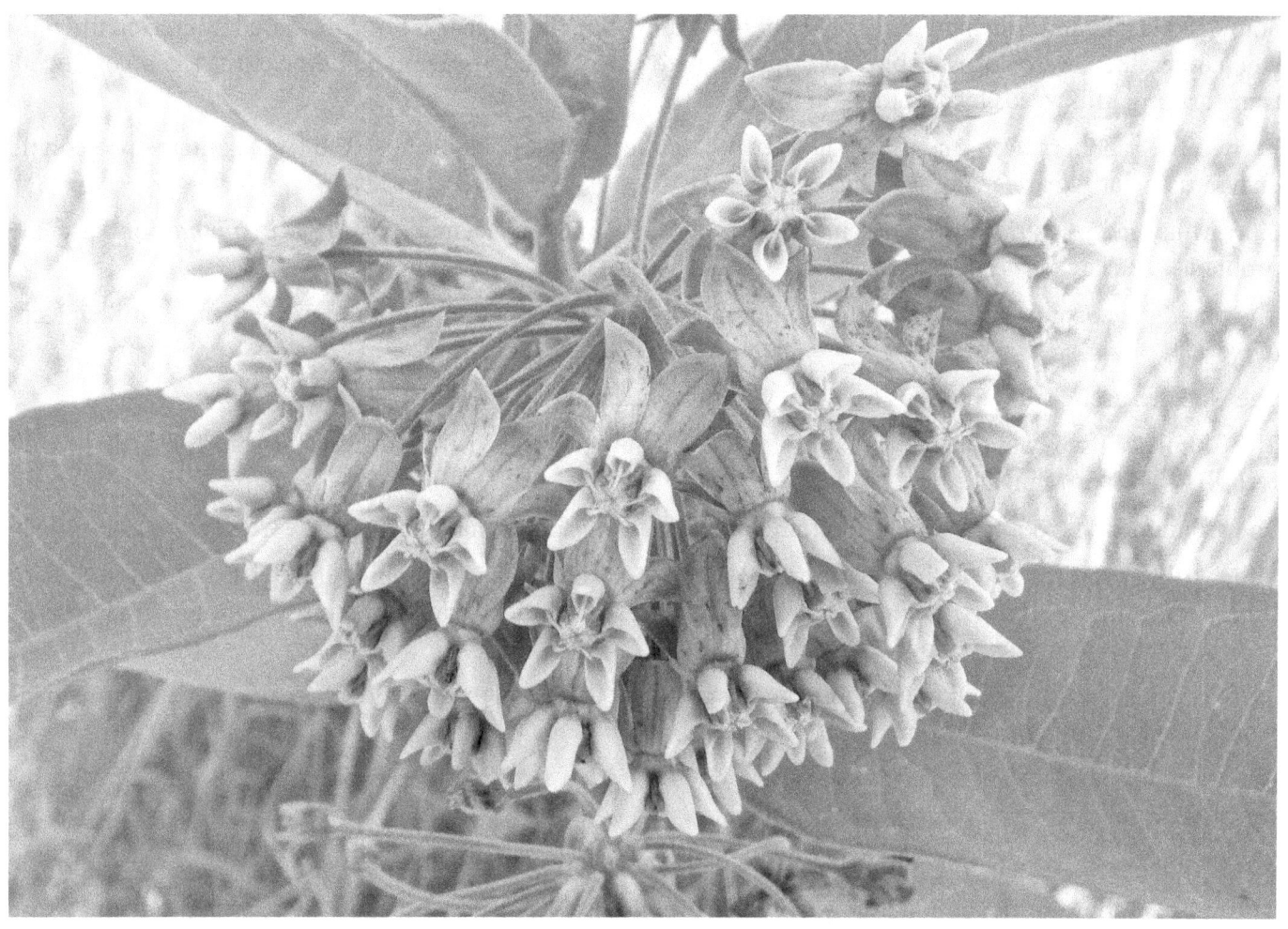

SWAMP MILKWEED

The mature plant was called "owl spoon", due to their resemblance to the common utensil. The milky juice of the broken leaves was allowed to harden and chewed as a gum. It is initially bitter and the juice is spit out, but later becomes sweet.

Various tribes used the powdered roots as a sedative, and for asthma. The fresh roots were reserved for bowel disorders, including worms; kidney and bladder water retention problems, as well as a temporary contraceptive.

The Thompson tribe decocted the roots for "general out-of-sorts feeling and emaciation" and headaches.

The Blood tribe of Alberta used plant extracts for reducing inflammation and swellings.

The Flathead of Montana decocted the roots for stomach aches. Some native tribes boiled the seeds to draw out snakebite poison, or powdered the seeds for skin ointments.

The Shoshone used the latex sap to remove corns, and calluses; and as an antiseptic on ringworm and syphilitic sores, and even poison ivy rashes.

The Dakota name **PANNUN'PALA** translates as "two little work bags of women." Both Dakota and Lakota ate the flower blossoms for food.

Likewise the Paiute and Shoshone who ate the stems, leaves, flowers and young fruit after boiling to remove bitter sap.

Some Okanagan and Salish used the stem fiber as a substitute for Dogbane, but considered it inferior and only when other fibers were not available. It was nicknamed "Coyote's Indian Hemp" alluding to the legend of Coyote transforming Milkweeds by urinating on them.

Early cattle ranchers used the milky sap to make temporary livestock brands. The latex contains proteolytic enzymes, including asclepain.

Silky Milkweed (*A. syriaca*) root was infused by the Cheyenne with clematis root (*C. virginiana*) for backache problems. The latex was applied to warts.

The plant was considered laxative, and taken for gravel and dropsy. The Cheyenne name means, "milk, pieces of wood."

The Natchez used root decoctions for kidney trouble, including Bright's disease.

The Chippewa used cold root decoctions in food to encourage post-partum milk production. They call the root **INI'NIWUNJ**, or Man-Like.

They combined the root with root fibers from Boneset (*Eupatorium perfoliatum*) to make whistles for calling deer.

Other tribes used root decoctions to prevent conception. The Mohawk combined one fist of dried herb with three Jack-in-the-Pulpit (*Arisaema triphyllum*) rhizomes in a pint of water for twenty minutes. One cup per hour was taken to induce temporary sterility.

The Cherokee used **U NA DI** to treat sore breasts, to purify the blood of weak elders, treat backache of pregnant women and attempts to overcome venereal disease.

The young sprouts, as they appear in spring, are much prized as a potherb, and cooked like asparagus. Ironically, the boiled roots also taste similar to asparagus.

The Omaha and Pawnee, when they first saw cabbage grown, called it Whiteman's Milkweed.

The buds and flowers can be added to soup. The dewy flowers exude a sweet sugar on summer mornings. The Onondaga call the plant **TGANOHAMSAHI'S** meaning, "milk comes out."

The early French Canadian settlers made a kind of brown sugar from the flowers.

The Métis call it **DILET NARBAAZH** or **TOHTÔSÂPÔWASHAW**.

In *Medicines to Help Us* written by Christi Belcourt, she quotes Métis Elder Olive Whitford. "The roots were boiled and the tea was drunk three times a day for kidney problems."

Thomas Jeffrys (1760) wrote, Silky Milkweed (*A. syriaca*) "is crowned with several tufts of flowers; these are shaken early in the morning before the dew is off of them when there falls from them with the dew a kind of honey, which is reduced to sugar by boiling".

The juice when applied to the skin forms a tough adhesive film for covering ulcers and recent wounds. The dried pods make handy spoons.

The root, according to Jethro Kloss, is very effective for gallstones. Equal parts of milkweed and marshmallow root are steeped in boiling water, and taken three cups daily, and one hot upon retiring. At the same time fomentations are applied to the liver region, and in a few days, the gallstones will pass.

Silky Milkweed seeds contain cis-vaccenic acid, which acts as a growth stimulator in laboratory rats.

Peter Kalm, the Swedish naturalist observed in his diary (1749): "The pods of this plant (*A. syriaca*) when ripe, contain a kind of wool, which encloses a seed, and resembles cotton, from whence the plant has got its French name (le Cotonier). The poor collect it and fill their beds, especially their children's, with it instead of feathers."

Eight to nine pounds of silk were sufficient to stuff a coverlet and two pillows.

One early explorer noted indigenous people used milkweed floss to cover "the secret parts of maidens that never tasted man."

Plant fiber can be modified for paper production. Iuliana Spiridon, *Ind Crops and Prod* 2007 26:3. Aphids on plants produce honeydew that is harvested by ants. Of course, cardenolide content, which does not affect aphids, does have antagonistic effect on ant survival.

The milkweed fiber has low cellulose content, and their slow degradation is an advantage in fresh and salt water applications in high density oil spills.

Whorled Milkweed (*A. verticillata*) is common to southern Manitoba on the Canadian prairies. Twelve fluid ounces of root decoction is said to cause an anodyne and sudorific effect, followed by a gentle sleep.

This is not surprising, as the plant will send sheep on a death dance, ending with the animals banging their heads into the earth in violent convulsions. Clark et al, *Vet Human Toxicol* 1979 21:6 431.

Whorled Milkweed root, was prepared as decoction by the Choctaw, as a sudorific and stimulant. It was chewed in the southern United States as a remedy for bites and stings from snakes and venomous insects.

Infusions of the whole plant were drunk by the Hopi and Lakota, for scanty milk flow in nursing mothers.

The Navaho used the plant for nose and throat problems in an unspecified manner.

Studies on the verticillosides, isolated from plant, showed no inhibition of breast cancer cell lines. Araya JJ et al, *Phytochemistry* 2012 78: 179-89.

Green Milkweed (*A. viridiflora*) was named **HU CINSHA**, meaning spoon shaped stem, by the Lakota. They crushed the roots for children with diarrhea, or tea of the whole plant was given to new mothers with low milk production.

The Blackfoot chewed the root for sore throats, or applied the masticated material to swellings and rashes, including diarrhea rash and the sore gums of a nursing baby. The name for this species is **ONNIKIISAIKIMSSKAAN** meaning, "milk oozing out."

The roots were added to winter soups, for a spicy flavor.

Low Milkweed (*A. ovalifolia*) is common in east-central Alberta, and up into the Peace Country. I spotted a small patch near Mill Creek ravine in Edmonton during the summer of 2005 that continues to thrive.

Desert Milkweed (*A. subulata*) is a perennial shrub of Arizona, California and New Mexico.

It is known as Rush Milkweed and Ajamete. The root was used by various indigenous healers of the Sonora desert, including Seris and Pima tribes, for the treatment of sore eyes, gastrointestinal disorders and cancer.

Bloodflower Milkweed (*A. curasavica*) is known in its native West Indies as "Bastard Ipecacuanha." The root and expressed juice are emetic. On the island of Dominica, where I spent some time on the black sand beaches in the early 1970s, the roots were decocted to treat fevers.

In Jamaica, the root is used in a manner similar to Pleurisy root, but will act on the bowels, unless combined with some diffusive stimulant for lung complaints.

It is cathartic and vermifuge in small doses, the juice made into syrup and given to children with worms.

In Mexico, the flowers were traditionally ground up and put into tortillas as a remedy for rabies. In parts of Mexico it is known as *Yerva de la Culebra*; while in El Salvador it is called *Bivorna Sangris*.

The plant has insecticidal properties, especially against fleas. When rooms are infected they are swept with weed brooms to rid it of various pests.

On the Solomon Islands, the leaves were rubbed on the head to cure headaches.

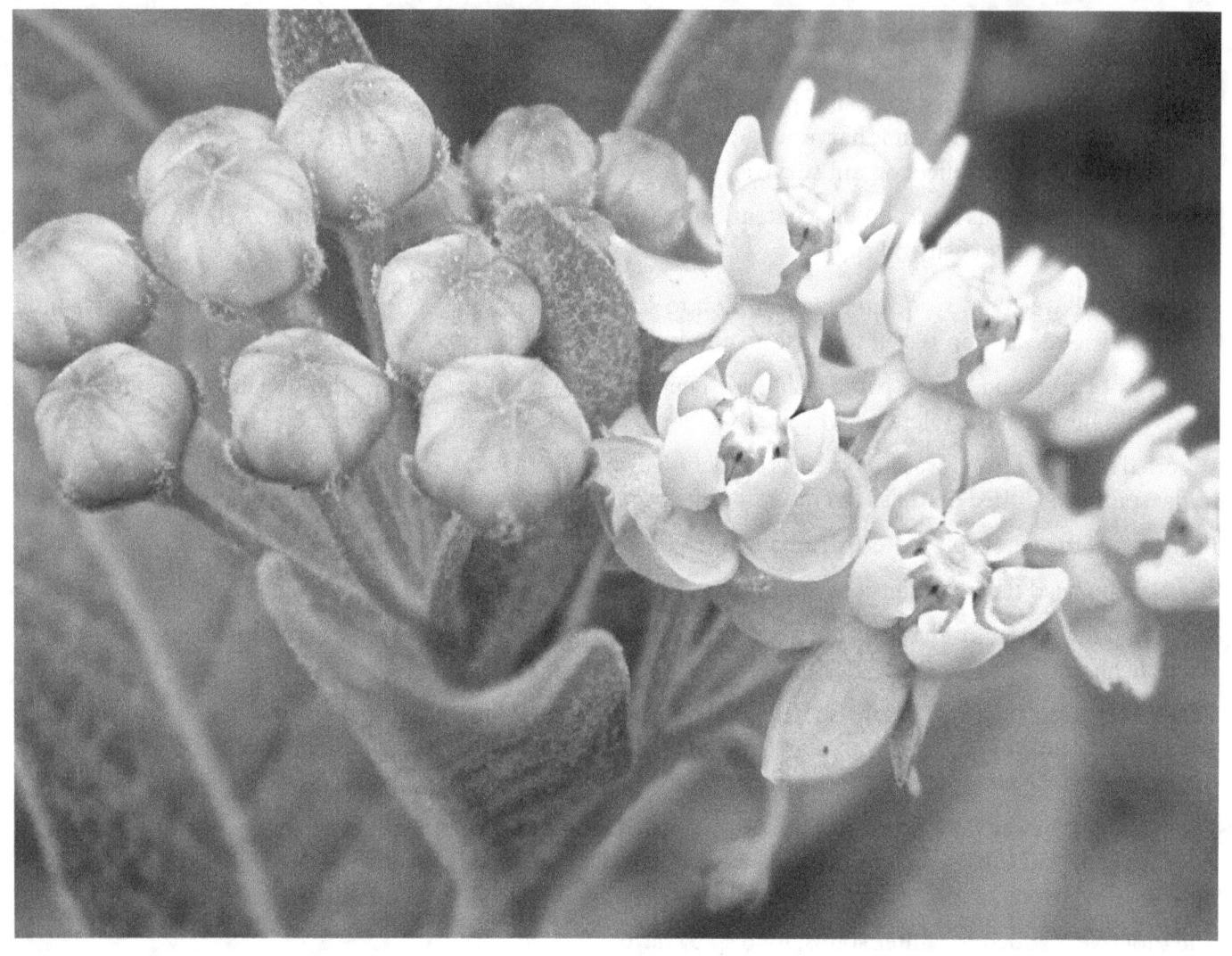

LOW MILKWEED

It has become naturalized in many parts of Australia, but here in Alberta the plant is a garden annual, or houseplant.

Milkweed species, especially *A. incarnata and A. syriaca,* have been investigated for their rubbery latex. During World War II, over 500 acres were seeded near Ottawa, to work on extraction of resin rubber gum from common Milkweed. Using various quantities in tire tread compounds resulted in improved tack, increased tear resistance, a drop in both tensile strength and modulus, a drop in resilience, and considerable improvement of flex life.

Milkweed seedpod fluff can be used like cattail fluff for beds, duvets and pillows. Eight pounds of the seed coma occupies up to six cubic feet of space. Milkweed floss is six times as buoyant as cork, and it was soon discovered that a life jacket containing 26 ounces could support a 150 pound man in the sea, for up to 48 hours.

Back in 1635, the French produced silk-like fabric from milkweed fiber.

During World War II, a call went out from the government for milkweed pods. In Michigan, milkweed farms were established to grow the suddenly valuable plants.

The fiber can also be mixed with wool or flax for weaving; as they are too short to work with on their own. It is warmer than wool, and six times lighter. Both in France and Russia, it has been used in textiles. It is naturally vermin and bacteria resistant.

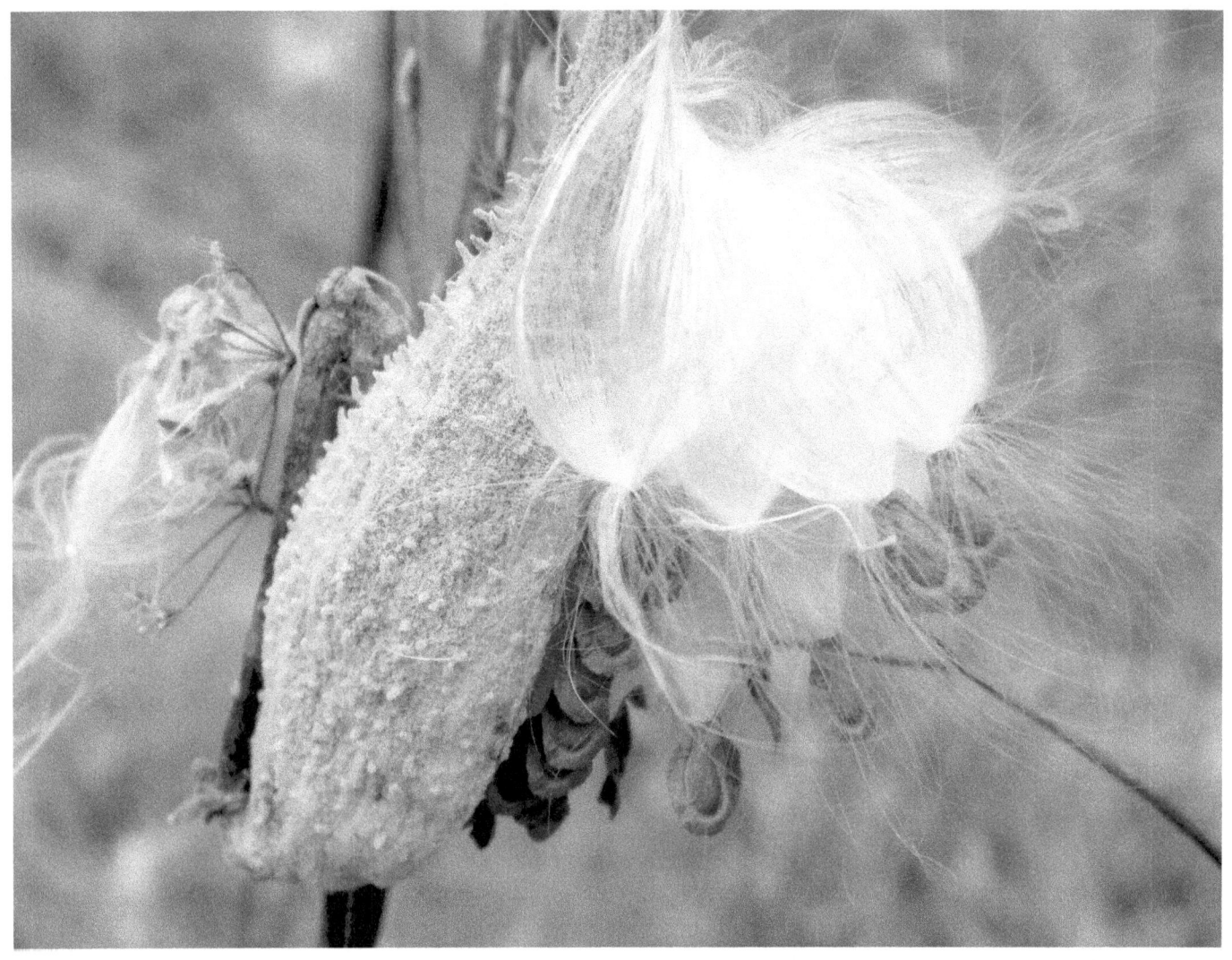

MILKWEED POD AND SEED FLUFF

Natural Fibers Corp, a Nebraska company currently processes more than 3,500 pounds of floss each year with down as a filling for comforters, jackets and pillows. It is the same density as goose down, with even better insulating factor and 20% warmer per unit.

One blend of 80% goose down and 20% milkweed wicks moisture about 30% faster than down alone and 70% faster than synthetic pillows.

Milkweed can be planted and cared for with traditional row crop equipment. Black spot fungus and a bacterial blight are two natural enemies that require control. It companion plants well with Goldenrod, Dill, and Penstemon.

The Green Milkweed pods are harvested with a modified New Idea Uni-system ear corn picker at 70% moisture, and before they open to release their floss and seed. The pods are cracked open in a roller mill and dried to 30% moisture in portable tanks. Once dried, the pods are processed using a modified 1940 model combine, a cleaning apparatus and a hopper. The floss is vacuum bagged from the hopper

Hats made with it are very light and soft. Candlewicks apparently burn clearer, and produce less offensive smoke than cotton wicks.

Herb Knudsen, the owner, says "several years ago, we ran preliminary tests on blending fibers for making facial tissue. Blended tissue soaked up moisture faster, and Kimberley Clark alone could use tufts from 10 million acres of Milkweed."

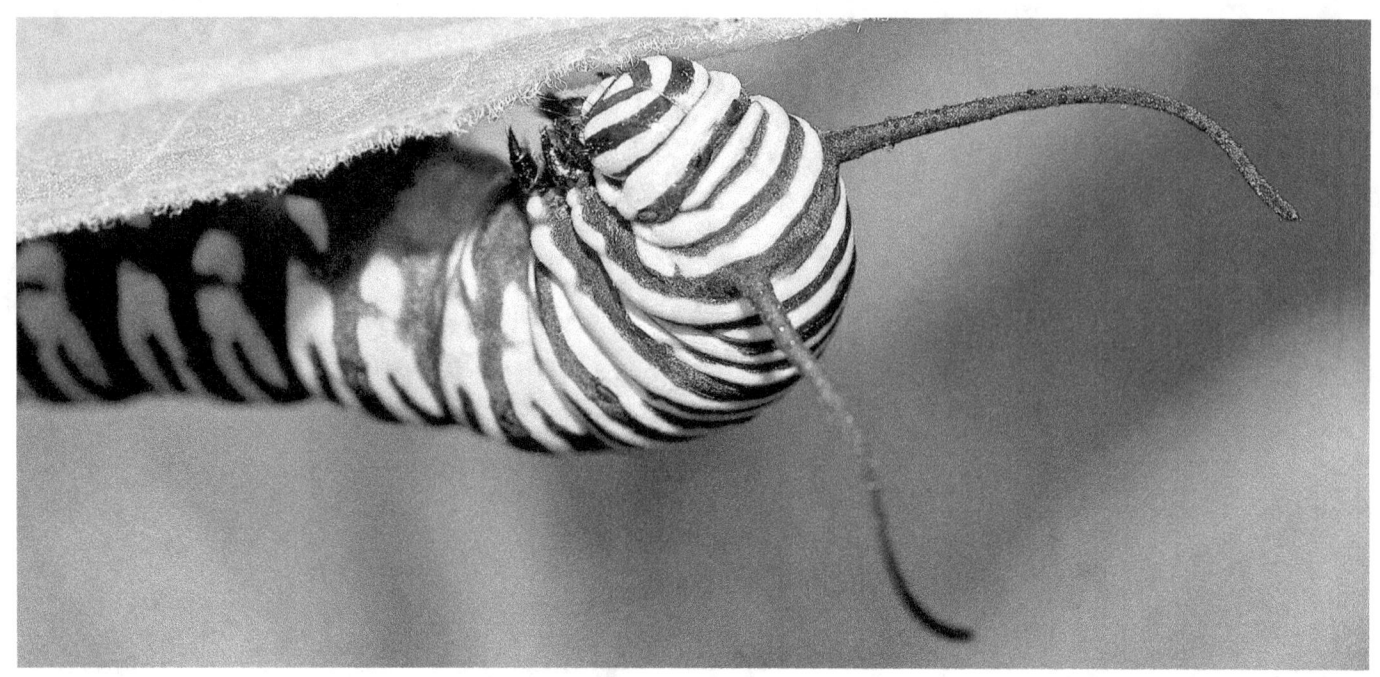

MONARCH CATERPILLAR ON MILKWEED

The floss is "non allergenic cellulose fiber; with a fill power of about 350 cm^3 which is comparable to high quality goose down; white in color; 50% more breathable than down; 20% more durable than down; and 10% warmer per unit of weight than down.

The seed meal left over contains cardenolides that produce heart palpitations, and cannot be used for animal feed.

Scientists in Peoria, Illinois have found the seed meal kills nematodes and fall armyworms. In one field study, milkweed seed meal killed 97% of nematodes on potatoes, and it is now thought that incorporating the meal into the soil may be a safe alternative to methyl bromide.

The Monarch butterfly feeds, almost exclusively in the larvae stage, on Milkweed. They retain strong concentrations of the glycoside (the females 24% more than males). Research conducted at Amherst College shows that birds dining on the Monarch suffer poisoning, and vomiting for up to 30 minutes afterwards.

In fact, the butterfly and plant are so intertwined that when milkweed was introduced to the Solomon Islands (now Hawaii) in 1840 there were no Monarch butterflies. Three years later the first ones appeared and began to breed.

A freak snowstorm in central Mexico, in January 2002, killed as many as 270 million Monarch butterflies. Their annual journey of nearly 5,000 kilometers is one of the wonders of the natural world. Fortunately, as a species, they have remarkable ability to come back.

Milkweed discourages other insects, hanging them by their tongues if they try to steal nectar, or coating the feet of ants with milky sap that hardens and cripples. The pollen sticks to bumblebees so tenaciously that when they try to fly away, a leg or two may tear off.

Both neurological and cardiotoxic/ gastrointestinal syndromes have been observed in sheep and goats ingesting various species of milkweed.

Both *A. tuberosa* and *A. speciosa* presented no abnormalities when fed deliberately to livestock. All species produced mild to moderate pulmonary changes including congestion and edema; and many produced death within 48-72 hours.

That being said, seed protein may be used as a thickener, protein extender and for adhesives and paint emulsifiers. Hojilla-Evangelista et al, *Indust Crops Prod* 29:2-3.

MEDICINAL

CONSTITUENTS- *A. syriaca-* aerial parts contain alpha and beta asclepiadins, alpha and beta amyrin and their acetates and butyrates, beta sitosterol, uzarigenin, xysmalogenin, aspecioside, syriogenin, lupenyl acetate, and syriobioside.

The root contains asclepione, a resinoid, 20 pregnane glycosides including ikemagenin, 12-O-nicotinoyllineolon, 5alpha, 6-dihydroikemagen, 12-O-tigloylisolineolon, and their aglycones; caoutchouc, fixed oils, tannins, glucose, a bitter principle, gum, starch and volatile oils.

seed- acyl-acyl carrier protein (ACP) desaturase. Also rich in palmitoleic and cis-vaccenic acids, as well as EFAs. Also contain cinnamic acid cardenolide ester, condurangin, cymarose, desglucouzarin, rhamnose, syrioboside, syriogenin, uzarigenin and xysmalogenin.

sprouted seed- nicotine, beta sitosterol, asclepiadin, alpha amyrin

latex- asclepians

leaf only-alpha resorcylic, vanillic and chlorogenic acids; anti-tumour polyphenols.

leaves and flowers- p-hydroxybenzoic, p-coumaric, protocatechuic, and caffeic acids;

flower only- gallic acid, kaempferol, kaempferol 7-0-beta-glucoside, kaempferol 3-0-beta-galactopyranoside, kaempferol-3-0-beta-glucopyranosyl (1—>2)-beta-galactopyranoside, iso-rhamnetin, isorhamnetin 7-0-beta-glucoside, etc.

A. speciosa- stems- 1,4 beta D glucans, arabinogalactan protein, ascecioside, alpha and bata amyrin acetate, beta sitosterol, pseudo taraxasterol, syriobioside, urosolic acid

A. incarnata root- two cardenolides, frugoside and gofruside, three 12-0-acylated pregnane glycosides, and 29 various oxypregnane glycosides, including tri- and penta- glycosides of isolineolin, ikemagenin and 12-0-acetyl lineolon.

aerial parts- 34 pregnane glycosides, including lineolon, isolinelon, ikemagenin, 12-0-nicotinoyllineolon, deacylmetaplexigenin, metaplexigenin, rostratamine, 12-0-acetyllineolon, 15beta-hydroxylineolon, and 15beta-hydroxyisolineolon as their aglycones, and 2,6-dideoxyhexopyranose, gluco-pyranose and allopyranose as the sugar components. Leaves contain seven flavonoid compounds.

A. subulata- aerial parts- cardenolide glycosides including 12,16-dihydroxyicalotropin, calotropin, corotoxigenin 3-O-glucopyranoside, desglucouzarin.

A. curassavica- the leaf contains calotropin, corotoxicenin, calotropagenin, uzarigenin, coroglaucigenin, asclepogenin, clepogenin, ascurogenin, and curassavogenin.

root- asclepin

A. tuberosa root- cardiac glycosides of cardenolide type including asclepin, calotropin, calcitin, gomphoside, syriogenin, syrioside, uscharidin, uscharin, uzarigenin and afroside, 16 pregnane glycosides including ikemagenin and lineolon; tuberogenin, 5,6-dideydrotuberogenin; gums and resin galitoxin.

aerial parts- flavonoids including rutin, kaemperfol, quercitin and isorhamnetin; triterpenes including friedalin, alpha and beta amyrin, lupeol, and viburnitol; choline, sugars, amino acids, caffeic and chlorogenic acid, resins, choline, essential oils, and bitters (asclepione); tuberosides A-L, tuberogenin, as well as 20 plus steroidal and pregnane glycosides of 8,14 seco-pregnanes including ikemagenin, lineolon, pleurogenin, with attached sugars ranging from tetraosides to heptaosides.

Cardiac glycosides of all Asclepias species are present in every plant part with descending amounts in the latex, stem, leaf and root.

Swamp Milkweed (*A. incarnata*) flowers, leaves and stems extracts (ether and saline), show activity against both Gram-positive and negative bacteria.

The root is a relaxant and mildly stimulating, according to Dr. Cook. Its principal use has been as a mild cathartic in worm preparations, often combined with *Chenopodium or Artemisia* for this purpose. Professor Tully recommended the herb for dry asthma.

Early Eclectics considered it similar to digitalis without the irritating gastrointestinal effects.

Dr. Ellingwood (1922) wrote. "It may be given in coughs and colds, rheumatism from cold, painful stitches in the chest with threatened inflammation of the lungs and pleura, asthma, chronic gastric catarrh, diarrhea, dysentery, dropsy, worms, erysipelatous diseases. It improves digestion, and is a good remedy in chronic catarrh of the stomach, and in catarrhal inflammation of the respiratory organs".

Showy Milkweed root can be dried and chopped as a medicine. When needed, a weak decoction can be drunk, and a poultice prepared from the plant residue for relieving sore breasts, cases of mastitis, and engorged painful breasts from too much milk production.

The root stimulates both urine and perspiration, softens bronchial mucus, dilates bronchial tubes, and encourages expectoration.

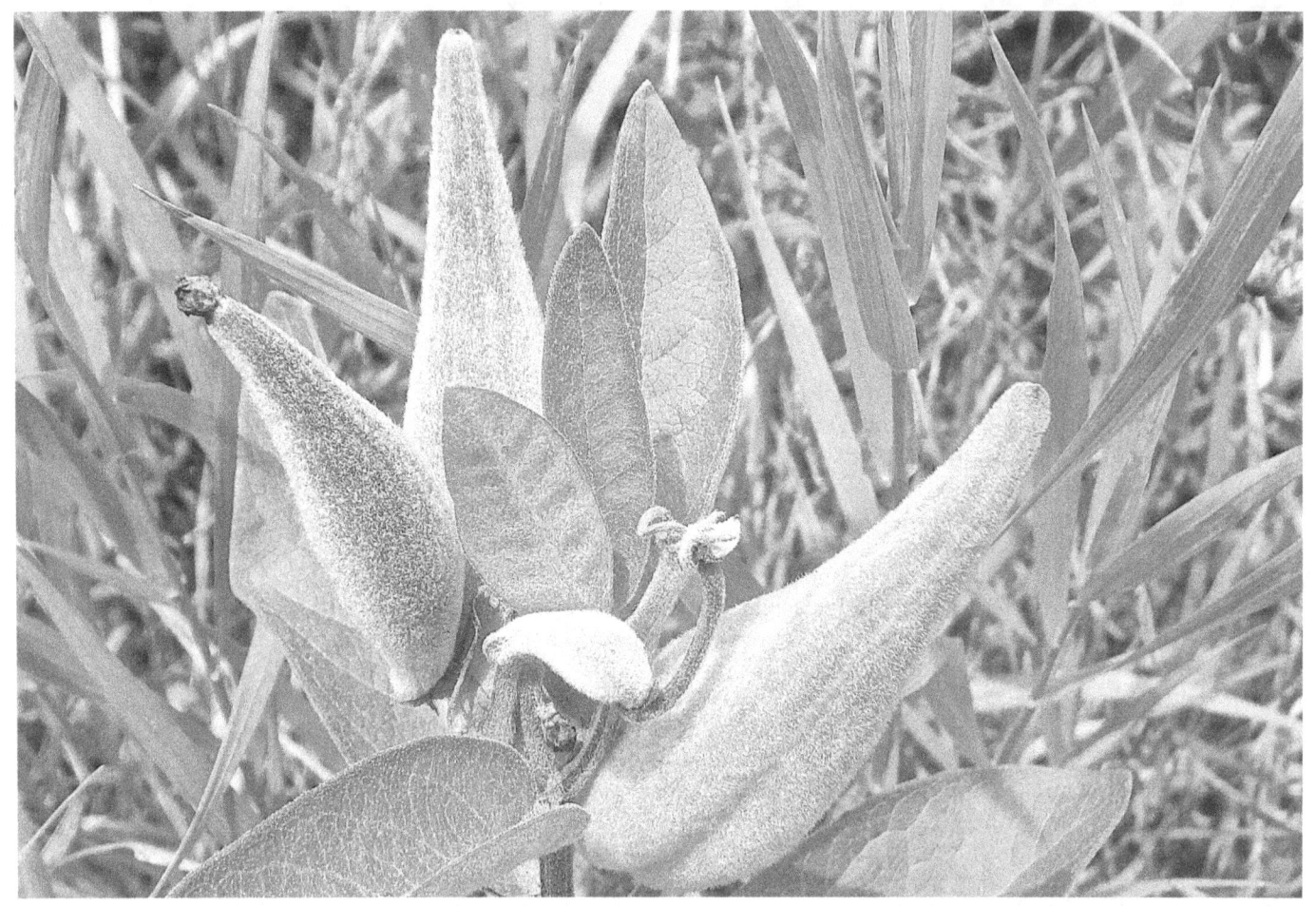

LOW MILKWEED PODS

As a diuretic it increases both the volume and solids passed in urine and aids chronic kidney weakness. Use half strength for kidneys, full for lungs.

Michael Moore relates a story of a dear friend who used one tsp of root with one tablespoon of marshmallow root, decocted slowly for one hour in pint of water for gallbladder attacks. "I have no idea why it helps so well but it does, and in fact, it is rather more effective than such traditional herbs as *Lobelia inflata, Chelidonium majus* and leptandra."

Common or Silky Milkweed dried root can be made into a tincture (see below). It is a valuable diuretic, increasing both the solid and watery constituents of the urine. It is also diaphoretic, not by stimulating, but by lowering the action of the heart.

It is thought to act directly upon the vaso-motor system, lessening local congestion. This is true as well in uterus stagnation, delayed menstruation, labor pains and retained placenta.

The drying root contains anodyne, or pain relieving properties not fully understood as yet. Grieve suggests that it is as efficient as Pleurisy root (*A. tuberosa*) for cases of asthma, relieving coughs and painful lung conditions. I'm not sure.

The flower infusion is taken hot for asthma and nasal catarrh, while cold root infusions are best for chronic kidney weakness with lumbago, especially in morning, edema, urinary gravel and Bright's disease.

It was placed formerly in the *United States Pharmacopoeia*, and recommended by the *Eclectic Dispensatory* as a fluid extract, in cases of amenorrhea, dropsy, retention of urine, asthma, dyspepsia, cough and difficulty in breathing.

Dr. Bastyr used the root for viral pharyngitis, in 60 drops doses three times daily.

Silky Milkweed is often combined with marshmallow root in the treatment of gallstones.

Also known as Inmortal Root, the herb's main action involves the circulation associated with the heart and lungs.

It is both relaxing to spastic bronchi, as in the case of asthma, but also useful in expectorating excessive mucous and phlegm in pneumonia and pleurisy.

The root helps resolve lymphatic congestion (taken cold) and cold, chilly flu-like symptoms, when taken hot.

The leaf of Silky Milkweed contains several polyphenols with anti-tumor activity comparable or more potent than standard chemotherapy preparations such as thiotepa, methotrexate, melphalan, and cyclophosphamide. Rotinberg et al, *Rom J Physiol* 2000 37.

More recent work identified new compounds and tested them against various breast cancer cell lines, including MCF-7, T47D and Sk-Br-3. Araya JJ et al, *J Nat Prod* 2012 75(3): 400-7.

A double linked cardenolide glycoside inhibits DU145 prostate cancer cells. Zhang RR et al, *Org Biomol Chem* 2014 12(44): 8919-29.

Work in India found various extracts of this herb showed cytotoxicity against human colon adenocarcinoma cell lines. Baskar AA et al, *Redox Rep* 2012 17(4): 145-56.

Michael Moore wrote extensively about southwest medicinal herbs. He suggests the rubbery latex, gathered by slicing the sterile green stems is a good chewing gum for dry, irritated coughs. It is bitter and stimulates saliva production.

"The root works well as an expectorant-diaphoretic when you are just getting sick, with a dry heat in the sinuses or across the chest, and the sense that your skin is not quite big enough to contain you—or less fancifully, when you toss and turn, hot, fretful and are not quite sure exactly how sick you are but know that you're coming down with something in your head and chest…The tincture seems the best way to use the roots; cups of the boiled tea can upset the stomach, whereas the small amount of tincture doesn't."

Desert Milkweed contain cardenolide glycosides induce apoptosis in A549 cancer cells. Rascon-Valenzuela LA et al, *J Ethnopharmacology* 2016 193: 303-311. The aerial parts, extracted with alcohol, showed significant activity on A549 (lung), and PC3 cancer cell lines, in study by same group. *Pharm Biol* 2015 53(12): 1741-51.

Bloodflower or Bloodflower Milkweed is a valuable medicinal plant, with a long tradition of use in China.

It is known as **MA LI CHIN** or **MA LI JIN**. The aerial part is known in some texts as **LIAN SHENG GUI ZI HUA**.

The entire plant is used for its bitter, acrid flavour and cold properties. It has several important actions, including dispersing inflammation, invigorating the blood circulation, and controlling bleeding.

It is used in tonsillitis, pneumonia, bronchitis, and urethritis. It is valued for stopping external bleeding, and chronic leucorrhea.

The herb is used in India to treat hemorrhoids, gonorrhea, roundworms and abdominal tumors.

The plant contains cardiotonic effects that are similar to strophanoside. This is probably due to the mild cardiac glucoside, asclepiadin, present in all the milkweeds. Work by Patnaik et al, has shown that asclepin, a glycoside, showed increased force of contraction, and was found more active than digoxin or strophanthin, with a wider safety margin. *Arzne Forsch* 1978 28. Asclepin is reported to exhibit a more powerful activity towards weak cardiac muscle.

Cysteine protease, derived from the latex, exhibits strong pro-coagulant and thrombin-like activity. Shivaprasad HV et al, *J Ethnopharmacol* 2009 123(1): 106-9. This appears to validate traditional use of sap to stop bleeding on fresh cuts.

Plant extracts stimulate mammalian CNS, causing an increase in serotonin and noradrenaline concentrations. Del Pilar, *An Inst Farmacol Espan* 1971 20.

In vitro, the constituent calotropin has been shown to inhibit human nasopharyngeal carcinoma. This anti-carcinogenic effect probably extends to human health as well.

It was tested in the early 1970s as a potential chemotherapeutic drug.

Calotropin, from this species, has been found to inhibit and induce apoptosis in cisplatin-induced resistant non-small cell lung cancer (A549)cells. Mo EP et al, *Biochem Biophys Res Commun* 2016 478(2): 710-5.

Caltropin inhibits the growth of K562 human chronic myeloid leukemia cancer cell lines and induces apoptosis. Wang SC et al, *Cell Biol Int* 2009 33(12): 1230-6.

Another compound asclepiasterol may be a modulator that reverses P-gp-mediated multidrug resistance in over-expressing cancer variants including MCF-7 and HepF-2, resistant to doxorubicin and rhodamine. Yuan WQ et al, *Oncotarget* 2016 7(21): 466-83.

Asclepin and 12beta-hydroxycalotropin show strong cytotoxic activity against HepG2 and Raji cell lines, in work by Li JZ et al, *Bioorg Med Chem Lett* 2009 19(7): 1956-9.

The sap has been shown to inhibit the growth of *Candida albicans*. It appears that the sap acts on the cell wall of fungi; and probably consists of terpenes, cardenolides, and enzymes including glucanases. Koike et al, *Chem Pharm Bull* 1980 28.

The sap or latex is thrombin-like and promotes coagulation of external wounds. Shivaprasad et al, *J Ethnopharm* 123:1.

Beta sitosterols, isolated from the herb, are cytotoxic to human colon adenocarcinoma cancer cell lines. Baskar AA et al, *BMC Complement Altern Med* 2010 10:24.

Dr. Cook suggested the roots are in all respects similar to Pleurisy root. It should be combined with a diffusive stimulant, as otherwise, the action on the bowels is quite pronounced, especially when used fresh as a relaxing emetic.

Pleurisy root (*A. tuberosa*) was first used by various Native groups, and recorded historically in Samuel Stern's *American Herbal* in 1772. Early settlers observed natives chewing on the raw root to relieve lung conditions.

From 1820-1905 it was official in the *US Pharmacopoeia*. The herb found its way to Germany, and into the literature there as early as 1787.

The plant prefers sandy and gravely soil. Dr. Brown (1867) even suggested that *A. tuberosa* grown on sandy soil is twice as effective as that on fertile. The dried root it bitter at first, but later has a nutty flavor similar to parsnips.

As the name suggests, the root is a specific for lung ailments of various sorts, including bronchitis, or any lung condition with congestion, inflammation and difficult breathing.

This cold, drying, bitter root is one our best relaxing and sedative expectorants. It may be considered a parasympathetic nervous system stimulant.

Pleurisy root is best suited for chronic conditions with stagnation, dry phlegm and hot, dry skin. For bronchitis and pneumonia it is best used in the acute stage.

Pleurisy, an inflammation of the pleura of the lungs, is an extremely serious medical condition that requires constant vigil. The lining of the lung dries out and sticks together, causing the pleuritic stitch, a sharp pain made worse by movement. The lungs are damaged and cannot release and re-circulate fluids.

The top of the lungs dry out, and the bottom collect fluid and stagnation.

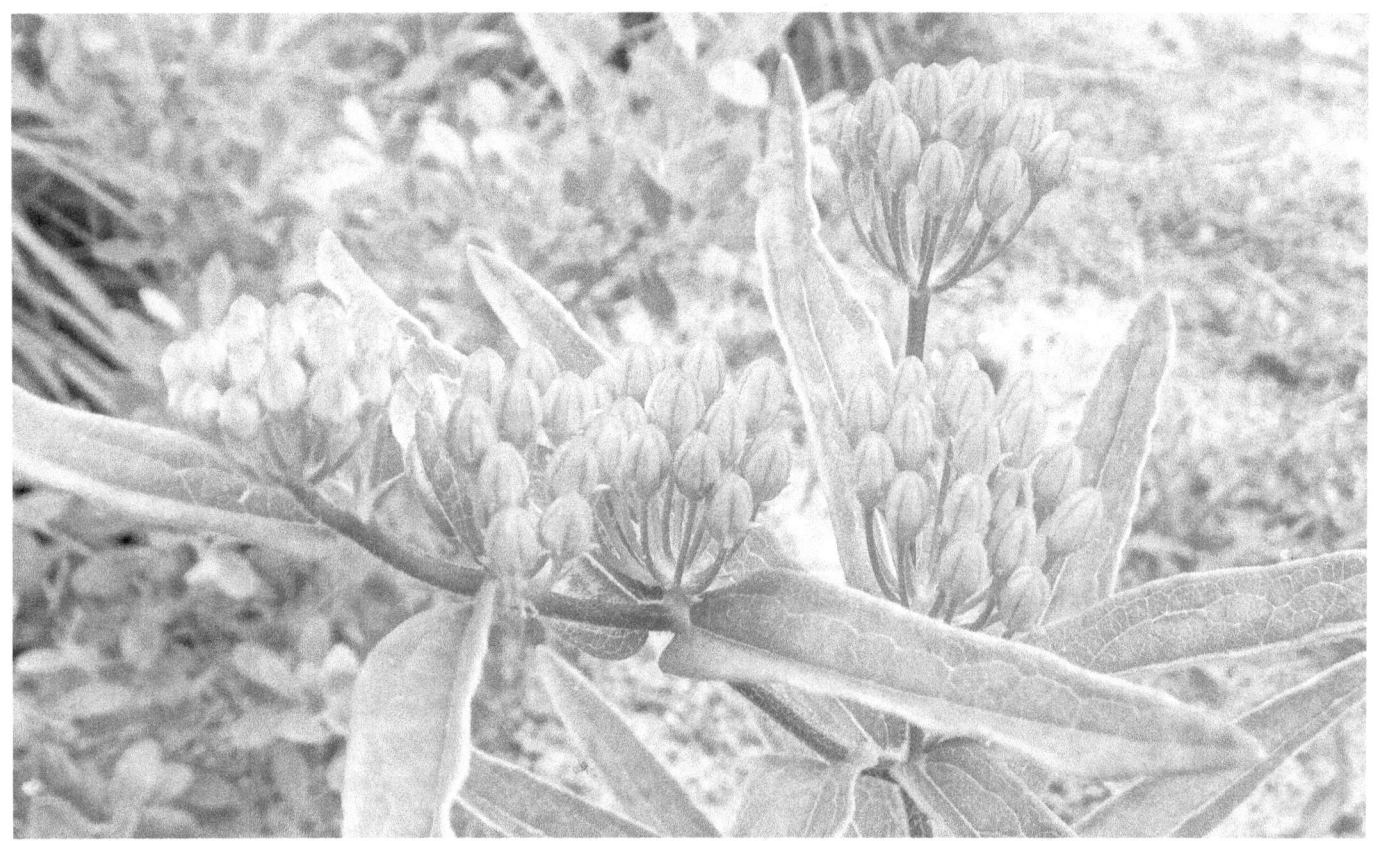

PLEURISY ROOT UN-OPENED FLOWERS

There is little expectoration, and even the skin is very dry. Warm pleurisy root tea stimulates the vagus nerve, increases cholinergic function, producing perspiration, expectoration, and bronchial dilation. Lymphatic drainage and increased fluid circulation help reduce both pleurisy and pulmonary edema. It may also be used with young children in small doses, and if there is a great deal of restlessness, combine with scullcap, until perspiration appears.

Add small amount of lobelia for any bronchial constriction associated with asthma.

Be careful when combining pleurisy root with goldenseal as it may intensify the drying effect, and create dehydration, as well as act hypotensively.

This could be quite dangerous and even life threatening in the extreme.

In TCM, this condition pattern is known as Lung Phlegm Heat, and Wind Heat Invasion.

Matthew Wood, in *The Book of Herbal Wisdom* writes.

"It is a remedy which disperses the chi and fluids of the lungs to the skin and disseminates them downward to the kidneys. It increases the perspiration in acute diseases and brings up phlegm in chronic cases.

It is for people who have a cold that settles in the lungs and causes a weight on the heart."

There is intercostal pain when taking a breath, that is relieved by bending forward. Acute pain is worse with motion. Spasmodic asthma with dry, hot mucosa, poor expectoration and non-productive pulmonary cough also fit the picture.

It combines well with lobelia for hot, spasmodic coughs with difficult expectoration; with American ginseng and calamus root for phlegm heat of the lungs; and with grindelia and know mother root for very dry cough with thick, yellow and obstinate mucus and phlegm.

For chest pain due to heat stagnation and bloody sputum combine with bugleweed.

It is useful in various digestive disorders, including diarrhea, and dysentery. A lesser known, but important usage, is for peritonitis, a serious infection and inflammation of the intestines. For all of these, take cold.

The powdered root can be applied to wounds, to stop bleeding. The fresh root can be grated and applied to bruises, rheumatism, and other inflammations, including lameness in the lower extremities. Both root and aerial parts contain pregnane glycosides that cause human fibroblasts to proliferate. Warashina et al, *Phytochemistry* 72:14-15 1865-75.

It is useful when bursa of the body are inflamed and painful, just like the lungs. Combine with black cohosh for inflamed joints, bursa and rheumatic pain made worse from motion.

Certain uterine problems are relieved due to the presence of estrogenic compounds. The root possesses estrogen-like activity. Costello and Butler, *Journal of American Pharm Assoc Sci Ed* 1950 39

The flavonoid kaempferol demonstrates estrogenic activity, as well as anti-spasmodic action; something shared with lupeol.

Lupeol possesses anti-arthritic properties that may help arthritic joints and intercostals rheumatism.

It is therefore, contraindicated during pregnancy, as even low dosage can cause uterine contractions.

In dry eczema, the use of Pleurisy root may be indicated, where lymphatic congestion and low-grade fevers are present.

Peter Holmes suggests its use in acute fever, as well as dry, stagnant eczema.

Because Pleurisy root contains cardiac glycosides, with effect on the electrical and muscle system of the heart, it may interfere with heart drugs. Asclepin helps strengthen heart contractions, but care must be exercised. Dr. Christopher suggested its relaxant properties act upon the capillaries, and give the heart a rest when burdened by undue tension.

Charles Kane suggested, " a key indication for the plant's use is a strong, bounding pulse in febrile conditions. Used in conjunction with elevated temperatures Pleurisy root often lowers blood pressure and slows the heart rate…The plant should be considered a constitutional medicine for individuals whose skin is chronically dry, injures/reacts easily, and heals poorly. Typically these people will be adrenalin stress types prone to allergic skin sensitivity, and constipation."

Proliferation of skin fibroblasts was noted in work by Warashina T et al, *Phytochemistry* 72(14-15): 1865-75. This would be as an external wash.

The cardiac glycosides increase the force of heart contractions, while decreasing the heart rate, likely through inhibition of Na/K-ATPase in cardiac myocytes. This in turn promotes influx of $Ca2+$, increasing contractibility of heart muscle. They appear to decrease the conduction velocity in the arterio-ventricular junction according to Eric Yarnell, a very fine teacher, author and professional member of the *American Herbalist Guild*.

The French herbalist, Bruneton suggests the glycosides inhibit the renin-angiotensin-aldosterone system, thereby exerting diuretic and diaphoretic activity.

Large doses may interfere with hormonal therapies and when medicines like MAO inhibitors are used for depression.

Water extracts of the stems exhibit activity against mycobacterium. However, the roots show poor inhibition of *Mycobacterium tuberculosis*. Green E et al, *J Ethnopharm* 2010 130(1): 151-7.

Dr. William Mitchell, Jr. suggested, "Asclepias tastes how I imagine the forest would taste if were tinctured. It is very bright tasting and feels green in your mouth." A very apt description! The aerial parts are toxic, only root is used.

Whorled Milkweed (*A. verticillata*) extracts show activity against both gram positive and negative bacteria.

HOMEOPATHY

Pleurisy root (*A. tuberosa*) has its chief action on the chest muscles.

Respiration is painful, especially at the base of the left lung. The cough is dry, the throat constricted. There may be a pain or pleuritic stitch between the shoulder blades or in the heart region.

The spaces between the ribs close to the sternum are tender and painful.

Expectoration is little and usually yellow and sticky. Lower eyelid appears ulcerated.

Stools are moss green and like rotten eggs, the stomach full of pressure, with flatulence.

The extremities and joints are rheumatic and give the sensation as if adhesions are breaking up when bending. Pain worse after a cold or after becoming cold.

Unusual elevation of spirits and cheerfulness towards evening, followed by fretfulness and peevishness. Dreams of the countryside, reckless boasting, and singing of political songs.

Craving for lemons and seasoned food.

DOSE- Tincture to 1st potency. The original proving on one male was the effect of two drops of tincture for 42 days, recorded by Savary in France in 1856. Nichol in Canada in 1865 used the tincture and 1x dilution.

Swamp Milkweed (*A. incarnata*) can be useful in cases of chronic gastric catarrh and in leucorrhea. It may also give relief in dropsy and difficulties breathing.

DOSE- Tincture and low potencies.

Silkweed (Silky Milkweed) *Asclepias syriaca* seems to act especially on the nervous system and urinary organs. It is a specific remedy for dropsy, hepatic, renal, or cardiac conditions.

It causes diaphoresis, and augments the urinary secretion.

Silky Milkweed may be helpful in acute rheumatic inflammation of the large joints.

It may also be of relief in intermittent, pressing down uterine pain.

The head feels as if a sharp instrument were thrust through from temple to temple. There may be forehead constriction, or a nervous headache.

After suppressed perspiration, increased urine flow with increased specific gravity may occur.

The mind is calm with quiet feeling. There is lack of confidence, a feeling that something will happen, or dreams of being in daily contact with famous people.

Increased appetite with craving for farinaceous food and nuts. Tongue feels swollen with speech difficult.

Shiny zigzags in a semi-circle in left field of vision. Extreme dryness of mouth in morning.

DOSE- Tincture to 30c doses. The mother tincture is made from the fresh root. Proving of fresh infused root was done by Clerbone and Potter. A more recent proving was done by Renate Muller at 30c in 1996.

ESSENTIAL OIL

Milkweed (*A. syriaca*) has been analyzed by headspace, with 2-phenylethanol and benzyl alcohol the most abundant. While mosquitoes found milkweed extracts attractive, they did not respond to synthetic blends of these compounds when tested in a dual port olfactometer. Also present were (E)-beta-ocimene, benzyl alcohol, nonamal and (E)-2-nonenal.

PLANT OILS AND RESINS

All the Milkweeds contain oils, latex, and rubber from their milky leaves and stems, and from their seeds.

Swamp Milkweed contains about 4.7% oil in the whole, dry plant. The rubber content is 0.3-2.6%; and the seed oil is 27% of the seed by weight.

Silky Milkweed contains 4.3% oil of the whole dry plant, latex 1-2% and rubber of 0.5-2.3%.

Whorled Milkweed (*A. verticillata*) is 4.5% oil (by dry plant), and between 1.2 and 2.4% rubber.

SEED OIL

The seed oils of Asclepias species contain mainly C-18 triglycerides that are 92% unsaturated. The oils possess high viscosity and excellent moisturizing properties.

Silky Milkweed (*A. syriaca*) seeds have been analyzed in Canada, by Watson and Levetin. The seeds are rich in oleic acid (51.8%), and linoleic acid (43.8%).

The seed oil contains 20-30% of a highly unsaturated oil having unusual fatty acids. The triglycerides have been oxidized by *in situ* performic acid to the poly-oxirane and polyhydroxy-triglycerides.

Vaccenic acid has been found to stimulate growth-promoting factors in rat studies. This could lead to a new industrial crop. Harry-O'kuru et al, *J Ag Food Chem* 2002 50:11.

Standard Oil of Ohio conducted studies on Milkweed as a source of synthetic oil in the late 1970s. Melvin Calvin, a Nobel laureate, and other scientists projected that billions of barrels of synthetic crude oil could be recovered from milkweed biomass.

It proved, at the time, to be economically unfeasible, but oil was only $20 per barrel in those days.

The seeds of *A. speciosa* contain 23% triglycerides by weight, with 50% linoleic, 34% oleic and 1% linolenic acid, as well as 0.1% squalene.

The defatted meal shows anti-nematode activity in both greenhouse and field trials. Holser RA, *Industrial Crops and Products* 2003 18.

FLOWER ESSENCES

Low milkweed flower essence is related to uniting the male and female nature of ourselves.   **PRAIRIE DEVA**

Butterfly Weed flower essence works with two dynamics in the personality; love and freedom. It allows for more maturity and deeper relationship. It is an excellent essence to take during family or couples therapy. Many sexual problems such as frigidity, impotence as well as genital disease and sexual addictions are helped. Cats and dogs who develop problems of urinating in the household benefit from this essence. It can be used by animal breeders to increase fertility.   **DALTON**

Silky Milkweed flower essence helps extract one from emotionally complex situations, and creates mental clarity, objectivity, and spiritual consciousness. There may be grief, despair, despondency and fear of death.
PEGASUS

Pleurisy root flower essence is for stress and anxiety that may cause ulcers. Suppressed rage and grief are alleviated. The third chakra and emotional body are balanced. It may help issues dealing with the mother image.
PEGASUS

Showy Milkweed essence is for establishing a working relationship with the spiritual aspect of self.
ROCKY MTN

Milkweed essence is helpful for periods where a powerful shift in consciousness brings about a deeper understanding of the essential nature of things.   **LIGHT MOUNTAIN**

SPIRITUAL PROPERTIES

Milkweed imparts a deep sense of nurturing in some individuals. It can be difficult at times for men to understand the nurturing or loving side of themselves. And women may sometimes struggle against this, as if in taking care of others they neglect to to take care of themselves.

The ability to release problems and truly love another individual and oneself is enhanced. This involves a deep set of psychic abilities that is very helpful for development of many other capacities. The Lemurians discovered a technique by which the watery substance of milkweed could be vibrationally changed. The sound vibrations allowed Milkweed to become easily assimilable by a person. This allowed energy of the Earth to permeate into a person's body, yet it had a certain nourishing capacity as well. Only small quantities of it were necessary, but the vibration has changed in a similar way that cooking is now used to change various herbs, plants, and food substances so they are assimilabile, by humans. The life stream was affect, and the devic spirits associated reflected on what was happening to the plant and what was working then for humanity. The question asked was "What can be contributed?" It was seen that this nurturing ability would be useful in the future, so the plant and associated nature spirits willingly took on the task of developing this nurturing ability in mankind. This is the karmic purpose of Milkweed.   **GURUDAS**

A. curassavica is associated with the response of the physical mind to the supramental light. That is, the physical mind is eager to understand and be transformed.   **THE MOTHER**

Few things produced by insects are more beautiful than the chrysalis of the Monarch. As I saw it that morning on the maple twig, it was jade green and decorated with a black line and dots of purest shining gold. Within this husk of chitin, the pupa lived and breathed, a half-creature neither larva nor butterfly but something between.   **E.W. TEALE**

PERSONALITY TRAITS

But not only to the mind of the artist and poet does the milkweed appeal. It is also beloved of the scientist. No other plant, except the strangely over-developed orchid and the gruesome little carnivorous plants, has received as much attention from scientists as the milkweed.

The scientific account reads like a modern horror and crime story with a beautiful friendship to add enrichment. One may read pates of scientific detail on how the milkweed traps small insects, hanging them by the tongue until they die a frightful death, because they tried to steal the nectar made for larger insects; how the milky juice repels the visits of marauding ants and small crawling bugs, coating their feet as they climb the stalk and eventually crippling them by hardening so they cannot remove it; and most interesting of all, the relationship between the milkweeds and the monarch butterflies, those beautiful orange and black butterflies so common in our gardens, which are always found hovering about a clump of milkweed.

How far along the road of evolution has this highly organized flower traveled from those first simple flowers which produced their pollen in such amazing quantities that they could trust an erratic breeze to carry it to its destination!

The monarch butterfly has a tongue perfectly adapted to the needs of the milkweed, and so does the work of fertilization for it. In return, the milkweed's leaves nourish the grubs of the butterfly and its acrid juice is so distasteful to birds that both grub and butterfly are immune from the attacks that so diminish the grubs of other species.

Moths and butterflies, those ethereal beauties who should thrive on sunlight and nectar are, alas for our sense of fitness, quickly attracted by a vile and putrid odour. Since all the flower's efforts are to attract these butterflies, the milkweed's fragrance enters into neither poetry nor art.   **A. BROWN**

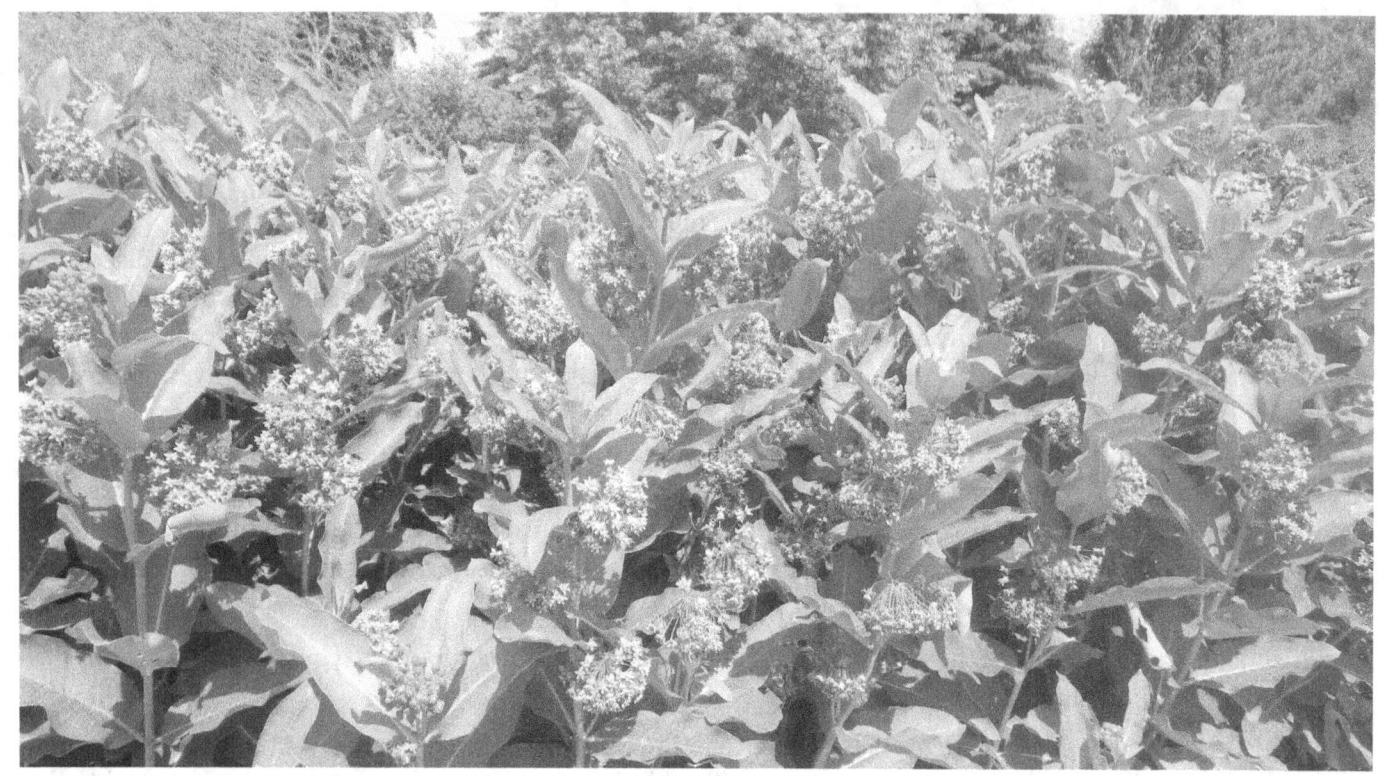

SWAMP MILKWEED PATCH

Pleurisy Root, as a gestalt, tends to stimulate skin and mucosal circulation, sebaceous secretions, and sweat; therefore it can be used with great success in tonic formulas for both dry skin and hair, frequent nighttime urination and generally poor adaptability to changes in heat and humidity. This all derives from our body's tendency to balance everyday fluid mechanics and blood chemistry between the lungs, kidneys and skin. Pleurisy root shifts dominance to the lungs and skin and away from the kidneys. Folks with a pattern of adrenalin stress and blood sugar ups and downs often manifest dry skin and mucosa and somewhat compromised pulmonary function. Pleurisy Root acts as a tonic for this by shifting energy to the lungs and surface membranes, i.e., strengthening weaknesses, a proper tonic effect. **MICHAEL MOORE**

DOCTRINE OF SIGNATURES

Asclepias is the perfect picture of a cooling diaphoretic herb, with its many arms of bushy green leaves reaching up to release heat in an explosion of bright orange flowers at its fingertips. What better metaphor could one find to describe a plant that draws heat out through the surface?

The explosive quality of its flowers can also be seen in that of the seed pod – bursting open to release its white tailed seeds upon the wind – and is indicative of the dispersing, diffusive qualities this plant processes as medicine…The transformation of these fire colored flowers to small compacted seed pods opening and releasing their silvery contents to the wind is almost metaphorical for the drying and cooling transition this plant ensues within the lungs. **DANIELLE CHARLES**

MYTHS AND LEGENDS

Like Jesus, Asklepios was born of a divine father and mortal mother. He, too, spent his time…walking through the countryside followed by his disciples, offering healing and succor to anyone who asked. Like Jesus, he was a manifestation of the archetype of the wounded healer and savior who knows our suffering because he has experienced it.

Apollo, the god of light and truth, medicine and music, fell in love with "lovely gowned Koronis". (She) was unfaithful to the god after he impregnated her.

Her unfaithfulness was reported to Apollo by the crow...originally white. In a fit of rage, Apollo turned the crow black.

Apollo named this baby Asklepios and gave him to Chiron, "that idyllic kentaur, that friend to man".

Chiron passed all his knowledge of the healing ways to his charge Asklepios, who in time surpassed him in skill.

This transfer from powerful but inadequate birth father to accessible mentor is another necessary aspect of the healer's development. Robert Bly likens a mentor to "the male mother".

The archetypal healer, planted and grounded in the human feminine, must partake of both mortal compassion and the dispassionate reason provided by the god. Too little humanity makes a healer unavailable to the relationship that heals. But err on the side of being "too human" and the healer may be so overwhelmed by feelings and personal issues that he or she is unable to heal others effectively. Asklepios, as archetypal is "the divine physician, who combines light and helpfulness in his personality".   EDWARD TICK

BOTANICA POETICA

Pleurisy Root for pleurisy
Its name is no surprise
A quite specific herb
A pulmonary prize
If you have pneumonia
Or bronchial congestion
For your mucous membranes
Reduces inflammation
A diaphoretic and expectorant
Useful for the flu
Helpful for a cough
Antispasmodic too
It's not for pregnancy
Nor to be eaten fresh
Dry and make a tincture
For pulmonary stress!

SYLVIA CHATROUX MD

RECIPES

COLD INFUSION- 2-4 ounces up to three times daily.

DECOCTION- root- One tsp to one pint of water. Decoct ten minutes. Drink from 2-3 ounces as needed several times daily. Use half dosage for kidney weakness. Inhale through nostrils at body temperature for congested sinuses.

The leftover root can be crushed and applied to painful breasts as poultice.

TINCTURE- *A. tuberosa, A. subulata* or *A. incarnata* root – Ten to thirty drops as needed. The fresh tincture is prepared at 1:2 or 1:3 at 70% alcohol; dry at 1:5 and 45%. Begin with low doses, 5-10 drops and increase as needed. Use larger doses of 30-60 drops up to five times daily for fever, and acute catarrhal conditions.

PLEURISY- Induce vomiting. Steep one teaspoon of pleurisy root in one cup of boiling water for 45 minutes. Take two tablespoons every two hours.

The fresh root is gathered in full plant vigor, before seed is mature, and dried, chopped and pounded to a pulp. It is mixed with two parts by weight of alcohol (45%) and mixed and left to stand for at least eight days. After straining, the tincture has a light, yellow-orange colour, with a bitter, astringent taste, similar to half ripe butternuts. For dry root use a 1:5 ratio of 45% alcohol. This is the preferred method for *A. cornuti and A. incarnata.*

For children 1-5 drops in water. Combine with skullcap if restless.

CAPSULES- *A. tuberosa-* 1-3 "00" capsules three times daily, or as needed

CAUTION- Do not use any of the milkweeds during pregnancy, or combined with existing heart drugs. There is also potential for interaction with MAO inhibitors, and anti-cholinergic drugs but nothing definitive. Caution is advised with diuretics. Do not take for an extended period of time.

PROPAGATION AND HARVESTING- Pleurisy root, or other Milkweed can be started from seed or root divisions, with a bud, in spring or fall. Fresh seeds require a cool damp stratification by mixing with peat moss and refrigerating at 41° F for 2-3 months. Older seeds can be sown directly in ground in the fall where you wish. They do not transplant well. Milkweeds will not grow on boron deficient soils.

Dry sandy soil with a pH of 4.5 to 5.5 is best, with a full sun suiting them fine. Pleurisy root will not flower the first year, putting its energy into root production. Once established, it can survive dry soils, and is very drought tolerant. If the flower buds are pinched off, the plant will branch out and sustain a longer blooming period.

Harvest the second year or older roots after aerial parts have died back in fall; or the following spring. Break off the bud, and replant it to replace the plant. Wash and cut into long strips to dry, or tincture immediately.

You can also propagate from stem cuttings before the plant flowers.

LEWIS' MOCK ORANGE
(***Philadelphus lewisii*** Pursh.)
(***P. gordonianus*** Lindl.) not accepted
GOLDEN MOCK ORANGE
(***P. coronarius*** L.)
PARTS USED- leaves, blossoms

We were made fools of.
And the scent of mock orange
Drifts through the window.
How can I rest? How can I be content when there is still that odor in the world?   LOUISE GLUCK

A white lie
growing bigger___
mock orange.   REV. ROTELLA

Philadelphus links the plant with one of the Ptolemy's of Egypt, who was devoted to his brother and given the surname Philadelphus, or *Brotherly Love*, by the Greeks.

Lewisii is in honour of Captain Meriwether Lewis of the famous Lewis and Clark expeditions. The plant is the state flower of Idaho.

It was previously placed in the *Syringa* genus, occupied by lilacs. The stems of both were easily hollowed and made into flute like musical instruments, and thus **SYRINX**, from the Greek meaning flute.

In Germany, it is sometimes referred to as "Deutsches Jasmin", or "Pfiefenstrauch".

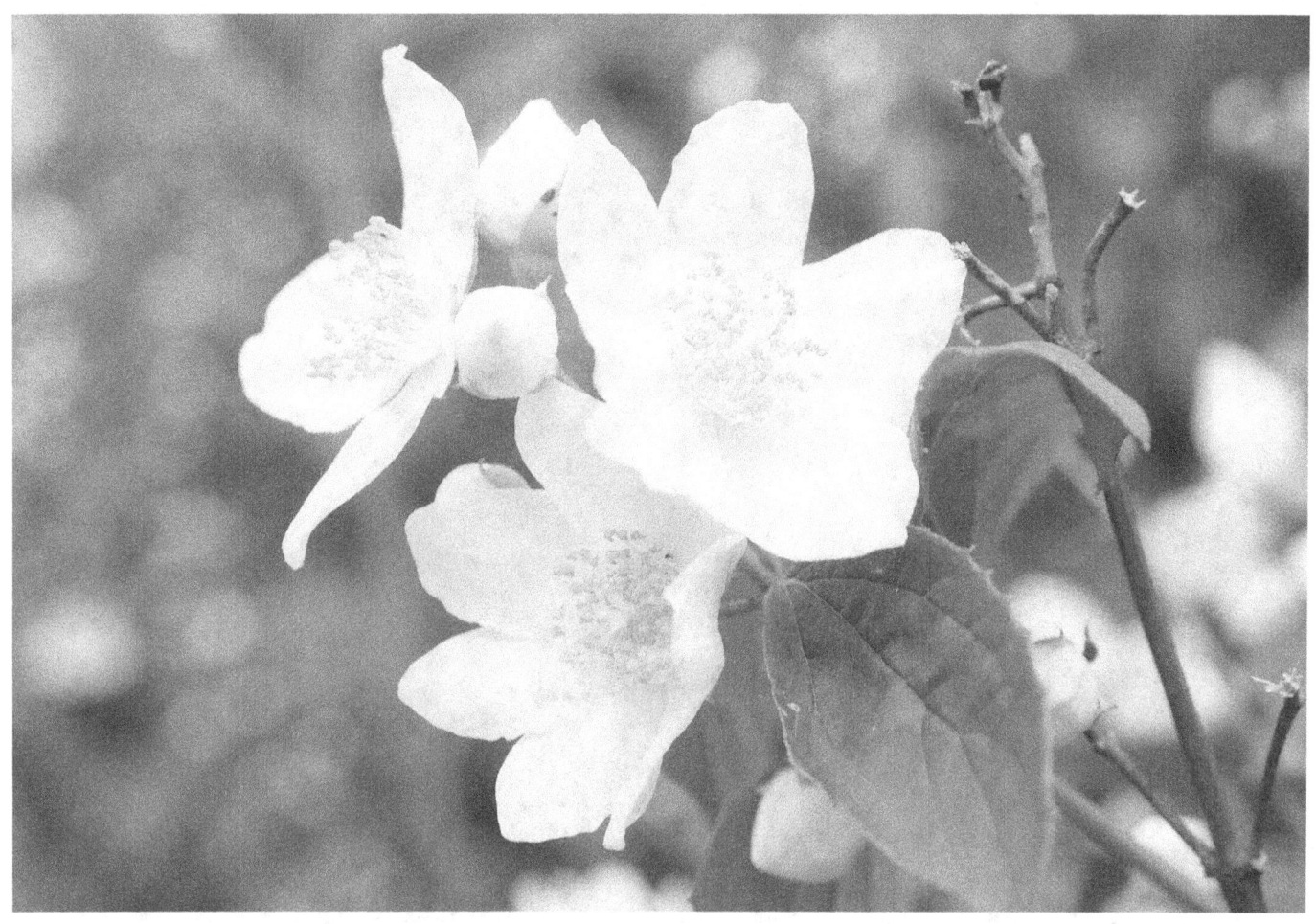

LEWIS' MOCK ORANGE

Mock orange shrubs are native to the Waterton National Park area of Alberta but hybridized, and hardy to zone two elsewhere in the country.

Golden Mock Orange is an introduced European plant, commonly found in gardens, and hardy to zone 3B.

The aromatic blossoms give the plant its common name.

In India, the Hindus put mock orange blossoms over the bodies of the dead before cremation. Corpses are burned quickly in that hot climate, but even four or five hours requires the masking of the smell of decay.

The related Mexican Mock Orange blossoms were used by the Aztecs to make garlands and distill cologne. They crushed the leaves in pulque to make a remedy for adult colic.

Francisco Hernandez reported in the 16th century that the leaves as a poultice were effective "beyond belief" in dissolving tumors.

In Mexico today, the blossom tea is used to treat nervousness and melancholy.

The wood is hard, strong, and never warps, bends or cracks. The Secwepemc of southern British and Saanich on Vancouver Island, used the wood for arrows, digging sticks combs, knitting needles, fish spears, bearpaw shoes and breast bone decoration.

Fire hardened tips of dogwood were sometimes attached as the arrowhead.

The Flathead of Montana, and Thompson of British Columbia made combs, pipes, bows and arrow shafts from the hard, flexible wood.

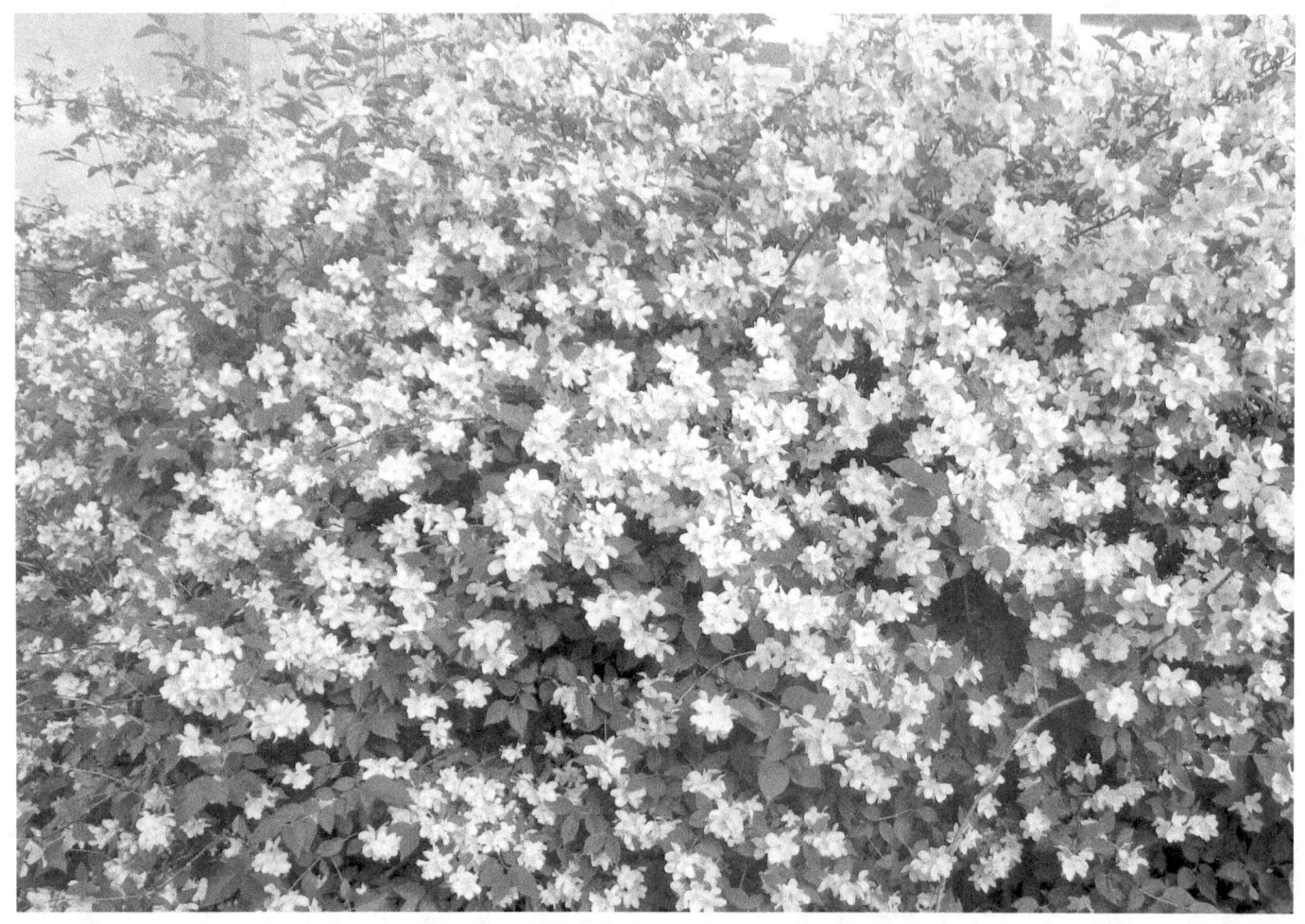

MOCK ORANGE BUSH IN FULL BLOOM

The wood was burned for charcoal that was then crushed and combined with spruce pitch or bear grease for sores.

The leaves were dried and used in the same way. The fresh leaves were mashed into a poultice for healing infected breasts, such as cases of mastitis.

Even the branches, sometimes with blossoms attached, were boiled by the Thompson to make medicinal decoctions for eczema or bleeding hemorrhoids externally, or taken internally three times over a period of time for a sore chest (pulmonary?).

The fragrant flowers, as well as leaves when crushed and rubbed, lather and foam into a soap substitute. Lather can even be obtained from the bark, by soaking it in warm water.

The leaves are very mucilaginous, and have been used for shining up old furniture, and polishing wood. They are edible.

Willow extracts increase efficacy of rooting from mock orange cuttings.

MEDICINAL

CONSTITUENTS- *P. lewisii-* flavonoids, saponins, epi-13-manool (fresh flowers)
Leaves- monoterpenoids such as myrtenol, nopinone, linalool, sesquiterpenoids such as (E)-beta-ionone and (E, E)-alpha-farnesene.
P. coronarius- leaves- uvaol, umbelliferone, scopolin, stigmasteryl-3 beta-D-glucoside, and 3 beta, 28-dihydroxyoleanane-11(12),13(18)-diene. Leaves contain 0.01% flavonoids and 0.70% phenolics; branches yield 0.63% and 3.25% respectively.

Very few studies have been done on the medicinal value of our local Mock Orange.

Myrtenol, derived from the leaves, acts as a positive allosteric modulator at synaptic and extrasynaptic GABA-A receptors, suggesting benefit as a sedative and anti-anxiety compound. Van Brederode J et al, *Neurosci Lett* 2016 628: 91-7.

It also exhibits gastroprotective effect, possibly due to GABA-A receptor activation and anti-oxidant activity. Viana AF et al, *J Pharm Pharmacol* 2016 68(8): 1085-92.

Scopolin exhibits 90.8% ulcer protection, and anti-*Helicobacter pylori* activity. Awaad AS et al, *Phytother Res* 2015 June 10. Scopolin is memory-enhancing and exhibits significant acetylcholinesterase inhibitory activity. Malik J et al, *Nat Prod Res* 2016 30(5): 578-82.

Earlier work found scopolin increased acetylcholine concentration in rat brain by 300%, nearly twice as effective as the control drug galanthamine. Rollinger JM et al, *J Med Chem* 2004 47(25): 6248-54.

The compound reduced the clinical symptoms of rat adjuvant-induced arthritis by inhibiting inflammation and angiogenesis in synovial tissue. Pan R et al, *Int Immunopharmacol* 2009 9(7-8): 859-69.

The fresh bark may be decocted as a mild laxative, while the root tea is steeped and drunk hot to reduce fevers.

A hot poultice of the fresh or dried leaves may be applied to mastitis.

Work by Jantova et al, *Phytotherapy Research* 2000 14:8 showed anti-microbial activity from *P. coronarius* and *P. microphyllus,* in the southwestern United States.

Work by Valko et al, *Biomed Pap Med Fac Univ Olomouc Czech Rep* 2006 150(1): 71-3 found water extracts of leaves and branches from *P. coronarius* cytotoxic against MCF 7 breast cancer cells. Over time, the extracts exhibited activity against skin melanoma A431.

The branches show moderate activity against *Saccharomyces cerevisiae*. McCutcheon et al, *J Ethnopharm* 1994 44.

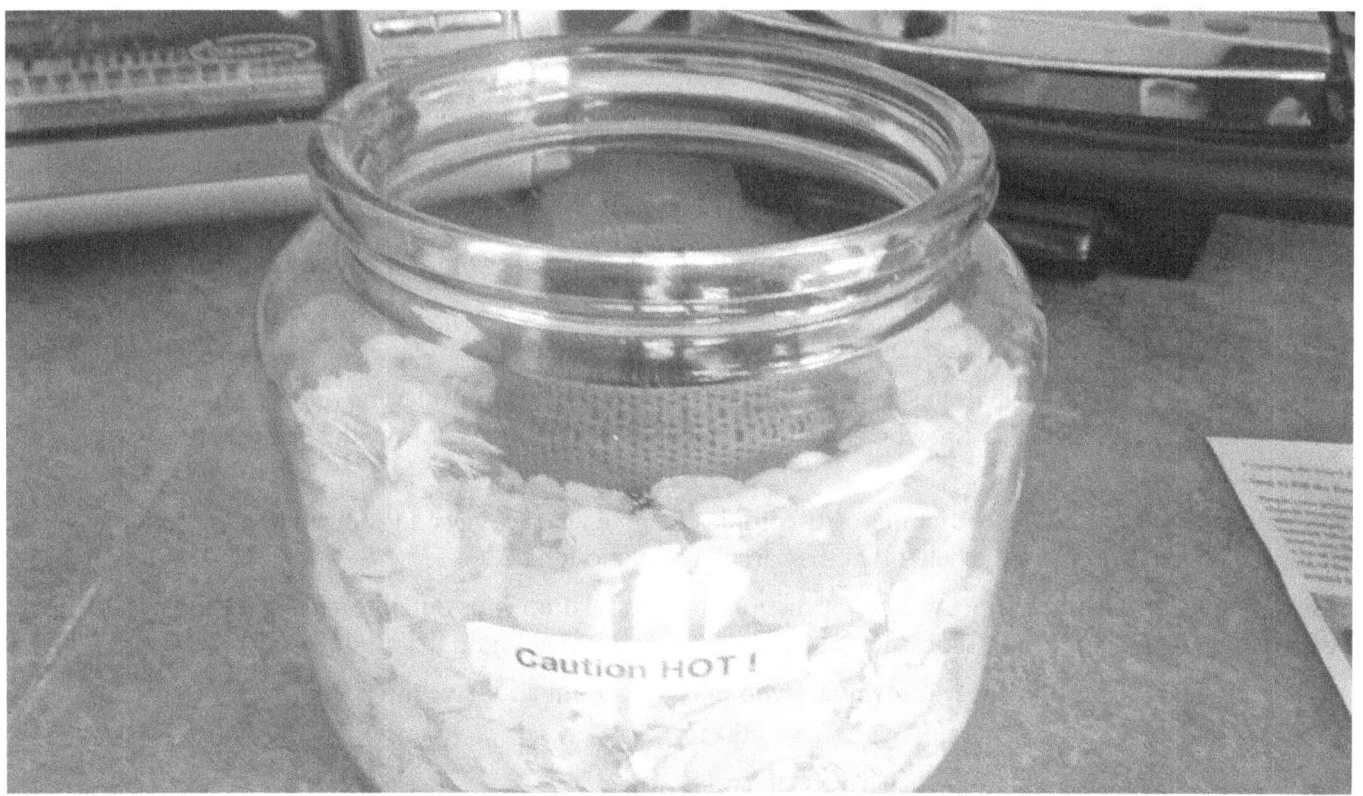

MOCK ORANGE PETALS READY FOR MICROWAVE DISTILLATION

ESSENTIAL OIL

An absolute can be obtaining from the flowers in full bloom.

This is done with petroleum ether, producing 0.237% of a concrete, which washed with alcohol, yields 52%.

The absolute is a viscous reddish-brown liquid, with a strong fruity, somewhat harsh odour, reminiscent of the flowers, such as jonquil and narcissus.

If the concrete is steam distilled, it gives 2.5-9% of a yellow distillate with a powerful odour similar to the flowers. Specific gravity of the oil is 0.912, and acid number of 25.2.

An ether extraction gives a yield of 1.4-1.8% of a brittle concrete red brown in colour. The yield of absolute was 25-27% of a thick red brown liquid with a whitish deposit. One dilution, a fine odour reminiscent of the flowers is observed.

The oil probably contains methyl anthranilate.

The absolute give 9% of an essential oil from the absolute, yellowish in color.

An essential oil is apparently available in small amounts, as it is used in the perfume, *C'est la Vie.*

It is one of the flowers I distilled in the summer of 2016. Using a microwave distillation unit from www.oilextech.com I "cooked" the flowers for six minutes and ended up with a few drops of essential oil and a wonderfully fragranced hydrosol.

The related *P. coronarius* essential oil contains 20% acetophenone, four linalyl oxides totally 11.5%, and indole 10%, with trace amounts of jasmone, 2-aminobenzaldehyde and benzothiazole.

WAX

A brown wax, with a slight odor resembling jasmine, is obtained from the petals of sweet mock orange, when extracted with petrolic ether.

The wax acids have a high molecular weight (398) indicating the presence of cerotic acid. The iodine number is 52, with a saponification value of 65.8.

The wax melts at 57 degrees Celsius and has a small yield (0.0784%).

FLOWER ESSENCES

Mock Orange flower essence is useful for stress reduction. In increases the ability of individuals to coordinate in deep states of relaxation and meditation.

This can be useful for the formation of new ideas, including dreams.   **PEGASUS**

Mock orange essence can help us to accept ourselves as we are. It helps us overcome the need to look or perform like someone else. It takes away the worry of not being good enough. It takes away the pressure of always having to put on show.

Mock Orange is the antidote for an inferiority complex. People who are gay and suffering, might find that Mock Orange can free them from the belief that they aren't good enough.   **JADE MOUNTAIN**

Mock Orange is for women who love too much, or remain in relationships out of fear, desperation or false hope. Positive qualities include faithfulness to oneself, trust, deep intimacy, and devotion.   **CAN FOREST TREE**

Mock Orange essence is for those individuals who need to get out and have more fun.

ROCKY MOUNTAIN

Mock Orange flower essence helps rebalance all female organs.   **CHOMING**

Mock Orange releases cellular emotions and allows old patterns to change, similar to the healing from dancing, chanting, drumming and other rituals.   **TREE FROG**

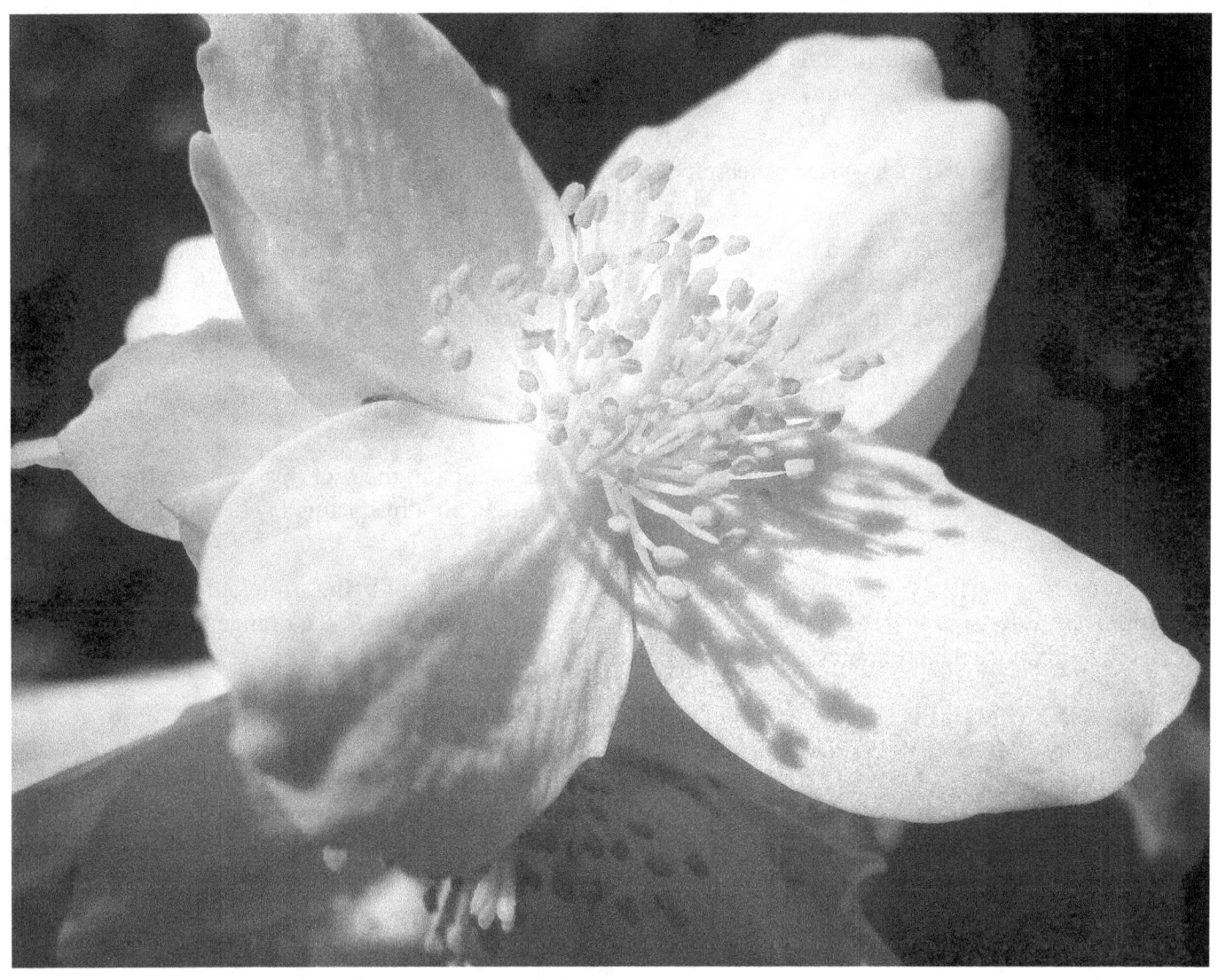

MOCK ORANGE

SPIRITUAL PROPERTIES

The Egyptian princess, Arsinoe was famed for her beauty and charm. Her brother, Ptolemy II, loved her as his sister and later as his wife. For since pharoahs cannot marry beneath them in rank, it was the Egyptian custom for the pharoah to marry one of his sisters. Arsinos died suddenly in 270 BC, and Ptolemy was grief-stricken. He deified her as Philadelphus, by naming a shrub in her honor. The Greeks carried on the tradition, by naming one of their shrubs Philadelphus in his honor.

When Linnaeus, that great namer of plants, sought a name for our shrub that would fit its beauty and sweetness, he remembered Arsinos and named it Philadelphus. **GUILLET**

PERSONALITY TRAITS

Pan and Bacchus came laughing through the woods and surprised two pretty wood nymphs at play. Startled, the nymphs ran from them down a woodland path. They ran swiftly but at a turn in the path, they were stopped by a broad stream. Their pursuers were close upon them and the besought the water nymphs to aid them.

The nymphs hastily aroused the river god from sleep. Quickly he changed one nymph into a reed growing on the river bank, and the other into a Mock Orange shrub to shelter it.

Pan was not to be cheated. He broke off the reed and put it to his lips to caress it and there came a mournful sigh. He blew stronger and there came forth sweet music. Bacchus broke off a branch from the Mock Orange and placed it to his lips but no sound came. So he bit a hole in the branch and cleared out the pith and lo, the first whistle.

Ever since, the Mock Orange has been called pipe tree or whistle shrub.   **GUILLET**

Here by the mock orange hedge was a bee, a honeybee, sprung from its hive by the heat. Instantly I had a wonderful idea. I had recently read that ancient Romans thought that bees were killed by echoes. It seemed a far-fetched and pleasing notion, that a spoken word or falling rock given back by cliffs- that airy nothing which nevertheless fore and spread the un-comprehended impact of something- should stun these sturdy creatures right out of the air...

It was wandering listlessly among dried weeds on the stony bank where I had sat months ago and watched a mosquito pierce and suck a copperhead on a rock.

Hello! I tried tentatively: Hello! faltered the cliffs under the forest; and did the root tips quiver in the rock? But that is no way to kill a creature, saying hello. Goodbye! I shouted; Goodbye! came back, and the bee drifted unconcerned among the weeds.   **ANNIE DILLARD**

Mock orange is a perfectly real flower she is only called mock because of being understudy to true orange blossom. Her perfume is a close second to the perfume of the blossom of southern orange groves; one hardly notices the difference in appearance of real or mock.   **EMILY CARR**

BLUE MONKEYFLOWER
ALLENGHENY MONKEYFLOWER
(*Mimulus ringens* L.)
RED MONKEYFLOWER
PINK MONKEYFLOWER
LEWIS' MONKEYFLOWER
(*M. lewisii* Pursh.)
YELLOW MONKEYFLOWER
MIMULUS
(*M. guttatus* DC.)
(*M. rivularis* Nutt.) not accepted
(*M. tenullus* Nutt. ex A. Gray) not accepted
SMALL YELLOW MONKEY FLOWER
(*M. floribundus* Lindl.)
MUSKY MONKEYFLOWER
(*M. moschatus* Douglas ex Lindl.)
SMOOTH MONKEYFLOWER
ROUNDLEAF MONKEYFLOWER
(*M. glabratus* Kunth.)

LARGE MOUNTAIN MONKEYFLOWER
SUBALPINE MONKEYFLOWER
(*M. tilingi* Regel)
BREWER'S MONKEYFLOWER
(*M. breweri* [Greene] Coville)
PURPLE MONKEYFLOWER
KELLOGG'S MONKEYFLOWER
(*M. kelloggii* [Curran ex Greene] Curran ex A. Gray)
ORANGE MONKEYFLOWER
STICKY MONKEYFLOWER
(*M. aurantiacus*) not accepted
(*Diplacus aurantiacus* ssp. *aurantiacus* [Curtis] Jeps.)
SCARLET MONKEYFLOWER
(*M. cardinalis* Douglas ex Benth.)
HAIRY MONKEYFLOWER
FALSE MONKEYFLOWER
(*M. pilosus* [Benth.] S. Watson)
PARTS USED- aerial

Mimulus is the diminutive form of the Latin **MIMUS**, a mime, actor, or buffoon. Some say Monkeyflower is so-named from the resemblance of the flower to a grinning ape's face. Guttatus means spotted, or drops, from the Latin **GUTTA,** referring to the tiny red drops on the yellow flowers lower lip. Lewisii is named after the famous explorer Meriweather Lewis; while breweri is named in honour of W. H. Brewer, a 19th century American naturalist. Ringens means, "gaping", in reference to the mouth opening of the flower. Luteus means yellow. Kelloggii is named after Dr. Albert Kellogg, a physician and northern California botanist. Aurantiacus means orange, cardinalis means red.

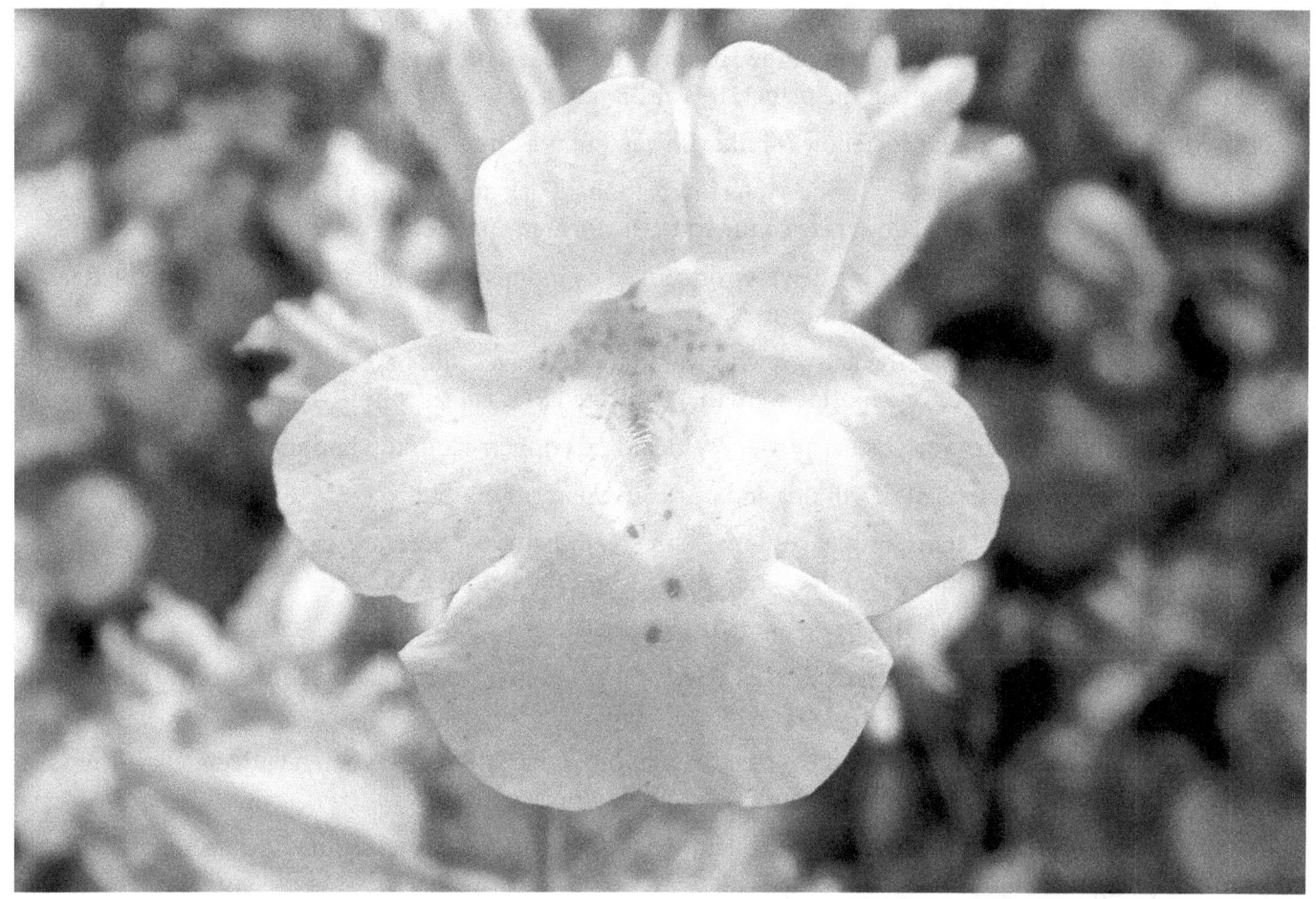

YELLOW MONKEYFLOWER

Blue Monkey flower is a native perennial found in the wet woods of Manitoba, and rarely along the Red Deer River of west central Saskatchewan. It should more properly be called Purple Monkey flower, as the flower color is more in that spectrum.

When found in areas with invasive, but useful, Purple Loosestrife (*Lythrum salicaria*), the pollen and seed numbers decline.

Yellow Monkey flower is a native annual with round leaves and bright yellow flowers.

It is restricted in Alberta to the extreme south of the province, growing all the way to Mexico, where the water conditions are pristine.

The plant produces small seeds, which when ripe, fall into running water. They float for a few days and then become waterlogged, and germinate underwater. They then resurface, later, as seedlings and float to where they can take root and grow. They also propagate vegetatively, growing small rootlets at each stem node. The torn stem pieces are carried by seasonal floods to new higher ground, and thus establish their home.

Red Monkey flower is a foothill annual, often found on moist montane slopes. It releases various volatiles, including d-limonene, beta myrcene and E-beta-ocimene to attract bumblebees for pollination.

Small Yellow Monkey flower is an annual that grows in wet places in the montane, but at lower elevations.

Musk Monkey flower has rather slimy and hairy leaves, and once had a musky scent, and hence its name. It was widely grown in England after its introduction by David Douglas, who took back seeds in 1828. Its scent was said to rival the perfume of the famous Mignonette (*Reseda odorata*).

In a strange case of morphic resonance, both the flowers in England, and in North America lost their scent at the same time. This is indeed reminiscent of the Hundredth Monkey [flower], a colorful tale spread to explain coincidence and synergistic action on the planet. It is also known as Sheldrake's theory of morphic resonance.

Smooth Monkey flower is similar to Yellow Monkeyflower, but is a larger plant found in east-central Alberta.

Large Monkey flower is found rarely in the Waterton National Park and Cypress Hills region; while Brewer's Monkey flower and its red purple flowers is confined to the former, and is somewhat rare species.

Yellow Monkey flower was traditionally eaten raw, or cooked by indigenous residents, and early settlers. It tastes like lettuce, or corn silk, with a tinge of bitterness.

The leaves were a source of salt to the natives, who would tie the leaves into balls and place them on flat rocks to burn. The ashes, high in sodium chloride were then collected as a salt substitute.

The plants have a tolerance to various heavy metals, including copper, cadmium and nickel.

The stems and leaves were applied to wounds and burns in the form of poultices.

The Kawaiisu decocted the stems and leaves for use in steam baths for soreness in the chest and back. The Shoshone crushed the leaves into a poultice for applying to wounds or rope burns.

The Haida call it **SGAAL TS'IIT'IISGA** meaning bee's-coat/jacket.

The Karuk name **IKSHASSAHANNIHICH IIFTIHAN** means, "one who grows up in little brushy places." The aerial parts were infused fresh to reduce fevers.

The Iroquois used Blue Monkeyflower root as part of compound decoctions for women with epilepsy. They also decocted the whole plant with others as a wash to counteract poisons.

The flower stems and leaves are edible and can be added to soups and stews; while the flowers make a colorful addition to spring salads.

Scientists have found that changing one gene in monkey flowers is enough to increase nectar flow, and double visits by hummingbirds. Another small gene change altered the flower's pigment and reduced visits by bees by 80%.

When *M. guttatus* and *M. tilingii* were crossbred, the hybrid seeds were less than 1% viable.

MEDICINAL

CONSTITUENTS- *M. guttatus-* neoxanthin, de-epoxy-neoxanthin, and mimulaxanthin, sodium chloride, verbascoside, phenylpropanoid glycosides.
M. glabratus- 6-chlorohalleridone, halleridone
M. luteus- halleridone, dihydroalleridone, alpha dunnione (naphtoquinone), ursolic acid, beta sitosterol.
M. lewisii- flowers- antheraxanthin, violaxanthin, neoxanthin, de-epoxy-neoxanthin, mimulaxanthin.

The leaves and stems of all species can be poulticed on cuts, wounds, burns and insect bites, in the manner of plantain.

The energy is neutral to cooling, with slight moistening properties.

The fresh plant tincture or dried plant infusions can be useful in relieving pain associated with anxiety, irritability, depression as well as physical nerve pain.

Neoxanthin is a xanthophyll (carotenoid) also found in sea buckthorn leaves, and spinach. It inhibits the initiation stage and promotion stage in two-stage carcinogenesis, and may be a useful chemopreventative agent. Chang JM et al, *Nutr Cancer* 1995 24(3): 325-33.

According to Janice Schofield, the greens can be added to chickweed and plantain oils for creating skin salves and body lotions. Agreed.

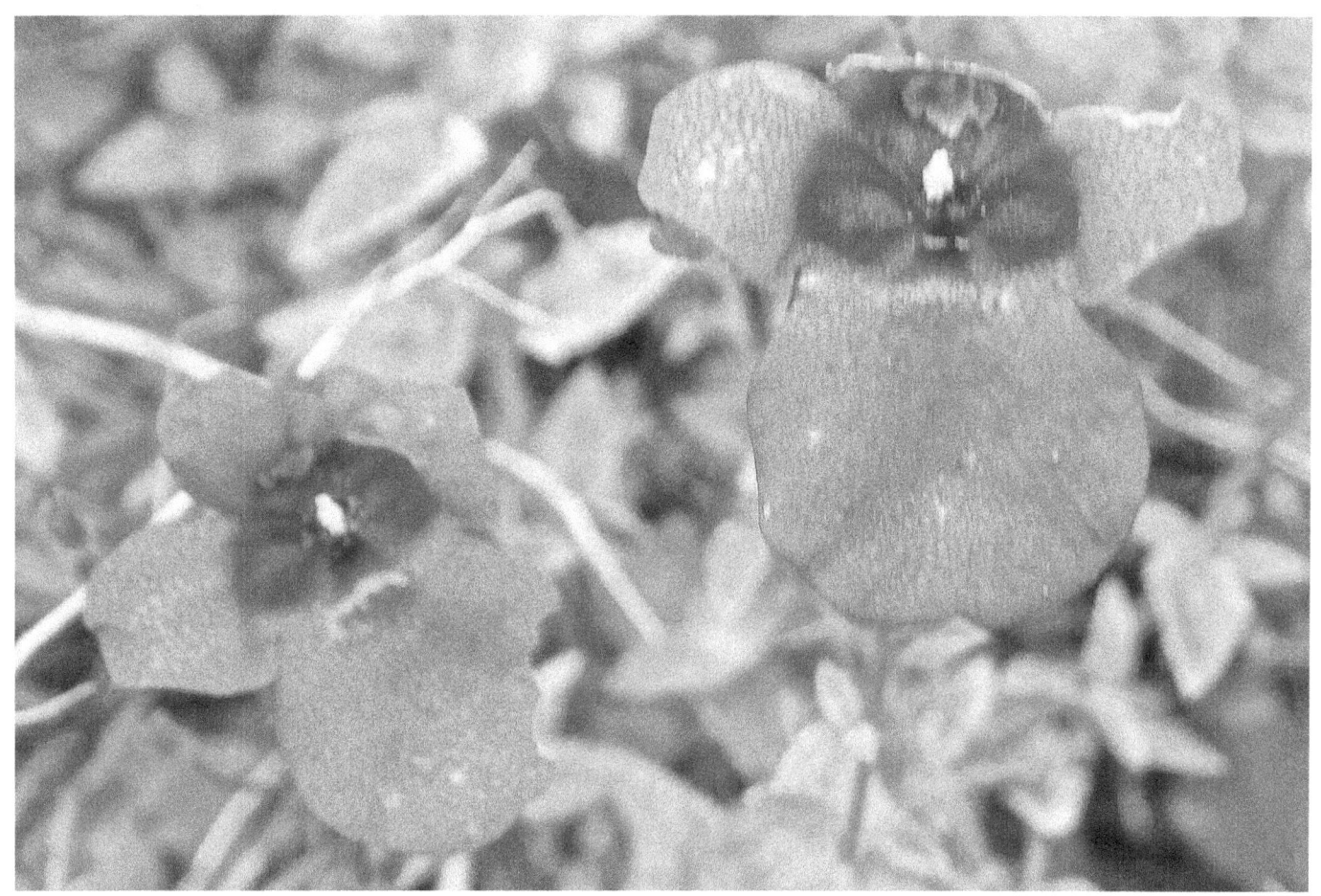

RED MONKEYFLOWER

Verbascoside (acteoside) is found in mullein (*Verbascum thapsus*) and other important medicinal herbs. It has a multitude of activity including anti-inflammatory, anti-viral, immune modulating and xanthine oxidase inhibition.

Halleridone is a cytotoxic constituent found in *Cornus controversa*. Nishino C et al, *J Nat Prod* 1988 51(6): 1281-2.

Dunnione ameliorates cisplatin toxicity through modulation of the NAD(+) metabolism. Kim HJ et al, *Hear Res* 2016 333: 235-46.

Angular-series naphthoquinones such as dunnione inhibit cell proliferation of human leukemia HL-60 cells. Inagaki R et al, *Chem Med Chem* 2015 10(8): 1413-23.

Alpha dunnione shows a mixed-type inhibition of both acetylcholinesterase and butyrylcholinesterase, suggestive of benefit in Alzheimer's disease. Cespedes CL et al, *Food Chem Toxicol* 2013 Oct 25.

Ursolic acid is found in a plethora of medicinal herbs, and has shown anti-inflammatory, anti-tumor, analgesic and a multitude of other health benefits. There are over 1700 citations for ursolic acid on PubMed.

Blue Monkeyflower (*M. ringens*) has been studied for biological activity. Both ether and acidic extracts of the whole plant show activity against Gram positive bacteria.

Red Monkeyflower (*M. lewisii*) can be used as a mild sedative.

Smooth Monkeyflower (*M. glabratus*) shows selective cytotoxicity against KB (nasopharyngeal), HEp-2 (larynx), HF-6 (colon), MCF-7 (breast), PC-3 (prostate) and Ca Ski (cervix) carcinoma cell lines. Moreno-Escobar JA et al, *Pharm Biol* 2011 49(12): 1243-8.

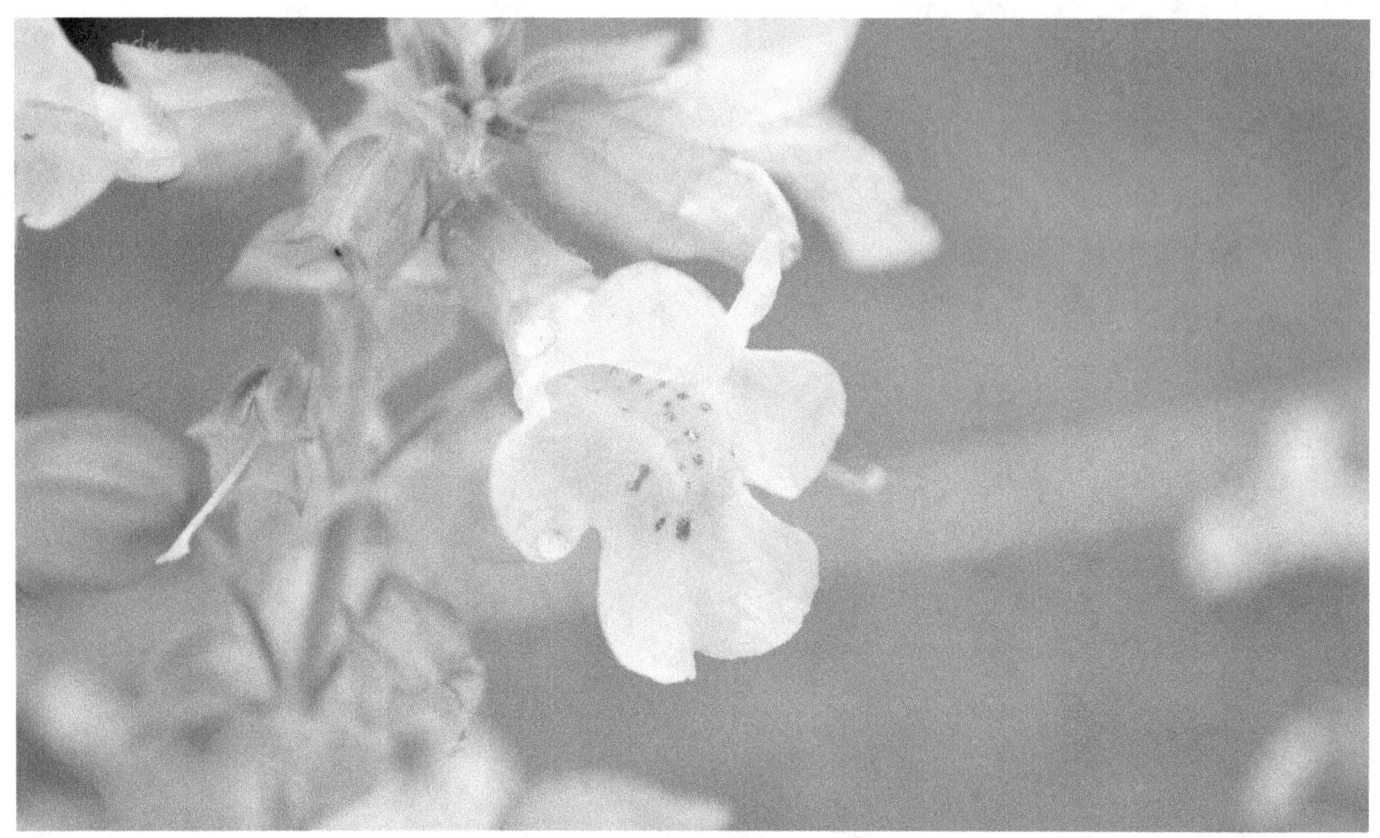

YELLOW MONKEYFLOWER (*M. GUTTATUS*) FLOWERS

Dr. King investigated the activity of Hairy, or False Monkeyflower (*M. pilosus*), a small annual native to California, but grown elsewhere. According to King, "it is probable that some of the other species of Mimulus possess similar properties", which are:

"A local application of the plant, in the form of a cataplasm, made either by bruising the leaves, or by steeping them in hot water, is reputed very efficient in local inflammations and painful affections, as in rheumatism, neuralgia, erysipelas, burns, etc.

A tincture of the plant, in the dose of from 3 to 10 minims, repeated 3 or 4 times a day will likewise be found beneficial in rheumatism, neuralgia and other painful disorders.

In cardiac affections, the sequence of rheumatic attacks, it has proved very serviceable, in several cases.

In obstinate bronchial and laryngeal affections, I have derived much benefit from the use of a tincture, made with diluted alcohol, in the form of a spray".

Combine with Melissa and Hypericum for seasonal affective disorder or SAD; golden corydalis and California poppy for nerve pain, restless gloom and nervous tremors; sweet clover for sciatica and neuralgia; green oats for heat and nervous exhaustion associated with irritated nerves; and vervain for headaches, moodiness and neck and shoulder pain.

Mimulus species contain flavonoids that may be useful against bladder infections. Wollenwever et al, *Z Naturforsch C J Biosci* 2000 55.

Chickweed Monkey Flower (*M. alsinoides*) contains sodium chloride salts. It is astringent and can be used for poultice on burns and wounds.

The related *M. bigelovii* showed anti-parasitic activity against *Trypanosoma brucei brucei*. Salem MM et al, *Phytother Res* 2011 25(8): 1246-9.

FLOWER ESSENCES

Pink Monkey flower (*M. lewisii*) flower essence is for feelings of shame, guilt and unworthiness; fear of exposure, rejection, the hiding of your essential self from others and masking one's own feelings. The essence helps emotional openness and honesty, and the courage to take emotional risks with others.
FLOWER ESSENCE SOCIETY

Lewis Monkey flower works more with the mental body assisting in changing belief systems and directions in life with relaxed open-mindedness—-more of a listening. **HIGH SIERRA**

Mimulus (*M. guttatus*) is for fears of the known nature, of everyday life, and shyness. The flower essence is to give courage and confidence to face life's challenges. **BACH**

Scarlet Monkeyflower (*M. cardinalis*) is for the soul's fear of its own 'shadow self' or lower emotions. There is fear or repression of intense feelings, and the inability to act upon issues of anger and powerlessness.
FLOWER ESSENCE SOCIETY

Sticky Monkeyflower (*M. aurantiacus*) flower essence heals those who are challenged in their efforts to understand and affirm their true sexuality. They may have a deep fear of intimacy, or mask their fear with over-compensation, choosing numerous superficial sexual relationships. **FLOWER ESSENCE SOCIETY**

Blue Monkeyflower (*M. ringens*) essence is related to anxiety around the expression of new ideas. Albert Einstein once said that Creative thinkers are always violently opposed by individuals with mediocre minds. The throat like flowering opening and blue colour both represent the fifth chakra, of communication and expression.

Blue Monkeyflower helps develop hope and trust in those who have lost faith in themselves and their ideas. It helps one voice their inner thoughts in a non-confrontative manner.

This essence is for those who fear ridicule or resentment due to creative expression, be it in the areas of art, education, or science. **PRAIRIE DEVA**

When you're scared of many things, but it's quite specific, instead of terrified, you will feel terrific, if you stock up on Mimulus, you won't feel so shy. You'll find you're getting bolder as the days go by.
D. CUMMINGHAM

For fear of people, beast or bird, for fear of dark or pain, take drops of golden Mimulus and be yourself again.

For every fear which you transcend an understanding grows, until with calm, courageous care you greet your former foes. **NORA HARRISON**

Mimulus alsinoides is excellent for when we have forgotten how to release joy, to feel joy, to express playfulness. We may be wearing a mask of how we feel we "should" be. This essence allows us to be who we are. Teaches us how to laugh again. **NETTLES AND MORE**

PERSONALITY TRAITS

On account of the high price of musk, and its liability to adulteration, Dr. Hannon (Journal de Pharm, 1854) sought for a vegetable substitute, which he thinks he has found in a Columbian plant, cultivated in Belgium, *Mimulus moschatus,* which plant yields an action on the intestinal canal, and on the brain. In a state of health it caused vertigo, cephalgia, dryness in the fauces, epigastric weight and eructations. He believes it may replace the animal musk, and may be given in hysteria and analagous complaints, in doses of from 2 to 4 drops in 24 hours. He calls it vegetable musk. **DR. KING**

Like a diver holding his breath, Mimulus can survive for some time under water- another reason why the water must be pure and well-oxygenated. The Mimulus type can be associated with breathing, or rather the lack of it. They stop breathing when frightened, and generally breathe in a shallow way, filling only the top part of the lungs. Like the Mimulus plant, these people learn to survive in the flood of feelings, overcome and swept away. It it remarkable; they are both delicate and determined. **J BARNARD**

The Monkey-flower or mimulus,
The mimulus, or musk,
That grows beside the Immulus,
The Immulus or Usk,
Is humble and subfimulus
Is modestly subfuse....

CHARLES JEFFRIES

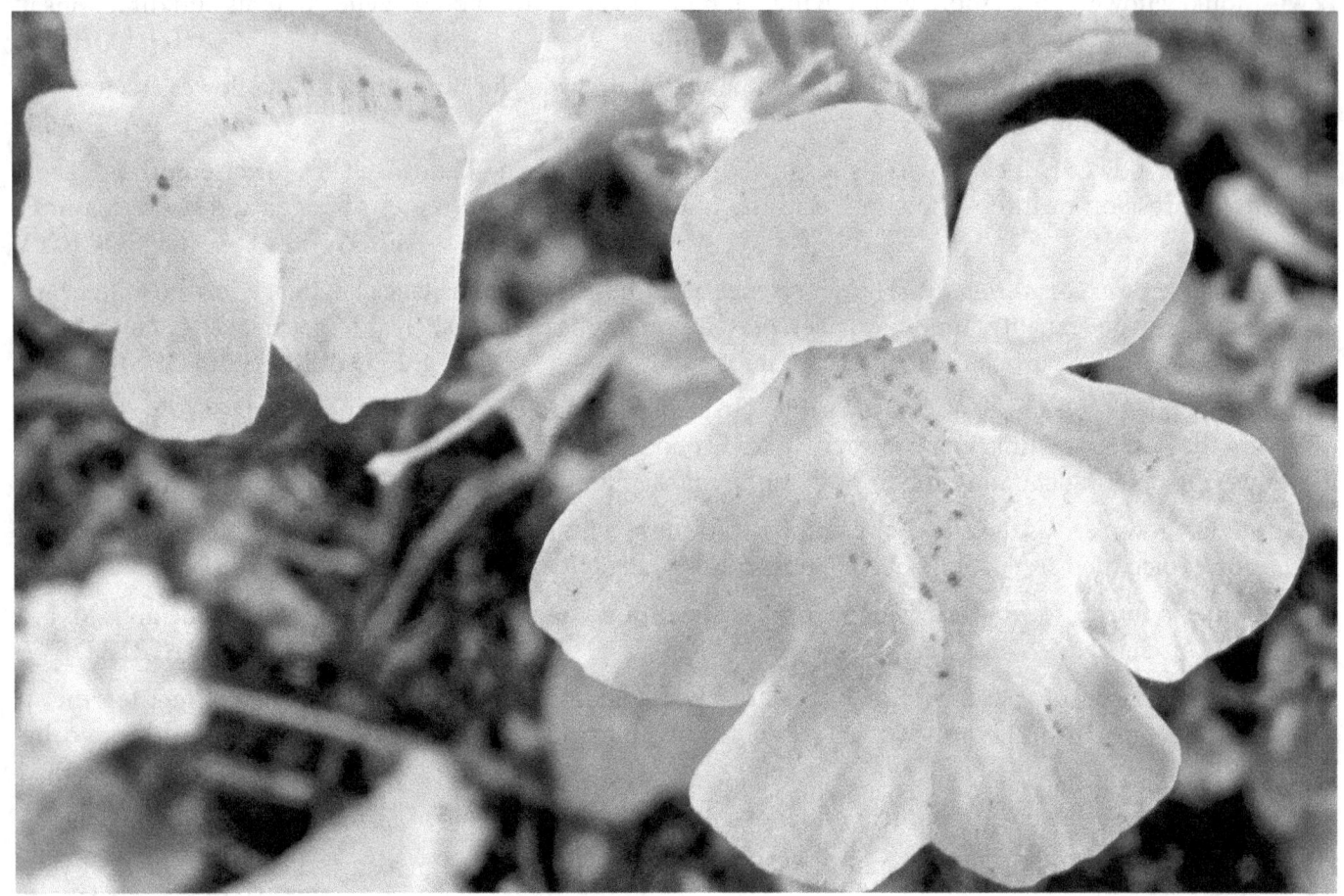

YELLOW MONKEYFLOWER

DOCTRINE OF SIGNATURES

The most prominent signature of monkeyflower is that it grows in or near flowing water.

Water represents emotions, moods and feelings. The fact that the flower prefers flowing waters demonstrates movement and cleansing of feelings and emotions.

The hairiness and stickiness of this plant represents the kinds of sticky situations that we find ourselves in, yet with help from flowing waters, or by letting our emotions flower with our feelings we have the capability to let go of whatever it is we feel stuck in.

The lobes of the flowers taste bitter, yet at the deep end of the tube that joins the flower's petals is a sweet nectar. The bitterness represents our own emotional bitterness, which can be overcome when we go back into our past to heal what was lost or stuck. Through the healing process, we are able to tap into our own sweet nectar, regaining personal power, compassion, strength, courage and a passion for life.

As a member of the snapdragon family, the funnel like part resembles a throat that opens into a mouth, giving it a signature for communication and expression- the fifth chakra center.

The yellow colour of the flower (*M. guttatus*) refers to the solar plexus; it deals with thought patterns associated with feelings, such as uncertainties, fear, emotional upsets, and mood changes. The reddish, orange spots indicate a connection with the earth as well as with fire and water, and demonstrate strength and courage. The spots get smaller as they go deeper inside the tunnel and eventually become hidden, resembling how we have to seek deep within ourselves to gather our courage and strength.	**PALLASDOWNEY**

MONKSHOOD
MONKS HOOD
VENUS' CHARIOT
(*Aconitum napellus* L.)
(*A. vulgare* DC.) not accepted
MOUNTAIN MONKSHOOD
(*A. delphiniifolium* DC.)
WESTERN MONKSHOOD
(*A. columbianum* Nutt.)
BICOLOR MONKSHOOD
HYBRID MONKSHOOD
GARDEN MONKSHOOD
(*A. X cammarum* L.) not accepted
(*A. neomantanum* Willd.) not accepted
(*A. X bicolor* Schult. [pro. sp.])
YELLOW WOLFSBANE
PYRENEES MONKSHOOD
(*A. lycoctonum* L.)
(*A. lycoctonum* ssp. *vulparia* [Rchb.] Nyman)
AZURE MONKSHOOD
CARMICHAEL'S ACONITE
(*A. carmichaeli* Debeaux)
FISCHER MONKSHOOD
(*A. fischeri* Rchb.)
PART USED- whole plant, root

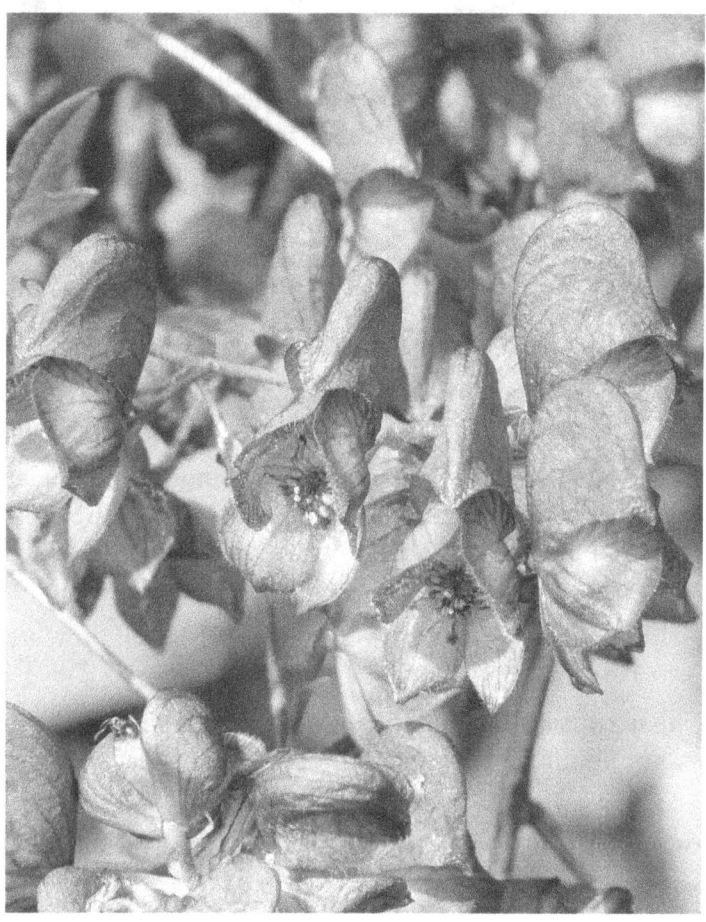

MONKSHOOD

Oyntment for flying here I have,
Of children's fat stolin from the grave,
The juice of smallage and nightshade,
Of poplar-leaves and aconite made…

	SHADWELL

That poisonous stalk of Aconite,
Whose ripened fruit hath ravish't
All health, all comfort of a happy life.

	JOHN FORD, 1633

For him Medea mixed, with murderous thought.
A draught of Aconite, from Scythia brought,
From Cerber's teeth the plant was grown.

	OVID

Aconite is from the Greek **AKONTION** meaning a dart, in reference to the use of the plant as poison for arrows and spears. Others believe it is from the Greek **AKONITOS** without a struggle, or without dust; or **AKONE**, for rock or cliff. It may also be from the Black Sea port of **AKONAI**, which the 3rd century naturalist, Theophrastus, explained. "It grows everywhere, and not only at Akonai, from whence it gets its name".

Casselman, in his excellent Canadian Garden Words, suggests that **AKONITON** is a dialect variant of **LYKOKTONON** meaning "wolf killer".

DELPHINI is derived from the Greek meaning "dolphin" and refers to the similarity, in shape of the flower and mammal. Napellus means "little turnip", and refers to the root shape.

In Medieval times, Monkshood, so named for its resemblance to a monk's cowl, was called **THUNG** a name given to any poisonous plant. Although named for its flower shape, it was also associated with political intrigue in the Vatican. The previous pope was Polish, and in that country it is called Slippers of the Blessed Mother.

In fact, the flower symbolizes fickleness; and has been long associated with the birth date of August 17th. It has been used in painting to symbolize death, and in the language of flowers is associated with crime. The hooded flowers are symbols of secrecy and secret sects.

The root was crushed and slipped into water holes to poison the supply of pursuing armies. It was used to put criminals to death; and was named by Pliny the Elder as "plant arsenic". Ancient peoples gave it the title The Queen Mother of Poisons.

It was used on the Greek island of Chios, for euthanasia of the old and terminal.

Greek legend has it that aconite originated from the hill of Aconitus, where Hercules brought Cerebus, the three head dog from the underworld. Saliva from the dog's mouth dripped onto monkshood, making it a deadly poison.

Hecate, the Greek goddess/witch of the moon, and Queen of the Underworld used aconite to poison her father, hence the original name for the plant **HECATEIS**. In mythology, Monkshood formed the cup that Medea prepared for Theseus and may have been the poison of choice in Shakespeare's, Romeo and Juliet. Certainly, the "tooth of wolf" mentioned in the witches' brew in Macbeth refers to this plant.

Aconite is also associated with spiders. Ovid tells how Athena sprinkled aconite on Arachne, transforming her into a spider.

The herb has a long history of use for ritual and psychoactive intent. It has been called Hat of Jupiter, Venus's wagon, Wolf's Plant, Hat of the Troll, Odin's hat and other suggestive names.

Nero ascended the throne in ancient Rome after his wife, Agrippina poisoned Claudius, by tickling his throat with a poison dipped feather. The High Priest Alcimus may have shared a similar fate.

Its widespread use by professional poisoners, led to cultivation of the plant becoming punishable, as a capital offense.

Monkshood is associated with the 14th Norse Rune called Peorth.

According to the Doctrine of Signatures, the eye-like fruit suggested its use in vision problems.

Only witches dared use it and they were said to smear the roots on their broomsticks before flying. Witches and broomsticks as known today came from the smearing of aconite and other herbs, including henbane, as an ointment on sticks inserted vaginally. This was done to increase the rate and intensity of absorption of the herbal mixture, without any sexual connotation.

In the Harry Potter series, Professor Snape brews aconite to assist Remus Lupin in his transformation to werewolf.

The entire plant, but especially the root and the leaves before flowering are extremely poisonous. This put aconite in the category of "drug-like" and a plant that requires respect, and intelligent use; like any powerful medicine.

It is considered a perennial, but in fact, the root only lives one year, and is replaced by "daughter" roots surrounding the original. It is propagated by root division, or from seed.

Aconitine was used on poison bullets by the Nazis during WWII.

The Newfoundland actor Andre Noble died from aconite poisoning in 2004, after mistaking the plant for an edible.

Yellow Wolfbane (*A. lycotonum*) is hardy to prairie gardens, with unusual creamy yellow hooded flowers in mid summer. It grows wild in the mountains of Sweden, Austria, and Siberia.

It has been employed since classic times as a sure method to dispose of an unwanted spouse. On the Greek island of Chios, officials prescribed the herb for euthanasia of the infirm and aged.

The Roman Emperor Trajan forbade the growing of Aconitum by law, probably in fear of his own demise.

A decoction of the powder of the root was once used to destroy flies and other insects. In France, the root powder was added to paste and toasted cheese to kill rats and mice.

It is also eaten in some parts of Sweden, being milder than most of this poisonous species, but not recommended. The ancients believed that it was fatal to those who slept under it.

Taxonomists are keen to re-classify Aconitum subgenus Lycoctonum. Hong Y et al, *PLoS* 2017 12(1).

The plant *A. carmichaelii* is a circumpolar native of northwestern China. It is one of the most popular garden varieties, due to its densely packed and rich violet-blue flowers.

FU ZI or **TZU** is the treated lateral root tuber; Fu meaning affiliated, and Tzu, son, suggesting it is a son affiliated with the mother root.

CHUAN WU is the root tuber. It was first mentioned in Traditional Chinese medical literature about 200 AD.

The Japanese call it **BUSHI**, and the Koreans, **KYEONG-PO BUJA**. Both cultures used treated root for weak digestion. Tibetan physicians refer to the herb as the "king of medicines."

Aconite leaves are smoked by yogis, and sadhus in India, in particular by the aghoris devotees who worship the goddess Kali. Poisonous plants, such as aconite, are processed by an Ayurvedic method known as Sodhana.

The Ainu, native peoples of Japan, tested the potency of the fresh root by making a small cut in the thenar below the thumb and holding it there. The thumb became numb and temporarily paralyzed and the duration of its effect indicated the potency.

The Lepchas of Sikkim used a root paste of *A. spicatum* on their arrows to kill game. The root paste of a *Rubus* species is applied afterwards to the flesh of the area to neutralize the arrow poison.

Fischer's Monkshood was possibly used as a hunting poison in the Aleutian Islands and Kodiak Island region, principally to hunt whales. Bisset NG, *Lloydia* 1976 39(2-3): 87-124.

Aconitic acid, found in Monkshood as well as Yarrow species, is converted to itaconic acid and was at one time used as a plasticizer, for rubber and plastics.

Both Mountain Monkshood and Western Monkshood are found in Alberta into British Columbia. The latter has palmitate leaves and the hoods are higher than wider when viewed from side. Both contain aconitin.

Aconite root extracts promote hair growth, externally, by triggering the activation of Wnt/beta-catenin signaling pathway and stimulation of bulge stem cells. Park PJ et al, *Life Sci* 2012 91(19-20): 935-43. Topical aconite preparations can create systemic toxicity through the skin and epidermis, especially in injured tissue.

MEDICINAL

CONSTITUENTS- *A. napellus* root- major alkaloids vary from .2% at higher elevations to 1.5% at low. Major constituents include aconitine, aconine, pseudoaconitine, neoline, sparteine, benzoyl-aconitine, napelline, isotalatizidine, karakoline, senbusine, taurenine; aconitic, itaconic, succinic, malonic and caffeic acids; ephedrine, benzaconitine, as well as various sugars and starches.
Aconitum delphinifolium (Mountain Monkshood) contains delphinifoline, and other diterpenoid alkaloids (1.7%) such as 14-0-acetylbrowniine, 14-0-acetylsachaconitine, 14-0-acetyl-talatisamine, browniine, condelphine, delcosine, gomandonine 13-0-acetate, and siotalatizidine.
A. lycoctonum- root- magnoflorine, corytuberine, lycoctonine, lycaconitine.
A. carmichaeli lateral root tuber- 122 compounds including C19-C20 diterpenoid alkaloids, aconitine (0.01%), hypaconitine (0.048%), mesaconitine (0.006%), dl-demethylco-claurine (higenamine); fuziline, hokbusine, senbusines A, B, and C; carmichaeline; salsolinol; crassicauline A, benzoylaconine, neoline, fuziline, songorine, talatisamine, honokiol, pinoresinol, salicylic acid, karakoline
root tuber- above as well as talatisamine, chuan-wu base A&B.
flower bud- 8-0-cinnamoylneoline
A. columbianum root- diterpenoid alkaloids mainly talatisamine, cammaconine, sachaconitine and derivatives.

In the dried root the aconitine decomposes into picro-aconitine, and aconine. As little as three grams of the root can kill a grown adult. The smallest piece will produce heart palpitations.

The roots and lateral roots of Aconite species contain water-soluble polysaccharides that possess anti-tumor and immune-stimulating activity, including nonspecific immunity, cellular and humoral immunity.

Aconitine alkaloid works by reducing the ion selectivity of sodium channels, which leads to more up-take of sodium and other ions that results in cardiac arrhythmia and respiratory depression.

The tincture is used in minute amounts as part of decongestant cough syrups, often combined with sundew, gumweed, or senega root.

Low doses stimulate the CNS, pulse rate, and peripheral motor system, while large doses paralyze, reduce heart contractions, leading to cardiac arrest and arrhythmia.

Aconitine, extracted from the root, is used in France (0.1 mg. granules) for facial neuralgia. Recent work on aconitine treated mice, suggest it may be useful in inhibiting the progression of disease and ameliorate the pathologic lesion of systemic lupus erythematosus. Li X et al, *J Pharmacol Sci* 2017 133(3): 115-121.

Aconitine induces cell apoptosis in human pancreatic cancer cells, in mouse model. NF kappaB decreased with aconitine treatment, but cell apoptosis increased. Ji BL et al, *Eur Rev Med Pharmacol Sci* 2016 20(23): 4955-64.

In the past, monkshood has been used as a heart and nerve sedative as well as for feverish conditions. It works well for local nerve inflammation and heat, in the form of external liniments.

A small dose is used for fever or chills with hot dry skin.

Aconite, in tiny doses, may be useful in some cases of agoraphobia and claustrophobia.

In China, the root of *A. carmichaeli* is prepared by special salt water and drying techniques that remove much of the toxicity. In this form, called **YAN FU ZI**, it is one of the most potent metabolic stimulants available in the plant world. It is considered the most yang of plants and good for cold, yin conditions, with extreme fatigue and weakness. The fresh root is called **WU TOU**.

Studies have found that traditional methods to reduce toxicity reduce alkaloid content by over 85%. Zhang DK et al, *Chin J Nat Med* 2017 15(1): 49-61. The team developed a novel one step method with same detoxification effect with only 30% loss of alkaloids.

Higenamine, one of the constituents of the lateral root has been found to possess cardiotonic action at dilutions of 1 in 10 to the ninth (10^9). Very dilute.

Fu Zi, the lateral root tuber, is considered an emergency remedy for prostration due to asthenia of the vital energy, with profuse sweating, coldness of extremities, abdominal pain, diarrhea and edema.

Chuan Wu, is considered more anti-rheumatic, and analgesic, but also considered for pathogenic cold conditions.

The mother root of *A. carmichaelii* is a potent anti-inflammatory that may act through the k-opioid receptor via dynorpin release and inhibition of transient receptor potential vanilloid type 1 ion channel. Wang C et al, *J Transl Med* 2015 13: 284.

Higenamine protects against type 11 collagen-induced arthritis, through heme oxygenase-1 and PI3K/Akt/ Nrf-2 signaling pathways. Duan W et al, *Exp Ther Med* 2016 12(5): 3107-3112.

Salsolinol, from the lateral root of *A. carmichaeli*, exhibits both cardiac and hypertensive activity. Aconitans A-D exhibit hypoglycemic effect. Hikino et al, *J Ethnopharm* 1989 25.

Mesaconitine is one of the three most important alkaloids in *A. carmichaeli*, with very strong analgesic activity that works through the noradrenergic system. Mesconitine suppresses histamines and blocks inflammation.

A double blind placebo controlled study on heart failure was conducted on 35 patients with left ventricular failure. In addition to various medications, 250 milligrams of prepared aconite tuber was given four times daily for seven month. Improvement was statistically significant for herbal therapy. Chen et al, *Am J Chin Med* 1990 18:1-2.

An earlier non-randomized study of 15 patients with left ventricular dysfunction given higenamine, a component of aconite root, was also significant, and comparable to isoproterenol when given as diluted injection. Liu et al, *Eur J Nucl Med* 1983 8:6.

Higenamine shows valuable therapeutic value in a variety of cardiovascular disorders including positive inotropic and cronotropic effects, activating slow channel effect, vascular and tracheal relaxation, anti-thrombotic, anti-apoptotic, anti-oxidant, anti-inflammatory and immune modulating effect. This suggest the need for further study in heart failure, disseminated intravascular coagulation, shock, arthritis, asthma, ischemia/reperfusion injuries and erectile dysfunction. Zhang N et al, *J Ethnopharmacology* 2017 196: 242-52.

It combines well with Astragalus to treat spontaneous sweating and chills related to deficient Yang. For extremely cold extremities, and diarrhea with undigested food, combine with licorice root.

In China, the tincture is used as a local surgical anesthetic.

Liniment of Aconite is a valuable pain reliever in myalgia and nerve pain. It has been used with success in ovarian neuralgia and delayed menstruation that has been brought on by cold. For this purpose it is applied three to four times daily. Work by Luo et al, *Phytotherapy Research* 1991 5:5 showed that aconite root extracts were equal in potency to hydrocortisone and indomethacin when applied against angiogenesis in chronic inflammation.

Monkshood stimulates and then depresses the central and peripheral nervous system; and is a depressant in high blood pressure with cardiac origin. Aconitine, mesoconitine and hypaconitine reduce the ion selectivity of sodium channels, with the resultant increased uptake of sodium and other ions via these channels. The result, in even small amounts, is cardiac arrhythmia and respiratory depression.

The tincture is sedative and analgesic and of value in trigeminal neuralgia, dental and ear inflammations; all as external application near affected areas.

Applied externally, it is active against *Streptococcus* and *Staphylococcus* bacteria skin infections; but not on open wounds.

Symptoms of overuse include slight trembling. External applications relieve the nerve pain of shingles (herpes zoster). Apply the tincture when the pain first begins, and let it dry.

Processed aconite, and its active compound neoline may alleviate Oxaliplatin-induced neuropathic pain. This platinum-based anti-cancer drug causes acute and chronic peripheral neuropathy, including cold and mechanical hyperalgesia. Suzuki T et al, *J Ethnopharm* 2016 186:44-52.

A few drops enhance arthritic or gout formulas, and can be added to footbaths.

The roots of our local Mountain Aconite (*A. delphinifolium*) have similar activity to others around the world. Condelphine, for example, is similar to methyllaconitine as a curare-like neuro-muscular blocker with hypotensive activity. It is used clinically in Russia for a number of various neurological conditions.

In Russia, aconite roots are boiled down to a black mass, and used in folk medicine for curing cancer. Anti-carcinogenic properties of aconite were roots spoken of in Solzhenitsyn's "Cancer Ward". He started with one drop of the alcoholic extract in glass of water on first day.

The next day he added two drops, the next, three until he could drink ten drops daily. After a week he gradually reduced down, and repeated it several times.

Recent work suggests the diterpenoid alkaloids show promise for the treatment of lung, stomach and liver cancers. Ren MY et al, *Molecules* 2017 22(2).

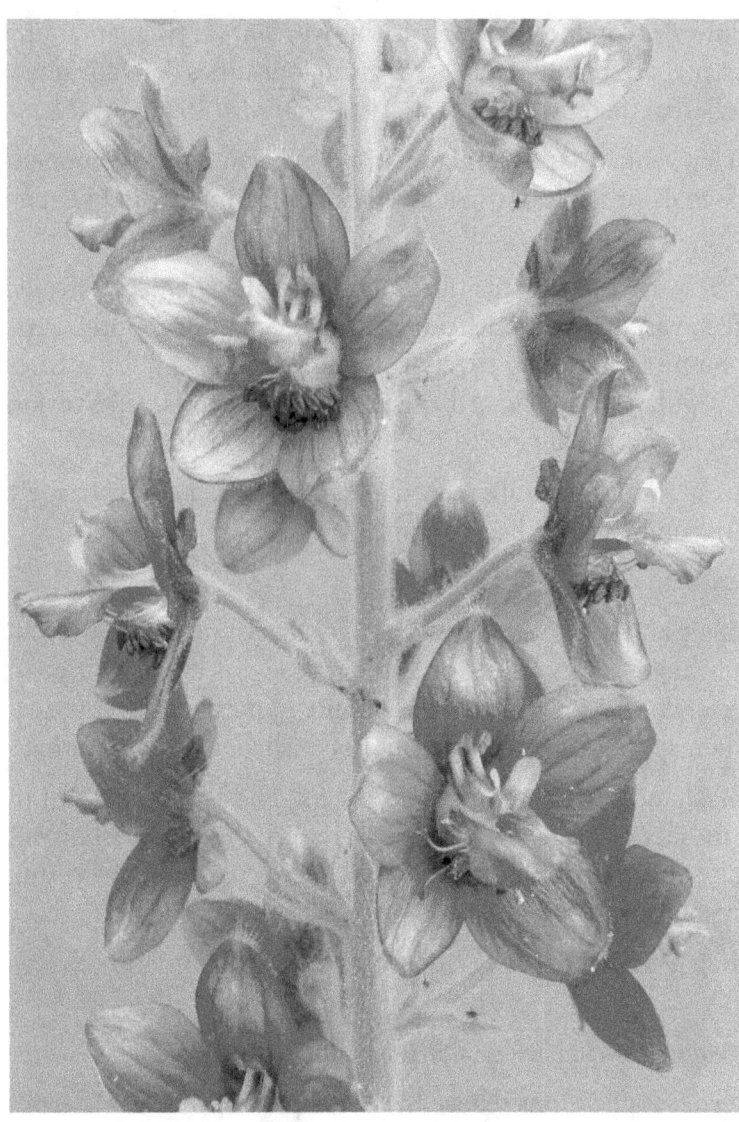

MOUNTAIN ACONITE

Five compounds from *A. carmichaeli*, oxonitine, deoxyaconitine, hypaconitine, mesaconitine and crassicauline A, show cytotoxicity against leucocythemia, breast and liver cancer. Gao F et al, *Molecules* 2012 17: 5187-94.

Most of the compounds with anti-cancer activity are C_{19}-diterpenoid alkaloids.

The processed root protects hepatocytes against acetaminophen induced toxicity, by inhibiting mitochondrial dysfunction. Park G et al, *Environ Toxicol Pharmacol* 2016 42: 218-25.

It is contra-indicated internally and externally during pregnancy. Do not use if tired, run down or cold. Aconite helps to moderate the excess symptoms of fever but not the actual cause of the fever.

Western Monkshood is not one of the more toxic aconites, but care is nonetheless advised.

Michael Moore writes. "The fresh herb tincture can be used internally, but be careful not to take excessive quantities; take only 3 to 6 drops at a time!

It should be used by the strong and vigorous with acute inflammation; not by the tired, depressed, or those with chronic disease. The small doses help to modify fever that includes pain, irritation and inflamed mucosa and eyes and is accompanied by a rapid, wiry pulse.

The few drops may be repeated every three hours as long as you feel hot and excited; when you feel better, stop its use…the first symptom of taking a little too much is a sense of slight tingling in the mouth and fingers… This is the herb, not the far stronger root, and the amount recommended is easily a tenth of the dosage formerly used as a cardiac sedative."

The seeds are a parasiticide, useful in hair washes for lice and concentrated oil infusions for scabies.

A. carmichaeli is considered in Traditional Chinese Medicine to be a hot drug.

An interesting study by Hwang et al, *Korean Journal of Pharmacognosy* 1999 30:2 looked at the effect of so-called hot and cold drugs like Goldthread (*Coptis ssp*) and their effect on MAO activity.

MAO, or monoamine oxidase, plays a main role in the metabolism of many neurotransmitters including serotonin.

Both Coptis and *A. carmichaeli* elevated MAO activity, especially *in vivo* MAO-B activity. The root of *A. carmichaeli* contains salsolinol, which exhibits both cardiac and hypertensive activity.

This species increases the secretion of interleukin-1b, tumor necrosis factor-alpha and interleukin-6 in human mononuclear cells. Chang et al, *Planta Medica* 1994 60.

Delcosine is insecticidal and poisonous to cold-blooded animals.

In vitro, MAO-A activities were increased by hot drugs like Aconite, whereas *in vitro* MAO-B was inhibited. Cold drugs, like Coptis, inhibited both enzyme activities *in vitro*. There are implications here, not only for herbal-drug interactions, but also the folly of some *in vitro* experiments.

Yellow Wolfsbane (*A. lycoctonum*) is native to Europe, and across the north regions to western Asia.

The compound lycoctonine inhibits acetylcholine reception at post-synaptic sites in neuromuscular junctions and has an action similar to curare. These compounds are found in Delphinium species.

The roots contain lappaconitine that is the basis for the Russian cardiac anti-arrhythmic drug Allapinin.

The roots of *A. septentrionale* are used in Uzbekistan, as a source of lappaconitine hydrobromine; which is the basis for the above cardiac anti-arrhythmic drug.

Work by Ono et al, *Japan J Pharmacol* 1991 55 identified lappaconitine as a central acting non-opioid analgesic that inhibits pain via action of substance P and somatostatin, on both first and second pain phases.

Lappacconitine irreversibly blocks heart sodium channels. Wright et al, *Mol Pharmacol* 2001 59:2.

High levels of 18:2 and 18:3 fatty acids have been found in the root lipids. Research by Khomova et al, *Chemistry of Natural Compounds* 1996 32:5 has found the content of fatty acids in processing root wastes comprising nearly 40% neutral lipids enriched with essential fatty acids.

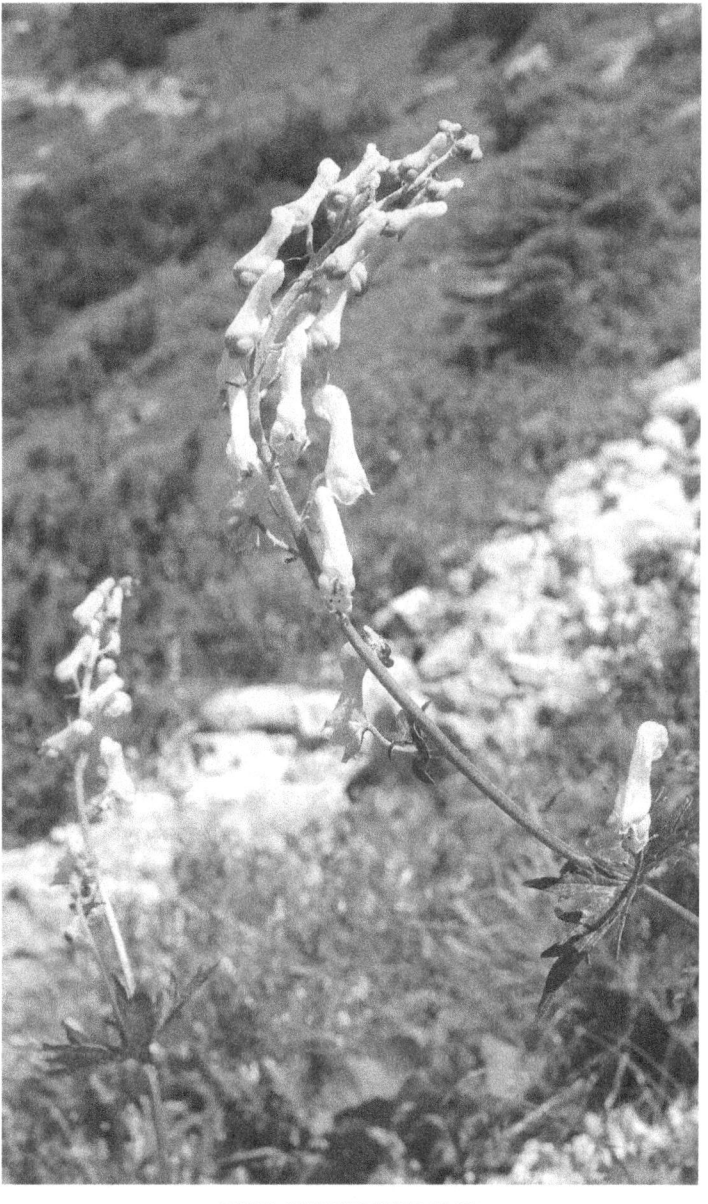

YELLOW WOLFSBANE

Research shows that other species possess anti-viral, anti-bacterial, anti-pyretic and anti-tumor activity.

Alkaloid content of *A. napellus* decreases with altitude. Napelline stimulates the regeneration of hemopoietic tissue in cytostatic myelosuppression, suggesting need for further exploration. Bone marrow suppression due to chemotherapy is too common, and any leads to preventing or reversing would be useful. Zyuz'kov GN et al, *Bull Exp Biol Med* 2013 155(4): 439-42.

Flower buds of *A. carmichaeli* contains an alkaloid that is 1/30th the toxicity of mesaconitine and 20 times that of benzoylmesaconine.

Endophytic fungi, on roots of this species exhibit anti-viral effect against strains of HINI. Zhang SP et al, *Fitoterapia* 2016 112: 85-9.

Recent work suggests transdermal dosage may soon be a practical and safe way to use this herb. Lin et al, *Zhongguo Zhong Yao Za Zhi* 2007 32:3. Maybe.

A decent review of the phytochemistry, pharmacology and toxicology can be found in article by Nyirimigabo E et al, *J Pharm Pharmacol* 2015 67(1): 1-19.

HOMEOPATHY

Monkshood (*A. napellus*), in diluted doses, is one of our most valuable remedies.

It is valuable in first aid, where high fever and accompanied inflammatory conditions arise. In infectious concerns, accompanied by hot and dry skin, the Aconite encourages perspiration and diverts toxins from the blood. Hot flushes at menopause, for example, often respond to the tenth potency. When perspiration has begun, the aconite has done its job and you can move on to other remedies.

The symptoms of Aconite come on quickly, violently and intensely. They may begin after exposure to cold, or experiences of fright, anger or shock. The patient may fear death, darkness or being in large crowds.

Aconite patients are usually very restless, physically and mentally. Light, noise and light touch can irritate them.

If the symptoms are stomach pains, they will be irritated by cold drinks.

All mental operations as if taking place in pit of stomach.

I often use Aconite at the first stage of flu like systems; and it seems to strengthen and often help the patient avoid colds and flu that could result.

Children can benefit from Aconite when teething pain is accompanied with fever, and where there is much tossing and turning in their sleep, or biting their fists and screaming.

Newborn babies who arrived in the world in a shocked state due to a fast labour, will relax and urinate with assistance from Aconite. A randomized, double-blind, placebo-controlled study on 47 infants, looked at post-operative pain. Homeopathic aconite significantly relieved agitation in children undergoing sub-umbilical surgery. A single dose, found 19 showed improvement within 15 minutes compared to eight in placebo. Alibeau et al, *Pediatrie* 1990 45:7-8.

Aconite is used by the strong and vigorous when there is acute inflammation.

The shock of Aconite is the exact opposite of Arnica. Aconite's action in fever and inflammation is similar to Lady's tresses (*Spiranthes species*).

DOSE- In the acute stage, it may be repeated frequently, even every hour. In neuralgia, the tincture can be applied externally, and the 30th potency taken internally. Five drops of the third potency in water every hour, if useful until perspiration appears or symptoms abate. The 200X potency can be tried to those suffering extreme fear or panic attacks, single dose and repeat if needed.

Higher potencies, such as 1M, should be administered by an experienced practitioner.

MOTHER TINCTURE- This is prepared from fresh root and plant of *A. napellus*, when beginning to flower. The expressed juice is mixed with equal parts of pure alcohol, and allowed to settle. The clear liquid is pour off. One drop is shaken twice with 99 drops of alcohol to obtain 1X.

First proving by Hahnemann with eight males and three females with juice of whole plant, thickened in sun and mixed with equal parts of wine in 1805. Poisoning cases cited by Reil in 1860. Proving by Hencke with four males and tincture in 1841. Proving by Gerstel with 16 provers with tincture, 1X, 2C, and 3X in 1843.

Hybrid Monkshood (*Aconitum X cammarum*) is useful for headache with vertigo and tinnitus. Cataleptic symptoms, with tingling and prickling of the tongue, lips and face.

Blue swollen lips, skin dry and icy cold.

Apathy and indifference to whole world. Uneasiness due to tickling sensation all over compelling constant movement. Restless.

DOSE- Proving by Schroff with 4-5 male provers and extract of root in 1853. Doses as above.

Aconitine (Aconitinum) is used for heavy feeling as of lead, pain in the supra-orbital nerve, ice-cold sensation creeping up and hydrophobia symptoms. Crawling sensation as if face is scaling off. Pupilary dilation and contraction is present, along with sudden heat of the face and head, accompanied by perspiration.

Flow of ideas is sluggish, long reflection is impossible, and the power of attention impaired.

For *tinnitus aurium* use 3X. Tingling sensation.

DOSE- Self-experimentation by Heinrich and Dworzack with small doses of alkaloid in 1853. Self-experiment by Hottot with alkaloid in 1863 and clinical effects observed in patients by Harley with alkaloid in 1860s.

Yellow Wolfbane (*A. lycotonum*) is used for Hodgkin's disease, with swelling of the cervical, axillary and mammary glands. It is often accompanied by itching of the nose, eyes, anus and vulva.

The skin of the nose is easily cracked, with a taste of blood in the mouth.

The consumption of pork leads to diarrhea.

DOSE- as above. Proving by Petroz in France in 1852.

MATERIA POETICA

Aconitum napellus

Oh *Death*, I beg you with full force
I know my time is up
But please don't take me yet, Oh *Death*
I'm panicked but of course
My heart is racing, I can't breathe
I'm suffocating with a wheeze
Anxiety becomes my flesh
Please stay away from me, Great *Death*
I beg you here with widened eyes
I've had my share of shock
And now my hour of demise
The wind my head doth mock
I don't feel well
My eyes a sting
The wheezing worse
The clock does bring
'Tis one o'clock and I do scream
Get me out of this bad dream!
Oh Aconite is what I need
Death let me go
For I am freed!

SYLVIA CHATROUX

FLOWER ESSENCES

Mountain Monkshood (*A. delphinifolium*) has an energy field with a strong vibration of calm, and a focus on sound energy.

The flower essence helps use look into the depths of our soul, while retaining our connection with the higher self. Issues of fear are dealt with, as we let go of some of our inner anxieties.

We are better able to allow others into our lives. Group work, where there is intense, interpersonal dynamics, is helped by allowing each person to better define their boundaries, while still working for group objectives.

ALASKA

Northern Monkshood (*A. delphinifolium*) flower essence is for inner vision. It is for tapping into the source of wisdom to guide us, as we contemplate our life and the illusions that we may have accepted as reality. It is a lifeline during any great period of change and growth.

CANADIAN

Monkshood (*A. napellus*) flower essence is the remedy that helps to unlock old tension burdens in the mind and body. Long standing illness that has roots in the distant past is relieved. The remedy is most useful for helping one accept adult responsibility for the past and get on with living.

BAILEY

Monkshood integrates aspects of the lower and higher self. The flower essence can be used with obsession and extreme emotional imbalances, including schizophrenia. It is for the person that may need a period of retreat to resolve emotional problems.

PEGASUS

Monkshood (*A. columbianum*) is for repression of spiritual capacities due to fear of psychic opening, often associated with traumatic memory of near death or related threshold experiences; paralysis of spiritual forces due to prior trauma or cultic abuse; hidden cultic or sexual behavior.

FLOWER ESSENCE SOCIETY

SPIRITUAL PROPERTIES

"Even a man who's pure at heart and says his prayers at night, can become a werewolf when the wolfsbane (monkshood) blooms, and the moon is full and bright".

ANON

Taking this remedy heals memories of trauma which have been locked in the body at a cellular level, so that shock symptoms are no longer re-stimulated at the slightest stress. The remedy dissolves states of panic and fear. You no longer feel terrified at the thought of death, although the fact that the experience is by its very nature unknown, will inspire awe in you.

LORIUS

PERSONALITY TRAITS

Vital, vigorous, extrovert, robust people who are yet exquisitely sensitive to mental shock, such as an earthquake, being trapped in an elevator, lights going out in a tunnel, accidents, or a weaker person suffering from a big shock. Clairvoyant.

They act as if death is imminent; fear of death is very strong…ask "when will this happen?" They answer, "Now!" Intense claustrophobia, evening driving in a car on the freeway or motorway, as well as in elevators.

PETER CHAPPELL

A woman recovering from aconite poisoning put words to what it feels like to be in an Aconitum state. When her breathing became easier, she said that it felt like coming out 'of a narrow, dark, hot room into a well-lighted one'.

HUGHES

The wet from Valais snow-melt and rain flowed down alpine meadows and just before it trickled into the stream by the cabin it licked the clump of monk's-hood. Hooded, helmeted flower contraptions of sprung lids, blue as an old police box, they signaled the presence of *Aconitum,* a notorious poison of wives and wolves. In that stone cabin with a scythe hanging from the ceiling, a sorcerer read a Persian text* and went in search of the mouse immune to monk's-hood, a theriac to use as an antidote. Too late, the neurotoxin unlocked a path which led him from the sky deep into the mountain where there were others huddled on a corner, hoods up against CCTV cameras.

PAUL EVANS

* Guy de Vigevani (1335) wrote of the archive of a Persian scholar, Avicenna or Ibn Sina (980-1037), which recommended searching for the mouse antidote to *Aconitum poisoning*. From De Cleene and Lejeune, *Compendium and Ritual Plants of Europe* (2003).

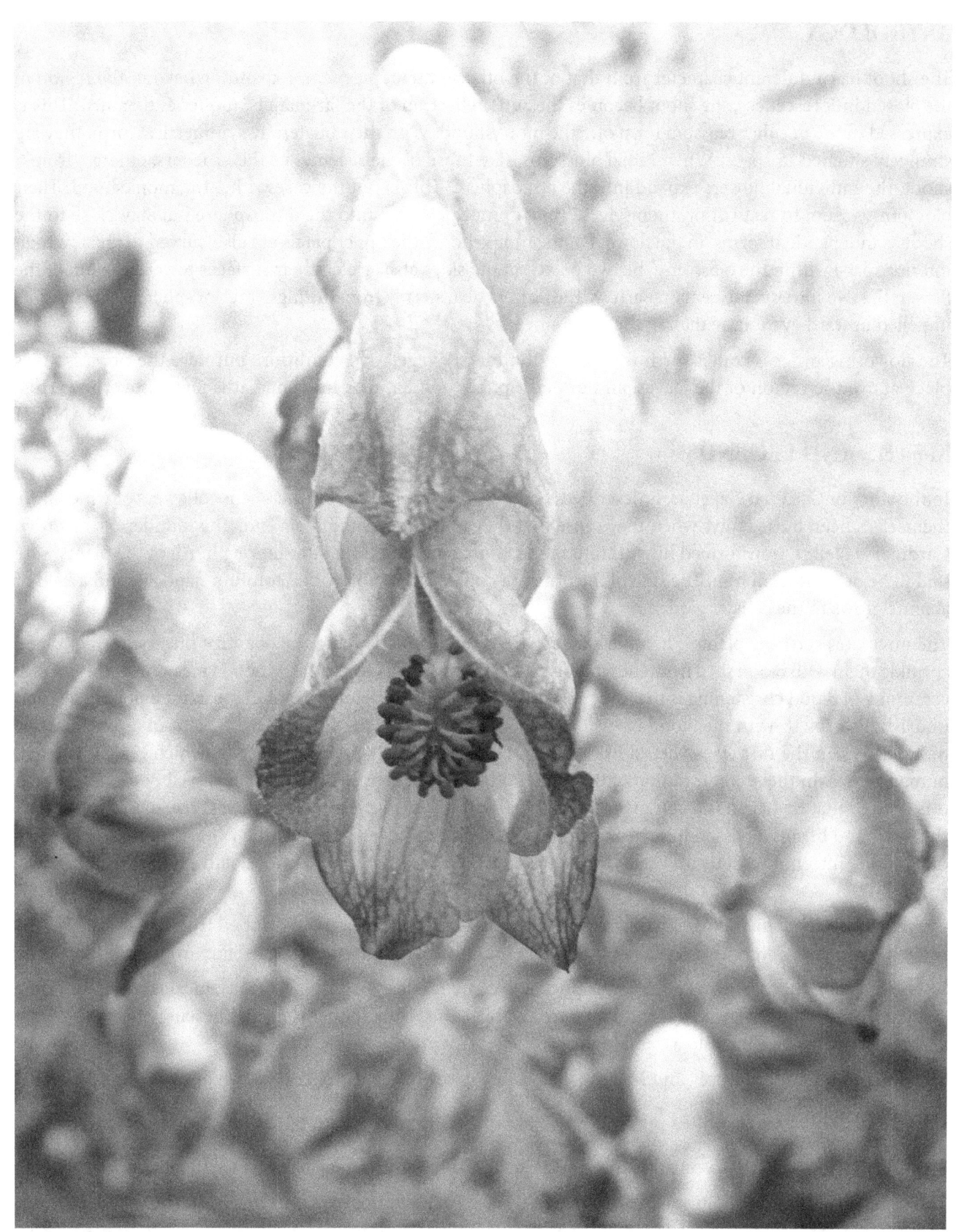

BICOLOR MONKSHOOD

ASTROLOGY

The shoot has a different character from that of the other buttercup genera. Expanding beyond the region of the closed inflorescences, the shoot becomes the sun's reflection of the far planets, Jupiter and Saturn. This is expressed in the peculiar blossom form of…the monkshood. With their bilaterally symmetrical form, they are strangely situated in space. When radial blossoms, like those of the racemes of the crucifers, emerge, from a shoot, the individual flowers expand into the atmosphere. This is not the case with…the monkshood. Their blossoms…seem to rest within themselves. They do not push out into the atmosphere but stay close to the shoot as independent forms. In the flowers of the monkshood, the upper petals are also curved to create a high interior space within the blossom. The two petals on the sides also stretch their surfaces toward the top of the flower; the two lower petals remain narrow. The flowers turn sternly from the high interior sphere to the outside, impelled upward even more than in the larkspur.

The flowering process comes forth from a predominately vegetative condition, but here the process takes place above the region of the leaves, and under Jupiter's and Saturn's influence, it is almost overpowering.

KRANICH

MYTHS AND LEGENDS

In the story of Cardinal Napellus, is described a sect "known as the blue brothers", the followers of which have themselves been buried alive when they sense that they are approaching their end. The founder of the order, Cardinal Napellus, transformed himself into the first monkshood flower after his death. All of the plants were said to be derived from him. The sign of the order, of course, is the flower of Aconitum napellus, and a field of aconite grows in the cloister garden.

The novitiates start the plants when they are accepted into the order, and they baptize these with blood and sprinkle them with blood shed from the wounds produced by flagellation. "The symbolic meaning of this strange ceremony of blood christening is that the person should magically plant his soul in the garden of paradise and nourish his growth with the blood of his desires". The brothers in the order use the plant in a psychoactive manner. When the flowers withered in the fall, we collected their poisonous seeds, which resemble small human hearts. In the secret tradition of the blue brothers, these represent the mustard seed of faith, of which it is written that he who has it can move mountains, and we ate of these. Just as their terrible poison changes the heart and brings a person into a condition between life and death, so shall the essence of faith transform our blood- into miraculous power in the hours between the gnawing pain of death and ecstatic rapture.

GUSTAV MEYRINK

According to Greek mythology, Aconitum napellus arose from the drool that dripped from the mouths of the three-headed dog. Cerberus-hell's gatekeeper- when the Greek hero Hercules dragged him from the underworld.

It was also thought to be the source of the poison used by Medea, on of the great mythical sorceresses of the ancient world. As the story goes, Medea prepared a poisonous drink for her stepson Theseus, who stood in the way of her own son's chance to ascend to the throne of Athens.

The deception failed, however, and Medea was forced to flee Greece with her own son in tow. **FOSTER**

RECIPES

TINCTURE- Fresh herb tincture is made in a 1: 4 alcohol dilution. The dried herb is a 1:10 ratio in 70% alcohol.

The lethal dose of pure aconitine is 3-6 mg for adult so only a few grams of plant material can be very dangerous.

DOSE- 3-5 drops as needed. Stop when improvement. Fluid extract- one drop. For trigeminal neuralgia 5 drops several times daily; in meningitis affecting the spine and brain, 5-10 drops as needed.

It is advisable to initially increase the dose and then decrease. More is not better! Five mls of tincture can be fatal.

If the patient does not die, recovery occurs within 24 hours.

For overdose, take activated charcoal, and then GI lavage or emetic or cathartic. Use stimulants such as coffee.

It is interesting to note, that in Traditional Chinese Medicine, licorice root is almost always used in conjunction with Aconite. When the amount of licorice in a preparation containing aconite and ginger was increased, a corresponding reduction in the amount of aconitine that could be extracted from the decoction was observed. Miaorong and Jong, *Proc. 40th Ann Conf, Beijing U of Chin Med* Aug 1996 Beijing University Press.

Chinese rhubarb (*R. palmatum*) appears to affect pharmacokinetics of fu zi alkaloids, by enhancing effects and reducing toxicity. Li Y et al, *Eur J Drug Metab Pharmacokinet* 2016 June 29.

Paeoniflorin from peony root reduces the acute toxicity of aconitine, at least in rat studies. Fan et al, *Fitoterapia* 2011 Sept 9.

When combined with panax ginseng the toxicity is reduced, by restricting intestinal absorption of alkaloids, without influencing other active components. You Q et al, *Chin J Integr Med* 2015 August 14.

EAR OIL- One part Aconite, four parts oregon grape root/goldthread, and four parts mullein (*Verbascum*) tincture. Four drops in the ear up to four times daily.

LINIMENT- The dried above ground herb in 1:2 ratio in 90% alcohol, and dissolve 5% camphor crystals weight to volume. That is, if you make 100 ml of the tincture, then dissolve 5 grams of camphor. Like arnica, do not use aconite tincture or liniment near open wounds. Moisten cloth with liniment and apply to affected area for few minutes. Use care to avoid eyes, nostrils or lips. Laws in England restrict external use to 1.3%.

OINTMENT- Mix one tablespoon of dried root powder in 500 grams of a natural ointment base, such as unpetroleum jelly. Apply twice daily to affected areas.

FU ZI (aconitum preparata)- Most yang of all medicines. Soak the whole roots n vinegar for one month; then in salt water for one month. Repeat this three times.

FU TZU- another process consists of cleansing the herb and immersing in cold water, that is changed 2-3 times daily until the paralyzing and pungent taste is removed. It is then decocted in licorice root and black beans until there is no whiteness in centre. Then it is sun-dried.

DOSE- 3-6 grams of processed slices. The prepared root is decocted for 30-60 minutes before other herbs are added.

CAUTION- In cases of poisoning, use vomiting, keep patient warm, and use atropine to fight bradycardia, and lidocaine to relieve arrythmia. Do not give opiates. Be careful of emetics, as they can cause cardiac failure. Recent work suggests flecainaide or amiodarone may be more useful for ventricular dysrhythmia. There may be a role for mexiletine, procainamide and magnesium sulphate (Epsom salts). Coulson JM et al, *Clin Toxicol* (Phila) 2017 55(5): 313-321.

Do not use during lactation or pregnancy, or in cases of severe debilitation and weakness (asthenia).

It was traditionally contraindicated with *Bletilla striata* rhizome. Not recommended. A recent study suggests that water extracts of *Veratrilla baillonii* may attenuate sub-acute toxicity. Yu Y et al, *Phytomedicine* 2016 23(13): 1591-8.

Aconitine, administered with P-gp substrate drugs may cause drug-drug interactions. Caution is advised.

CANADIAN MOONSEED
YELLOW PARILLA
VINE MAPLE
(***Menispermum canadense*** L.)
(***M. angulatum*** Moench.) not accepted
PARTS USED- bark

Menispermum means Moonseed, as the fruit is shaped like the crescent moon. Canadense means of Canada. Parilla comes from its superficial appearance to the Smilax species; ie. sarsa parilla.

Moonseed, or Yellow Parilla is of the Moonseed family, a mainly tropical grouping with 78 genera and over 500 species.

It is related to Pareira, which is used for curare, an arrow poison in South America, Calumba root, and *Cocculus indicus,* another important homeopathic plant. In fact, it is used as a bitter tonic in a manner very similar to Calumba root due in large part to its berberine content.

Our Moonseed is a vine up to three meters long, found in the woods of Manitoba.

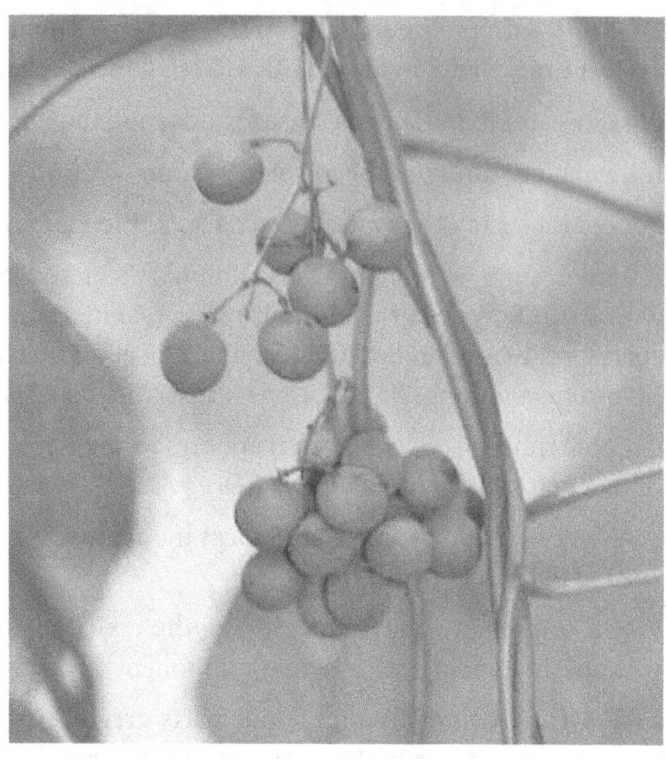

CANADIAN MOONSEED FRUIT
(Courtesy of Walter Muma)

It is hardy to the rest of the prairies, but cannot make it over dry, prairie soil, and needs trees for support. The plant has inconspicuous yellow-green flowers, that when both sexes are present, will produce fruit.

These grape-like berries are considered poisonous, and possibly fatal, to children. The berry has very sharp-ridged pits that can also be irritating or damaging to intestinal tissue.

The Cherokee used the root for skin diseases, as a diuretic and laxative. It was prepared and taken by "weakly females", before or after childbirth, and for a weak stomach and bowels. It was called appropriately Moonroot, or **UDO SA NO E HI.**

The Delaware made a salve for use on chronic sores.

The Omaha Ponca call it Thunder Grapes, or **INGTHAHE-HAZI-I-TA.**

Another name among the Ponca was Grapes of the Ghost. The Pawnee went for the more obvious, less poetic Sore Mouth, or **HAKAKUT.**

At one time, it was used as a substitute for sarsaparilla in "root" beers.

The Blister Beetle, *Chauliognathus marginatus,* aggressively attacks and shreds *Potentilla* and other flowers for pollen and nectar. When it lands on the small flowers of Moonseed it carefully takes the pollen, and flicks the grains from the anther. It then licks nectar from the base of female flowers without injuring the ovary. Clever.

In Traditional Chinese medicine, the related *M. dauricum,* known as **BEI DOU GEN** is widely used for inflammatory conditions of the bowel, throat, muscles and lungs.

MEDICINAL

CONSTITUENTS- Alkaloids make up 2.2% of the plant by dry weight, and include in the rhizome; acutimine, acutimidine, daurinoline, dauricine, tetrandrine, N'-demethyldauricine, N'-methyl-lindcarpine; vinetine (oxyacanthine) and berberine. The plant contains berberine, dehydrocheilanthifolin, magnoflorine, N-desmethyldaurin, N-methylindcarpinmethiodide. The leaves contain (-)viburnitol. The seeds contain fat and protein.

Millspaugh noted that the use of Moonseed by early practitioners was very similar to sarsaparilla. It was an official drug in the *US Pharmacopoeia* at the turn of the 19th century, from 1882 to 1905 as a tonic and diuretic.

Earlier, various Native healers used the root for scrofula, or tuberculosis of the neck lymph glands; while early settlers used it as a diuretic for strangury in their horses.

Dr. King noted "indications seem to point to its probable value in leucocythaemia, especially when the spleen is prominently involved."

Dr. Brown, in 1875, noted that "yellow parilla seems to possess one virtue which is paramount to all others, it is essentially and particular anti-syphilitic, anti-scrofulous, anti-mercurial."

Dr. Cook voiced similar opinion, stating that "in small doses, its action is chiefly manifested upon the respiratory passages, where it increases expectoration and gives a feeling of stimulation to the lungs...the stomach is fairly improved by it, and the hepatic apparatus and smaller bowels distinctly influenced, whence it will lead to free discharge of bile and to fair evacuations of the bowels.

Its general glandular action makes it valuable in scrofula, secondary syphilis, mercurial rheumatism, indolent ulcers and similar low conditions...Most commonly it is combined with more relaxing articles such as *Rumex, Fraxinus, Celastrus and Arctium lappa.*"

Alma Hutchens, in her somewhat erratic book, notes that it is useful "for all diseases arising from inheritary or acquired impurities of the system. It exerts its influence principally on the gastric and salivary glands and is found expressly beneficial in cases of adhesive inflammation and where it is found necessary to break up organized deposits and hasten disintegration of unwanted tissue."

Bolyard, in his book on *Medicinal Plants and Home Remedies of Appalachia* gives the following recipe.

"One span of (Moonseed root) is boiled in a quart of water until one half pint of liquid remains. One half pint of whisky and a heaping tablespoon of sulfur is added to this. One spoonful is taken before each meal until it is all used".

Grieve, in A Modern Herbal, notes that Moonseed contains berberine.

"In small doses it is a tonic, diuretic, laxative and alterative. In larger doses, it increases the appetite and action of the bowels; in full doses, it purges and causes vomiting. It is a superior laxative bitter, considered very useful for scrofula, cutaneous, rheumatic, syphilitic, mercurial, and arthritic diseases; also for dyspepsia, chronic inflammation of the viscera and in general debility.

The herb has some influence on the spleen and may be of use in some forms of leukocytosis.

"Externally, the decoction has been applied as an embrocation in cutaneous and gouty affections... in powder is recommended as a nervine and is considered superior to Sarsaparilla taken in doses of 1-3 grains, three times daily."

She forgot to note that light increases in heart pulse will be noticed, in large doses as well.

Dauricine is used as an anti-arrhythmic agent in China. It has been shown to inhibit platelet aggregation in work by Tong et al, Yao Xue Xue Bao, 1989 24:2.

More recent work by Qian, confirms dauricine's effect in cardiac arrhythmia. *Acta Pharmacol Sin* 2002 23:12.

Dauricine is analgesic, hypotensive and relaxant of uterine and other muscle tissue. It is a dopamine receptor inhibitor, a calcium antagonist, and central nervous system depressant.

Like other isoquinoline alkaloid, dauricine induces autophagic cell death in drug-resistant cancers, including HeLa, A549, MCF-7, PC3, HepG2, Hep3B and H1299. Law BY et al, *Oncotarget* 2016 7(7): 8090-104.

Dauricine inhibits the proliferation of bladder and prostate cancer cells. Wang J et al, *Asian Pac J Trop Med* 2012 5(12): 973-6. It also inhibits human breast cancer angiogenesis by suppressing hypoxia inducible factor

1alpha protein accumulation and vascular endothelial growth factor expression. Tang XD et al, *Acta Pharma Sin* 2009 30(5): 605-16.

It was found to prevent or treat colon cancer through modulation of the NF-kappaB signaling pathway. Yang Z et al, *J Cell Physiol* 2010 225(1): 266-75.

Dauricine is an isoquinoline alkaloid with anesthetic, anti-inflammatory and weak curare-like activity. It is anti-arrhythmic and cardio-protective.

It is a platelet-activating factor receptor ligand.

Tetrandrine is an ACE inhbitor, analgesic, anti-anginal, anti-arrhythmic, anti-histamine, anti-inflammatory, anti-mitotic, antioxidant, antipyretic, anti-tumor, bradycardic, as well as a calcium antagonist and circulatory stimulant.

Tetrandrine may be useful, when combined with glucocorticoids for inflammatory and auto-immune conditions, where there is a desire to suppress the immune system. On its own, tetrandrine suppresses the phosphorylation of mitogen-activated protein kinase, and inhibits the secretion of pro-inflammatory cytokines. Xu W et al, *Eur J Pharmacol* 2017 April 11. Other work found it suppresses Th17 cell differentiation.

It combines well with cisplatin in resistant A547 (non-small cell lung cancer). Ye LY et al, *Cancer Cell Int* 2017 17:40.

It may also be useful for osteosarcoma, based on work by Tian DD et al, *Oncol Rep* 2017 37(5): 2795-2802. It prevents multi-drug resistance in osteosarcoma cell lines in other studies.

It may be useful in metastatic renal cell carcinoma. Chen S et al, *PLoS One* 2017 12(3).

Other studies suggest benefit in breast cancer (MCF-7), gastric, lung, colon, glioma, nasopharyngeal, and liver cancers.

A very good review of tetrandrine, as a potential candidate for cancer chemotherapy is by Liu T et al, *Oncotarget* 2016 7(26): 40800-15.

Tetrandrine is an L-type calcium channel blocker that helps reduce hypertension, and enhances sleep by suppressing the noradrenergic system. Huang YL et al, *Phytomedicine* 2016 34(14): 1821-29.

It may also be neuroprotective in chronic vascular dementia by reducing interleukin-1beta expression, N-methyl-D-aspartate receptor 28 phosphorylation at tyrosine 1472, and neuronal necrosis. Lv YL et al, *Neural Regen Res* 2016 11(3): 454-9.

Viburnitol is also present in yarrow, and high bush cranberry.

The alkaloid acutamine has been shown to inhibit growth of human T cells.

Oxyacanthine, also found in *Mahonia, Magnolia and Ranunculus* species, is anti-microbial to *Bacillus subtilis* and *Colpidium colpuda*, as well as an adrenalin antagonist and vasodilator. The compound shows significant cytotoxicity against HT29 cancer cell lines. El Hosry L et al, *Nat Prod Commun* 2016 11(5): 645-8.

Also found in Orgeon grape root, the compound is a potent inhibitor of keratinocyte growth, associated with psoriasis. Muller K et al, *Planta Medica* 1995 61(1): 74-5.

Daurinoline is a muscle relaxant.

It is one of the few bitter tonics that does not contain tannic or gallic acid.

HOMEOPATHY

Moonseed (*M. canadense*) is a remedy for migraine, and is associated with restlessness and dreams. There may be spinal pain, with a dryness and itchiness all over, and dryness of the mouth and throat.

The head has pressure from within outward, with stretching and yawning, and pains down the back. There may be sick headaches, with pain in the forehead and temples, moving toward the occiput. The tongue is swollen, with copious saliva.

The legs are sore, as is bruised, with pain in the thighs, elbows and shoulders.

They feel so weak, empty and hollow that is as if the whisper of death is heard.

Low spirited, but attend to business with rapidity. Quick tempered, irritable, surly, ill-natured and stubborn.

DOSE- Third potency. Taylor did self-experiment with tincture in 1867, and Graham with 1x trituration of menispermine in same year.

SEED OIL

The fruit seeds contain 16% oil composed mainly of octadecadienoic acid (46%), oleic acid, 29%, and octadecatrienoic acid (25%).

PERSONALITY TRAITS

A fundamental them of Menispermaceae is oversensitivity. Plants in general are sensitive to outside influences. Some plant families, like Menispermaceae, are more sensitive than most.

Menispermaceae are sensitive to numerous things such as emotions, pain, noise and touch..[and]…especially sensitive to the suffering of others and those who need care.

Generally, Menispermaceae have a strong sense of self-reliance and responsibility. They think everyone has the duty to take care of themselves, yet when confronted with the unfortunate, they can't help but to take on that responsibility too. Though weighed down by the duty, they would feel guilty if they didn't.

Taking on the responsibility of care and tending to those in need lead to emotional over-reactions. They are too caring, too concerned and too sensitive to the situation of seeing someone ill. They can't moderate or modulate their impressions and reactions. They have to react, to care, to move, to overdo, overextend and overwork.

The strain causes either outbursts of irritability or a complete collapse to the extent that they are now as ill and debilitated as they initially were driven to help. Only reducing the underlying sensitivity will allow them to moderate their reactions and offer the kind of assistance that is truly beneficial to all concerned, especially themselves.   **VERMEULEN**

MYTHS AND LEGENDS

Long ago it rained for many days and the land was flooded for miles around. The Indians has to go about in canoes and food was becoming scarce. They appealed to the Chief to know what to do. The chief said, "Make ropes of the Moonseed vine half as long as a boy can walk in one sun. Put the ropes in your canoes and get into them. Wait until the water gets as high as yon rocky height, then attach one end of the rope to the rock and the other end to the canoes".

The Indians fell to work twisting the fibers of the vine, but they grew tired and stopped when the ropes were still short. All but Goplobet, who worked on and on, until he had obeyed the chief's instructions.

He wound his rope up and it filled the canoe. The Indians waited until the water had risen to its highest, then tied their canoes to the rock. As the waters went down, one short rope snapped, then another, until all the canoes but Goplobet's, were adrift.

Soon the canoes were scattered all over the earth and that is why there are so many tribes of Indians. But Goplobet stayed in the same country and became a great chief and had many children.   **GUILLET**

RECIPES

TINCTURE- 10-40 drops as needed. For a bitter tonic take 5-10 in water before meals. The fresh or dry root tincture is made at 1:5 with 70% or 40% alcohol, respectively.

DECOCTION- 1-4 ounces three times daily.

DR. CHRISTOPHER'S ALTERATIVE COMPOUND- Take two parts each of red clover, moonseed and burdock root, and combine it with one part mullein leaf. Simmer in water, until reduced by half. Dosage is four ounces three to four times daily.

MOSS
HAIRCAP MOSS
(*Polytrichum juniperinum* Hedw.)
COMMON HAIRY CAP MOSS
GOLDEN MAIDEN-HAIR
(*P. commune* Hedw.)
PEATMOSS
(*Sphagnum species*)
CYPRESS-LEAVED FEATHER MOSS
(*Hypnum cupressiforme* Hedw.)
BROOM MOSS
(*Dicranum scoparium* Hedw.)
CUSHION MOSS
(*D. groenlandicum* Brid.)
BROOK MOSS
(*Fontinalis species*)
AQUATIC APPLE MOSS
(*Philonotis fontana* [Hedw.] Brid.)
STAR MOSS
(*Tortula ruralis* [Hedw.] Gaertn. et al)
SILVERY BRYUM
(*Bryum argenteum* Hedw.)
LONG NECKED BYRUM
(*Leptobryum pyriforme* [Hedw.] Wilson)
FERN MOSS
(*Cratoneuron filicinum* [Hedw.] Spruce)

HAIRMOSS
(*Ditrichum ssp*)
CORD MOSS
(*Funaria hygrometrica* Hedw.)
WOODSY LEAFY MOSS
WOODSY MNIUM
(*Mnium cuspidatum* Hedw.) not accepted
(*Plagiomnium cuspidatum* [Hedw.] T. Kop.)
OEDER'S PLAGIOPUS MOSS
(*Plagiopus oederiana*[Sw.] Crum & Anderson)
ROUGH MOSS
(*Claopodium crispifolium* [Hook.] Ren. & Card.)
TREE MOSS
(*Climacium dendroides* [Hedw.] Web. & Mohr.)
STEP MOSS
SPLENDID FEATHER MOSS
(*Hylocomium splendens* [Hedw.] Schimp. In B.S.G.)
YELLOW MUSHROOM MOSS
YELLOW MOOSE DUNG MOSS
(*Splachnum luteum* Hedw.)
RED MUSHROOM MOSS
BRILLIANT RED DUNG MOSS
(*S. rubrum* Hedw.)
APPLE MOSS
(*Bartramia pomiformis* Hedw.)
PARTS USED- aerial

In mosses...strength is mingled with humility, gentleness and charm, with elemental essence, reflecting the gladness of wind, sun and rain.
                                                                                    JOHN BLAND

And may at last my weary age find out the peaceful hermitage, The hairy gown and mossy cell, where I may sit and rightly spell of every star that Heaven doth show, and every herb that sips the dew till old experience do attain to something like prophetic strain.
                                                                                    JOHN MILTON

The sacred Virgin's well, her moss most sweet and rare against infectious damps.   **POLYOLBION**

A rolling stone gathers no moss.
While tenderly the mild, agreeable moss
Obscures the figures of her date of birth.

                                                                                    DOROTHY PARKER

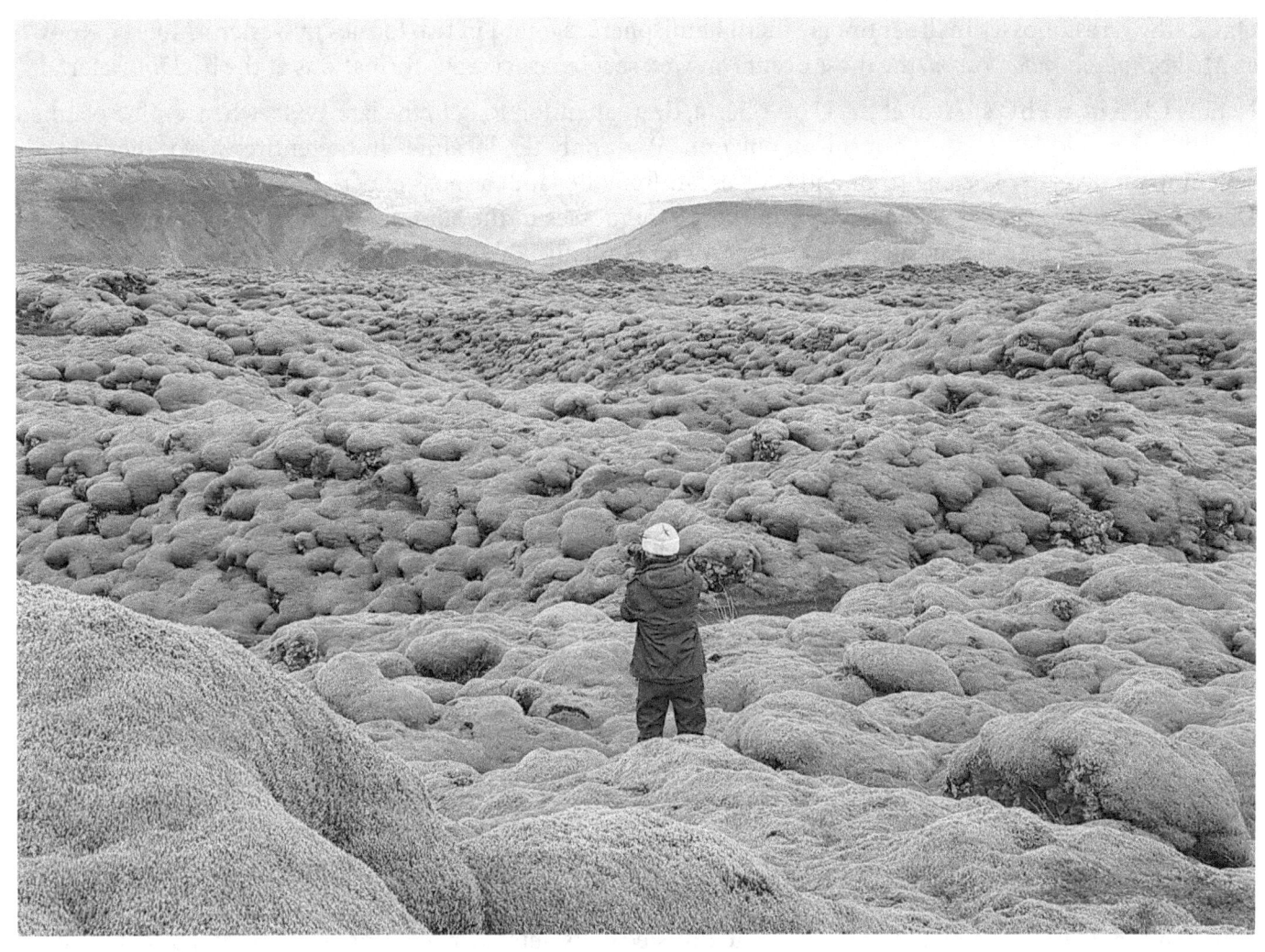

MOSS COVERED FIELD IN ICELAND

Moss is from the Old English **MÖS**, meaning a bog or the vegetation growing in it. It probably stems from the Latin **MUSCUS** and further back to the Indo-European base **MEU** for damp.

Hynum is from the Greek **HYPNOS**, to sleep. Bryum is derived from the Greek **BRYON** meaning, moss. Leptobryum means slender; pyriforme is pear-shaped, in reference to the sporophyte capsule.

Dicranum is in reference to the two forked teeth around the mouth of the capsule. These teeth control spore dispersal by opening and closing according to changes of humidity.

Funaria is from the Latin for a Cord, **FUNALE**.

Polytrichum refers to this plants appearance of having many hairs. This juniper-like moss is located all over the world except for some tropical locations.

The Japanese have long cultivated moss and lichen gardens, and the word **SHIBUSA** was invented to describe the venerable quality they help instill to a setting. Common hairy cap moss is the most widely used species in these moss gardens, alternating with *Pogonatum contortum*, found in British Columbia and elsewhere.

The most famous moss garden in the world is Kyoto's Kokedara meaning, "moss temple".

Moss covered boulders are the astute landscapers prize find, with half moss and half exposed rock considered ideal.

Polytrichum commune and *Bartramia pomiformis,* both common in Alberta, are widely used in moss landscaping.

One of the rarest mosses in the entire northern hemisphere is found in two locales in western Alberta. Known as *Mielichhoferia macrocarpa*, the moss occurs on wet, seeping calcareous formations at the back of waterfalls.

Natalie Cleavitt, a PhD student at the U of Alberta, drew attention to it, in the late 1990s when a mine planned a road that would have wiped out this population. With only ten localities in the entire world, the fight for retaining biodiversity became front and centre. Dr. Rene Belland, a moss expert from the U of Alberta and Devonian Gardens, found a small cluster of these rare mosses in the summer of 2007 near Jasper. Rene and I worked together for a short while on the *Adopt A Plant* initiative, after I was hired as the volunteer coordinator. I admit to being a difficult employee.

A close relative, the Copper Moss (*M. mielichhoferi*) has been widely used by prospectors as a determinate for heavy metal deposits.

Common Hairy Cap moss is a readily overlooked and yet valuable plant from the forest floor.

Hairy Cap tea was used traditionally to remove stones from the kidney and gallbladder; and to treat common colds.

It was gathered and well combed and becomes a beautiful chestnut colour when cured. The stalks were tied together and called Silk Wood, and used for dusting beds, curtains, hangings, and carpets.

Common Hair Cap Moss was made into brooms, brushes, plaited articles, mats, rugs, and baskets. A partially finished *Polytrichum* basket was found near an Early Roman fort near Newstead, England dated 86 AD.

Laplanders use Hairy Cap Moss for bedding. They would select a large patch of plants, cut out an area and separate them from the soil. This bed was rolled up and carried from place to place. In northern England, it was used to stuff mattresses and upholstery. Linnaeus recommended the *Polytrichium* mattress, as they didn't attract fleas and other pests.

Gilbert White wrote about "neat little bosoms which our foresters make from the stalk of the *P. commune*, or Great Golden Hair, which they call Silk Wood, and find plenty in the bogs.

When this moss is well combed and dressed, and divested of its outer skin, it becomes a beautiful bright chestnut color; and, being soft and pliant, is very proper for the dusting of beds, curtains, carpets, hangings, etc."

Today, it is used in Japanese bowl gardens; and is sold in nursery squares to create checkerboard designs. See recipes below for tips on growing moss gardens.

Decoctions and oil extractions of Hairy Cap were used to strengthen and beautify ladies' hair. This is probably due to the long hairs on the calyptra covering the capsule.

In New Zealand, the Maori call it Totara, and weave it into their cloaks for insulation and decoration.

According to Grout, the spore-filled capsules of *Polytrichum* might be eaten as a survival food. This author would probably find something else in the forest to eat first!

Long-Necked Byrum is found in a variety of conditions, from rotten wood to disturbed sites, and even greenhouses.

Cell cultures of the moss have shown the ability to synthesize EPA and other fatty acids.

Cypress-leaved Feather moss is used in France for window displays, and sold as sheet moss for nativity scenes. It has been used for bedding, and pillows due to being insect repellant and rot resistant. Other mosses used as green carpets for floral displays are *Rhytidiadelphus loreus*, *R. triquertus* and *Hylocomium splendens*.

Pillows stuffed with Hypnum species were supposed to help induce a special trance-like sleep.

Studies by Bargagli et al in Italy, found *H. cupressiforme* to be a most efficient accumulator of trace elements. This makes it an excellent determinant of heavy metal contamination from power plants, refineries, and chemical processors. Mosses in general, and Feather moss in particular, are a most suitable accumulative bio-monitor.

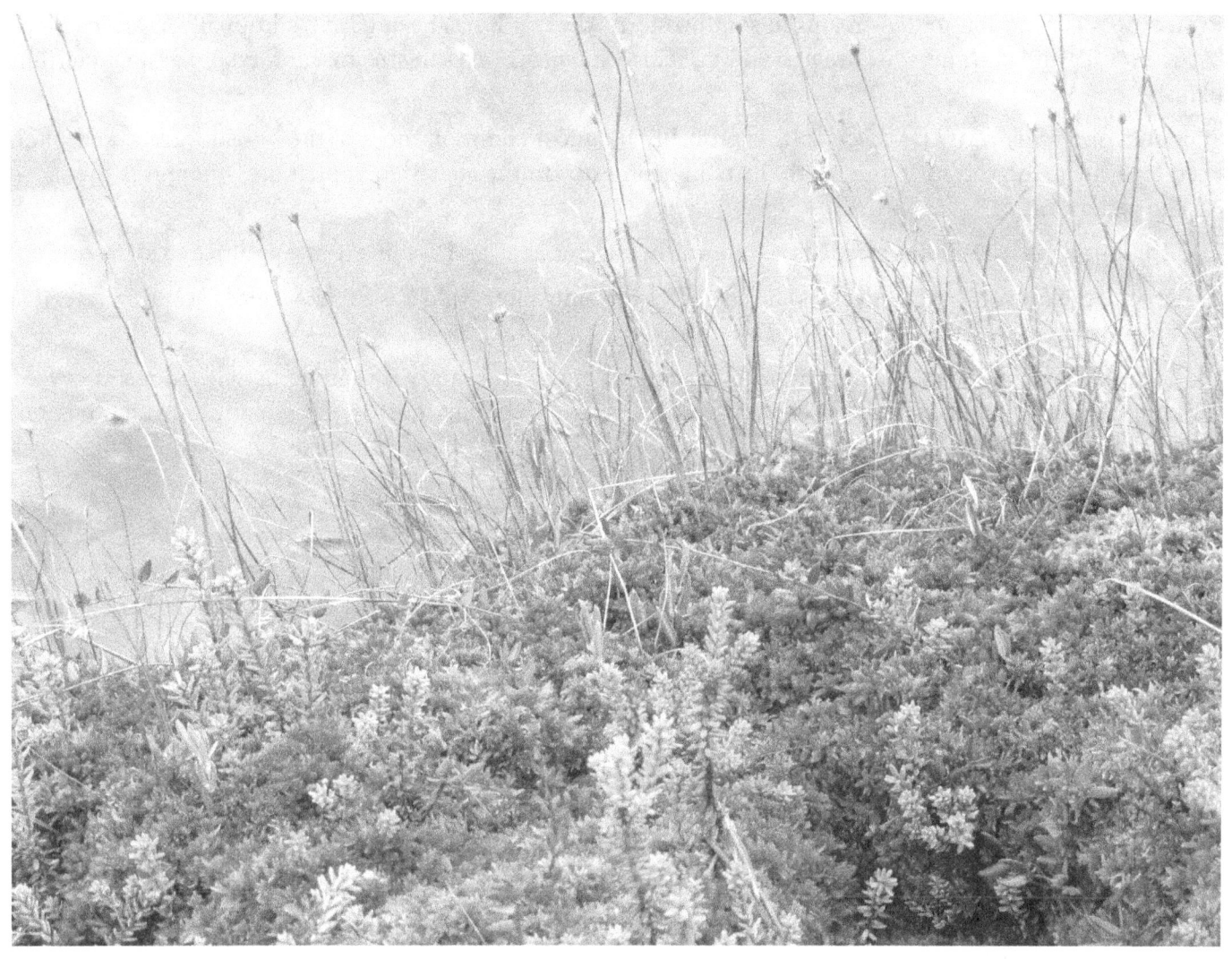

SPHAGNUM MOSS

Broom moss is used in shop windows as displays, moss gardens, and traditionally in bedding, mattresses, cushions and pillows.

Dicranum species, as well as *Racomitrium lanuginosum*, make superior wilderness wicks for candles.

Dicranum elongatum, known as **MANIQ** to the Inuit of Baffin Island, was prepared dry or in a broth for indigestion or sickness that requires bed rest.

At one time it was used as a diaper for babies. Broom Moss is usually a good indicator of acidic soils, whereas Silvery Bryum (*B. argenteum*) indicates alkalinity.

More specifically, Silvery Bryum is indicative of nitrogen from bird droppings, prairie dog urination, to the area around urban fire hydrants visited by dogs.

Silvery Bryum is probably the most common urban moss, on rooftops, and growing through cracks in sidewalks. Here it feeds on libations of feathery and furry animals, but mainly on the hair of Homo sapiens for the past 10-20 years. This moss is a major bonsai ground cover. It is being used in Antarctica to measure the effect of ozone radiation.

Cushion Moss was used by the Chipewyan, for its long parallel stems that absorb grease and make good wicks. They call it **NODHULE**.

Brook moss is common to the streams in southwestern Alberta. It has been used traditionally as an insulator between walls and chimneys for fire prevention. It also stabilizes weirs in streams, and is sold as an aquarium plant.

Stair step or feather moss (*H. splendens*) is probably the most common moss of the boreal forests, and often used to insulate log cabins in the north. Its name comes from the stair step annual growth, and is therefore easy to recognize.

The Thompson, or Nlaka'pmx steeped the moss as hot as possible, and applied it as a poultice to skin sores.

In Finland, the moss is bagged to assess heavy metal concentrations, and has a 55% water absorption rate. It is used by women in India, as a cushion to carry water vessels on their heads.

Woolly Moss (*R. canescens/R. lanuginosum*) is found on gravel and sandy sites in higher elevations. It is used for chinking cabins, and as lamp wicks by Labrador Eskimos. Woolly moss is also used in bowl cultivation, especially popular in Japan, for miniature gardens.

Tree Moss has been, in the past, dyed and used to decorate women's hats.

Red and Yellow Mushroom Moss are two of the most spectacular mosses of the north. They grow on moose dung in fens and bogs of the boreal forest, and resemble fairy rings. Flies and mosquitoes use the caps as landing pads, attracted by the scent of ammonia and butyric acid, and help disperse spores to the next dung pile. Pretty clever!

Rainbow trout and other mountain stream fish will eat *Scleropodium obtusifolium* when insects are scarce.

Native people mixed the green Sphagnum Moss with animal fats to treat cuts. It also was the first disposable diaper material, because of it's absorbency and disinfecting properties. Sphagnum moss is capable of holding 20 times its weight in water.

Both the Cree of Saskatchewan and Alberta call it **ASKIYAH** and use it for wiping as paper towels are used today; and traditionally for cleaning babies of mucous and blood after birth. The Chipewyan, further north, call it **TTH'AL**, and distinguish between the red and green varieties.

The Cree call Green Peat Moss **MASKWOSKWA**.

The Red was applied directly to cuts or skin infections, while the green was considered better for diapers (**TTH'AL DHETH**). The red peat moss was considered too irritating for babies.

Red Sphagnum is known as "moss that is red" by the Dena'ina of Alaska. It is used for any injury involving swelling, broken bones, blood poisoning or serious ear or eye problems. The red moss is boiled and afflicted area held over the steam and then the moss placed on the skin.

For ear troubles, hot rocks are surrounded by wet red sphagnum in a birch bark container and then placed on the patient's head so the steam enters the ears.

Red sphagnum is soaked in cold water and applied to headaches and lung problems.

White Sphagnum was used traditionally as baby diapers, toilet paper and menstrual pads. The species *S. magellanicum* is most prized by Johnson and Johnson for sanitary pads and diapers, due to its non-irritating properties.

It was sometimes put on fires to smoke meat or leathers.

The Crow of southern Montana call it **BEE MA GA SUT CHE**.

The Gwich'in, from the Mackenzie delta, used **NIN'**, or sphagnum moss for some of the same purposes. The wet moss was used for washing dishes, and wiping off fish tables, or put into a jar of water as a houseplant. For diapers, it was first hung in the lower branches of black spruce trees to dry and let the bugs crawl away.

Special houses were built to store the dried moss for winter diaper use. It was built of black spruce saplings bent to form a bent dome as for sweats, and tied together with split black spruce roots. The walls were filled in with spruce saplings stuck into the ground to form a dense wall. Boughs were placed on the ground, and then the dried moss was heaped on top.

Another unusual use, where plentiful, is the building of moss houses, or **NEEK'AN**. The houses were built of blocks of moss, cut in the fall, just after it starts to freeze. In the spring, the blocks were stored away until the next fall, when the good ones would be re-used. The blocks measured three feet by one foot wide and eight inches thick, and were packed between peeled poles that came together at the top. For a large, 3 family home, 20 poles would be used and it would take about one week to construct.

A fireplace was built in the middle, and gravel stones were built up about one foot. As the ground thawed, more stones were placed on the platform. If built carefully, the smoke would linger about six feet above people's heads. Smaller moss houses were sometimes built along trap lines.

Alaskan natives make a salve from mixing sphagnum moss with animal fats.

In China, it is used as a binder for iron and vitamins, as piglets are often born anemic.

Europeans used the powder or burnt ashes of sphagnum as a germicide; and during World War I it was used as surgical dressing on the battlefield. Towards the end of the war, about one million pounds of dressings per month were used. These dressings were cooler, softer and more absorbent than cotton. It absorbs three to four times as much liquid three times faster.

The natural acidity contributes to the anti-microbial activity. The pH of water at the edge of a sphagnum bog may be 4.3, the equivalent of dilute vinegar. Work by Varley and Barnett, 1987 cites evidence from controlled testing that the amount of wound area covered by new epidermis doubled using Sphagnum dressing compared to none.

Laplanders used the moss for children's cradles. The use of sphagnum moss for spinning material has been attempted in Sweden; producing cloth and clothing. It is used in inner soles of hiking boots to absorb moisture and odour.

Today, sphagnum moss is used in menstrual pads, for the same purpose. It can absorb up to 30 times its weight in water.

It is used today to help clean up heavy metals, PCPs and toxic wastes, including oil spills, and dyes. It is very effective at removing nitrogen (96%) and phosphorus (97%) from river and wastewater. It absorbs up to twelve times its weight in petrochemical spills.

Many bryophytes are hydrophobic and lipophilic, meaning they repel water and absorb oils.

In the past it has been used to make alcohol, various chemicals, paper, paraffin, naphtha, bricks, life preservers, gunpowder, fireworks, paint, insulation and charcoal. One factory near Minsk, Russia produces mineral wax from peat and uses it for leather polishes, crayons and plastics. A cream is also made for the treatment of eczema, ulcers and burns.

Global warming may speed up the decomposition of northern peat, according to Dr. Kelman Wieder. This in turn could increase the amount of CO_2 into the atmosphere by as much as 10%.

Peat moss is a valuable commodity that is used primarily in dry form as a soil conditioner.

It is a very good medium for help germinate jack pine and stimulate the growth of tamarack or larch seedlings.

It is used by florists and horticulturists for cuttings to propagate orchids.

Alberta has 103,000 square miles of peat land, or over 16% of its land base. The provincial peat moss industry produces over $33.5 million of sales annually, with three quarters shipped to the U.S. Canada wide the annual figure is about $130 million. In Canada, there is more energy in native peat than in the forest and natural gas reserves.

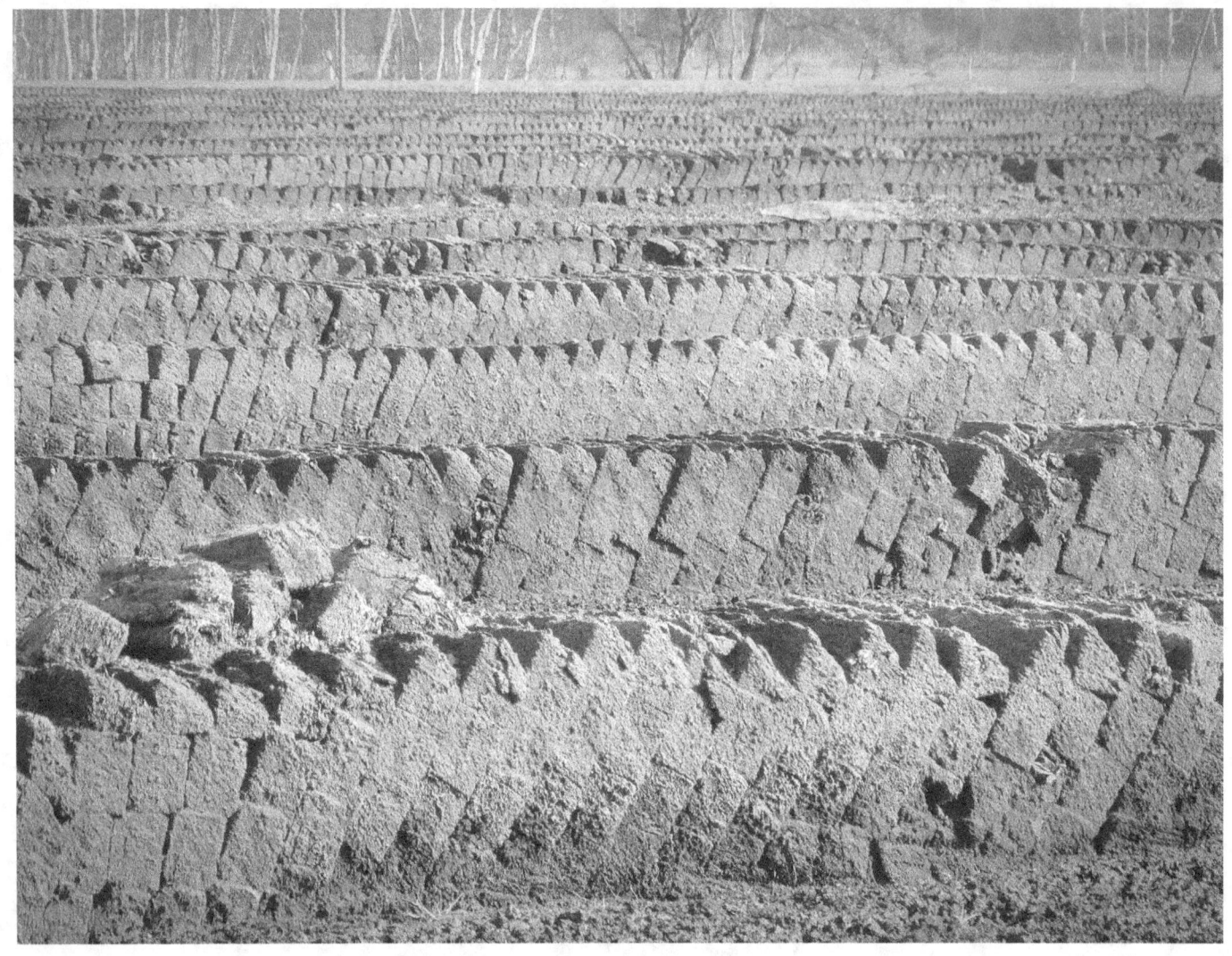

HARVESTED PEAT MOSS

Peat moss is best suited to production of methane, regenerates quickly, easily harvested, low sulphur content and heating value is superior to wood.

Peat lands, when drained and neutralized of acidity, are prolific producers of leaf and root vegetables. Over 100,000 acres throughout Canada are under agricultural use, supplying a large amount of produce for Toronto and Montreal.

The moss, *Campylium stellatum* is often found in fens as a dominant on hummocks. In northern Indiana, floating islands have been formed in ponds with this moss a major part of the mat formation.

Star Moss grows abundantly throughout Western forests. It is being investigated by Mel Oliver, for its relatively untapped gene pool, that may lead to more drought resistant crops.

As soon as a few drops of water are poured on the dry moss, what seemed like a brown brillo pad, becomes a lush green with individual star-like branches.

Viewed through an electron microscope, the dried moss shows massive cell damage that is repaired within minutes. Oliver envisions lawns, rangelands and pastures that could do the same.

"We're talking about using genetic engineering to create a grass that can approach the capability of the star moss to completely dry up, turn brown, and recover quickly when it rains."

He reasons that clues to the drought-repair gene begin with those proteins that increase during the recovery period. He has found 74 proteins that increase significantly within two hours of re-wetting.

Oliver is pleased that what was once an academic interest, while teaching at the University of Calgary, may now change forever the meaning of crop drought tolerance.

Mosses bio-accumulate heavy metals such as Pb, Fe, Zn, and Ni in high concentrations.

Fontanilis species show ability to hyper-accumulate cadmium, and absorb up to 43% of phenols in a water environment.

Racomitrium species remediate diesel fuel spills. *Drepanocladus fluitans* is able to concentrate copper up to high levels, while *Orthotridum obtusifolium* reacts negatively to hydrogen fluoride and is a good bio-monitor. Likewise, *Hylocomium splendens* is a good monitor of heavy metals.

Pleurizium schreberi has been found to reduce the number of seed capsules it produces under increased acidic environments, making it a good candidate for study of acid rainfall, etc.

MEDICINAL

Traditional Chinese medicine uses about forty bryophytes and mosses to treat illness of the cardiovascular system, skin disease, burns, tonsillitis, bronchitis, tympanitis and cystitis.

Mosses contain a number of biologically active compounds that protect them from fungi and other microorganisms as well as insects, slugs and other predators. In a way, the biochemistry helps make up for lack of thick bark or cuticle.

An extract of *Rhodobryum giganteum* has been shown to increase aorta blood flow by up to 30% in animal studies.

HAIR CAP MOSS
(*P. juniperinum*)

CONSTITUENTS- lunularic acid (stilbenoid)

Hair Cap moss's main attribute is as a powerful diuretic. In some individuals, it has been shown to remove twenty to forty pounds of water in a twenty-four hour period, according to the Eclectic physician, Dr. Ellingwood.

Taken as a strong infusion it possesses very little smell or taste. It never produces nausea or any disagreement with the stomach.

It is useful for removing uric acid and phosphate-based gravel from the system. And is effective in lessening urinary obstructions and suppression due to a chill or "cold in the kidneys."

Ascites, anasarca and hydrops, especially of cardiac origin are likewise relieved.

Fevers and inflammations are likewise treated with infusions of hair cap moss.

Enlargement or inflammation of the prostate is helped by use of an infusion or tincture. Dr. Cushing recommended a tincture or infusion for old men suffering an irritable or prolapsed bladder, enlarged prostate, or prostatitis.

It may be safely used in dysuria associated with pregnancy and helps relieve urethra pain during urination.

It was used in the past for acute gonorrhea with severe burning pain upon urination.

Lunularic acid shows inhibition of thromboxane synthase, 5-lipoxygenase and calmodulin. It is anti-fungal and often found in liverworts, but rarely in mosses. It is also present in fresh celery.

Laboratory studies have shown plant extracts to have weak anti-tumor effects against sarcoma 37. Belkin et al, *Journal of the National Cancer Institute* 1952 13.

HAIR CAP MOSS

CONSTITUENTS- allantoin, sphagnol, silicon dioxide, communins A-B, benzonaphthoxanthenone, ohioensin H.

Hairy Cap Moss (*P. commune*) is useful in fevers states, and to help alleviate cuts and wounds by staunching the bleeding and encouraging clotting and regeneration of tissue. It makes a useful mouth rinse in gingivitis.

Allantoin is found in corn silk, lungwort, comfrey and other Symphytum species. It is a cell regenerator, useful for repairing epithelial cells. Sphagnol is antiseptic.

It is used in TCM for fever, to staunch bleeding, uterine prolapse and lymphocytic leukemia.

Ethanol extracts show anti-tumor and apoptosis against cultured leukemia L1210 cells, suggesting traditional use for leukemia was based on empirical observation. Cheng X et al, *J Ethnopharm* 148(3): 926-33; Cheng X et al, *J Ethnopharm* 2012 143(1): 49-56.

Ethyl acetate extracts damage the membrane system and triggered Ca(2+)-dependent mitochondrial apoptosis, suggesting new insights into its efficacy against human leukemia cells. Yuan W et al, *J Ethnopharm* 2015 172: 410-20.

It is specific in pulmonary tuberculosis, as well as the common cold. The moss infusion has been used to help dissolve kidney and gallbladder stones. Gulabani et al, 1974.

In the *Materia Medica* it is mentioned for prostate gland swelling, and amenorrhea.

The latter is based on work of J. P. Bonnafoux, who in 1831 reported twelve cases of amenorrhea cured, using an infusion of this moss in milk.

Common Hairy Cap Moss (*P. commune*) is the largest unbranched moss in western Canada. Extracts show inhibition of *Trametes versicolor, Botrytis allii, Fusarium bulbigenum* and *Pyricularia oryzae*. Wolters et al, *Planta Medica* 1964 62 88-96.

Other *Polytrichum* species of moss have shown cytotoxic activity. *P. ohioense* contains ohioensins A-E, which exhibit activity against 9PS murine leukemia and certain human tumour cells, including MCF-7 *in vitro*. Zheng GQ et al, *The Journal of Org Chemistry* 1993 58.

Work by Cassady JM et al, *J Nat Products* 1990 53(1): 23-41 identified this moss and rough moss below as potential anti-cancer agents.

Ohioensin F has been isolated from *Polyerichastrum alpinum*. The compound exhibits anti-inflammatory activity and protective effects on atherosclerotic lesions. Byeon HE et al, *Life Sci* 2012 90(11-12): 396-406. Ohioensin F and G exhibit anti-oxidant activity. Bhattarai HD et al, *Z Naturforsch C* 2009 64(3-4): 197-200.

P. pallidisetum contains five novel compounds, mainly benzoaphtho-xanthenones and cinnamoyl bibenzyls cytotoxic against several human cell lines, RPMI-7951 melanoma and U-251 glioblastoma multiforme; as well as anti-tumour activity against murine P-388 lymphocytic leukemia. Zheng GQ et al, *J Nat Products* 1994 57(1): 32-41.

Rough Moss (*Claopodium crispifolium*) is found on the coast of British Columbia, but also in southeastern parts of Alberta. Studies by Suwanborirux et al, at Purdue in 1990, isolated ansamitocin P-3 from the moss. Subsequent trials found this to be a potent cytotoxic substance active against human solid tumor cell lines A-549 and HT 21. *Experientia* 1990 46(1): 117-20.

Work by Spjut et al, *Economic Botany* 1998 42:1 found activity against both P388 lymphocytic leukemia and KB cell cultures. The blue green algae Nostoc was found present on the samples with highest levels of activity. This suggests that Nostoc may be the source of bioactivity, or it precipitates allelopathy.

Tests conducted by the *National Cancer Institute* in 1986, on 184 mosses, identified this one as possessing the strongest anti-tumor activity. No follow-up has been done that I am aware.

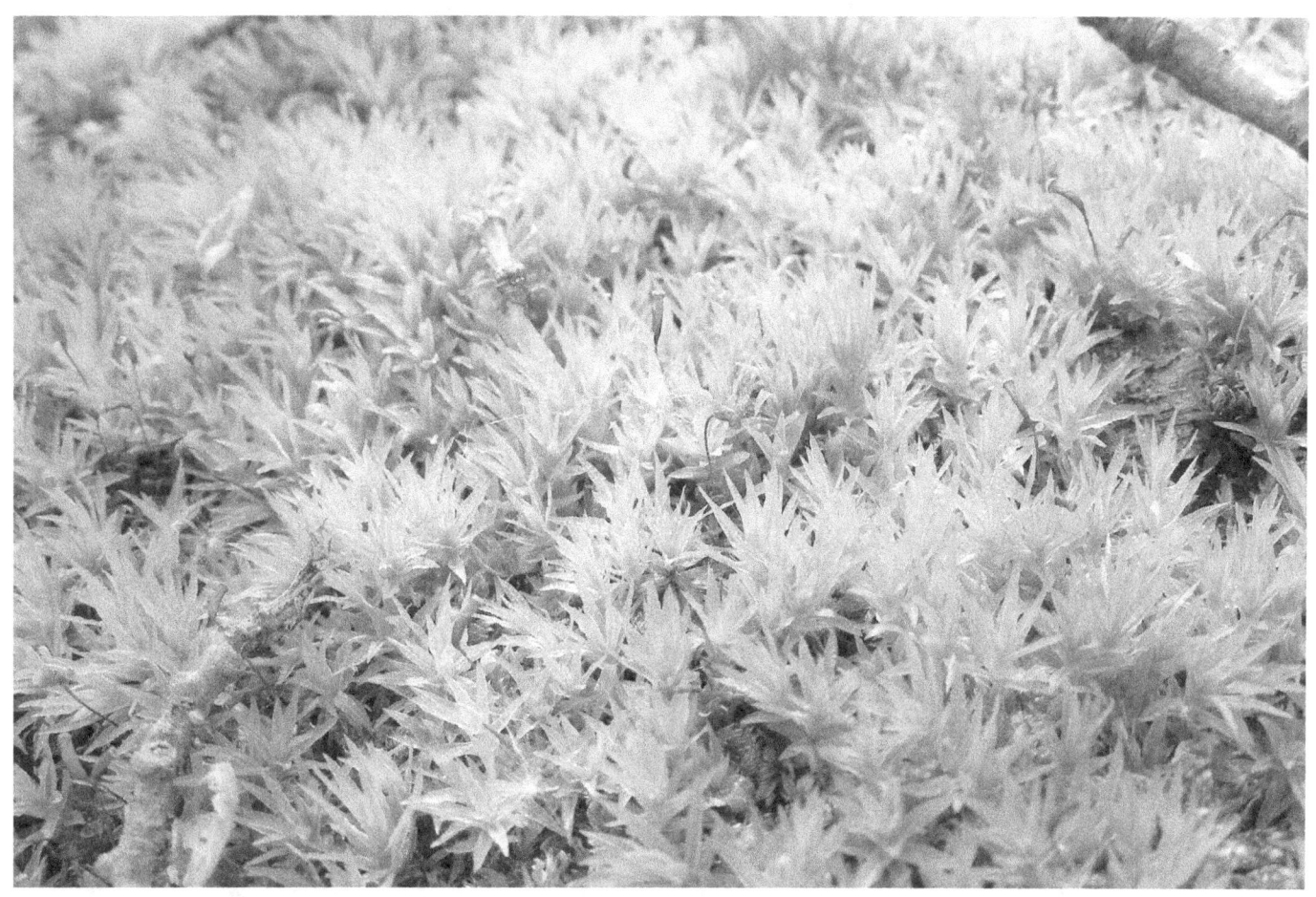

CLIMACIUM SPECIES

Tree Moss (*Climacium dendroides*) looks like little trees, and is all over the prairies, save for the driest areas of southeastern Alberta and southwestern Saskatchewan. On the west coast, it is a common yard weed, but on the prairies it is found in fens and calcareous tundra conditions.

Research by Nerlo et al, *Acta Pol Pharm* 1977 34(1): 89-95 identified sterol content in the moss.

Various *Plagiochila* species contain natural pesticides, including the sesquiterpenes, hemiacetyl and plagiochiline, which are a potent poison to mice.

SPHAGNUM
(*S. squarrosum* Crome, and others.)

CONSTITUENTS- terpenoids, flavonoids, essential oils, carotenoids, fulvic acid, sphagnol, iodine.

Sphagnum moss is sold in herbal shops in China; and decoctions are used to cure acute hemorrhages and eye diseases.

Studies conducted in Belarus in 1995, by Dolidovich et al, found sphagnum moss alcohol extracts possess anti-inflammatory, anti-bacterial and anti-viral activity.

Sphagnol, extracted from peat moss, is used for hemorrhoids, and various skin problems such as psoriasis, eczema and acne.

T. J. Painter in *Journal of Ethnopharmacology* 2003 88:2 found sphagnum dressings 3-4 times more absorbent than cotton dressings. The herb pectins react chemically against various proteins, immobilizes whole bacterial cells, as well as enzymes, exotoxins and lysins secreted by various pathogens.

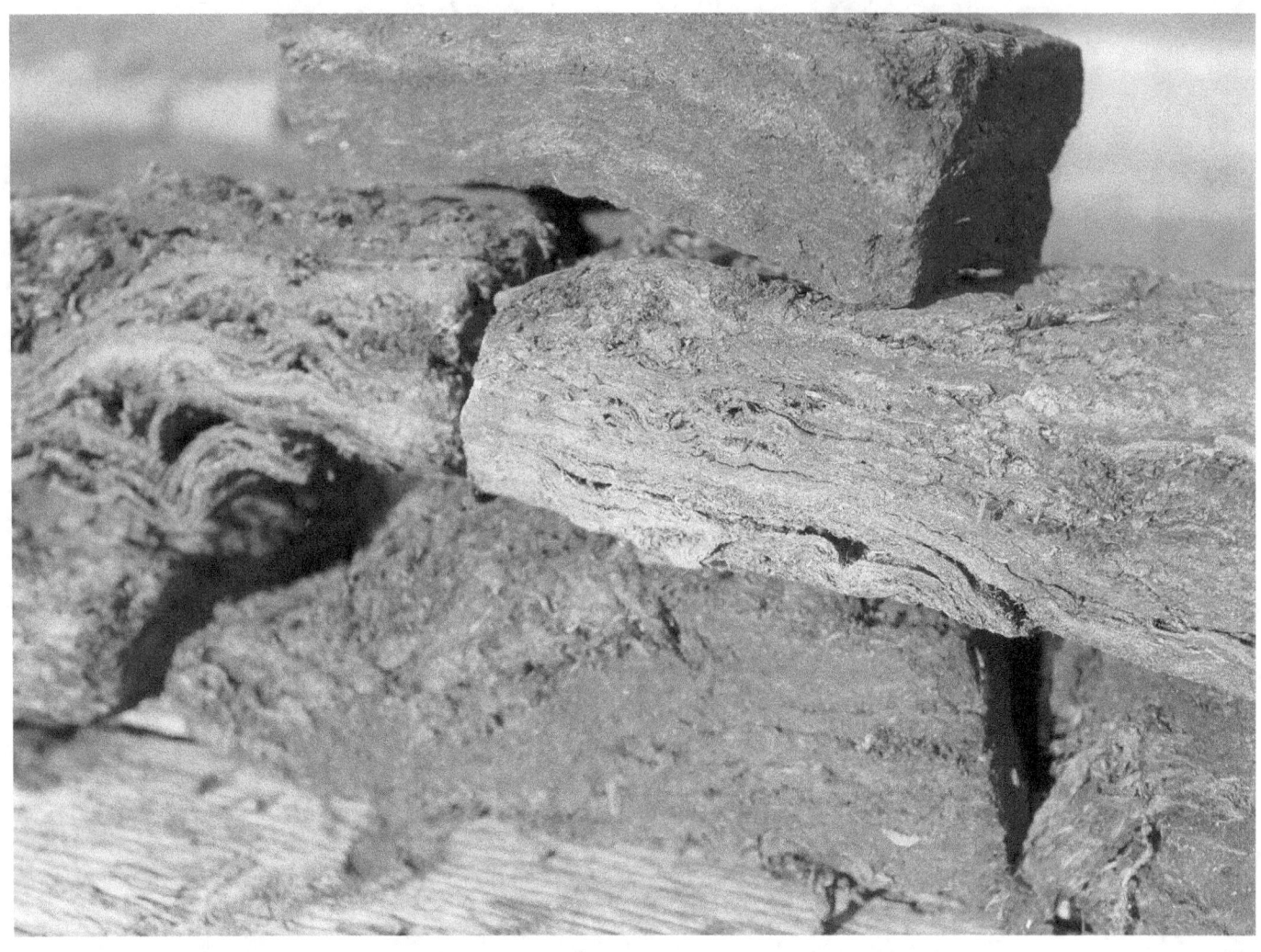

PEAT BALES

PEAT

The antiseptic properties of peat tars date back to as early as 1902; from distilled tars at an Irish peat fueled generator.

It was used extensively in military hospitals during World War I, for fighting infections.

Studies on Sphagnum species by Efimenko and Dzenis in 1961 showed an extract to have an anti-bacterial activity, at dilution of 1:40,000.

Work conducted in Ireland by Corrigan et al, has shown that six *Shagnum* species possess activity against both Gram positive and negative bacteria.

Shagnum peat has been investigated as a source of stimulants for microbial fermentation processes.

The main medicinal product made from peat is Torfot, a Soviet preparation developed at the *Ukrainina Research Institute of Eye Diseases* in Odessa. Its main application is the treatment of ophthalmic conditions like progressive myopia, myopic chorio-retinitis, opacification of the vitreous humour, opacification of the cornea resulting from keratitis, and early retinal degeneration. For these purposes it is administered both topically and subcutaneously.

More recently, it is being used in anemia, hepatitis, and various skin, nerve and reproductive diseases. Torfot's active principles are probably phenols and amines.

Preparation TK2, derived from reed sedge peat and administered orally, has favorable effect on asthma patients. Ugorski and Tolpa (1974) both have isolated Gram positive and negative antagonists.

In the same year, Christeva et al, reported peat preparation counteract the phytotoxic effect of various thiophosphates and chlorinated fungicides.

The healing properties of hot peat baths are well known in health spas throughout Europe. From muscle injury to infertility, peat baths are taken at high temperatures that would be close to scalding as water.

Of long-term importance, maybe peat derivatives of steroid and triterpenoid content, with beta sitosterol and beta sitostanol, account for half the steroids recovered from peat.

The other half is partially examined, with small amounts of estrone, estradiol, and estriol present.

Dr. Nebel, a German physician uses the high temperature peat baths for both injured athletes and amputees. "In peat, heat is transferred molecule to molecule, not by convection the way it is in water. Thus, a temperature of 45-48 degrees Celsius can be tolerated, which would be unbearable to a person bathing in water. After thirty minutes in a peat bath, a patient's body temperature rises one degree, dramatically increasing circulation of blood to injured areas and reducing pain."

Dr. Rudolph Steiner suggested in the 1920s that substances from peat could offer protection and healing to humanity. Dr. Hauschka in the 1940s began to manufacture peat products to help people who are suffering under chaotic environmental change. This includes stress associated with electromagnetic radiation.

Solum uliginosum is produced by collecting peat liquid, storing it in a dark incubating chamber for seven days, exposing it rhythmically to the sun rising and setting. It is then stored for 2-3 months, to help dissipate the sulphur odor.

The fiber remaining can be carded and spun with silk or wool. Johannes Moss has a small factory in Rydoebruk, Sweden where for over thirty years he has harvested peat scraps and forms a fiber that is woven into garments in Copake, New York.

Sphagnum peat contains fulvic acid that has been found useful in prevention and treatment of allergic disease. Yamada et al, *Biosci Biotech Biochem* 71:5. It also contains humic acid, that shows activity against the polio virus.

A rat study found fulvic acid a good source of iron, and both fulvic acid and humic acid increased manganese concentration in hair. Szabo J et al, *Acta Vet Hung* 2017 65(1): 66-80.

Sphagnum fimbriatum and *S. nemoreum* solvent extracts show activity against *Coniophora cerebella*, *Trametes versicolor*, *Fusarium bulbigenum* and *Pyricularia oryzae*. Wolters et al, *Planta Medica* 1964 62 88-96.

CAUTION- Fungal caused sporotrichosis is a hazard to nursery workers and sphagnum harvesters. It can be dangerous to use as a bandage, and pulmonary sporotrichosis (a fungal lung infection) can result. Be careful.

If the fungus enters a cut, it can create a slightly nodular sore in 1-10 weeks. The fungus then travels up the lymph leaving a red streak and series of nodules on the arm's skin. In some people it finds a way to the joints and bones. It can be treated with potassium iodide and other anti-fungal medications, including Usnea tinctures and creams.

CYPRESS-LEAVED FEATHER MOSS
(*Hypnum cupressiforme*)

This is a common ground covering moss that covers much of western Alberta from north to south. Extracts have been reported to possess anti-microbial and anti-viral activity. Recent studies in Germany indicate aromadendrin-derived flavonoids may play a role. It has been used in pillows like hops, to induce sleep.

It possesses both anti-bacterial and anti-fungal activity.

It accumulates up to three times, concentrations of zinc, copper and cadmium.

Methanol extracts show activity against *Trichoderma viride*, *Aspergillus niger*, *A. flavus* and *Penicillium funiculosum*. Veliljic et al, *Arch Biol Sci* 2009 61 225-9.

BROOM MOSS
(*Dicranum scoparium*)

Broom moss extracts have been shown to test strongly against *Bacillus cereus, B. subtilis, B. stearothermophilus, Staphylococcus aureus* and *E. coli*. Borel et al, *J Nat Prod* 1993 56:7. A compound, identified as dicranin, when isolated, was found inactive against *E. coli*. The strongest effect was observed against *Streptococcus faecalis*.

Work by Pavletic and Stilinovic (1963) found Broom Moss strongly inhibited all bacteria tested except for *E. coli*.

Dicranin exhibits 15-lipoxygenase inhibition, suggestive of anti-oxidant activity.

Guichardant et al, at the Nestle Research Centre, found dicranin a new inhibitor of platelet aggregation, when induced by either thrombin or arachadonic acid. *Thromb Res* 1992 65(6): 687-98.

Studies by Ichikawa et al, have reported the presence of prostaglandin-like fatty acids in Broom Moss.

Various fractions, including unsaturated fatty acids, of this moss were tested for anti-proliferative activity against HeLa cell lines. Strong activity was noted in this work. Abay G et al, *Comb Chem High Throughout Screen* 2015 18(5): 453-63.

The related *D. fluvum* showed marginal activity against P388 cancer cell lines.

BROOK MOSS
(*Fontinalis sp.*)

In medical testing, brook moss has been shown to decompose up to 43% of phenols at low concentrations. It has also been used as a bio-indicator of excessive ethylene glycol in the water.

Fontinalis species are bio-accumulators of uranium, iron and cadmium.

Fontinalis antipyretica organic solvent extracts showed activity against *Aspergillus parasciticus, A. flavus* and *A. fumigatus*. Savaroghu et al, *J Med Plants Res* 2011 5.

Generally speaking, Fontinalis species are good monitors of water pollution. Devitalized moss, through oven drying is recommended for biomonitoring of aquatic environments.

AQUATIC APPLE MOSS
(*Philonotis fontana*)

Apple moss has been used by the Gasuite natives of Utah to alleviate burn pain by crushing into a paste and applied as a poultice. It can be used for covering bruises and wounds; or a padding under splints to set broken limbs.

In the Himalayas, the moss is burned into an ash and mixed with fat and honey for cuts, burns and wounds.

It is antipyretic and antidotal for cases of adeno-pharyngitis and boils.

FEATHER OR STEP MOSS
(*Hylocomium splendens*)

Hylocomium splendens is the most common moss of the boreal forest.

Studies have found it to possess significant P388 lymphatic leukemia activity.

Work by Kang et al, *Fitoterapia* 78:5 found this moss to show great activity against Gram positive bacteria.

The moss is commonly used in Bryometers, which are really just a bag of moss hung to monitor pollution.

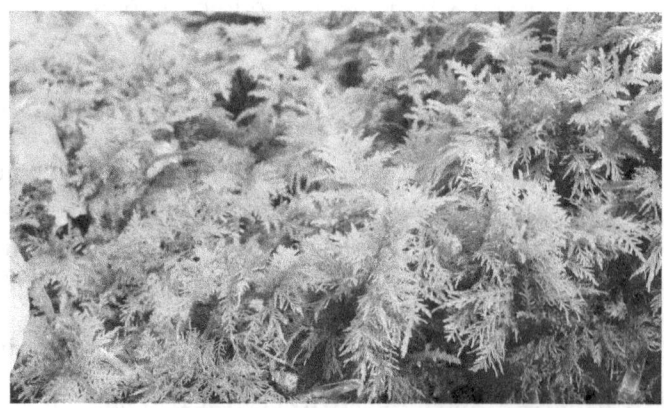

FEATHER MOSS (HYLOCOMIUM SPECIES)

Most species, including this one are injured in 10-40 hours at 0.8 ppm of sulfur dioxide. I wonder how well a Bryometer would survive downwind of one of the Athabasca Tar Sands projects?

Apple Moss (*B. pomiformis*) possesses some P388 anti-tumor activity, as well as activity using the astrocytoma (ASK) assay that measures both cytotoxicity and microtubule inhibition.

Star Moss (*T. muralis*) possesses cytotoxic activity as measured by P388.

Various other mosses have potential as both medicinal and aromatic use.

Bryum argenteum, or as the name suggests, Silvery Bryum is a compact, silver moss, due to lack of chlorophyll in the upper leaves.

The plant is useful in fevers, and is antidotal in cases of rhinitis with bacterial involvement. It contains the interesting compound isoscutellarein-7-glucoside.

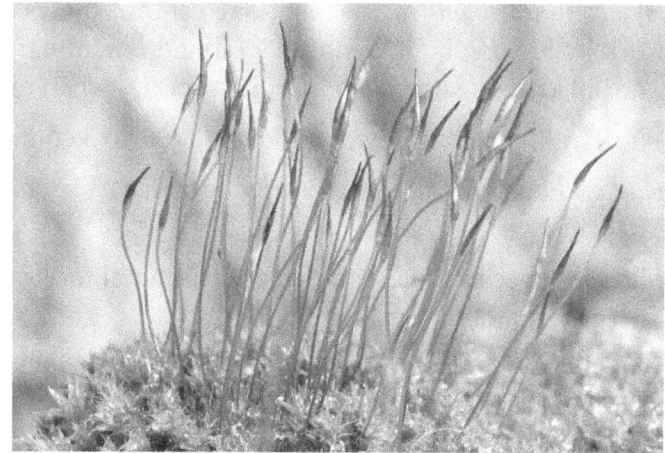

TORTULA MURALIS

Work by Sabovljevic et al, *Fitoterapia* 77:2 144-5 found ethanol extracts of the moss effective against a variety of bacterium and fungi, including *E. coli, Bacillus subtilis, Micrococcus luteus, Staphylococcus aureus, Aspergillus niger, Penicillium ochrochloron, Candida albicans,* and *Trichophyton mentagrophyes.*

Various solvents of moss showed activity against *A. niger, Fusarium moniliformae* and *Rhzoctonia bataticola*. Bodade et al, *J Med Plants* 2008 7 23-28.

This moss is used in Antarctica to monitor effects of ozone layer.

Cratoneuron filicinum is often found in the northern prairies on calcareous rocks. It is a specific remedy for *malum cardis*, meaning a bad heart.

Funaria hygrometrica is everywhere, and like *Byrum argenteum*, can be classed as a "weed of the world". It is fond of 1-2 year old campfire sites, with the various nutrients available. Medicinally, it is used for hemostasis, pulmonary tuberculosis, hematenesis (vomiting of blood), bruises, athlete's foot, and other dermatomycosis.

Plagiopus oederi is a fairly common moss of the Eastern Rockies, growing on moist, calcareous cliffs. It is a sedative, useful in epilepsy, apoplexy and cardiopathy.

Various Hair Mosses (*Ditrichum* species) have been used for convulsions, especially in infants.

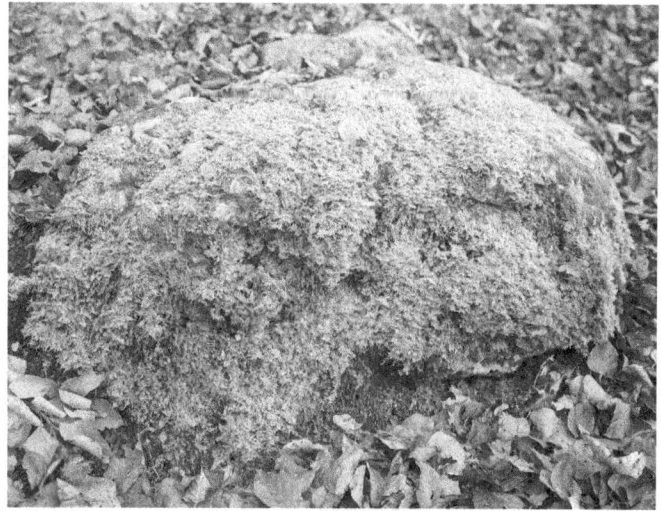

CRATONEURON FILICINUM

Rose Moss (*Rhodobyrum roseum*) is used in Traditional Chinese Medicine for angina and other cardiovascular conditions. One study on white mice showed an increase of blood flow in heart aorta by over 30%.

The six species of *Mnium* in Western Canada are rich in arachidonic acid, used to treat fat deficiency associated with vitamin F, and used to treat eczema in dogs and hogs. It also inhibits LOX associated with inflammation.

Work by Singh et al, found *M. marginatum* active against five Gram-positive and six Gram-negative bacterium, as well as eight fungi species. *Fitoterapia* 78:2. They contain various ferulic and m and p-coumaric acids.

More recent work by Singh et al, *Pharm Biol* 2011 49:5 identified this moss as having the highest inhibition of *Staphylococcus aureus* of many bacteria tested.

Work by Behera et al, *Fitoterapia* 77:3 found *Graphis* species inhibit tyrosinase and xanthine oxidase activity, as well as scavenge superoxide. Xanthine oxidase inhibition is beneficial in cases of gout and rheumatic conditions.

Hylocomium splendens, as mentioned above, shows activity against a variety of Gram positive bacteria. This work by Kay et al, *Fitoterapia* 78:5 found *Bartramia pomiformis, Ceratodon purpureus* and *Neckera douglasii* were all active against *Staphylococcus* species when exposed to UVA irradiation.

Work by Spjut et al, *Economic Botany* 1986 40:3 contains great detail about moss anti-tumor activity.

Haplocladium microphyllum is used to treat cystitis, bronchitis, tonsillitis and tympanitis in Traditional Chinese Medicine.

Fissidens species are used as an anti-bacterial for swollen throat and other symptoms of bacterial infections. There are about ten species in Alberta.

Work by McCleary and Walkington, 1983 found eighteen mosses with antibiotic properties, including *Atrichum, Dicranum, Mnium, Polytrichum* and *Sphagnum* species, which were the most active against Gram positive and negative bacteria.

Atrichum undulatum inhibited all bacteria tested except *Aerobacter aerogenes* and *E. coli.* In anti-fungal studies by Sabovjevic et al, *J Med Plants Res* 2011 5 656-71, the moss showed activity against *Aspergillus versicolor* and *A. fumigatus,* and a DMSO extract active against *Penicillium funicolosum* and *Trichoderma viride.*

Work by Wolters et al, 1964 found solvent extracts active against *Botrytis allii, Coniophora cerebella, Trametes versicolor, Fusarium bulbigenum* and *Pyricularia oryzae.*

Atrichum undulatum possesses anti-oxidant activity. Chobor et al, *Z Naturforsch* 2008 63:7-8. This species and *Pleurozium schreberi,* also known as Big Red Stem Moss, show anti-oxidant activity.

Big Red Stem (*Pleurozium schreberi*) also shows significant anti-fungal activity. Veljic et al, *Pharm Bio* 46:12.

Plagiomnium venustum shows activity against P-388 cells; as does the Big Red Stem (*Pleurozium shreberi*) found all over northern boreal forests.

Barbula species were found to possess high Gram positive and negative anti-bacterial activity. Singh et al, 1971.

Homalia trichomanoides contains 3-beta-methoxyserrat-14-en-21beta-op, atranorin, methyl 2,4-dihydroxy-3, 6-dimethylbenzoate. Wang et al, *Chem Biodivers* 2005 2 139-45 found compounds in this moss active against *Candida albicans.*

Tortella tortuosa is a moss found on calcareous rocks in the montane regions, but also on stream and lake banks in the higher altitude boreal forest. Acetone extracts show activity against *Candida albicans.* Elibol et al, *Afr J Biotech* 2011 10 986-9.

Oligotrichum hercynicum is found on west side of Rocky Mountain divide and along the British Columbia and Washington coastlines, usually at higher elevations. Solvent extracts exhibit inhibition of *Fusarium bulbigenum* and *Pyricularia oryzae.*

Plagiothecium denticulatum is widespread on swampy soil and in grassy fens at base of trees or fallen logs. Extracts show inhibition of *Botrytis allii, Rhizoctonia solani, Trametes versicolor* and *Fusarium bulbigenum.* Wolters et al, *Planta Medica* 1964 62 88-96.

Pogonatum urnigerum extracts show inhibition of *Trametes versicolor* and *Botrytis allii* in cited work by Wolters above.

Physcomitrella patens is circumpolar and although not yet found in Alberta, was identified in British Columbia in 1978.

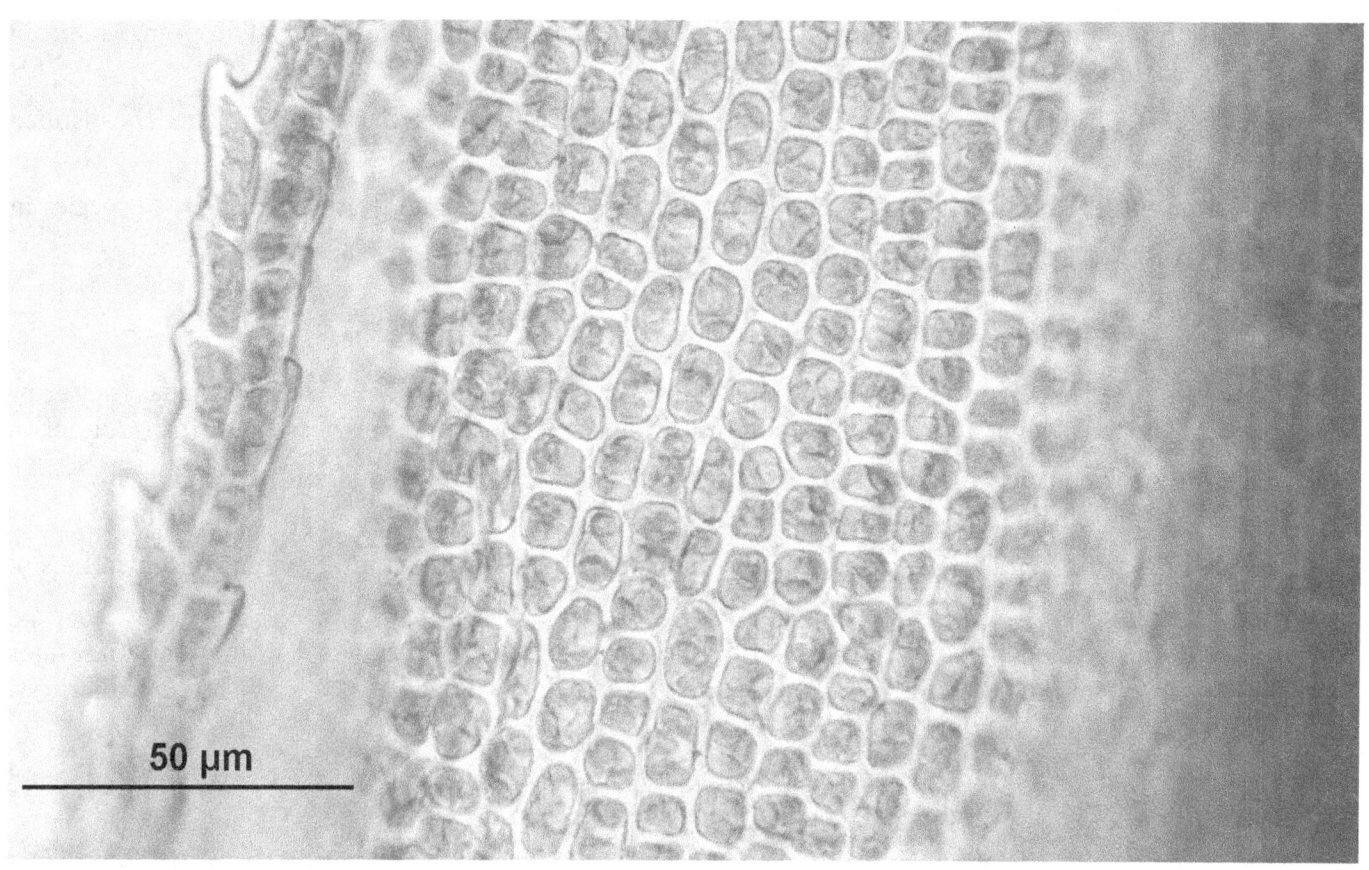

CLOSE UP OF BARTRAMIA POMIFORMIS

It is being used in moss bioreactors to produce human protein. Dr. Eva Decker explains. "With the complement factor H we have produced a protein in moss that otherwise occurs only in blood and is important for the immune system. Not enough of this protein in older people is the main cause of blindness for 50 million people worldwide.

This age-related macular degeneration is a problem, particularly in industrialized countries." (*Science Daily* July 23, 2010).

Transgenic *Physcomitrella* is used to produce blood clotting factor IX, for treatment of haemophilia B.

HOMEOPATHY

Polytrichum juniperinum is THE remedy for painful urination in older people. Urinary obstruction, suppression and prostatitis are all relieved by the use of this plant.

DOSE-mother tincture- 5-10 drops as needed in water.

ESSENTIAL OIL

The dried *P. juniperinum* was extracted with benzene and yielded 0.34% oil consisting mainly of a waxy ketone, 12-tricosanone.

Distilled oil produced from sphagnum moss tar is called "Sphagnol". This is very useful for external application in eczema, psoriasis, skin itching, mosquito bites, hemorrhoids, chilblains, acne and scabies. It is very similar to Cade oil from juniper in usage for skin problems.

Many mosses have aromatic characteristics that would be useful in perfumery.

Some *Frullania and Porella* species have strong turpentine odour, similar to conifer needles.

Plagiochila and *Frullania* emit mysterious sweet mossy and woody odors highly esteemed by European, American and Japanese perfume companies.

Plagiothecium undulatum is a large, complanate moss in humid forests, especially northern Idaho. The distilled oil contains (+)-dauca-8, 11-diene and two butenolides.

Polygodial, present in Smartweed (*Polygonum hydropiper*), has been isolated from several *Porella* species in rates from 10-30%.

Funaria hygrometrica possesses a unique, sea star like aroma.

Lophozia species also have a pleasant aroma.

Splachnum luteum and *S. rubrum* are two of the most interesting looking mosses of Western Canada. They grow on moose dung, in fens, bogs and trails throughout northwestern Alberta and northeastern British Columbia.

Despite their source of nutrients, both contain interesting volatile oils, including octanol, 3-octanone, 3-octanol, trans-2-octenal, 1-octen-3-ol, 1-octanol, and 2-octen-1-ol.

S. rubrum has much higher levels of octanol, with the male gametophyte containing large concentrations of valeric and isovaleric acids.

Tortula muralis essential oil is very complex, with 42 compounds representing 74% of the total oil. Major compounds are nonanal 18.3%, tetradecanal 4.3%, oleic acid 4.2%, 2E, 4E-decadienal 2.4%, and hexahydrofarnesyl acetone 2.2%.

Hypnum cupressiforme contains 29 compounds including nonamal 12.5%, E-2-tetradecen-1-ol 6.9%, tetradecanol 6.3%, pentacosane 5.7%, alpha cadinol 3.5%, beta germacrene 3.3%.

Pohlia nutans contains 45 compounds including nonanal 7.8%, E-2-tetradecen-1-ol 7.1%, 2-E, 4E-decadienal 6.2%, beta elemene 5%, neo-intermedol 4.6%, and hexahydrofarnesyl acetone 3.7%.

The above three oils show activity against fungi. Ucuncu et al, *Turk J Chemistry* 2010 34 825-34.

PLANT OILS

Sphagnum moss contains long chain hydrocarbons and fatty acids. The lipid content, explains, in part, the absorbency of these mosses and their usefulness as surgical dressings.

Studies by Corrigan et al, reported in *Planta Medica* 29 found six Sphagnum species contain activity against both gram negative and positive bacteria.

Some peat humic acids possess anti-viral activity against herpes simplex 1 and 2, as well as polio.

WAX

One of the most valuable by-products of peat is a wax with relatively high melting point. Peat yields 9.4% of a crude wax with a melting point of 73 degrees Celsius.

MOSS ESSENCES

Hair cap moss essence is for those who hold all their emotions inside. At times they feel they could explode, but continue to suppress their tears. Crying is difficult, and oddly enough frequent urination may provide an outlet for this emotional build-up.   **PRAIRIE DEVA**

Sphagnum moss is for releasing the need for unbalanced or harsh judgment of one's healing journey; creating a space of unconditional acceptance in the heart so that cores issues can emerge and heal.   **ALASKA**

Sphagnum moss essence is the call to life, to helping understand the evolving journey of life and inner growth. It is for those whose past is emerging; with understanding and release of deep core issued experienced. It brings new levels of freedom and a greater expression of self.   **CANADIAN FOREST**

Water Moss (*Sphagnum palustre ssp*) essence helps when you are avoiding intimacy- appearing open and able to give, but only on a material and superficial level. The symptoms may manifest as intolerance towards others or appearing superior or aloof.

Extreme cases may manifest as phobias, inertia, or reclusive behavior- concealing weaknesses rather than confronting, revealing and healing them.

Water Moss lets you learn to exist for yourself, moving from survival as a way of being; it's all about communication. Throat, ears, thyroid, mouth, teeth, gums and neck problems may all be eased.

Realignment with this essence means reaching for the stars, uniting in spiritual goals, a true feeling of belonging, and an absolute sense of connection. **OLIVE**

Dicranella heteromalla essence is to help those who fear light and freedom in their lives. In particular, for those who have ' dark spaces' within them. Within these dark spaces there is a fear of joy and freedom and the responsibility that comes with them.

With such people there is not overall gloom, but small dark spaces that nevertheless seriously affect their lives. Some of these areas may be very guilt-laden from old conditioned patterns. **BAILEY**

Thuidium recognitum essence is for the love of life. It is for nourishing the old places that have become crippled; bringing rebirth, growth and joy.

It brings a zest for living, discovery and expansion; and the desire to seek and search for new paths, a trust in oneself to experiment and be open to the unknown. **CANADIAN FOREST**

Tortula ruralis essence is useful where the Soul is lost and disconnected, and receptivity is to be enhanced and reconnection found.

This is essential for the inner growth of the soul and our attunement to all life and will allow one to see life as you never have before. **CANADIAN FOREST**

Goose Neck Moss or Frightened Cat-tail Moss (*Rhytidiadelphus triquetrus*) essence is the restoration. It clears deep blocks and trauma not known on the surface. It restores at the core and cellular level, bringing deep shifting and new freedoms. It can help create profound changes within the individual. **CANADIAN FOREST**

Member of the *Fissidens* genus symbolize seclusion. **CARTER**

Leptobyrum pyriforme essence addresses Core issues. It is the anchor to your source. It is for cutting through fear and illusion, reviving your deepest goals.

It brings about freedom and strength to fulfill oneself through connection to one's core. **CANADIAN FOREST**

Polytrichum piliferum essence helps one to see good and beauty if ones thoughts have been negative. It gives another starting point and rest. **MARIANA**

PERSONALITY TRAITS

Sphagnum bogs also produce methane gas: often a hollow rod inserted into a bog will nurture a flame. Small clouds of released methane sometimes spontaneously ignite, producing those mysterious, hovering "bog-lights", or "will of the wisps" seen over a bog at night. **J. EASTMAN**

I love listening to a bog, the papery rustle of dragonfly wings, the banjo twang of a green frog, the occasional hiss of sedges moving in the breeze. On a hot summer day, if you're very quiet, you can witness the smallest discernable sound I know- the "pop" of Sphagnum capsules. It's hard to imagine that a sound emitted by a capsule only one millimeter long could be audible...the heat of sun builds up air pressure inside the capsule, until the top blows off, propelling the spores upward. **KIMMERER**

Some people, myself included, could never live in a city. I go to the city whenever I must and leave as soon as I can. Rural folks are more like *Thuidium* (species). We need a lot of room and shady moisture to flourish, choosing to live along quiet brooks rather than busy streets. Our pace of life is slow and we are much less tolerant of stress. In a city, that lifestyle would be a liability.

On the streets of New York City the *Ceratodon* style is much in demand, fast paced, always changing, and making the best of the crowds. ...And everywhere beneath your feet is *Bryum argentum*. **KIMMERER**

[Moss appears] where the cosmic forces bring to life only the uppermost layer of the Earth and where the life of Earth itself is reduced to a minimum. The mosses spread a tundra carpet all over the Earth and build a second plant world under and among the normal vegetation…Mosses are closely related to the mineral earth. They are a kind of transition stage between dead mineral and live plant, as can be seen by those species which continue to grow above whilst becoming peat below…

A single moss plant would be an absurdity, for only in a mass, a carpet, are they a viable whole. **GROHMANN**

In the *Dicranum* clan, there are family roles that could easily apply to sisters in any big family. *D. montanum* is the unassuming one, you know the type- nondescript, overlooked, with her short curls always in disarray... Moist shady rocks are also the habitat of the glamorous *D. scoparium*, the one who draws the looks with long, shiny leaves, tossed to one side....*D. flagellare*, with leaves trim and straight, like a military buzzcut, remains aloof from the others, choosing to live only on logs in an advanced state of decay. She's the conservative one, celibate for the most part, foregoing family in favour of her own personal advancement by cloning.

Solitary and intensely green, *D. viride* has a hidden fragile side, with leaf tips always broken off like bitten fingernails. *D. polysetum,* on the other hand, is the most prolific mother of the family...Then there's the long, wavy-leafed *D. undulatum*, capping the tops of boggy hummocks, and *D. fulvum*, the black sheep of the family. **KIMMERER**

True mosses belong to a watery world that is in transition to a terrestrial one. Earth and water mix together. Their production of soil called peat is telling of the themes of this group of plants.

They also affect the urinary system and are diuretic. Water and minerals again collide in their effect on bladder and kidney stones.

[It] is interesting in consideration of mosses own ancient heritage from algae, bypassing the more common developmental route that gave plants vascular structure and a root system, both of which mosses lack. **VERMEULEN**

RECIPES

INFUSION-Prepare with one ounce of fresh, or dried, hair cap moss to one pint of boiling water. Steep for twenty minutes. Drink two ounces every half hour in sever cases. Otherwise five to sixty drops every one to three hours. Drink warm, not hot.

TINCTURE- One to two ml of mother tincture three times daily. The mother tincture is made from the whole plant above ground of hair cap moss.

Moss tincture is prepared fresh at 1:4 and 70% alcohol.

MOSS MILKSHAKE- Take moss and place in blender with a quart of buttermilk and whirl to a green froth. Paint this mixture on rocks to yield a coating within two years. Other recipes use yogurt, egg whites, brewer's yeast, or any substance that provides nutrients and adhesive quality.

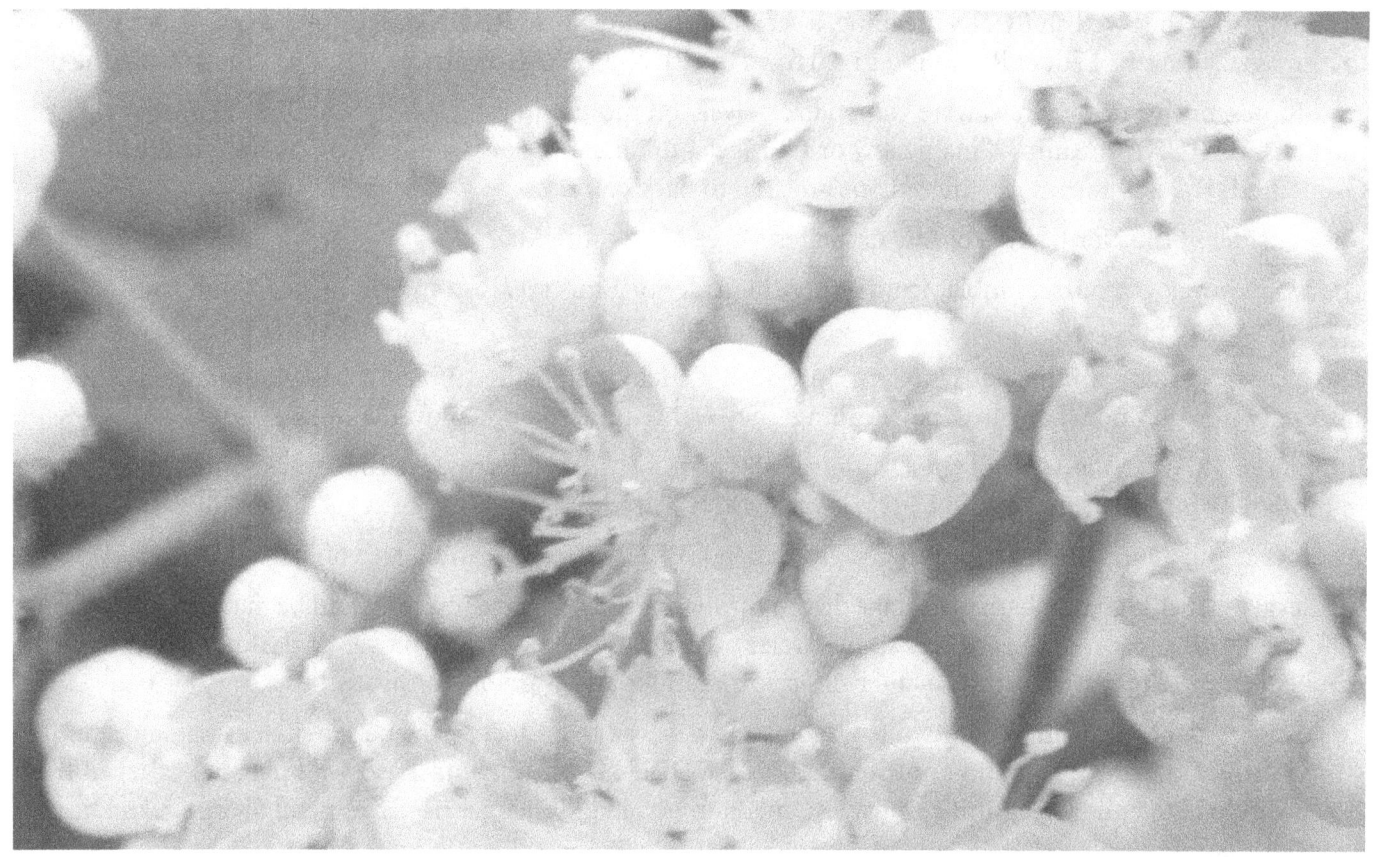

WESTERN MOUNTAIN ASH

WESTERN MOUNTAIN ASH
ROCKY MOUNTAIN ASH
GREENE'S MOUNTAIN ASH
(*Sorbus scopulina* Greene)
AMERICAN MOUNTAIN ASH
(*S. americana* Marshall)
NORTHERN MOUNTAIN ASH
(*Pyrus americana* DC.) not accepted
(*S. decora* [Sarg.] C.K. Schneid)

SITKA MOUNTAIN ASH
(*S. sitchensis* M. Roemer)
ROWAN TREE
EUROPEAN MOUNTAIN ASH
(*S. aucuparia* L.)
SERVICE TREE
SORB APPLE
(*S. domestica* [L.] Spach)
PARTS USED- berry, flower, twigs, root

By the magick of this rowan wise
I ask the faeries to bless my eyes
With their wings and gift of flight
I beckon you this very night.

ANON

SORBUS is derived from French **SORBE** with same root as sorbic acid, first isolated from the mountain ash berries. It may originally come from a Greek name for oak.

Scopulina is from the Latin **SCOPULA** meaning, little broom and **INA** for resembling. Aucuparia means bird catching and derives from the use of hair nooses baited with mountain ash berries, used to trap small birds in Germany and elsewhere. It is derived from the Latin **AVIS** for bird, and **CAPERE** to catch.

Ash is derived from the Old High German **ASK**, due to leaves similar to Ash.

Rowan is from the Swedish **RUNN** meaning, a secret or the Old Norse **RAUN** or **RUNA** a charm, both referring to its magical powers. Ladder Rungs is derived from the **RUN-STAFAS** or mysterious staves made from the tree.

And Runes, or mystical secrets, were carved exclusively on mountain ash trees in Scandinavia. It may be from the Sanskrit **RUNA** meaning, "magician", or Old Icelandic meaning "to whisper" or "secret". It may be from Gaelic **RUDHA-AN** meaning, "the red one", related to bark color.

It is considered the Nordic Tree of Life or Genesis Tree of Ask, the Man.

The woman was, of course, Embla, from either the Alder or Elm tree. Rowan is associated with the 10th Rune of Norse mythology, Nyd Not.

The berries were steam distilled, in Germany, until a sticky pulp called Volelbeerol was obtained. This was smeared on trees, and when birds came calling, they were captured and enjoyed as a pie.

It represents the second letter of the Druid tree alphabet L (luis), and provides the "quickening" of energy set in motion by birch, the first tree.

Another name, Quickbeam is from the Anglo-Saxon **CWIC-BEAM** meaning tree of life.

Medieval folk believed the sharpened stake driven through the heart of a vampire should be made from mountain ash. The Druids planted it near their stone circles as protection against the power of darkness, and used the smoke from fires to initiate a trance and call up spirit guides and warriors for protection.

The tree was associated with serpents and dragons, and believed to protect earth energies in ley lines and standing stones. In Ireland, the tree is still known as **FID NA NDRUAD**, the Druid's Tree. Walking sticks carved from Rowan are said to enhance intuitive ability and meditative walks. Twigs are used for metal divining, and known as witch wands.

In Irish legends, the tree bore the berries of immortality. The tree was guarded by a Fomorian Giant, with one fiery eye in the middle of his forehead. This myth is similar to the Cyclops of Homer's *Odyssey*, blinded in his single eye by a sharpened stake.

The tree was associated with Brigid, the goddess of poetry and inspiration. Brigid is the daughter of Dagda, the Irish Lord and Guardian of Nature. She is associated with fertility and spring and shot blazing arrows of rowan wood through the seasons, following the arc of the sun. February 1st, the author's birth date, is also the Celtic festival of Imbolc, sacred to Brigid, who kindles the divine fire of inspiration and visions.

Later Christian myths had her nursing the baby Jesus, and they incorporated her into the Feast Day of Saint Brigid. Of course!

The rowan berry, when cut, like hawthorn and apple, contains a five-pointed star, or pentagram, the ancient symbol of protection. The number five is associated with the White Goddess, protector of pastoral people and livestock. A necklace of the berries was believed to increase intuition and protect from evil.

The Celts considered the tree associated with divine inspiration and creative arts. Mountain ash symbolizes intellect, and associated with the birth date of September 4th. An ancient Celt name for the tree is "delight of the eye".

The rust-red berries and green leaves are believed the inspiration for many tartans of Celtic clans. Once again, Brigid the goddess of spinning and weaving, was associated with preparing the never-ending fabric of life. It is no surprise the hard wood was used to make spindles and spinning wheels.

In Scotland, the tree symbolized death and afterlife. Making love under a Rowan tree was said to result in a male child.

The Irish romance of Fraoth speaks of a dragon guarding the berries that contain the nourishment of nine meals.

In Greek legend, the tree was born from the blood and feathers of an eagle. It fell to earth as the divine bird fought demons to save the cup (Holy Grail?) from which the gods drank nectar. The red berries and feathery leaves are a symbol of the sacred eagle's blood and spirit.

In Greek mythology, the goddess of Youth, Hebe gave rejuvenating ambrosia to the gods from her magical chalice. When she lost the cup to demons through carelessness, the gods sent an eagle to recover it.

Rowan is a widely planted ornamental tree in prairie cities that can grow over ten metres.

The Rowan tree represents creativity, and has been used to divine future love and mates. It is planted by homes for protection from evil spirits. In Poland, it was considered a sin to cut down a mountain ash, as it was a woman turned into a tree by a mean mother-in-law. Another folktale suggests hanging a branch over the bed of a young man or woman with "immodest desires".

The Welsh once brewed an ancient beverage that contained mountain ash berries. Today, it is used in various European liqueurs, including one from Poland called Rowan Brandy. The French make ciders, juice and vinegars.

The berries were once dried and used as a flour substitute in parts of northern europe, according to Grieve.

In Austria, horticultural research has developed rowans that produce berries with higher sugar and vitamin C content.

Annual yields on mature trees of 15-30 kilograms are common. In Bashkortostan, over 15 tonnes of dried *S. aucuparia* berries are gathered each year for medicinal purposes.

The berries of both trees are much sought after by birds, particularly after fermentation. There are numerous stories of waxwings and other birds eating the fermented berries and falling off their perches. In the morning they are sometimes found dead on the ground, with post-mortems indicating they were severely drunk when they died, some with acute alcoholic liver disease. Morner and Segerstad, *Journal of Wildlife Diseases* 1995 31.

It is claimed when native and european species are grown side by side, birds will eat the native fruit first.

Do not eat the raw fruit due to its content of parasorbic acid. This acid possesses activity against gram-positive bacteria but is extremely irritating.

Parasorbic acid is an unsaturated lactone, that when hydrolyzed gives a 2,4-hexadienoic acid, called sorbic acid. It appears in fruit as a glycoside, parasorbaside. Sorbic acid is non-toxic, whereas parasorbic acid can irritate the mucosa of GI tract, leading to salivation, vomiting and gastroenteritis.

Studies have found consumption of 90 kilos of berries would be needed to reach a lethal dose for 50 kg humans. The drying and boiling of fruit destroy parasorbic acid.

Steaming the stems and bark releases the acid that clears catarrh, and treats migraines and other headaches.

The fruit can, and should, be collected after repeated freezing as it improves the flavour a great deal. Otherwise, the fruit is astringent and sour, as well as mealy. It is best stewed and lightly sweetened, but can be used in pies, and jams without adding commercial pectin. A wild rowan jelly produced in northeast Scotland uses rowan concentrate from Holland.

In Poland, a berry liqueur called **JARZEBIAK** is still available today. An alcohol is produced in parts of Germany called Vogelbeerschnaps. The berries are picked after first frost and from 100 litres of mash only 1.5 liters of alcohol are obtained.

The berries show anti-tumor and anti-metastatic activity, in vitro. Razina TG et al, *Bull Exp Biol Med* 2016 162(1): 93-97.

The leaves are a potential source of novel compounds specific to gram negative bacteria. Turumtay H et al, *Biomed Chromatogr* 2016 Nov 17.

The berries can be made into astringent facemasks for combating wrinkled skin. The berries contain sorbitol, which is a natural humectant that helps retain moisture in the skin. Sorbitol is increasingly used as a sugar substitute in diabetic diets, but is also used to make sorbose, vitamin C and propylene glycol, or antifreeze. The latter is non-toxic and used in the dairy industry and brewing business, to inhibit undesirable yeasts and molds.

Sorbitol is used in processing leather and printing, manufacture of tobacco, and take bitter edge from artificial sweeteners. It is used to increase absorption of vitamins and nutrients across the stomach wall into the bloodstream.

American Mountain Ash is native as far west as southeastern Manitoba.

Western mountain ash is a tall shrub that grows up to four metres, has sticky twigs and orange to red fruit. It is native to Alberta and British Columbia.

Northern Mountain Ash (*S. decora*) is native from southern Greenland to Manitoba.

Sitka mountain ash grows in the foothills, has non-sticky twigs, and red to purple fruit.

The Cree of southern Saskatchewan call western mountain ash, Bear Berry Tree, or **MASKWAMINANAHTIK**. The bark is decocted for bones, while branches are decocted for the heart and unspecified parts for treating cancer.

The Woods Cree call it **MASKOCISK** and used inner bark decoctions from local trees without berries, to treat backaches and rheumatism.

The Chipewyan name is **NAIDI DECHENE,** Medicine Stick.

The stems are boiled to make a tea for colds, coughs, headaches, sore chest, kidney pain, back pain, and rheumatism. The root and stem are used together to treat tuberculosis.

The Dena'ina of Alaska use bundles of the twigs for steam bath switches, in preference to any other tree. The dried inner bark and fresh/dried berries are decocted for sore throat, laryngitis and tonsillitis, difficult urination and tuberculosis.

The leaves are decocted for the flu. The inner bark was chewed or boiled for constipation.

To the Northern Cree it was sometimes the same name as red willow, **ATOSPIY.**

In Bush Cree, a red mountain ash branch is known as **COMIAYKWACHOOWASS-OOT.** Other Cree names are **MASKOMINANATIK** and **ESNIYWACHI-WAHTIK.**

It is also known as **ASINIYOCIYIPIYK.**

The Cree of Northern Alberta harvest the roots, then dry and grind them as a coffee substitute. They traditionally used branch bark for pleurisy and inflammatory disease; including internal bleeding.

Some tribes boiled the branches, and then steamed to relieve headaches and sore chests. The Cree of Wabasca, Alberta area use the root as part of diabetic and cancer treatments.

Various tribes used the bark for coughs, colds and fevers. The Mi'kmaq of the Maritimes boiled the bark to treat boils, and to treat "mother pains", and vaginal infections. They chewed raw bark to alleviate stomach pains, while the neighboring Maliseet infused the bark as a tea to relieve labor after pains.

The Montagnais tribe decocted the inner bark to stimulate appetite and purify blood, while the Tête de Boule drank the inner bark for depression.

The Forest Potawatomi used hot leaf tea to help patients vomit, remove excess mucus, treat colds, pneumonia and croup. They call it Bear Bush as they observe these animals eating the berries.

The Ojibwa infused the root bark to treat gonorrhea, while Hudson Bay Cree boiled young branches of *S. decora* for pleurisy and other inflammatory disease.

The Algonquin combined the small branches with those of white pine, the flowers of red elderberry (*S. canadensis*), and sweet wine. They boiled this for three hours, for a drink both fortifying and stimulating.

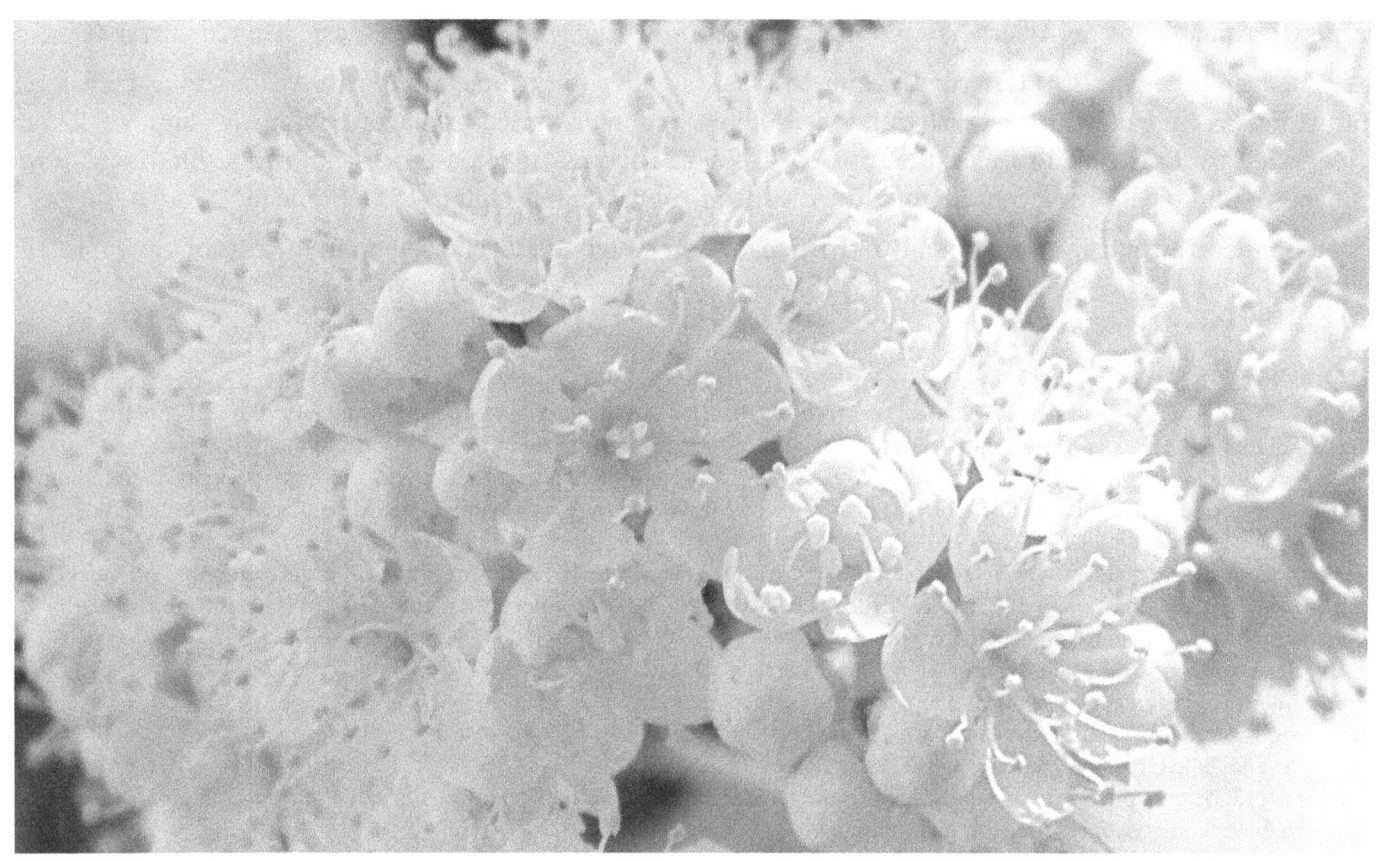

EUROPEAN MOUNTAIN ASH FLOWERS

Nancy Turner, in her excellent ethnobotanical book on Thompson of BC, relates the use of mountain ash branches as an infusion to treat someone with weak kidneys and frequent urination.

The Wet'suwet'en of northern British Columbia call the tree **DICIN ILHTSIN** meaning, "smelly wood" or "stinkwood". The inner bark was infused for bad colds and flu, or mixed with devil's club, fir, and black twinberry bark for whooping cough. It was combined with yellow pond lily root for tuberculosis.

The Gitksan use the bark in very similar manners, not surprising considering their close proximity. It is known as **SGANSA ANGITL'**.

The leaves contain prussic acid, and are considered poisonous, although some native tribes chewed the leaves to induce vomiting. Natives of North Carolina, probably the Cherokee, crush the leaves as a wash for cleansing after-birth.

The leave and bark are used in tanning, producing a black dye. The compact wood from the European species is highly esteemed by wood turners and engravers; and traditionally used to make barrel hoops due to its elasticity.

Hildegard de Bingen suggested, "throw the earth from around the root of this tree into gardens, strewing it where caterpillars and butterflies eat and devastate the vegetables. When they are troubled by this, they withdraw and can no longer flourish there."

The USDA-ARS National Clonal Germplasm Repository in Corvallis, Oregon has gathered more than sixty different mountain ash from around the world. One of the more interesting is a Soropyrus, a mountain ash and pear cross.

The fruit is about the size of a small peach, with a pale yellow speckled skin with reddish blush. The yellow flesh has a sweet mild taste of a pear.

A newly available tree in Alberta is a mountain ash from Russia, with berries that taste like red currants.

Service tree (*S. domestica*) is hardy to zone 2-3, and is native to Europe and North Africa. It has inch-long brownish-green fruit, with a reddish tint, that is edible, and mainly used for flavoring liqueurs, and previously cider. Like fruit of related species, they are left to freeze and almost rot, a process known as bletting, before preparation into jellies and condiments. The distilled fruit product is high in (R)-limonene.

It accumulates arsenic in environment on drier years, and molybdenum and selenium in years of more rainfall.

MEDICINAL

CONSTITUENTS- *S. aucuparia-* fruit parasorboside (bitter), forming parasorbic acid through cell destruction (lactone of the (5S)-hydroxyhex-2-en-acyl-1) 0.1-0.3% of the fresh weight. This is destroyed or volatilized through drying and cooking. Only traces are found in the cultivated variety. The fruit contains tartaric acid before ripening and citric and malic acid after. Galacturonic acid, pectin (including galactose, arabinose, glucose) sterols (cholesterol,aucuparin, methoxy-aucuparin, dimethoxy-isolariciresinol, stigmasterol and sitosterol), malic acid (3-5%), tartaric acid; 7 fatty acids (myristic, palmitic, palmitoleic, stearic, oleic, linoleic and linolenic).
Benzoic and cinnamic acid as well as D-sorbitol (10%) are also present. Small amounts of prunasin in the fruit pulp. Vitamin C is 0.03-0.13%, and bioflavonoids 1262 mg%. Phenolics in sweet rowanberry cultivars vary from 550-1014 mg/100 grams of fresh berries, mainly chlorogenic and neochlorogenic acids.
L-Iditol, an unusual sugar alcohol is only found in the berries.
Iron content is 35 mg/kg, manganese is 33 mg/kg, and copper 5 mg/kg.
heartwood- aucuparin, 2'-methoxy-aucuparin, 4'-methoxyaucuparin, 2'-hydroxyaucuparin, and isoauruparin.
leaves- cyanogenic glycosides, flavonol aglycones.
Flowers- 11.83% total phenolics, including 4.3% chlorogenic acid, 5% proanthocyanidins, and 1.28% flavonoid aglycones.
Seeds- 0.2-0.5% amygdalin, cyanogenic glycoside.
S. domestica- seed- magnesium
Bark- calcium, zinc.
S. decora- bark- 23-hydroxybetulin, betulinic acid, uvaol, alpha amyrin.
Stem bark- 23,28-dihydroxyursan-12-ene-3beta-caffeate; 23,28-dihydroxylupan-20(29)-ene-3beta-caffeate; 3beta,23,28-trihydroxy-12-ursene, triterpenoids, catechin, epicatechin.

Both leaves and fruit are used in traditional medicine for hemostatic action. The fresh leaves can be applied to the skin to treat fungal infections, and various skin allergies.

Russian medicine uses fresh berry juice for gastritis and hypertension. Golubenko et al, *Sovetskaya Med* 1967 30:4 used *S. aucuparia* berry preparations. It was found as effective as anti-coagulants in patients with myocardial infarction and angina pectoris.

Decoctions of the dried fruit without seeds are useful for reducing bile duct inflammation, as well as passage of kidney and gallstones.

Because of the vitamins A and C, and trace minerals, the fruit tea is useful in anemia, emaciation, anorexia, and various vitamin deficient conditions.

The fully ripened fruit may be eaten fresh, as juice or jam, to reduce cholesterol in the blood and prevent heart disease. The fruit tincture may be used to elevate prothrombin levels in blood and help prevent strokes, according to herbalist, Darcy Williamson. The fruit stimulates bile and relieves gall bladder colic and irritation.

The berries can be used for a gargle in sore throat and inflamed tonsils. Juice the ripe berries and make ice cubes.

Gargling with the juice will help keep the vocal chords smooth and supple, a good tonic for singers and speakers.

Infusions of berries can be used in retention enemas, for tonic and astringent properties in soothing hemorrhoids; or drank internally for slow and painful urination.

Western mountain ash berries in water extract show activity against mycobacterium. The berries of the Rowan tree possess cytotoxic activity.

The fresh fruit will increase labour contractions and speed birthing.

Decoctions of fruit are used for heart health, helping reduce blood pressure, fibrillation and angina pain. This is due to the hexanoic form of parasorbic acid, which is a potent beta-adrenergic blocker, according to noted botanist, Diana Beresford-Kroeger.

The introduced rowan tree berries have been well researched. Extracts with acetone, alcohol and water reveal activity against gram-positive bacteria, and viruses. Recent work by Kylli et al, *J Ag Food Chem* 2010 58:22 identified various cultivars with activity against *Staphylococcus aureus, Salmonella typhymurium, and E. coli.*

Either the glycoside or parasorbic acid formed by enzymatic hydrolysis shows antibiotic effect. This is found in both fresh and dried fruit. Protozoa and gram positive bacteria are susceptible to parasorbic acid.

The berries are used in Europe for kidney problems, as well as disorders of uric acid metabolism and dissolution of uric acid deposits (gout). The berry is used for catarrh, internal inflammations, menstrual complaints, and alkalization of blood. Remove seeds prior to using the fruit for food or medicine.

Sweet rowan berries, cultivated since the 19th century in Czech Republic, and in various Russian breeding programs, contain chlorogenic acid, a powerful antioxidant associated with decreased risk of type 2 diabetes and other health concerns. Hukkanen et al, *J Ag Food Chem* 2006 54.

In fact, the berries inhibit alpha glucosidase as effectively as the pharmaceutical drug, acarbose. Boath AS et al, *Food Chem* 2012 135(3): 929-36.

Recent work by McDougall et al, in same journal 2008 56:9 found activity against cervical and colon cancer cell lines at low concentrations, from this berry as well as raspberry, lingonberry, cloudberry and strawberry fruits.

A puree of berries is used for diarrhea, and the freshly pressed juice for lung and pleura conditions associated with fever. The fresh juice contains parasorbic acid that in very large quantities leads to gastroenteritis, vomiting, and kidney damage; but is fully destroyed upon cooking. Therefore, the raw berry juice is a mild laxative; whereas the high content of pectin and tannins means boiled fruit will treat diarrhea.

The D-sorbitol is sweet to the diabetic, and breaks down to carbon dioxide without a glucose reaction. Industrially, it is used to make ascorbic acid, and added to toothpastes.

Sorbitol is the starting material for wetting and emulsifying products such as Tween.

Glen Blouin, in his beautiful book, *An Eclectic Guide to Trees*, mentions that one of the two fruit sugars relieve eye pressure in patients suffering glaucoma.

Ethanol extracts of *S. decora*, found in the eastern boreal forest increase glucose uptake in skeletal muscle cells and reduce insulin sensitivity *in vivo* in manner similar to drug metformin. Vianna et al, *Evid Based Compl Alt Med* 2011;2011:237941.

The anti-diabetic gene flavonol synthase is higher in leaf and bark, in northern latitudes, of both *S. decora* and *S. americana*. Bailie A et al, *Peer Journal* 2016 4:e2645.

The stem bark contains a caffeate compound that significantly enhances glucose uptake in C2C12 cells. Guerrero-Analco JA et al, *J Nat Prod* 2010 73(9): 1519-23.

Uvaol in the bark inhibits phosphodiesterase-4D, helping reduce inflammation. Tan BX et al, *Nat Prod Res* 2017 March 10:1-6. Uvaol is a triterpene also found in olive oil and black cherries.

Decoctions of dried bark were used for diarrhea and in vaginal douches for vaginitis and leucorrhea. The fresh bark tincture has been used as a tonic in fevers of the malarial type, similar to dogwood, where it was used as a cinchona substitute.

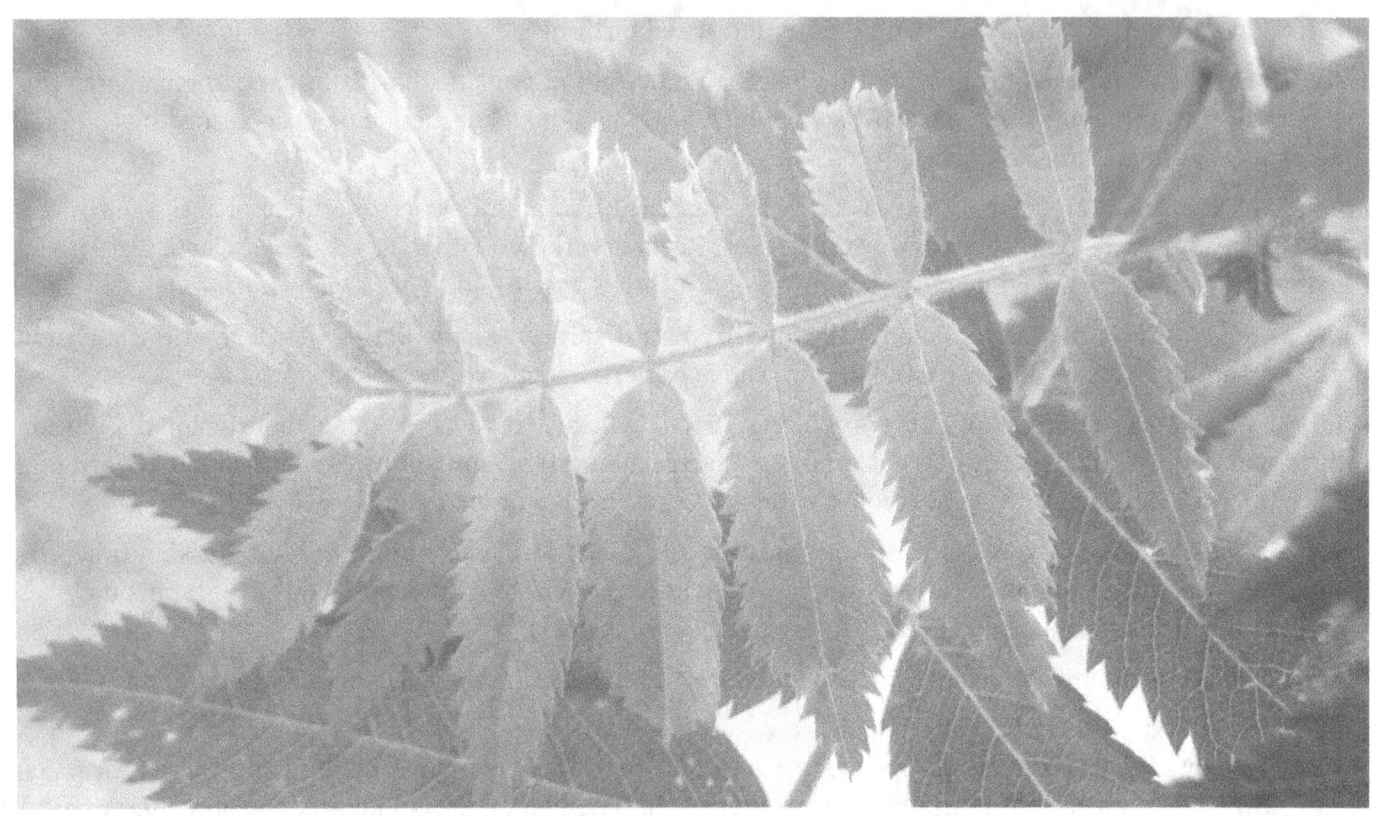

YOUNG MOUNTAIN ASH LEAVES

The fresh leaves contain similar properties and can be used interchangeably. Traditionally, the leaves were burned and the fumes inhaled for asthma. Early work by Bergeron et al has shown dichloromethane extracts of both stem bark and young stems effective against *Candida albicans, Bacillus subtilis* and *E. coli.*

Stem and root decoctions are used to treat tuberculosis, and possess fungicidal activity.

Russian herbalists recommend flower decoctions for liver problems; helping reduce fatty livers, and stimulating liver metabolism. As well, they soothe persistent coughs, and prevent goiter formation in women.

Flower tinctures are recommended for hemorrhoid treatment.

Work by Olszewska et al, *Nat Prod Res* 2009 23:16 identified nearly 12% total phenolics in flowers, suggesting anti-oxidant and other health benefits.

Extracts show anti-cancer activity. Goun EA et al, *J Ethnopharm* 2002 81 337-342.

Heartwood affected by fungal infections produces phytoalexins, which are anti-fungal and worth examination.

Mistletoe from *S. aucuparia* has been analyzed and found to contain twelve components, the main one being salicylic acid, at 39.55%.

The fruit of *S. domestica* has been found to prevent diabetic complications due in part to inhibition of aldose reductase. Termentzi A et al, *Pharmazie* 63(9): 693-6

The related *S. rufopilosa*, a tsema rowan, as ethanol extract, has been found to possess anti-oxidant activity and inhibit proliferation of HT29 cancer cells by inducing cell cycle arrest and apoptosis. Oh YN et al, *J Cancer Prev* 2016 21(4): 249-256.

The twigs of *S. alnifolia* have been used traditionally in Koreas for neurological conditions. An alcohol extract protects dopaminergic (DA) neurodegeneration and recovers diminished DA neuron function, suggesting its possible use for Parkinson's disease. Cheon SM et al, *Pharm Biol* 2017 55(1): 481-486.

The stem bark of *S. commixta* contains sorcomic acid, that potently induced NGF secretion from C6 glioma cells. Kim CS et al, *Lipids* 2016 51(8): 989-95.

Tinctures of the cortex appear to prevent development of atherosclerosis. Sohn EJ et al, *Biol Pharm Bull* 2005 28(8): 1444-9.

HOMEOPATHY

Mountain ash (Pyrus) is used for irritation of the eyes; or whenever there is a constriction around the waist. It relieves spasmodic pains in the uterus and bladder; and is a mild diuretic.

There may be a sensation as if cold water were in the stomach; extending up into the esophagus. It is recommended in catarrhs and diarrhea.

It is useful in various neuralgias and gouty pain in the big toe. It contains malic acid, an active factor in the citric acid cycle.

Patients are gloomy and discouraged but unable to cry. Sad, weeping mood, heart aches from deep sorrow. Thinks she is clairvoyant, thinks the blood dark blue. Thinks she is looking down at her own body.

DOSE- Third to 6X potency. The mother tincture is prepared from the bark. Proving by Gatchell on self, two lads and a married woman with a tincture of the bark around 1878.

A case report from George Loukas concludes. "Pyrus could also be recommended in cases of schizoid personality. These people are peculiar, eccentric with odd appearance and behaviour, strange way of talking, thinking and perceiving. When someone describes the typical feeling of going out of the body and traveling, we must think of Pyrus."

GEMMOTHERAPY

Rowan (*S. aucuparia*) or Service Tree (*S. domestica*) buds are used as the major regulator of venous circulation, and overcoming congestive conditions. The glycerite increases the tone of the venous walls. It is particularly suited to the female patient with circulation disturbance during menopause, venous hypertension, phlebitis, varicose veins and heavy leg syndrome.

May be useful in deafness, ringing in ears, tinnitus and related auditory disturbances.

DOSE- 15-30 drops up to three times daily of the 1D glycerin macerate.

ESSENTIAL OIL

When mountain ash berries with seeds are used to prepare malic acid, a pungent odour is noticed. Upon condensing of the vapor, a color-less oil with pleasant odour is obtained. The amygdalin is decomposed with water at high temperatures into hydrocyanic acid, oil of bitter almonds (benzaldehyde) and glucose.

Also present in the volatile oil is parasorbic acid (a lactone of $C_6H_8O_2$).

The mature or nearly mature berry only is most suitable for distillation. Whereas the immature berry contains malic acid only, the ripening berries contain sorbin oil and the malic acid disappears. At the same time sorbinose ($C_6H_{12}O_6$) and sorbite ($C_6H_{14}O_6$) result. Sorbic acid (2E,4E)-hexadienoic acid) was first found in the oil of un-ripened mountain ash berries.

Studies by Kubo and Lee, *J Ag Food Chem* 1998 46:10 conducted at Berkeley, showed the fungicidal activity of sorbic acid was increased by 6400% in combination with polygolial derived from Smartweed (*Polygonum Hydropiper*). This synergistic activity is due to inhibition of plasma membrane H+-ATPase.

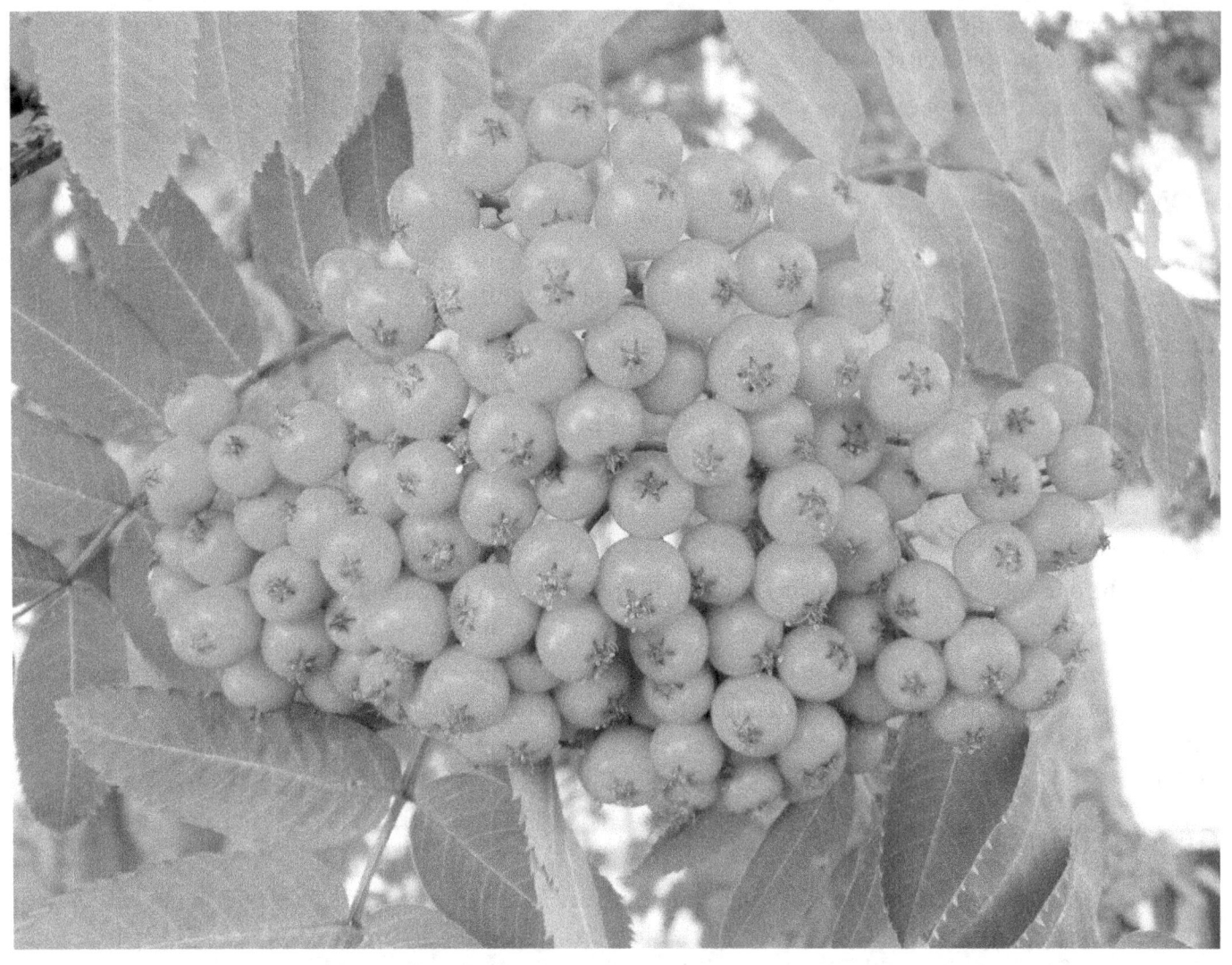

RIPE MOUNTAIN ASH BERRIES

SEED OIL

The seeds contain 21.9% fatty oil that has a sweetish taste, with a slight yellow colour. However, considerable amounts of hydrocyanic acid make it unsuitable for human consumption.

It dries quickly upon exposure to air with iodine value of 128.5 and specific gravity of 0.9137.

WAX

A methanol/petrolic ether (1:1) extract was made of dried residue left after alcoholic extraction of ripe mountain ash berries (*S. aucuparia*).

From this an insoluble wax-like substance precipitated, which was found to contain carotenoids.

FLOWER ESSENCES

Rowan (*S. aucuparia*) flower essence is for forgiveness. It helps us to let go of resentments and to heal old wounds. As we learn to forgive ourselves, and others, we can heal the past and have reconciliation.

It is indicated whenever we are clinging to old behaviour patterns, judgment, avoidance, self-pity, shame, defensiveness, self-destructive patterns, or resentment.

It present opportunity for forgiving oneself and other, to learn from past experience, resolve karma, and face deep repressed emotions.

Rowan essence addresses our attachment to habitual, inherited or karmically acquired emotions/ patterns.
FINDHORN

In vibrational medicine, Essence of Rowan attunes us to the energies of nature, broadening perspectives and allowing a deeper understanding of our place in the universe.
GIFFORD

Rowan flower essence is for judgment, and when you are not discerning enough. The essence protects against enchantment, and helps you use your own instincts to help you.
OGAM

Rowan leaf essence helps restore energy and repair damage after surgery. It assists in tissue repair and shortens the recovery period after general anesthetic.
FALLING LEAF

Rowan essence helps one to get rid of long existing anger towards others.
MIRIANA

Mountain Ash (*S. scopulina*) flower essence is most useful to those who have too great a need to please others, and in the process lose track of their own selves. This essence is particularly important in group settings, team sports, and even family structure, where an individual is willing to relent to "make things smoother". They fail to realize the consequence of blindly following others; and give too much of their own individual power and identity away.
PRAIRIE DEVA

SPIRITUAL PROPERTIES

Thus Rowan, known among modern Druids as the Tree of the Bards opens our higher senses to subtle processes and connects us with the realms above. It makes us resistant to the spells of the world by connecting us more strongly with our Higher Self, the source of true, authentic inspiration.

Rudolf Steiner described Thor as the archangel who brought the powers of will power and self-awareness, to the people. So, by rescuing Thor, Rowan helps to maintain the independence and individuality of the conscious self.
HAGENEDER

PERSONALITY TRAITS

An ancient Scandinavian legend related that the foundation of the world was the sacred ash which was named Ygdrasil. Three austere sisters, "Past, Present and Future", guarded the tree. Its trunk passed through the disk of the earth at its center and its three roots sank deep into hell where all was dark and still. From these roots flowed three springs, Force, Memory and Life.

Outside the earth's disk of land stretched the ocean and on the outermost rim lay the great serpent encircling the disk with its tail in its mouth. The wise serpent gave the world Continuity and Eternity.

Iduna, the goddess of life, plucked the red berries of the ash tree and threw them down to the lesser gods. The fruit gave them great strength and they taught the people how life pervaded everything, naming of man and beast brothers.

The great gialler horn is hidden beneath an ash tree and on the day of judgement it will sound all over the world. On that day, the heavens will open and mightly judge will descend. The sea will rush in with enormous waves; fire spirits will leap up from hell and fire will spread over the whole earth. But after the holocaust, the tree of life will grow again, the gods will return and men will live on a higher plane.
GUILLET

Rowan emphasizes the need for color and creative endeavor in our lives and encourages us to open our minds to creative inspiration. It also teaches us that we can draw on the forces of life to heal ourselves, and those around us. Rowan protects and gives courage and strength to those walking the path of spiritual growth and enlightenment.
GIFFORD

RECIPES

TINCTURE- Chop and pound the fresh fruit pulp without seeds. Add two parts by weight of 60% alcohol and mix thoroughly. Store for eight days in cool, dark place. The tincture is a reddish brown, with a slight bitter taste.

INFUSION- Take one teaspoon fresh or dried berries to one cup of water. Bring to boil, let cool, and strain. Take one third cup three times daily.

FRESH JUICE- One tablespoon three times daily before meals. For gastritis, take one tsp twenty minutes before eating. Use with caution.

BITTERS- Fresh mountain ash berry juice is added to gin, and tastes exactly like Angostura bitters.

JELLY- Four part berries are boiled with 3 parts green apples and just enough water to cover until the juice is red and bitter. The juice is then strained through a jelly bag overnight, and boiled with sugar (between 16-24 ounces per pint of liquid until it jells. Certo is not necessary if the apples are young enough.

The berries make a tasty addition to venison dishes.

ROWAN JELLY- Pick 8 cups of berries after frost. Bring to boil with three cups apples or crabapples with water to cover for hour. Strain through jelly bag. For each cup juice add one cup of sugar or 20% less honey. Boil over high heat until jelly stage, about one hour. Add half-cup whiskey (your choice) after half hour. Bottle and store.

CAUTION- Seeds and bark contain hydrocyanic acid that is destroyed by drying and heat. Do not use during pregnancy, thrombophlebitis, any viscous blood conditions or history of myocardial infarction associated with blood clots.

The berries of various Sorbus trees, particularly *S. decora*, have the potential to affect the CYP2C and 3A4 mediated liver metabolism and may interfere with bioavailability and pharmacokinetics of pharmaceuticals.

MOUNTAIN AVENS
WHITE DRYAD
(*Dryas octopetala* L.)
(*D. hookeriana* Juz.)
YELLOW MOUNTAIN AVENS
YELLOW DRYAD
(*D. drummondii* Richardson ex Hook)
PARTS USED- whole plant

Dryas is from the Greek **DRYAD**, meaning a wood nymph. Dryades were daughters of Zeus, and nymphs of the oak. The leaves of some species were thought by early botanists to resemble tiny oak leaves, a bit of a stretch in my opinion.

Drummondii is named after the Scottish naturalist that accompanied Franklin on a search for the Northwest Passage. He was also the earliest botanist to study the Berland River country more than a century ago. Octopetala means 8 petals.

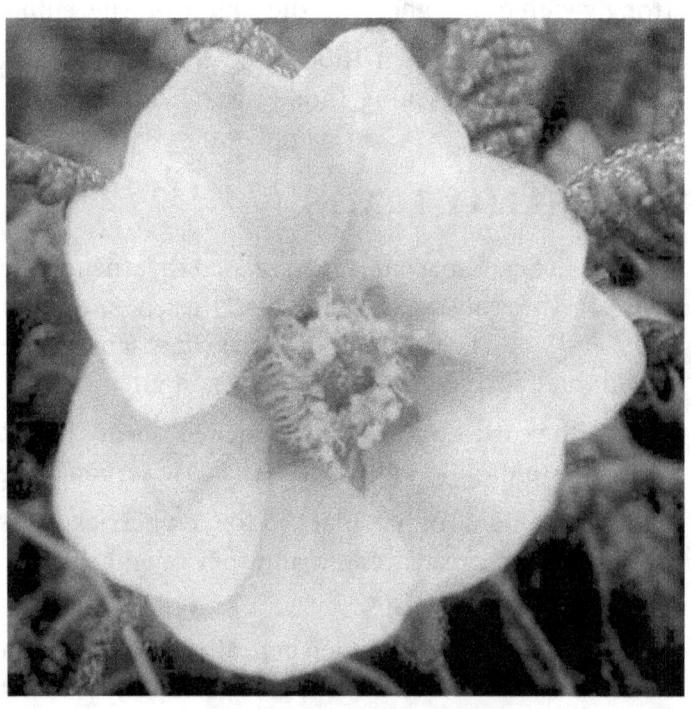
MOUNTAIN AVENS FLOWER

Mountain Avens is a dwarf under shrub with white flowers. It is circumpolar and found on alpine slopes; and the floral emblem of the former North West Territories. The Inuit call it **MALIKAAT**, which means the follower, because it follows the sun around the sky. This is known as heliotropic, something shared by sunflowers and other plants. In the case of mountain avens, because the flowers always face the sun, they act like solar collectors to attract insects for pollination and to speed up their own seed production.

Many commercial varieties have been developed from the related European stock.

The related *D. integrifolia* is also known as White Dryad, making for some confusion. This plant is known to the Inuit as either **MALIKKAAT**, because the plants follow the seasons, or **ISURRAMUAT** referring to the tracking of the sun. When summer is coming they fold out one direction and when winter is coming they fold in and twist in another.

Yellow Dryad is commonly found in the foothills, and at higher elevations. The plant seed clusters unwind and then rewind, signaling the moon of Akulliruut in Nunavut. This was the signal that caribou skins were in prime condition for making winter clothing.

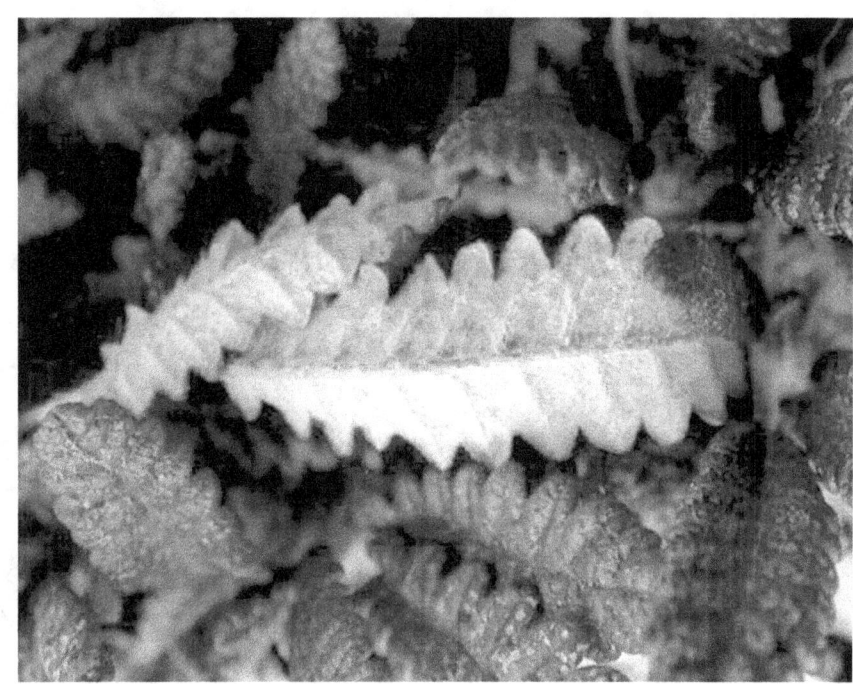

WHITE UNDERSIDE OF WHITE DRYAD LEAVES

By growing close to the ground, they are protected from the cold, drying winds of summer and covered by snow in winter. The rolled, evergreen leaves help reduce water loss, and in early spring they can begin producing food immediately.

The flowers are also close to the ground, to help in seed formation, and by always facing the sun they can direct the sun ray's like a parabolic lens on the stigma, increasing the temperature by up to 3.6 Centigrade.

The plant helps enrich the soil with nitrogen, by means of bacteria around the roots, helping encourage other plant growth.

MEDICINAL

CONSTITUENTS- aerial parts- ent-epicatechin and six flavonol glycosides including; 3-0-alpha-L-arabinofuranosyl-8-methoxy-quercitin;3-0-beta-galacto-pyranosyl-8-methoxykaempferol; 3-0-beta-galacto-pyranosyl quercitin (hyperin); 3-0-alpha-L-arabinofurano-sylquercitin (avicularin); 3-0-beta-L-arabinopyrano-sylquercitin; 3-0-beta-D-galactopyrano-syl-8-methoxyquercitin.

Hyperin is a common phenolic compound. Research has found it is anti-oxidant, anti-inflammatory and inhibits ACE (angiotensin 1-coverting enzyme) associated with cardiovascular health. Huang WY et al, *J Food Sci* 2017 82(5): 1239-46.

The compound may be useful in the treatment of thrombotic disease, preventing hydrogen peroxide damage. Liu XX et al, *Int J Mol Med* 2016 37(4): 1083-90.

Hyperin inhibits inflammation by inhibiting TLR4 and NLRP3 signaling pathways. It may be beneficial in treatment of sepsis-induced acute kidney injury. Chunzhi G et al, *Oncotarget* 2016 7(50): 82602-8.

The use of cisplatin for chemotherapy caused kidney damage. Hyperin protects against this effect by inhibiting inflammatory and oxidant damage, at least in mice. Chao CS et al, *Int Immunopharmacol* 2016 40: 517-23.

Avicularin is a potent anti-fungal, present in various Polygonum species. In one study it showed strong activity against *Candida albicans*. Da Silva Sa FA et al, *Molecules* 2017 22(7).

The compound has a role to play in the treatment of Helicobacter pylori, binding to the arabinose 5-phosphate site. Cho S et al, *Eur J Med Chem* 2016 108: 188-202.

FLOWER ESSENCES

Yellow Dryas flower essence gives support to those who are exploring the edge of the known. It helps one maintain an energetic connection to one's soul family during dynamic cycles of growth.   **ALASKA**

White Mountain Avens essence is for dealing with directness, calling a spade a spade.

ROCKY MOUNTAIN

SPIRITUAL PROPERTIES

Dryas octopetala of the high mountains, with its flower and woolly bearded fruit would like us to believe that it is an anemone, but if one sees its rocky habitat and its clinging woody stems- the Dryas is in reality a stunted bush- one cannot doubt for a moment that one is dealing with a member of the rose family.

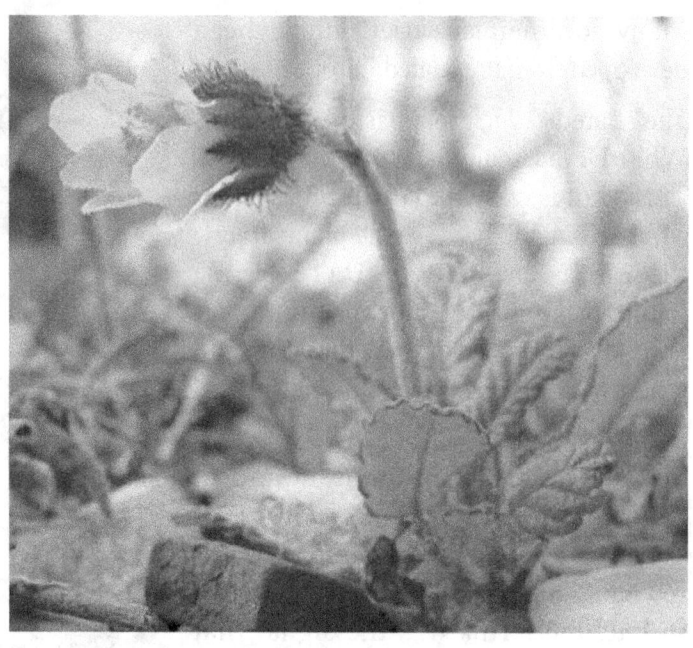

YELLOW DRYAS FLOWER

The very small evergreen leaves, silvery-white on the underside are not pinnate like the rose, but the indentation stops halfway so they are only deeply crenate.   **GROHMANN**

MYTHS AND LEGENDS

Dryad is a Greek version of a female "Druid" or tree nymph that lived in or near her special tree and would never die until the tree itself died.

It was believed by some that dryads could take on human or arboreal form when desired; explaining many of the ancient myths of maidens turned into various flowers and trees.

In Hindu mythology, tree nymphs are necessary to feed these trees.

Dryads also dwelt in the Holy Land under the name of Benat Ya'kob: Daughters of Jacob.

WALKER

Dionysus traveled with a merry retinue of nymphs, satyrs, centaurs...who were prone to frenzied fits of ecstasy and abandon. When they arrived in Thrace, King Lycurgus rushed at them with a cattle prod... and scared Dionysus so badly that he leaped into the sea.

Needless to say, Lycurgas paid for his transgression. Homer says that Zeus blinded him. Apollodorus reports that Dionysus made the king hallucinate so badly that he took an axe and chopped away at what he thought was a vine. When he came to his senses, he saw that he had hacked off the hands and feet of his son Dryas, thereby killing him.

HATHAWAY

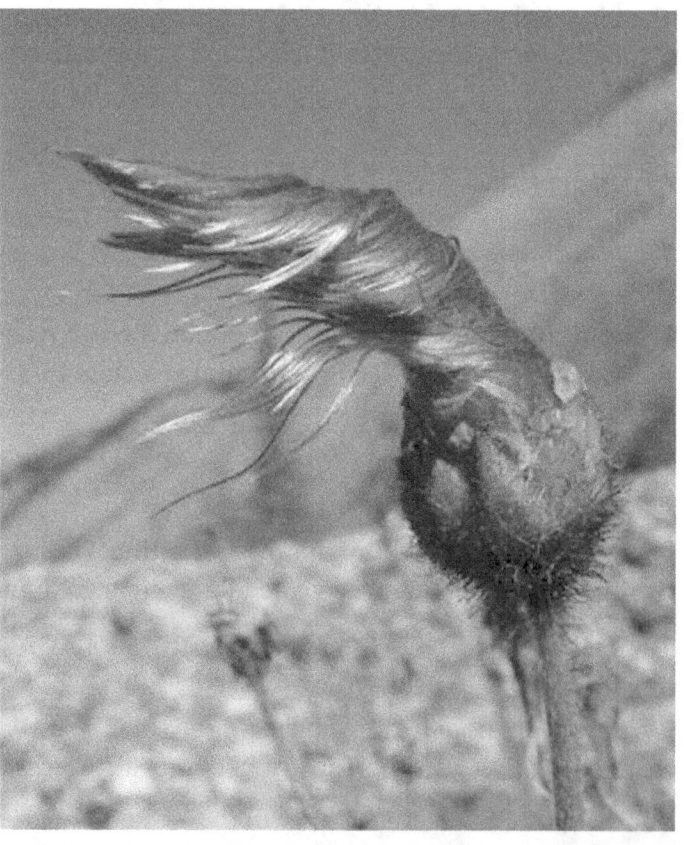

DRYAS DRUMMONDII

PERSONALITY TRAITS

As the last ice age was ending and the glaciers retreated, trees typical of cold climates, such as birch began to appear. Then their pollen was overlaid by that of the mountain avens (*Dryas octopetala*), a flowering herb of mountain sides and the far north. The trees had died, and the ground was carpeted with mountain avens, showing that the climate had suddenly grown much colder...

Because it was the discovery of its pollen that led to the realization of what had happened, the period is called the Dryas. In fact, it happened twice, so there is an Older Dryas, lasting from about 12,200 to 11,800 years ago, and a Younger Dryas, from about 11,000 to 10,000 years ago. During each Dryas, the glacial retreat halted and in places was reversed. Temperatures fell almost to their ice-age levels. **ALLABY**

WHITE MUSTARD
YELLOW MUSTARD
(***Brassica hirta*** Moench.) not accepted
(***B. alba*** [L.] Rabenh.) not accepted
(***Sinapis alba*** L.)
BLACK MUSTARD
(***B. nigra*** [L.] W. D. J. Koch.)
(***S. nigra*** L.)
BIRD RAPE MUSTARD
COLZA
(***B. rapa*** L.)
(***B. rapa ssp. sylvestris*** [L.] Janch) not accepted
(***B. campestris var oleifera*** DC.) not accepted
INDIAN MUSTARD
CHINESE MUSTARD
LEAF MUSTARD
BROWN MUSTARD
JAPANESE MUSTARD
MIZUNA
(***B. juncea*** [L.] Czern.)
(***S. juncea*** L.)
WILD MUSTARD
(***B. kaber*** [DC.] L. C. Wheeler) not accepted
(***S. arvensis*** L.)
PARTS USED- seeds, leaves

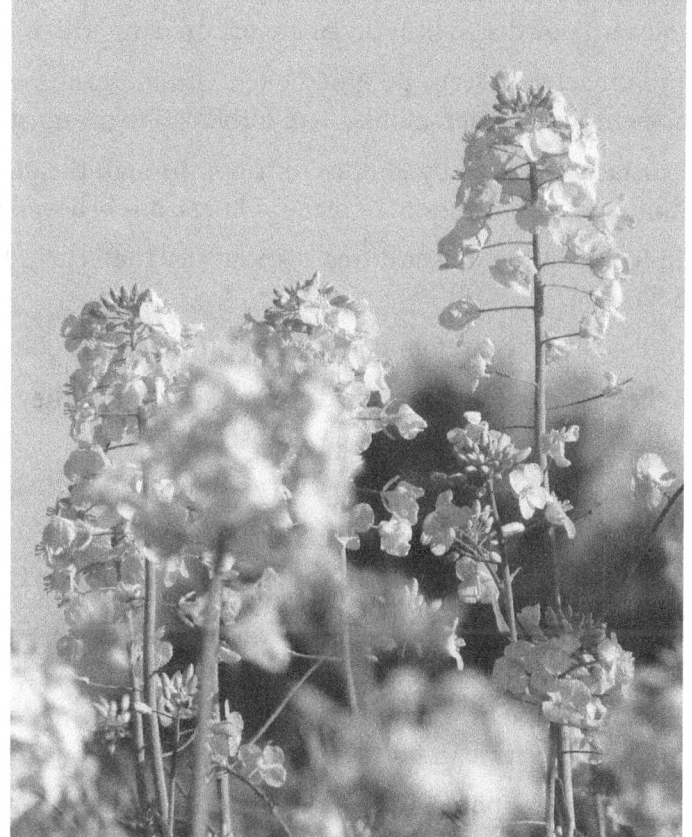

MUSTARD

Bottom: Your name, I beseech you, sir?
Mustardseed: Mustardseed.
Bottom: Good Master Mustardseed, I know your patience well: that same cowardly, giant-like ox-beef hath devoured many a gentleman of your house: I promise you your kindred hath made my eyes water ere now. I desire your more acquaintance, good Master Mustardseed. **SHAKESPEARE**

It is indeed possible to live without mustard. It's also possible to survive without music, poetry, or art- possible but not much fun. **BARRY LEVENSON**

I'm mad about mustard
Even on custard. **OGDEN NASH**

A tale without love is like beef without mustard. **ANATOLE FRANCE**

Mustard comes from the Latin *MUSTUS,* or *MUST*, the freshly crushed grapes, or new wine. Ardens means "burning".

MUSTUS ARDENS was the mixture of crushed mustard seeds mixed into a new wine sauce; later shortened to mustard. The Old French term for mustard, **MOULT ARDRE** means, "much burning". This phrase is probably an adaptation of **MOULT ME TARDE**, for "I ardently desire", and related to a motto on the gates of Dijon, placed by Philip the Bold, Duke of Burgundy in 1382.

Brassica is from the Celtic **BRESIC**, meaning cabbage due to the removal of leaves from the stems for horse or cattle feed.

Juncea is Latin for rush or seed; nigra means black.

I have to say that I've always loved mustard, the tangier the better. As a kid, I was first exposed to the American mustard, the kind most prevalent on hot dogs. Later, I noticed that my mom would add the dry Coleman's mustard powder to her special French dressing with oil and vinegar.

In France, they serve pommes frites with mustard mayonnaise, and its not bad either. This is in contrast to ancient times, when monks were forbidden to eat mustard, due to its stimulating effect on virility.

Mustard was used by Hindus to travel through the air, while Italian farmers sprinkle the seed around their doorstep for protection. In many cultures, it is believed that eating mustard seeds increases fertility in women.

In Sanskrit, the mustard tree is known as The Witch. Written Sanskrit texts mention mustard seeds around 3000 BCE.

A deposit of seeds, found at a site in Iraq dates to 3000 BC.

When ancient Hindus wanted to discover a witch, they lit lamps during the night, and fill vessels with water on which are placed drops of mustard seed oil.

At the same time, the name of every woman in the village is spoken, and if a female shadow appears in the water, it was a sure sign of condemnation.

Mustard is associated with Tuesday, the 18th of June, the planet Mars, and the astrological sign of Aries.

White Mustard originated in the eastern Mediterranean region, Brown types from the foothills of the Himalayas, and the Black seed from the Middle East.

Black Mustard flower buds, collected before they open, can be steamed like broccoli. The leaf and buds are a popular vegetable in Italy and other Mediterranean countries.

The green seedpods can be pickled in vinegar like capers. The seeds are small and difficult to harvest, averaging 1654 in one teaspoon.

Mustard seed is a major special crop of Western Canada, with 238,000 tonnes produced in 1998. The majority, 195.5 tonnes, is grown in Saskatchewan; with the United States the largest market, followed by Belgium, Japan, Germany and Denmark.

Alberta only produced 26,000 tonnes, but that was still worth over $15 million, of the yellow and brown or oriental mustard, seed combined. In 1999, Oriental mustard became the No.1 mustard seed grown in Saskatchewan, with over 265,000 acres harvested, with seed production of over 130,000 tonnes.

Mustard seed is widely used in pickles and relishes, but the main market its for prepared or powdered mustard for table use. Most Yellow Mustard is exported to the United States, for the manufacture of hot dog mustard, and blended with Black Mustard seeds to make typical English brands. Mustard flour is also used as a meat extender in the blending of sausages and prepared meats.

The seeds are ground into mustard powder by G.S. Dunn of Hamilton, the largest dry miller of mustard in the world. They process some 20 million kilograms each year, sold to the United States to be mixed with water, vinegar and tumeric, or to England for repackaging as Keen's Dry Mustard.

Brown mustard is used in France to produce the famous Dijon mustard. The plant grows 4-5 feet tall and lends itself well to mechanical harvest. It is then wet-milled in France, to which is added water, wine vinegar, salt and perhaps some herbs. It was first used in 1336 at the table of King Philip VI. The acidic juice of unripe grapes replaced vinegar in 1856.

Last year, Canada imported $6 million worth of prepared mustards from France very close to the value of the brown mustard seed we exported , to supply 90% of the world market. Poor economics on our part! Grey Poupon mustard originated in Dijon in 1866.

We could make our own mustard in this country, and even call it Dijon, as the name is not yet protected by the French government, nor the European Union. An appellation of origin was granted legal status in 1937, but is a geographic protection.

Black Mustard is sometimes planted in spring or fall as a cover crop to suppress weeds, some pests and bring up minerals for the next crop. Of course, it is important to clean up before going to seed.

Unlike in Europe, Japan and other markets, Oriental mustard seed is either milled directly or cold pressed to remove some of the cooking oil, followed by milling.

White Mustard, or Yellow Mustard as it is called in the United States (*B. alba*) is not as pungent as the other two, and is used a lot in American mixed mustards, some in English, but forbidden in Dijon.

In England, the former is sprouted for salads and sandwiches; while the latter is considered the White or Yellow Mustard grown specifically for seed. They are the same plant. White mustard is used for flavoring, black or brown for aroma. White mustard contains no sinigrin, and black mustard no sinalbin.

In all markets, the seed is reduced to a fine powder and then used as a spice. It is the perfect condiment for hotdogs, as mustard helps promote digestion, and its organic sulphur content counteracts the fat allergy or sensitivity that accompanies this pseudo-meat.

White mustard seed is a preservative, used in pickles, and to emulsify mayonnaise.

Try adding mustard seed one part, juniper berries one part, and peppercorns two parts to your peppermill. The seeds are quite rich in magnesium at 33 milligrams per tablespoon. By comparison, four ounces of oatmeal only contains 28 mg.

It is an excellent green manure, a crop that can be turned under to add organic matter and minerals to the soil.

Mustard requires just over 100 days to mature, with yields in the 2500-3000 kilos per hectare. Glucosinolate containing plants are being studied as a source of pesticidal, phytotoxic compounds that can replace synthetic approaches. Work by Borek et al, *J Ag Food Chem* 2005 53 found the crushed seed meal effective in controlling weed species, due to formation of ionic thiocynate from 4-hydroxybenzyl glucosinolate in the meal.

Scientists, working with mustard plants have identified the gene that directs the synthesis of cellulose. They now hope to make tiny alterations in the gene so that plants will make novel types of cellulose, including paper, or biosynthetic fibers that can be woven into 21st century fabric.

Excessive amounts of various Brassica in the human diet can produce goiter. Although not a problem in normal humans, under normal circumstance, excessive consumption can lead to problems in those with genetic or constitutionally inherited weakness of the gland.

Goitrin (1,5-Vinyl-2-thiooxazolidone), the major anti-thyroid principle was first isolated from seeds, and later fresh leaves. Thiocyanate and allyliso-thiocyanate are other goitergenic compounds. Rape and cabbage seed both contain goitrogens and growth depressants that are overcome in various ways.

Mustard waste precipitated hydrolysate has been found to improve astaxanthin production eleven-fold in presence of *Xanthophyllomyces dendrorhous*. Tinoi et al, *J Ind Micro Biotech* 33:4.

Bird rape Mustard (*B. campestris*) seed, when defatted and de-hulled, contains a protein efficiency level of 98%, which is higher than milk casein. Brassica seed protein is highly nutritious, due in large part to the high content of sulphur amino acids. Bird Rape or Flowering Chinese Cabbage is grown in the orient as a vegetable. Known as **YOU CAI**, meaning oil vegetable, or **CAI TAI**, vegetable moss, the plant is contraindicated in cases of patients recovering from measles and other eruptive skin diseases, as well as conjunctivitis and eye infections.

The flowering cabbage is juiced and taken for stomach pain and dysentery with bleeding, or crushed and applied like other cabbage to mastitis.

The Cree, among others, use Mustard plasters for bronchitis and other respiratory congestions. It is known as **KOTAWAHKAN**.

To make a mustard plaster, take one part ground mustard seed and four parts whole wheat flour and mix it with lukewarm water to make a paste. Do not let the mixture get hotter than 60 degrees Celsius, or the enzyme will be de-activated.

Spread this on a cloth and place on the chest that first had vegetable oil applied to it. Remove the cloth when burning sensation is felt, usually 5-15 minutes. Be careful not to blister the skin. If the mustard and flour are mixed with egg whites instead of water, the poultice will not blister, according to Jethro Kloss.

You can also apply mustard oil externally (see below) in concentrations of 0.5% or a little higher, up to four times daily. Both black and white mustard seed can be used for plasters, but the essential oils in white mustard seeds do not evaporate in a hot plaster.

Both seed plasters and teas kill many kinds of fungi that infect the skin.

The seeds can be ingested whole to help ease constipation and reduce stomach upset caused by acid indigestion.

Mustard plants have the ability to remove selenium from the soil. Five mustard crops in a row will pick up 50% of the soluble selenium in the top foot of soil, according to USDA researchers.

Recently, a bio-organic supplement has entered the health food marketplace, contains selenium or chromium, both sourced from Indian Mustard (*B. juncea*). The plants are grown in a greenhouse and fed mineral-enriched waters to increase the organic content transmuted by the plant. Other bio-products from *Integrated Health Technology* including zinc and multi-minerals, based on the same hyper-accumulation in selected Indian Mustard cultivars.

Indian Mustard is used in phyto-remediation, which is the removal of heavy metals from the environment. Because Indian Mustard lends itself to genetic manipulation, the development of transgenic lines that over-produce heavy metal binding peptides is possible.

Work by Eapen et al, found hairy root cultures of Indian Mustard remove uranium from water solutions, taking up 20-23% at concentrations of 5,000 microM. *Environmental Res* 2003 91:2.

Phytotech, a New Jersey remediation company, use mustard to clean up lead contamination at old battery manufacturing plants. Phyto-extraction involves metal accumulation from the soil, while phyto-stabilization is the use of plants to prevent toxic metals from entering ground water. Brown Mustard does both better than nearly any other plant. The use of soil additives can also make the toxins more easily absorbed.

In 1999, Professor Guardiola-Diaz and six undergraduate students sowed Indian Mustard on a former paint store site contaminated with over 7,000 ppm of lead. After only two planting and harvesting cycles, lead levels were cut by 66%. Today, the land is home to a neighborhood park and flourishing vegetable garden.

Phyto-remediation takes longer, but the cost is considerably less, environmentally safe, and 25-50% more effective than traditional permanent remediation technologies.

Traditional engineering approaches cost from $10-100 per cubic meter of soil, and up to three times if carted to a hazardous waste facility. Phyto-remediation, on the other hand, can cost as little as a nickel per cubic meter.

Field Mustard hyper-accumulates zinc and cadmium.

Black Mustard contains allyl isothiocyanate, a compound toxic to the potato cyst nematode *Heterodera rostochiensis*. AITC is toxic to wireworms and pea root rot fungus.

AITC from steam distilled *B. junea* seed has been tested as a possible preservative for modified atmospheric packaging.

Mustard greens (*B. juncea*) are a favorite in the southern United States, often boiled with salt pork and onions, and hot cornbread to sop it all up.

In Russia, the seeds are ground into yellow flour, known as Sarepta or Russian Mustard. The fixed oil is used much like olive oil.

Several sub-species include Chinese mustard greens, Gai Choy, and Pai-tsai. These are eaten raw in salads like lettuce or spinach, or steamed, in soups, or stir-fries.

Mustard greens are easy to grow, maturing in only 5-7 weeks.

The leaves of Mizuna are widely used in both Japanese and Chinese cooking, usually in stir-fries and steamed dishes.

It makes an excellent cream soup, garnished with Chinese chives.

The plant is both cold and wet resistant, and will sometimes survive the first snowfall. It also has the advantage of not going to seed in hot weather.

English mustard, made correctly with cold water and allowed to stand for ten minutes, is clean and pungent.

Then add vinegar to kill the enzyme myrosinase and you retain that degree of heat and flavour. Milk, wine and beer can be used, the latter giving a very hot product.

Worldwide there are over 1000 varieties of mustard.

Three places are worthy of note. In Mount Horeb, Wisconsin is a Mustard Museum, with over 3,122 prepared mustards to sample and purchase. See www.mustardweb.com.

In early spring, the annual Napa Valley Mustard Festival is held, with some 250 entrants from around the world. The website is www. mustardfestival.org.

And of course, if you ever visit Dijon, France, be sure to visit their Mustard Museum.

Mustard makes a good green manure, especially to deter wireworms that attack carrots and potatoes; and to ward off snails. Mustard powder sprinkled amongst daffodils is said to give them better color.

Wild Mustard (*S. arvensis*) pollen and nectar is used by bees as part of honey production on the prairies. In one study in Saskatchewan, the pollen was found in 55% of samples.

In parts of Europe, the seeds are used to make poor quality table mustard, and the greens eaten as a salad.

Mustard may be used as a substitute for sulfites in stabilizing semi-sweet wines. Work by Chalenko and Korsakova conducted in Russia in 1961, used 0.4 grams of mustard per liter of wine, with very good results.

It also works for stabilizing fruit juice, in this case using 11-22 ppm of mustard oil, to retard fermentation. Kosker et al, 1949.

Ice, containing 5% mustard powder, doubles the storage period of fresh fish.

Carrots, powdered with mustard, had a 92% survival rate after 160 days in sand, or 55 days in wood shavings.

White Mustard seed powder contains phenethyl isothiocyanate. Research by Lim et al, *J Ag Food Chem* 2008 56:21 found this compound has 48 folder greater activity than benzyl benzoate to control dust mites.

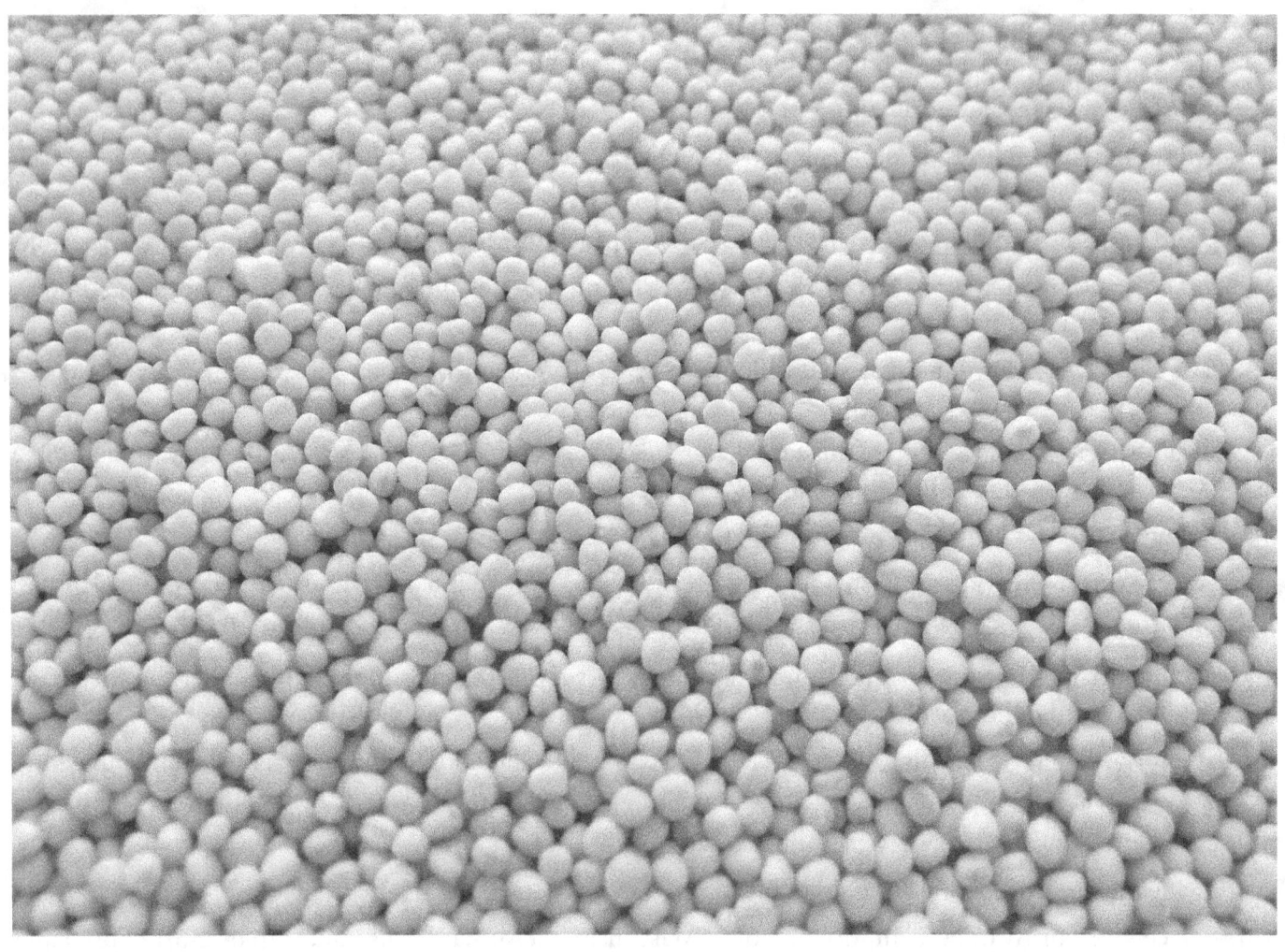

WHITE MUSTARD SEEDS

MEDICINAL

CONSTITUENTS- *B. alba* seeds- glucosinolates chiefly sinalbin; p-hydroxybenzyl isothiocyanate, fatty oils (20-35%), proteins (40%), phenyl propane derivatives including sinapine, the choline ester of sinapic acid (1.5%).
White mustard does not contain allyl isothiocyante.
B. juncea and *B. nigra* seed–sinigrin, allyl isothiocyanate, sinapic acid.
B. campestris seed- wild 26% protein, cultivated, 20%; glucosinolates- 0.92% wild, 1.13% cultivated.
S. nigra leaf- various phenolic acids including caffeic, p-coumaric, and protocatechuic acid; flavonoids including isorhamnetin, kaempferol, myricetin, myricetin-3-glucoside, quercitin, quercitin-glucuronide.

Both White and Black Mustard seed powders act as a counter-irritant to induce inflammation. This causes dilation of the blood vessels, thus increasing the flow of blood to the area. Used externally, mustard plasters are an age-old remedy for chest and bronchial problems. It also gives relief to cold, painful, arthritic joints of old age.

Acute cardiac pain, whether due to angina pectoris or not, is relieved by mustard plaster. See recipes below. The mechanism of mustard plasters and their effect on the immune system is not well studied. One possibility is that the active compound, sinapine thiocyanate, found it accumulates in the stratum corneum and that cytokines including interleukin 1beta and tumor necrosis factor alpha were increased.

Langerhans epidermal cells were significantly reduced in density and increased in shape factor. This may explain in part the use for asthma and bronchitis. Guo X et al, *Int J Pharm* 2013 457(1): 136-42. Or maybe it is simply the counter-irritant effect that moves more blood to the area.

Mustard baths at about 28° Celsius give a sense of coldness, according to Dr. King, "and even distinct chills may be felt in the limbs, abdomen and back. This continues until the person is removed from the bath, when stinging, glowing, and burning of the surface indicate that reaction is established."

The seed tea is good for colds, influenza and early stages of fevers. The tea will rapidly increase sweating, and thereby reduce any raised temperatures. It will sometimes help bring on a delayed menstruation, if due to cold or exhaustion.

For hypothermia, take a quarter of a teaspoon of mustard powder in some honey or a banana, to stimulate body heat. A commercial bath preparation, with mustard powder and various essential oils is on the market. Mustard baths are also useful in the treatment of paralytic symptoms.

Mustard footbaths are good for treating headaches by drawing congestion out of the head region. At the first sign of cold, sore throat, flu or fever, a bedtime footbath will help re-circulate blood flow, and give rapid relief.

Sinapic acid is a potent anti-inflammatory. Work by Yun et al, *J Ag Food Chem* 2008 56:21 found the compound suppressed iNOS, COX-2, TNF alpha, and interleukin IB via NFkappaB pathways.

Like Cayenne, you can sprinkle mustard powder into your socks or mittens for winter activities like skiing, ice fishing.

The Germans authorities approve of white mustard seed in the form of a poultice for helping joint and soft tissue complaints. An expert panel recommended mustard oils for acute uncomplicated respiratory tract infections. *MMW Fortschr Med* 2015 157(18):76-7.

White mustard seed is not as well flavored but the enzymes are strong and not as easily disturbed or damaged as *B. nigra*. It is strongly preservative, discouraging mold and bacteria; and for this reason used in pickles. It also aids emulsifying and helping prevent mayonnaise from "breaking".

Mustard gum has properties similar to xanthan gum for emulsion and stability in food products. It has a unique 1,4 beta glucan content that shows modest glycemic index in both normal and diabetic volunteers. Work by Begin et al, *Can J Physio Pharmacol* 1988:67 found yellow mustard gum significantly decreased postprandial insulin levels by slowing glucose absorption and delaying gastric emptying.

The gum also shows promise against colon cancers, in bird models.

Dr. Michael Eskin at the University of Manitoba has done a lot of work on the isolation, and health properties of mustard gums. A publication by the author in *Phytomedicine* 14:7-8 2007 found mustard mucilage deterred colon cancer cell development in rat studies.

Organic isothiocyanates inhibit tumor formation in breast, colon, lung and skin tissue in animal models. Tseng et al, *Pharm Res* 2002 19. This study also found dietary organic isothiocyanates inhibited the P-gp- and MRP1-mediated transport in multi-drug resistance-associated human cancer cell lines. For example, added to diet, the compounds inhibited the efflux of daunomycin and vinblastine in MDR human cancer cells, enhancing the efficacy of cancer chemotherapy.

Sinigrin inhibits HL60 human leukemia cell lines. Lozano-Baena MD et al, *Molecules* 2015 20(9): 15748-65.

The compound inhibits production of inflammatory mediators and has immune modulating effects. Lee HW et al, *Int Immunopharmacol* 2017 45: 163-73.

A review of sinigrin and its therapeutic benefits has been published. Mazumder A et al, *Molecules* 2016 21(4): 416.

Two compounds in white mustard have been shown to prevent induced benign prostatic hypertrophy in animal studies.

Black Mustard water extracts given to diabetic induced rats, showed reduce serum glucose levels, increased serum insulin, and release of insulin from pancreas, suggesting benefit in blood sugar elevation. Anand et al, *Exp Clin Endocrin Diabetes* 2009 117:6.

Black mustard seeds may be useful in the treatment and prophylaxis of malaria, albeit a mouse study. Muluye AB et al, *BMC Complement Altern Med* 2015 15:367.

The leaves of Indian Mustard (*B. juncea*) are used medicinally to treat various gastric, cardiac, bronchial and urinary disorders. Known in TCM as **GAI CAI** or **GAI JIE**, meaning mustard vegetable, both the seed and leaf are used.

The former will help induce sweating, while the seed is warming to the lungs and helps clear phlegm. The seeds should be used with caution in cases of fever or heart problems, due to their warming nature.

One study appears to indicate that Mustard greens can play an anti-oxidant role in high fat diets.

Khan et al, *Indian Journal of Experimental Biology* 1997 35:2 fed a high fat diet (20% coconut oil) along with 10% mustard greens to a group of rats. Their conclusion after a twenty-day supplementation was mustard leaf can prevent the formation of free radicals and maintain body tissues at a normal level, despite a high fat diet.

Indian Mustard seed appears to possess hypoglycemic activity. In a study by Khan et al, *Indian Journal of Biochemistry and Biophysics* 1995 32:2 the seed showed effect on carbohydrate metabolism by increasing hepatic glycogen and glycogenesis, and decreasing the activity of glycogen phosphorylase and gluconeogenic enzymes.

Work by Kim et al, identified anti-oxidant properties that appear to ameliorate the effects of diabetes. *Phytotherapy Research* 17:5.

Zou et al, *J Agric Food Chem* 2002 50 has found sinapic acid from *B. juncea* has an efficient peroxynitrate scavenging ability. This compound forms from a reaction of superoxide and nitric oxide, and is one of the most potent cytotoxic species known to oxidize essential proteins, lipids and DNA.

This compound is involved in various inflammatory conditions, as well as several gastrointestinal disorders.

Tyrosine, for example, will form 3-nitrotyrosine, which has been detected in various diseases, including atherosclerotic lesions in human blood vessels.

Sinapic acid may be useful for inducing hair growth and treatment of alopecia, via expression of various growth factors. Woo H et al, *Arch Dermatol Res* 2017 Mar 20.

Sinapic acid may protect from cadmium-induced nephrotoxicity, due to antioxidant, anti-inflammatory and anti-apoptotic potential. Ansari MA et al, *Environ Toxicol Pharmacol* 2017 51: 100-7.

It also mitigates gentamicin-induced kidney toxicity when taken concurrently. Ansari MA et al, *Life Sci* 2016 165:1-8.

Ethanol extracts of *B. campestris* seed, taken orally, reduce skin papilloma. Qiblawi et al, *Phtyo Res* 13:3.

Brassinosteroids found in many species of this genus has been found to inhibit breast and prostate cancer cell lines by arresting at G1 phase and induced apoptosis. Malikova et al, *Phytochem* 2008 69:2.

Fatty acid derivatives from pollen of *B. campestris* var. *oleifera* are aromatase inhibitors, suggesting benefit in prevention of hormone-sensitive cancers. Yang et al, *J Asian Nat Prod Res* 2009 11:2.

One unusual study involving white mustard seeds is for auricular acupressure. In one study, 49 female college students considered obese or overweight, were asked to stimulate five auricular points ten times at a rate of two times per second, thirty minutes before meals, three times daily for one month. Compared to control group, the mustard seed students shows significant decreases in weight and body mass index. Kim D et al, *J Altern Complement Med* 2014(4): 258-64.

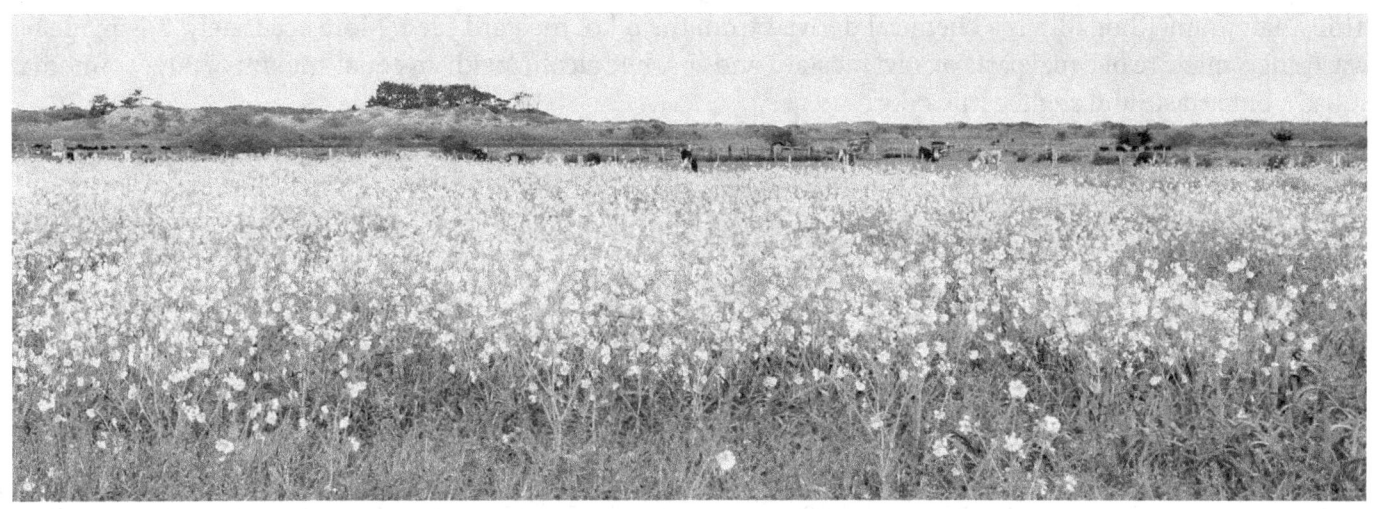

WILD MUSTARD FIELD

HOMEOPATHY

White Mustard (*S. alba*) is used when throat symptoms are pronounced, especially pressure and burning, with obstruction of the esophagus.

There may be a sensation of a lump in the esophagus behind the manubrium sternum with much eructation and heartburn. There may also be similar sensation in the anus.

Mind is easily distracted when reading, must make great effort to prevent thoughts from wandering and must read a sentence several times before understanding.

Dreams of journey and of dangers, falling from heights, of dead people, devils and thieves, of foreign countries and dangerous expeditions.

It is also indicated for coryza and hay fever. In the German monograms, *S. alba* is indicated for inflammation of the respiratory and gastro-intestinal tract.

DOSE- Third potency. The mother tincture is prepared from the ripe seeds. First proving was self-experiment by Bojanus in Russia with grain doses of triturated seeds and tincture. Clinical observation by Hering as well.

Black Mustard minds are irritable, cross, dissatisfied, provoked by the least unpleasant thing or wholly causeless; don't want to be spoken to, answers short and snappy. Mind works more rapidly at night, easier to study and perception is clearer.

Great desire to stay in bed. Sensations like weight below belly button, hot water in blood vessels, something stuck in trachea. Dry, short hacking cough worse from cold air and laughing; better from lying down and eating. Heart on the right side.

Mucous membranes are dry and hot, often no discharge from nose, worse in afternoon and evening.

DOSE- First to 30th dilution. First proving by Butler with one female and nine males at 1x, 2x, 15x, and 30x in 1871. Clinical observations by Hering are included.

Krichbaum writes in 1908. "Another striking and peculiar symptom which may spread sudden illumination in these all too common cases of catarrhal difficulties, is that the patient complains of or notes the odd fact that sweat appears on the upper lip and forehead. This symptom appeared in a patient of mine every time he ate mustard pickles, his scalp became hot and itching violently. These peculiarities plus an excoriating discharge which would blister almost instantly the part coming in contact with it, led me to prescribe this remedy in a case of Lupus Vulgaris, with prompt relief of the then acute activity of the disease."

Thiosinaminum-Rhodallin is a chemical derived from the oil of mustard seed. More accurately, it is made by warming a mixture of equal parts of allyl mustard and absolute alcohol with an equal amount of 30% ammonia. It has a bitter taste and slight garlic odor.

It is a resolvent, used both externally and internally, for dissolving scar tissue, tumours, enlarged glands, lupus, strictures, adhesions, cataracts, fibroids and scleroderma.

In veterinary medicine, it is used to minimize scar tissue.

It has been suggested for use by Dr. A. S. Hard for retarding aging.

Also a remedy for *Tabes dorsalis*, helping improve the lightning pains. For stricture of the rectum use 2 grains daily.

It is useful for tinnitus and otosclerosis vertigo; catarrhal deafness with cicatricial thickening; sub-acute suppurative otitis media, and formation of fibrous bands impeding free movement of the ossicles. Deafness related to fibrous changes in the nerve may be helped.

The mind is active and body sluggish. Contented with self, unaffected by unusual amounts of criticism. Delusions that body is thin (think Anorexia nervosa). Delusion that time is wasted, sensitive to odors. Like *Cochlearia officinalis*, dreams of being stuck and unable to move.

DOSE- Inject under the skin, or into a lesion as a 10% solution in glycerine and water; 15-30 drops twice a week.

Internally, in 4-8 grain capsules every other day. For obstinate otosclerotic conditions one half grain three times daily, never more.

For vertigo and arthritis, try 2X. Proving was by Tony Grinney on six females and three males at 6c, 30c, 200 and 1M in 1998. Clinical observations by David Riley, presented at Professional Case Conference IFH 1994.

Riley says. "The most striking cases in terms of consistent results were three cases of infertility secondary to pelvic inflammatory disease. The patients in these cases had several symptoms in common: the appearance of scarring (particularly pelvic scarring), in conjunction with depression, alternating moods, and aversion to consolation. They also had confirmatory symptoms of seasonal allergies and increased urination at night."

ESSENTIAL OIL

White Mustard essential oil exhibits characteristics quite the opposite of Black Mustard, with little odour and a very, sharp pungent taste.

It must be obtained by solvent extraction from the seedcake, because it does not contain a volatile essential oil. Prior to distillation, the seed cake must be hydrolyzed to release sinapine acid sulfate from the sinalabin glucoside.

In both white and black mustard, the aromatic components do not exist in a free state in the seeds, but are produced only as a result of myrosin decomposition of the glycosides when the crushed seeds are mixed with water.

An essential oil of the seeds contains 68 compounds, with 4-hydroxy benzene acetonitrile at 29.6%.

White Mustard seeds contain 33% dimethyl trisulphide, 10.5% heptadecane, and 9.1% methyl pentadecane.

An essential oil is produced from the black mustard seedcake, after the seed oil has been expressed.

Prior to distillation, it is necessary to hydrolyze the press cake to release allyl isothiocyanate from the sinigrin glucoside.

The essential oil is a clear, pale yellow, with a very intense odour having lachrymatory effects with relatively poor flavour. It has a specific gravity of 1.014-1.022; an allyl isothiocyanate content of 94%.

Black mustard essential oil is used extensively in flavouring sauces, and condiments.

This same essential oil has been proved to be more effective as a preservative, even at 0.1% against fungal infection of rape, Indian mustard, flaxseed, lentils, mung beans in natural storage than propionic acid; and with no phytotoxicity.

CAUTION- Never taste or smell undiluted oil. It is very toxic. Toxic mustard gases used during the war contain derivatives of allyl isothiocyanate, as do certain chemotherapy drugs.

SEED OIL

Take mustard seeds and crush. Add two parts of vegetable oil to one part of powder by weight, and gently simmer for one half hour. Strain and bottle. Use for cold, arthritic joints.

Commercial mustard oil is fatty oil obtaining by pressing the seeds of the Field Mustard (*B. campestris*), Rape (*B. napus*), and even *Turnip* (*B. rapa*) and other mustards.

In work conducted by Choudbury et al, 1997, it was found that mustard oil exhibits greater anti-carcinogenic effect in animals with arsenic induced chromosomal aberrations than garlic.

Fatty acids from mustard seed oil, both raw and heated, caused astrocyte maturation in serum cultures.

Astrocytes are involving in brain health and may be related to cognitive conditions such as dementia and Alzheimer's disease. Joardar et al, *Cell Mol Neurobiol* 2007 27:8 973-83.

The press cake contains about 5% mucilage composed of 15% glucuronic and galacturonic acids, 24% glucose, 14% galactose, 6% mannose, 3% rhamnose, 3% arabinose, and 1.8% xylose.

Gums used commercially are not normally extracted from oilseeds or the press cake. Paper Mate uses mustard oil in their Liquid Paper All Purpose Correction Pen.

Studies by Barber et al, in 1974, studied the gums from *Lesquerella* species for entrapment of mosquito larvae. Perhaps white mustard gums have similar application, combined with Shepherd's Purse seeds.

Black mustard seed yields 28.5% oil, consisting of 15.5% linolenic acid, 33.9% erucic acid, and glucosinolate concentration of 217 umol/gram.

Birds rape mustard seed yields 37% oil containing 9% linolenic acid, 47% erucic acid and 177 umol/gram.

Wild Mustard seed contains 25.8% oil, consisting of 13.6% linolenic acid, 21% erucic acid and 138 umol/g. The oil has been used traditionally to make soap, as a lubricant and as a cooking oil.

The latter use is not recommended, due to the content of glucosinolates.

Indian mustard seed yields 6.7% oil that has shown activity against a range of pathogenic organisms.

Optimal essential oil production from *B. juncea* were for two hours at 70 C, with a pH of 4.5, and 0.02 mg/gram of ascorbic acid.

The oil contains 14 components the main one being allyl isothiocyanate at 43.8%. Others are 3-methylthiopropyl isothiocyanate (9.4%), 3-butenyl iso-thiocyanate (4.8%), butyl isothiocyanate (4.7%), phenyl isothiocyanate (3.7%) and 2-phenylethyl isothiocyanate (3.7%).

A study reported in *Fitoterapia* 1993, showed the oil had significant effect on both Gram positive and negative bacteria; as well as fungi such as *Aspergillus flavus* and *A. niger*. It has greater anti-microbial activity than cinnamon, cloves or cassia. Blum et al, *Fruit Products Journal* 1943.

Mustard oil contains glycosides that provide anti-oxidant protection for oils and fats.

Plant breeding programs have been attempting to develop a canola quality *B. juncea* plant. The idea was to take the drought resistant of mustard and combine it with canola quality; much easier than the other way around from a breeding perspective.

Fifteen years ago, in Saskatoon, plant breeders at Agricultural and Agri-Food Canada (AAFC) started working on this plant, believing it would be classified as canola.

If the seed looked like canola, crushed like canola, and tasted like canola, there shouldn't be a need for separate registration.

But biotechnology and consumer concern over transgenic crops has changed this; even though Indian Mustard is not a transgenic crop.

Health Canada would like proof that canola quality *B. juncea* is non-allergenic. And of course, the pesticides registered on canola and mustards may need to be registered for use on canola quality *B. juncea*.

Internationally, the product would need to obtain GRAS status in the United States.

The fifteen years have produced seed oil equal to the higher oil yields of canola, with a similar fatty acid composition. The Saskatchewan Wheat Pool trademarked the new species, *Prairie Canola*.

Mustard oil by inhalation acts on the sensory nerve ending of the trigeminal nerve. It relieves pain in middle ear diseases, and in painful conditions of the nose, throat, nasal cavities and tonsils.

Mustard oil is used in Ayurvedic Medicine, and called **SARSAPA**. It is used for parasitic infections, itching, obstinate skin diseases. It is pungent, depleting and a digestive stimulant.

Black Mustard seed oil is used as an active ingredient in some commercial dog and cat repellants.

It is also used as a lubricant and illuminant in soaps.

HYDROSOL

The distilled water of the herb, when it is in the flower, is much used to drink inwardly to wash the mouth when the palate is down, and for any disease of the throat to gargle, but outwardly also for scabs, itch, or other the like infirmities, and cleanses the face from morphew, spots, freckles, and other deformities.
CULPEPPER

The distilled water of mustard flowers is good for pain in the teeth, cold gout and causing the flesh to grow again, according to Brunschwig.

Recent studies on diabetic-induced rats fed black mustard water, found lowered serum lipids and decreased glycosylated hemoglobin levels.

FLOWER ESSENCES

Mustard (*S. arvensis*) flower essence is for melancholy, gloom, despair and depression. It is as if a cloud has descended just on you, without any obvious cause.

The flower essence helps one re-find joy in life and more balance with the ups and downs of life. **BACH**
Mustard is prepared by sun method.

When depression drops like a cloud from the sky, you don't know where it came from, and you don't know why. You don't know how to cure it or how long it's gonna stay. If you take Mustard, it'll help it go away.
D. CUNNINGHAM

SPIRITUAL PROPERTIES

To dream of mustard means you have faith that all things are possible; or that you will soon be rewarded for past work.

To dream of eating seeds and feel them in your mouth, signals that you have done something for which you now feel sorry.

If you dream of eating unripe green mustard seeds, it shows impatience and a need for instant gratification. Farmers, dreaming of a field of yellow blossoms, are a sign of a successful crop and joy. **ANTOL**

PERSONALITY TRAITS

Mustard plants only develop when a field is left empty, the soil bare. The Mustard state follows disturbance of the settled pattern of life (ploughing) and only takes root in the mind because there is some inactivity in the will (an empty field).

So Mustard is an opportunistic pattern of interference, a form of possession, which takes up residence only because of the weakness of the host.

The image of an empty, ploughed field (or even upturned earth) invites such thoughts. There is something unnatural about land devoid of all plants. Today, when farmers spray fields with weed-killer, before planting and ploughing, there is cause to wonder about the effect on the psyche of the planet. Eradicate all plants from a field and what will enter?

The psyche of the planet may be too abstruse a concept, but the complex relationships of plant to earth, of biodiversity and subtlety in thought are the very things forced under by the bulldozer of materialism.

BARNARD

If I had to give it a human dimension, I'd say that the mustard plant would make a fairly agreeable houseguest. It wouldn't mind sleeping on the floor, would gladly cook for itself and would never use up all the hot water.

DEWEY

MYTHS AND LEGENDS

One of the better known phrases associated with this plant is "to cut the mustard." It is related to someone with the youth and vigour required to do something well.

In the early 1900s, phrases such as "up to the mustard", and "keen as mustard", were in common use. In the 1920s, to be mustard was to be very good at some enterprise, or if applied to a female, as in "she's real mustard", to connotate a hot tamale.

Lovers with robust bedtime maneuvers were said to really be "cutting the mustard". Today it is often used as a negative phrase, related more to physical or mental exertions.

After the passing of her only child, a woman sought medicine from the Buddha to restore her son to life. The Buddha instructed her to obtain a handful of mustard seeds from a house where no one had lost a child, husband, parent or friend. When she was unable to find such a house, she realized that death is common to all humankind; she buried her son, and took comfort in the teaching of the Buddha.   **MERCATANTE**

In a legend from India, a man was changed into a buffalo and sold by his evil wife, who had turned into a witch. A good witch changed him back, and gave him some magic mustard seeds, which he sprinkled on his wife, turning her into a horse.

Another Indian legend tells of a farmer and his wife who were unable to have children. One day he plowed over the ancient temple of a nymph known as Bakawali, and a mustard plant grew on the spot. When the farmer's wife consumed the mustard seed, she gave birth to a baby girl, who turned out to be the re-incarnated form of Bakawali herself.   **SMALL**

In Hindu myths, mustard seed enabled people to travel through the air, helping them locate treasures within the earth, and gave them the ability to effect transformations.

A farmer and his wife had tried for some time to have a child, but the woman did not conceive until she consumed some magic mustard. The farmer plowed a field over the site of an ancient temple where a nymph named Bakawali had lived, and mustard grew on the spot. Later, after his wife consumed the mustard seed, she miraculously gave birth to a baby girl. Even more miraculously, the baby girl appeared to be Bakawali herself, reincarnated in another form—transformed by the power of mustard.   **TAMRA ANDREWS**

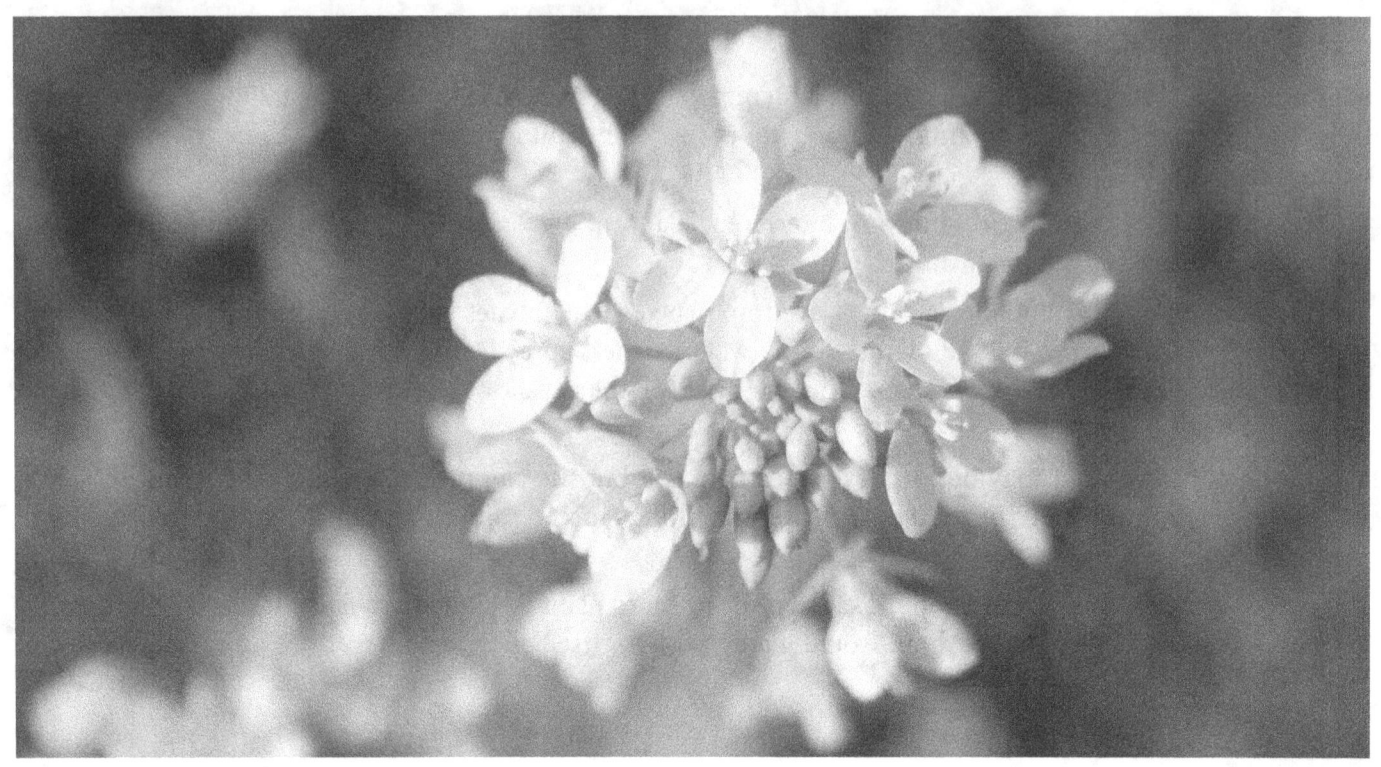

MUSTARD FLOWERS

BOTANICA POETICA

Here's an interesting seed
Growing wild as a weed
It's a spice that you might know
Stimulates the blood to flow
It's very hot and warming too
It can be taken for the flu
Breaks up mucous, clearing phlegm
Mustard is this little gem
If you need a fast emetic
Toss the cookies in an instant
A tablespoon of the seed
Is just the thing you might need
Mustard seed is really strong
For aching joints that have gone wrong
Use it as an application
It stimulates the circulation
When pneumonia has you flat
Rub it on your chest and back
Draw the toxins out of you
Decrease a fever as you do
Yes, indeed a Mustard plaster
Get the healing going faster
Burn the skin if you overdo
Aches and pains away with you!

SYLVIA CHATROUX

RECIPES

FOOTBATH- One tablespoon of mustard seeds to one litre of hot water.

Do not use mustard oil preparations, including plasters, in cases of severe circulation disorders, varicose veins and other vein problems.

MUSTARD PLASTER- Be careful with mustard plasters, as blistering, ulceration and tissue damage can occur if left on skin for too long.

To prepare, take one part of dry mustard to ten parts of flour. Add enough warm water to make a paste. Spread evenly on a piece of cloth and cover with another. Apply a vegetable oil to chest and apply for up to twenty minutes. A 1:4 ratio may be used for short period of time. Skin will turn pink, but not a raw, ugly red. Remove if too intense.

Cases of hyperthyroidism with goiter have been traced to the isothiocyanates in mustard preparations. Individuals with low-functioning thyroid should also avoid excessive use.

Health Canada restricts mustard oil content in liniments to 0.5-5%.

ORIENTAL KNEE BATH- Add one cup of mustard powder to a hot bath, deep enough to cover affected area. Bathe for 15 minutes, and then shower with cool water.

MUSTARD LEAF PICKLE- (*B. juncea*) The mustard plant is wilted dry, salted and pressed under a heavy stone in a jar. The liquid is drained off, more salt added and pressed again. It ferments 5-10 days at between 5-30°C. Repeat as before, then wash, and add garlic, ginger and cumin, pasteurize at 80°C for fifteen minutes, cool and package. It will keep six months at room temperature, used as a side dish.

NIGELLA
BLACK CUMIN
FENNEL FLOWER
BARAKA
(*Nigella sativa* L.)
(*N. indica* Roxb. ex Flem.) not accepted
LOVE IN A MIST
VIRGIN IN THE GREEN
STRAWBERRY CUMIN
DEVIL IN THE BUSH
(*N. damascena* L.)

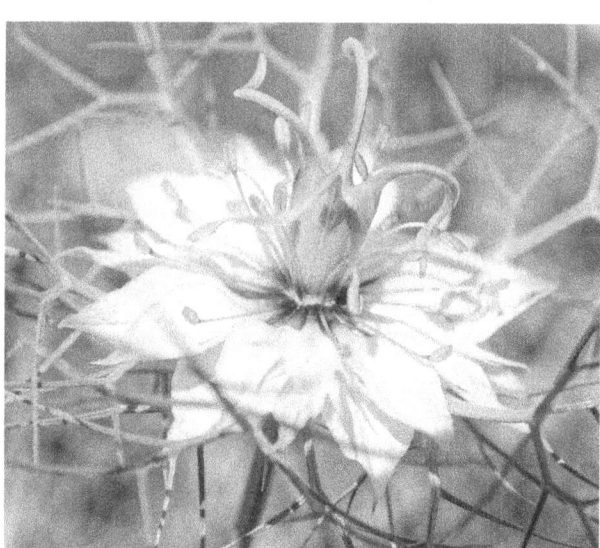

NIGELLA FLOWER

Their names were nymphs, and they were nymphs indeed
A whole mythology from pinch of seed,
Nemesia and Viscaria, and that
Blue as the butterfly, Phacelia;
Love in mist Nigella whose shining brat
Appears unwanted like a very weed.

V. SACKVILLE-WEST

Let all the black seed upon you, these contain cure of all diseases except death.

RASOOL ALLAH

Curative black cumin.

ISAIAH 28:25

Yet marked I where the bolt of Cupid fell:
It fell upon a little western flower.
Before milk-white, now purple with love's wound, and maidens call it, Love-in-idleness.

SHAKESPEARE: A MIDSUMMER NIGHT'S DREAM

Nigella is from the diminutive Latin **NIGER**, meaning small black, and referring to the seed colour and size.

Damascena refers the city of Damascus where the plant is believed to originate.

Both Nigella species are annuals that will complete their growth to mature seed on the prairies if they get enough heat. They require minimal moisture and love porous, sandy soil.

Love in a mist refers to the fine hair-like leaves surrounding the flowers. The fine hairs must have been suggestive, the French calling them "Chevaux de Venus", the Germans "Venushaar", meaning Venus Hair. Up until the 18th century, brides wore long hair decorations to demonstrate virginity. Another name was Capuchin's Beard.

In the Middle East, seeds are put into cakes and breads. The Syrian Book of Medicine suggests its main use is for headaches.

The German nickname, strawberry cumin, or **ERDBEERKUMMEL** does not really explain the flavour, which is more like pineapple when the seeds are crushed.

Gerard says that the seed drunk with wine is a remedy for shortness of breath. He suggested that Love in a Mist would "bringeth down the menses".

Egyptian ladies were said to eat them to produce stoutness.

Medicinally, it was combined with *Plumbago* root for digestive complaints and intermittent fevers.

It was a favoured medicine in India, to give new mothers after childbirth.

The seeds are often used to adulterate the more valuable black cumin, but the oil, which can be obtained in larger amounts, is also lower in active constituents.

The seed of *N. damascena* smells like grape soft drink when rubbed between the fingers. An early Latin name was *Papaver nigrum*, meaning Black Poppy, due to the narcotic effect of the alkaloid damascene.

It is dedicated to St. Catherine, and the patroness of spinsters. She was successful at converting folks to Christianity, and then ordered to death by Emperor Maxentius.

She met her death via a wheel stuck with spikes; and then beheaded. The linear foliage bears some resemblance to a wheel.

It has another side. If a young girl handed the flower to an admirer, it meant to leave her alone. It was used to send someone packing by placing it in a covered basket. In Victorian flower symbolism it stands for perplexity and "you puzzle me".

The flower is used in bread dough as a topping for decoration.

At one time, the seeds were burned to protect against fleas, gnats and other insects.

The flower has an ingenious hinged lid that keeps unwanted insects from stealing nectar.

Black Cumin is a popular spice in India, Turkey, Greece, and all over the Middle East, including Tunisia, and Egypt.

The seeds have a spicy, fruity taste, but were supplanted with the more recent popularity of pepper.

They smell aromatic, more like fennel than cumin with a touch of nutmeg or camphor. Others describe the aroma like lemony carrots with hint of nutmeg. Some authors say oregano-like with a peppery nutmeg taste.

It is popular in spreads and soft cheeses. A popular hot dog shaped croquette in the Middle East made with bulgar wheat and lamb is spiced with the ground seed.

Dioscorides called the pale blue flowered, black-seeded plant, **MELANTHION**, meaning Black Leaf. He recommended the seed for headache, toothache, nasal congestion and intestinal worms. The seeds were found buried with King Tut, suggestive of their value.

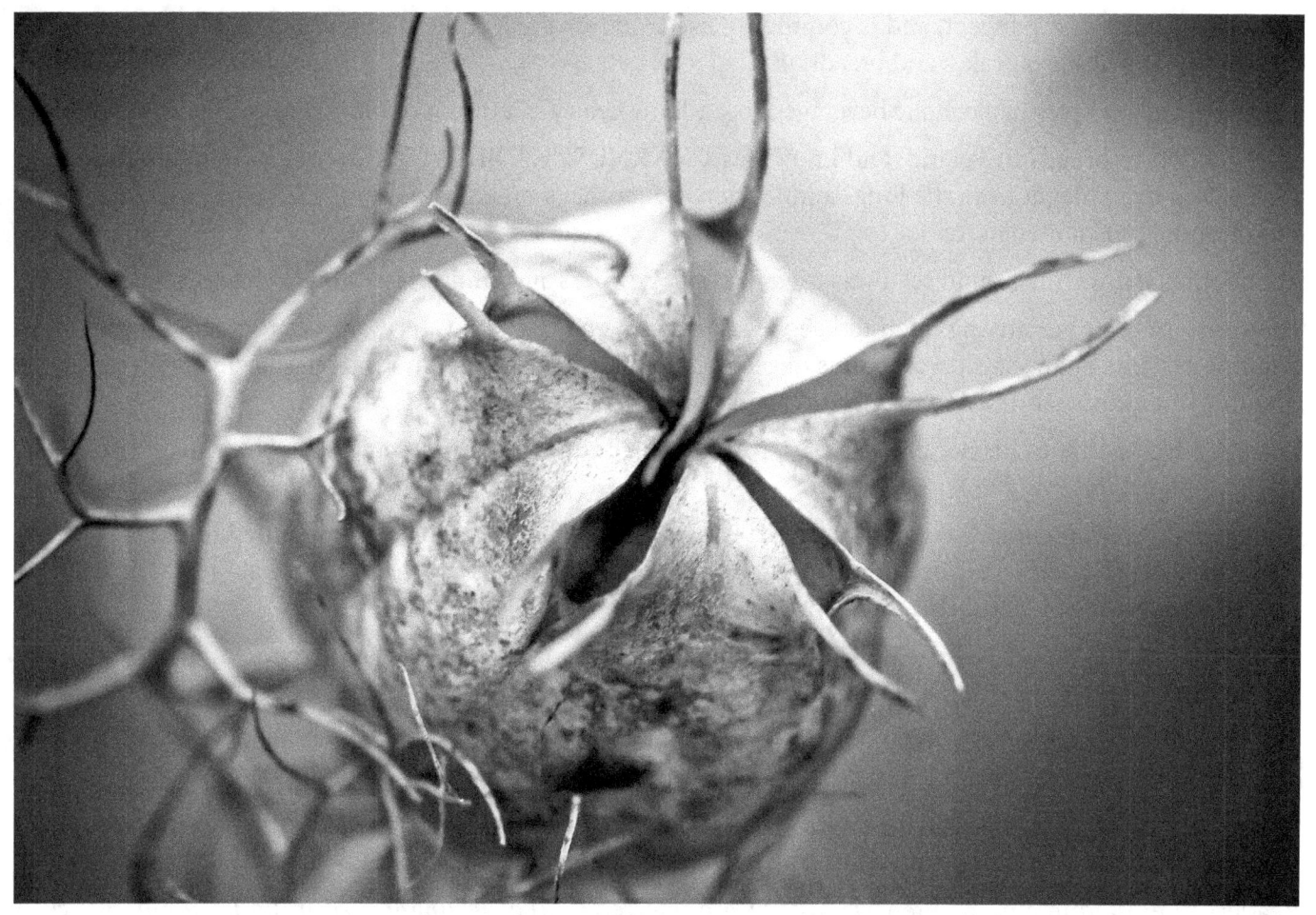

NIGELLA SEED POD

Greek physicians classified the herb as hot and dry to the third degree, meaning it warms up the center and opens the skin to release toxins.

In ancient Latin, the seed was called **PANACEA**, meaning cure all.

Arabic, Persian and Hindu physicians know Nigella as **HABBATOUSSOUDA, SIYAN-DANAH,** or **KALA-DANAH**, meaning Black Seed in all three languages. **HABBAT EL BARAKA** is an Arabic word meaning "seeds of blessing".

An ancient Syrian herb book calls it Black Tin-tir.

In the Old Testament of the Bible, it is called **FITCHES** from the Hebrew for vetch, **KETZAH**. See Isaiah 28:25-27.

Kala-Danah is a common Asian name associated with pre-European medicinal and religious plants, and associated with a number of plants. Pliny called it Git, similar to the Arabic Gith.

Its use medicinally goes back at least 3600 years. A recent archeological find in north central Turkey was a flask containing the seed mixed with propolis and beeswax.

Hildegard de Bingen, under its name **GITHERUM RATDE**, suggested crushing the seeds and combining with honey. This is smeared on the wall to attract flies that will taste it, sicken and fall dead.

The Romans used it for flavouring food; the French as a substitute for pepper, calling it **QUATRE EPICES**, or **TOUTE EPICE**.

The seed is spicy, and pungent, and is commonly used all over the Middle East and into India for flavouring curries and a sprinkle on cakes and breads.

In Ethiopia, it is a spice in alcoholic beverages, like adding celery salt to rim of Bloody Mary, on this continent.

It was added to breads in Poland, and known as **CZARNUSZKA SIEWNA**. The seeds were also added to wine to remove phlegm from the lungs and to increase mother's milk. It was combined with wormwood as a summertime mosquito deterrent.

At one time, the warm, ground seed was used in sweet powders and sniffed to restore a lost sense of smell.

The seeds are also put among linen to keep away insects, and used by veterinary doctors to strengthen the immune systems of animals (two pounds of seeds per each ton of animal food). It has been shown to reduce allergic symptoms such as asthma and eczema in horses, and prevent mastitis in cows.

When added to diet of broiler chickens, it proved to be both an economic and efficient growth promoter. Mahmood et al, *Int J Ag Bio* 11:6.

Akhtar and Javed, *Indian Veterinary Journal* 1991 68:8 found powdered seeds (suspended in 2% tragacanth gum) were as effective as Niclosamide in treating *Moniezia* infections in sheep. Essential oil activity against tapeworm was found comparable to piperazine.

Other veterinary uses include increasing milk production in ruminants, and as an anti-oxytocic during pregnancy and birthing to retain placenta. Lab studies suggest it is a more potent galactagogue than cumin seed.

The seed alone, or combined with *Thymus vulgaris* appears useful in raising healthy rabbits, with a high level of safety. Tousson et al, *Toxicol & Health* 2011 27:2.

It was traditionally used in medicine for dropsy and kidney complaints. In fact, the hard small black seeds look like kidneys in the doctrine of signatures, and even kidney stones they help eliminate.

Readers interested in a more intensive history, are referred to *The Healing Power of Black Cumin*, by Sylvia Luetjohann.

The seeds were one of the first into space, travelling on Sputnik III in 1958.

MEDICINAL

CONSTITUENTS- *N. sativa* seed- 21% protein, 38% carbohydrates, and 35% oil.
High levels of linoleic acid, alkaloids such as nigelline, nigellone, nigellimine, nigellidine, nigellicine, nigellamine A-C, and the glycoside melanthin, volatile oils, alpha hederin, kalopanaxsaponin I, thymoquinone.
Shoot, root- vanillic acid
N. damascena seed- 1-0-(2,4-dihydroxy) benzoyl-glycerol (phenolic ester); and three other phenolic compounds, triterpene glycosides Nigellosides A-D, 3,4-dihydroxy-beta-phenethyl alcohol; 2,4-dihydroxyphenylacetic acid, and 2,4-dihydroxyphenylacetic acid methyl ester; alkaloids, flavonoids, sesquiterpenes germacrene; damascenine, and elemene, sterols, saponins, polyols, and fatty acids.

Black Cumin (Nigella) has a long history of medicinal use in Islam countries, being exported to Malaysia; and by the Unani physicians of Pakistan, and area.

Various studies, *in vitro*, *in vivo* and some human clinical trials suggests the seed is anti-inflammatory, analgesic, anti-diabetic, anti-hyperlipidemic, anti-convulsant, anti-microbial, anti-ulcer, anti-hypertensive, anti-asthmatic and anti-cancer. Dajani EZ et al, *J Physiol Pharmacol* 2016 67(6): 801-817.

A systematic review of 23 clinical trials involving 1531 patients, found fasting blood sugar was reduced significantly in 13 of studies, including levels of glycosylated hemoglobin (HbA1c). Mohtashami A et al, *J Res Med Sci* 2016 21:3.

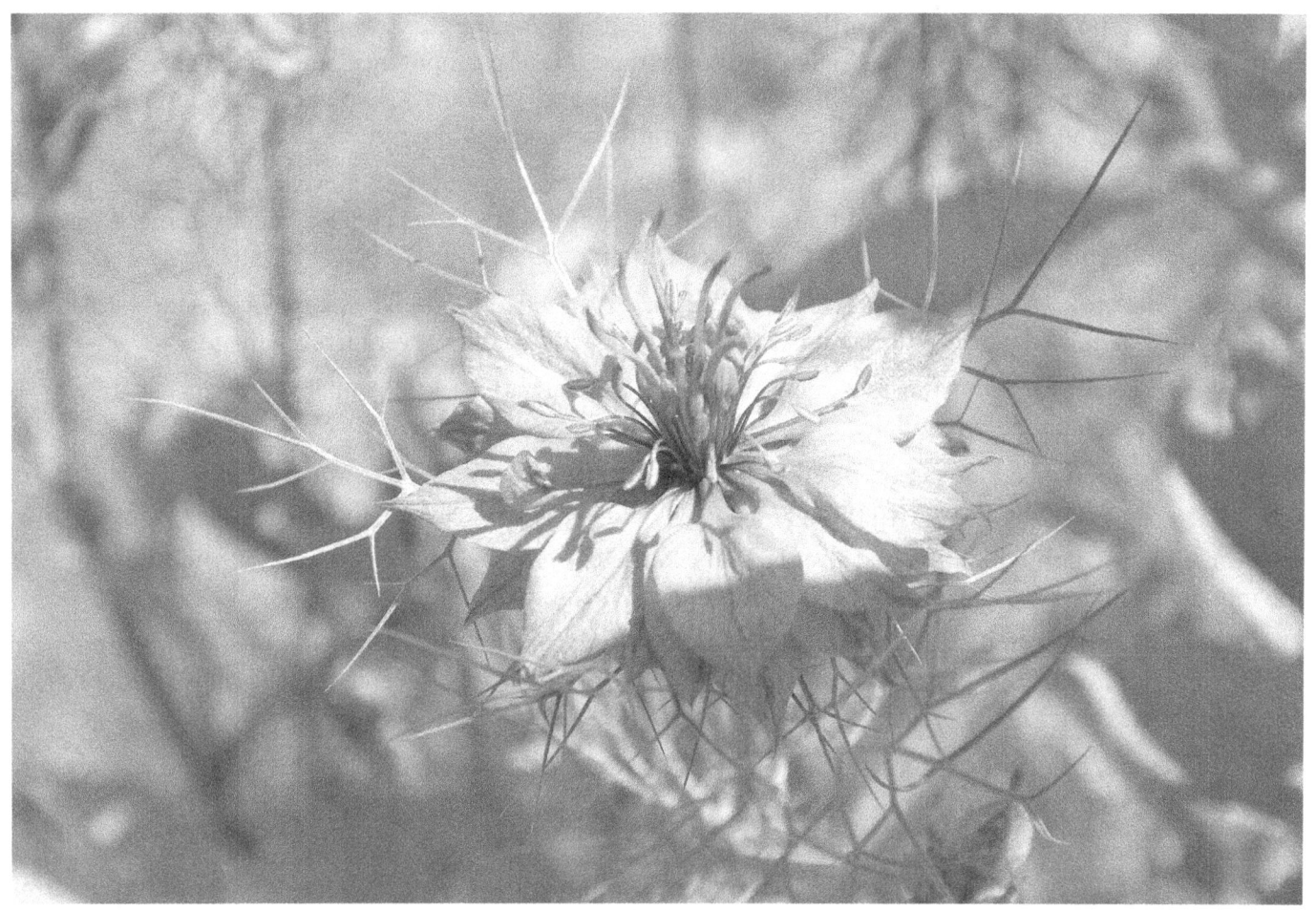

LOVE IN A MIST FLOWER

The seed is laxative, stimulates the uterus, increases lactation, reduces inflammation and improves digestion due to the bitter compounds.

The seed infusion reduces painful menstruation, and postpartum contractions. It combines well with demulcent herbs for various bronchial complaints, including asthma.

Combine Black Cumin seeds (3 parts) with licorice root (2 parts) for a great cold and flu tea.

Nigellone, in low concentrations, inhibits the release of histamine from mast cells. Chakravarty, et al, *Ann Allergy* 1993 70.

Decoctions of the ground seed help relieve airway constriction, but less than theophylline. Boskabady et al, *Phytomed* 17:10.

Work by Weinkotter et al, *Planta Medica* 2008 74:2 confirmed the antispasmodic and mucociliary clearance of nigellone.

Nigelline (damascenine) inhibits edema and is anti-pyretic in activity.

Work by Salem et al, *International Journal of Immunopharmacology* 2000 22:9 looked at the anti-viral effect of black cumin seed. It showed a striking antiviral effect against murine cytomegalovirus infection that may be medicated by increasing the Mphi number and function, as well as IFN gamma, or interferon production.

Black Cumin seed supports the metabolism, digestion, and helps lower blood sugar levels. Al-Awadi et al, *Diabetes Research* 1991 18:4.

Matthew Wood puts it well. "Thus, it [the seed] balances the inflammatory suppressant side of the adrenal cortex associated with high cortisone (high blood sugar, digestive heat, impotence) and on the other it controls excessive immune reaction associated with high aldosterone and androgens (hyperactivity, allergies, asthma, gum disease, food allergies, inflammatory and degenerative arthritis, skin eruptions)."

The seed powder was given to 40 patients with Hashimoto's thyroiditis (aged 22-50 years) for eight weeks, in a randomized controlled trial. Improved thyroid status and various indicators suggest benefit in nigella group, none in control. Farhangi MA et al, *BMC Complement Altern Med* 2016 16(1): 471.

Work by Meral et al, *J Vet Med A Physiol Pathol Clin Med* 2001 48:10 found Nigella may be useful in diabetic patients to prevent lipid peroxidation, increase anti-oxidant activity and prevent liver damage.

Ethanol extracts are an agonist of PPAR gamma and produce insulin-like stimulation of glucose uptake in skeletal muscles. Benhaddou-Amdaloussi et al, *Diab Obes Metab* 2009 September 25.

Studies conducted by Nabil et al, reported in the *1998 Pharmaceutical Biology Journal* 1998, found various fractions of Black Cumin were tested on rats vaccinated with Brucella vaccine (Rev 1).

Examination of lymph nodes revealed a remarkably consistent reactive lymph hyperplasia; and infiltration of the medullary sinuses with plasma cells, lymphocytes and macrophages.

One study, on cisplatin-induced toxicity in mice, found Black Cumin offered protection, and increased their lifespan from 150-200%. Reductions in leukocytes and hemoglobin were prevented. Cisplatin is a widely used, extremely toxic cancer therapeutic drug with devastating side effects in most patients.

If lab studies can be extrapolated, it appears that the toxic principles are somehow neutralized and are not present in the excreted urine.

Various *in vitro* and *in vivo* studies indicate some selective toxicity to certain cancer cells. One study by Abuharfeil et al, *Journal of Ethnopharmacology* 2000 71:1-2, found fresh plant water extractions have maximum natural killer activity (62.3%) against tumour cells at a 1:50 dilution.

Black Cumin contains 23 different plant sterols that fit hormone receptors in the human body. This may be one of the reasons relief from menopausal symptoms, prostate inflammation, and other hormone-related conditions is experienced by some individuals.

In one study, an ether extract of the seed at 1.8% concentration shows a more powerful galactagogue effect than one induced by 0.5 mcg of estrogen.

Various fractions including the volatile oil, ethanol extracts and polysaccharide compounds were effective; with the latter the most effective fraction of all. Alcohol extract of the seed was inhibitory of *E. coli* and *Staphylococcus aureus*.

Work by Hannan et al, *J Ajub Med Coll Abbottabad* 2008 20:3 found ethanol extracts inhibit *MRSA*, a particularly virulent form of the latter bacterium.

Petroleum extracts are effective against *B. subtilis, Micrococcus pyogenes* var. *aureus, Diplococcus pneumoniae* and *Streptococcus pyogenes*.

Thymoquinone shows activity against *Clostridium difficile*, a life-threatening diarrheal condition. Randhawa MA et al, *J Intercult Ethnopharmacol* 2016 6(1): 97-101.

A combination of approximately six parts *Nigella*, and one part *Phyllanthus niruri* showed significant improvement in the treatment of tonsil pharyngitis over seven days compared to placebo. Dirjomuljono et al, *Int J Clin Pharmacol Ther* 2008 46:6.

Gilani et al, *Journal of the Pakistan Medical Association* 2001 51:3 confirmed the anti-spasmodic and broncho-dilating effect of nigella seed, or **KALONGI**, as it is more well known. The mechanism is believed to involve calcium channel blockade.

Boskabady et al, *Fund Clin Pharm* 2007 21:5 suggested benefit in treating asthma.

Seed decoctions reduce inflammation in airways associated with asthma, but less effectively than theophylline. Boskabady et al, *Phytomed* 17:10.

Efficacy against allergic rhinitis was noted by Nikakhlagh et al, *Am J Otolarynol* 2010 October 12.

A single blind, placebo-controlled, randomized study of sixty asthma patients showed improvement of pulmonary function and inflammation. Salem AM et al, *Ann Saudi Med* 2017 37(1): 62-71.

Nestle scientists have found thymoquinone useful in food allergies and have registered a patent on a compound to treat and prevent. A huge cry went out across the web when some people speculated the company was trying to patent the plant. Not true.

Work published in *Biol Trace Elem Res* 116:3 found parathyroid hormone and nigella seed together were more effective than separately, in treating induced diabetic osteopenia.

A US patent was issued in 1996 for the use of *N. sativa* to stimulate immune competent cells in humans. However, as the patent has no specific proprietary processing method, the patent offers rather weak protection to the "inventor". One study found nigella seed enhances production of certain human interleukins and alters macrophages, suggesting changes in immune response. Haq et al, *Immunopharmacology* 1995 30:2.

In fact, black cumin is an immune modulator, helping to balance the body's response to under or over active conditions. One study found people treated with the herb had a 30% increase in natural killer cell activity.

Rheumatoid arthritis (RA), for example, is one auto-immune condition. Studies by Sajad et al, *J Comp Integr Med* 2010 7:1 found water and alcohol extracts of the seeds reduced inflammation in RA patients.

A combination of nigella seed and honey (alpha-Zam) was tested on six patients with HIV, by Onifade AA et al, *J of Herbal Medicine* 2013 13:99-103. Symptoms associated with infection disappeared within twenty days.

Cancer cells are controlled in four different ways, through stopping proliferation, stopping metastases, initiating apoptosis and enhancing effectiveness of chemotherapy.

The seed appears to induce apoptosis in HepG2 cancer cell lines. Hassan et al, *Integr Cancer Ther* 2012 11:4 354-63.

The seed extract induced apoptosis in SiHa human cervical cancer cells through both p53 and caspases activation. Hasan et al, *Nat Prod Commun* 2013 8:2 213-6.

It appears that persons of African descent are more sensitive to the anti-tumor compounds alpha hederin and its derivative kalopanaxsaponin I. Feller et al, *Planta Medica* 2010 76:16 1847-51.

By blocking cell receptors for androgen, it may be effective in preventing or treating prostate cancer.

The seeds increased splenocyte proliferation, decreased Th1 cytokines, increased Th2 cytokines, decreased macrophage inflammatory, and increased NK (natural killer) cytotoxicity. *Journal of Ethnopharmacology* 131:2.

The seeds reduce the toxicity of drugs used to treat pancreatic cancer, and increase tumor inhibition by 60-80% according to article in Cancer Research.

Cervical cancer cells are killed, *in vitro*, by the powdered seeds, in work published in Cancer Cell International.

Thymoquinone is one of the main bioactive components of seeds. It appears to specifically sensitize tumor cells to conventional therapies (radiation, chemo and immunotherapy), and also minimize therapy-associated toxic effects on normal cells. Mostofa AGM et al, *Front Pharmacol* 2017 8:295.

Black cumin seeds or thymoquinone reduced kidney toxicity induced by cisplatin in twelve studies. Cascella M et al, *Nutrients* 2017 9(6).

Work by Meddah, *J Ethnopharm* 121:3 found water extract of the seeds inhibit intestinal absorption of glucose, probably due to inhibition of alpha-glucosidase.

Khan et al, *Hamdard Medicus* 1998 41:3 found female patients with urinary tract infection had decreased pus cells in urine after taking *N. sativa* seeds.

Ethanol extracts of the seed appear to lower calcium oxalate levels and reduce their deposition, suggesting benefit in treating kidney stones. Hadjzadeh et al, *Urol J* 2007 4:2.

The same study found that men with normal blood pressure, showed decreased systolic and diastolic readings after taking the seed. Systolic pressure was depressed after one hour and continued for four hours. Diastolic was significantly depressed from two hours after ingestion onwards.

This may be due, in part, to thymoquinone that decreases heart rate.

A two-month randomized, double-blind (DB), placebo-controlled (PC) trial found seed extracts lowered systolic and diastolic blood pressure in hypertensive subjects, and decreased LDL cholesterol. Dehkodri et al, *Fundament Clin Pharmacol* 2008 22:4.

Work by Kocyigit et al, Saudi Med J 2009 30:7 found seeds supplemented in human diet increased HDL and lowered LDL cholesterol and triglyceride levels.

A study of 123 patients taking nigella seed found serum lipid levels, blood sugar, blood pressure and weight loss were all favorable over placebo. The small sample size did not make the difference statistically significant. Qidwa et al, *J Altern Complem Medicine* 2009 15:6.

A single-blind, randomized one year trial of seed supplemention on 114 patients found the black cumin group improved total cholesterol, arterial blood pressure and heart rate in type two diabetics on oral hypoglycemic agents. Badar A et al, *Ann Saudi Med* 2017 37(1): 56-63.

Work by Leong et al, *Evid Based Compl Altern Med* 2013:20732 confirmed lowering of both blood pressure and cholesterol in a human study.

Work by Parvadeh et al, *J Med Plants* 5 found thymoquinone effective as an anti-seizure compound due to its benzodiazapine receptor activity.

Akhondian et al, *Med Sci Monit* 2007 13:12 found water extraction from seeds show anti-epileptic activity in children with refractory seizures, in a double-blind crossover study involving 23 patients.

The seed may be useful in a number of neurological conditions. Beheshti F et al, *Avicenna J Phytomed* 2016 6(1): 104-16.

Thymoquinone crosses the blood brain barrier, and exerts neuromodulatory activity. In animal studies it demonstrates protection against ischemic brain damage; reduction of epileptic seizures; reduction of morphine tolerance; anxiety reduction, and oxidative injury to brain associated with toluene, lead and ionizing radiation. It also suppresses growth and invasion and induces apoptosis of glial tumor cells. Elmaci I et al, *Biomed Pharmacother* 2016 83: 635-40.

Animal studies suggest it may be useful in treating multiple sclerosis.

The seed shows activity against *Helicobacter pylori*, associated with peptic and duodenal ulcers. Salem et al, *Saudi J Gastroenterol* 2010 16:3.

A review of the seed's medicinal properties, identified in work from 1960 to 1998, was published by Khan et al, *Inflammopharm* 1999 7:1.

Both the root and shoots contain vanillic acid, the former more anti-mutagenic and the shoots more anti-oxidant in nature. Bourger et al, *CR Biol* 2008 331:1.

A review of clinical and preclinical effects was published by Gholamnezhad Z et al, *J Ethnopharm* 2016 190: 372-86.

One mouse study by Vahdati-Mashhadian et al, *Pharmazie* 60:7 found water extracts of the seeds toxic to liver cells. Do not feed your pet mice seed water until further studies are conducted. Pubmed lists nearly one thousand studies on the herb. I have not included all of them.

The seeds of *N. damascena* possess both analgesic and diuretic activity. Work by Agradi et al, *Phyto Res* 2002 16:5 found alcohol extract of seeds possess low phyto-estrogenic influence. Human application is unknown.

Work by Toma et al, *Rev Med Chir Soc Med Nat Inst* 111:1 found seed and leaf extracts active against *Leishmania promastigotes*. It may be a natural alternative to pentamidine and amphotericin B.

The seed is used in treatment of fevers and inflammation, to regulate menstruation and to expel tapeworms. However, the seeds, and its major alkaloid damascenine show liver and kidney toxicity, in mice studies. Bouguezza Y et al, *Interdiscip Toxicol* 2015 8(3): 118-24. It is not diuretic, like its more famous cousin.

The compound damascenine lowers body temperature and reduces inflammation.

Love in a Mist is used in the production of a hypertensive pharmaceutical.

Both plant and seed extracts are active against *Leishmania promastigotes*, and may be an alternative to pentamidine and amphotericin B. Toma CC et al, *Rev Med Chir Soc Med Nat Iasi* 2007 111(1): 285-9.

HOMEOPATHY

Nigella sativa symptoms include nervousness, anxious fearfulness, fear of death, discouragement, tendency to start and out of humor. The voice is anxious, hurried and interrupted.

Violent, darting stitches in occiput, and vertex. Intolerable pressure and digging in frontal eminences. Cutting in the middle of brain, with continual throbbing. Dullness of eyes with frequent obscuration of sight. Twitching of right upper eyelid. Tip of nose cold as ice, dryness of nose, face pale and bluish with pale lips. Scanty urine, soreness in vagina, with heat and dryness. Violent tearing pain in back. Legs feel paralyzed.

DOSE- 6x potency. Ruckert reported three cases cured with this potency. All cases concern inflammatory conditions brought on by cold. It was given after the inflammatory symptoms were first subdued by Aconitum (Monkshood) in homeopathic form.

ESSENTIAL OIL

CONSTITUENTS- *N. sativa* seed- 0.5 to 1.5% consisting of 15% p-cymene, 20% 38% trans-anethole, alpha thujene, alpha and beta pinenes, sabines, sabinen hydrates, thymol, carvacrol, 1,8 cineol, borneol, carvone (4%), d-limonene (4.3%), linalool, nigellone semohiprepinon, thymochinon, thymoquinone, (+) citronellol,
N. damascena seed- damascenine (8-10%), sesquiterpenes including beta elemene 59%, beta (12.8%) and alpha selinene (12%), beta caryophyllene and alpha humulene, as well as methoxy anthranylate of methyl esters 30% and 47 other compounds.

The essential oil of black cumin decreases blood pressure and increases respiration. It is used topically for hemorrhoids and skin conditions such as eczema and infections, diluted of course.

Chowdhury et al, *Phytotherapy Research* 1998, found the essential oil of *N. sativa* exhibited activity against various drug-resistant strains of *Shigella, in vitro*.

Synergistic action with streptomycin and gentamicin was found in work by Ferdous et al, *Phytotherapy Research* 1992 6:137.

Various bacterial and fungal conditions, including *Candida albicans* overgrowth, are inhibited by the volatile oils. Dental plaque be prevented and treated.

Gram-positive bacteria such as *Staphylococcus aureus*, and *Vibrio cholerae*, as well as *Streptococcus pyogenes* and *S. viridans* are most susceptible, with *in vitro* studies indicating activity comparable to ampicillin. The essential oil inhibits *Bacillus subtilis, B. anthracis, B. pumilis, Staphylococcus aureus, S. luteus, S. albus, E. coli, Salmonella typhi*, and *Pseudomonas aeruginosa*.

Methicillin and drug-resistant strains of *S. aureus* and *P. aeruginosa* also succumb to the oil. Salman et al, *Nat Prod Rad* 2008 7:1.

The oil inhibits various fungi, including *Candida albicans, Aspergillus niger, A. flavus, M. gypseum, Trichoderma viride* and *Curvularia lunata*.

In vivo activity against *S. flexneri* by the oil was also proven, fully curing infected monkeys within three days.

It is active against *Vibrio parahaemolyticus*, a virulent species related to cholera, and common in salt water regions. Manju S et al, *J Invertebr Pathol* 2016 136: 43-9.

Nigellone semohiprepinon, when inhaled or rubbed on chest, enlarges the bronchi, reduces cramps and raises the temperature, to quickly alleviate bronchial asthma, whooping cough.

Nigellone inhibits the release of histamine from mast cells; while thymochinon inhibits infection, is an anodyne, anti-oxidant and stimulates gall bladder function.

A study by Aqel and Shaheen, *Journal of Ethnopharmacology* 1996 May, tested the effects of Black Cumin essential oil on uterine tissue. Their results indicate the oil has anti-oxytocic potential.

Work by Badary et al, *Drug Development Research* 1998 44:2-3, found thymoquinone, a major component of the essential oil, induced significant decreases in the fasting plasma glucose concentration.

Thymoquinone is very potent, with approximate IC50 values against 5-lipoxygenase and cyclooxygenase of <1 and 3.5 μg/ml, respectively.

Thymoquinone possesses hepato-protective activity. Daba et al, *Tox Letters* 1998 95:1.

The essential oil has been found active against Jurkat T-cell leukemia cells, *in vitro. Intern J Pharmacognosy* 1995:33.

The essential oil suppresses cancer cell proliferation in colon mucosa, according to research by Salim and Fukushima, *Nutr Cancer* 2003 45:2.

Administration of the essential oils into tumor sites inhibits liver metastasis development and improved mice survival. Ait et al, *Braz J Med Biol Res* 2007 40:6.

A nanoemulsion of the essential oil significantly reduced viability of MCF-7 breast cancer cells, including apoptosis. Periasamy VS et al, *Ultrason Sonochem* 2016 31: 449-55.

Thymoquinone and alpha pinene affect benzodiazepine receptors associated with anti-anxiety. Raza et al, *J Herb Spice Med Plant* 12:1-2.

Oral ingestion increases levels of 5-HT and tryptophan in both blood plasma and brain, suggesting a mechanism reducing anxiety.

Toxicology testing on mice, at significant doses for up to ninety days showed no signs of toxicity. Acute oral administration gave an LD50 of 2.4 g/kg.

Water stress, while growing, increases the content of both seed and essential oil. Water stress produced by irrigating every 12th day increases thymoquinone content in distillation product.

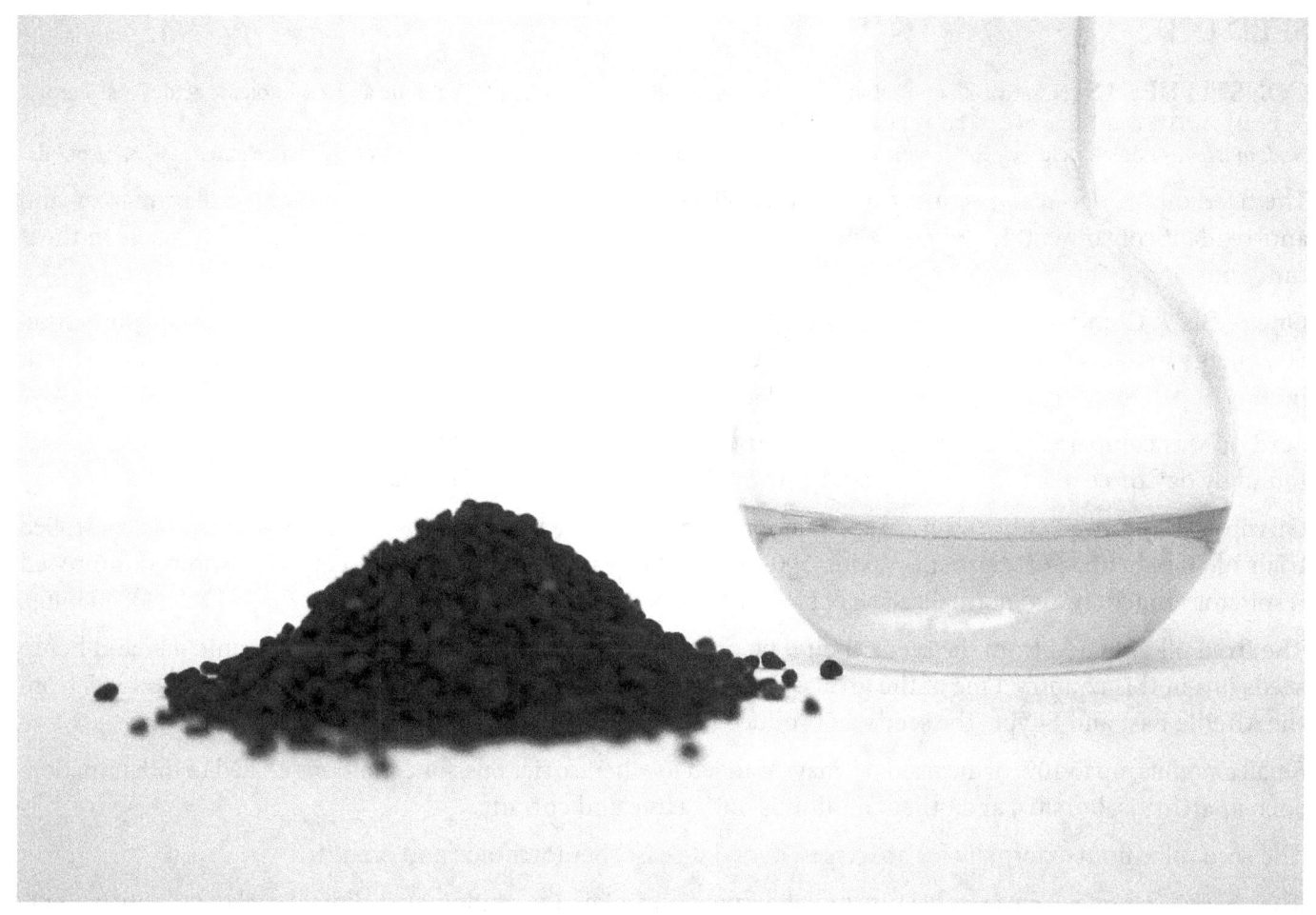

NIGELLA SEED AND OIL

The seeds of *N. damascena* are distilled to produce an essential oil of quite unique and interesting aromatic potential.

This oil is not as medicinal like its more famous cousin, but mostly used for the perfume and cosmetic industry. Elemenes are the most abundant volatiles (22-29%), as well as up to 30% methyl-3-methoxy-N-methyl anthanilate.

The oil is yellowish and intensely sweet-fruity, with a somewhat unpleasant odor when first distilled. This dissipates rather quickly, and on blotter paper shows a great tenacity, and very pleasant wine or brandy like character similar to ambrette seed oil.

The citrus, peach-like notes have been compared to the scent of wild strawberries. Sweet and fruity, the oil must be used in small amounts 0.2-0.5% to avoid that perfumery scent.

The oil, when diluted, has a blue fluorescence due to its content of damascenine.

Butanol extracts show activity against *Staphylococcus aureus* and *Pseudomonas aeruginosa.* Phytotherapy Research 18:6

The oil cannot be used in food work, as it loses its flavor in an acid medium, and grape and peach are usually presented as acidic flavors.

However, the oil can be used in lipsticks as well as fruity and floral perfumes, combining well with gardenia, jasmine, bergamot, neroli, etc.

It has a few medicinal applications, especially as a powerful anti-histamine and anti-allergenic for treating bronchial asthma.

SEED OIL

CONSTITUENTS- N. sativa- thymoquinone, 23-49% oleic, 38-55% linoleic, 12% palmitic and 2% linolenic acid; Total sterol content is 0.51% consisting of 63% beta sitosterol, 17% stigmasterol, and 15% campesterol.
N. damascena- linoleic acid (43-50%), oleic (14-23%), stearic (15-23%), and palmitic (10-12%) acids. Beta elemene is 73.2% of oils.

The fixed oil of *Nigella sativa*, like the essential oil, contains thymoquinone, a potent anti-inflammatory and anti-oxidant constituent. It also contains an unusual C20:2 unsaturated fatty acid that may play a role in these functions.

One of Black Cumin's strengths lies in its anti-allergenic, anti-histamine activity. One study from Munich on 600 allergy patients found 500 mg of black cumin oil twice a day for three months showed clear improvement in 85% of patients.

Seed oil was compared with control in 84 patients with asthma wheeze. Statistically significant difference was found by day three of a fourteen-day study. Ahmad et al, *Afr J Pharm Pharmacol* 2009 3:5.

Oil capsules improved asthma control and pulmonary function in a randomized, double-blind, placebo-controlled trials of 80 patients. Forty patients taking 500 mg of oil capsules twice daily for four weeks showed improved respiratory function, and normalization of blood eosinophilia. Koshak A et al, *Phytother Res* 2017 31(3): 403-409.

The fixed oil obtained from the seeds should be processed with the same care afforded organic flax and hemp seeds oils in this country. One of the great disadvantages at the present is the uncertainty of oil products from the Middle East and Egypt. The seeds do produce from 30-35% fatty oil, with over 60% linoleic acid.

Small amounts, up to 10% of the fixed oil, may be added to other carrier oils, for conditions related to inflammation, such as arthritis, bursitis, and other conditions both acute and chronic.

The seed oil is used externally for abscesses, dental disease, hemorrhoids and orchitis.

The seed oil in honey helps resolve functional dyspepsia in a DB, PC randomized clinical trial of seventy patients for eight weeks. Mohtashami R et al, J *Ethnopharm* 2015 175: 147-52.

The fixed oil and unsaponified portions show anti-fungal activity against *Fusarium solani, F. moniliforme, Helminthosporium turcicum, H. oryzae, Alternaria helianthi, Colletotrichum capsici* and *Pyricularia setariae*.

Work by Enomoto et al, *Biological and Pharmaceutical Bulletin* 2001 24:3 found methanol soluble portions of the fixed oil, shows inhibitory effect on arachadonic acid- induced platelet aggregation and blood coagulation.

Compounds in the oil possessing aromatic hydroxyl and acetoxyl groups had more potent activity than aspirin, as an anti-thrombotic agent.

A study by the *Amala Nagar Cancer Research Centre* showed evidence that a long chain fatty acid in the oil possesses potent anti-tumour activity. Salomi et al, *Cancer Letters* 1992 63:41.

The fixed oil has been shown to prevent chronic cyclosporine nephro-toxicity in work by Uz et al, *Am J Nephrol* 2008 28:3.

It reduces liver toxicity from tramadol. Omar NM et al, *Acta Histochem* 2017 119(5): 543-554.

The seed oil is safe, and comparable to topical diclofenac in the treatment of cyclic mastalgia. Pain scores were similar from application in this randomized, triple-blind, active, and placebo-controlled clinical trial of 154 women. Huseini HF et al, *Planta Med* 2016 82(4): 285-8.

The seed oil appears to alleviate the deleterious effects of highly active anti-retroviral drugs, reducing insulin resistance by stabilizing beta cells, and insulin activity at periphery of body. Chandra et al, *Can J Physio Pharmacol* 2009 87:4.

Thymoquinone reduces the release of inflammatory mediators in pancreatic cancer cells. Arafat et al, *Am Assoc Cancer Research*, Denver April 2009.

Thymoquinone is a promising agent in the treatment of neck and head cancer, via apoptosis and synergy with radiation. Kotowski U et al, *Oncol Lett* 2017 14(1): 1147-51.

Previous studies showed Nigella possesses anti-cancer effects on prostate and colon cancers. Afarat and colleagues compared thymoquinone with trichostatin A, an HDAC inhibitor that has been shown to ameliorate inflammatory associated cancers.

Thymoquinone and piperine (black pepper) act synergistically to target breast cancer, in vitro, and in vivo. The combination inhibits angiogenesis, induces apoptosis and shifts the immune response to Thelper 1 response. Talib WH, *Sci Pharm* 2017 85(3).

Inhibition of NFkappaB was noted as well. When animal models with pancreatic cancer were treated with thymoquinone, tumors shrank 67% and pro-inflammatory cytokines were reduced.

The oil shows efficacy against *Trichomonas vaginalis*, as efficiently as metronidazole. This suggests a vaginal suppository composed on this oil, and various essential oils may be a useful treatment. Mahmoud MA et al, *J Parasit Dis* 2016 40(1): 22-31.

The oil showed activity against MRSA infections on diabetic patient's wounds, albeit complete resistant to treatment in 11 of the 34 patients. Emeka LB et al, *Pak J Pharm Sci* 2015 28(6): 1985-90.

The essential oil strongly deodorizes methyl mercaptan.

FLOWER ESSENCES

Love in a Mist (*N. damascena*) flower essence assists in allowing free association of thoughts, feelings and ideas. It can be very useful in hypnosis or other trance work. For individuals who have difficulty with the Air elements, this essence helps one to achieve oneness with one's soul family. **PEGASUS**

Love in a Mist flower essence helps purify the aura, clarifies issues of etheric and auric boundaries, clearing out distracting energies. Use it as a ritual ablution or cleansing before prayer; it sets the intention of purity. **HUMMINGBIRD**

Love in a Mist, a very gentle flower essence, works on the strands between the heart chakra and other, smaller charkas of the body and encourages you to be both strong and courageous. A physical cleanser, Love in a Mist also clarifies your emotional motivations, helping to ease frustrations and allow clear choices to be made. **OLIVE**

ASTROLOGY

The flowers of the love-in-a-mist are surrounded by a group of pinnate leaves, so that they are hardly noticeable. Their petals are pointed as though in an intermediate form between the simple leaf and the sepal; they are like an early stage of the metamorphosis ending in the perfect petal…the development of the flowers is deeply rooted in the vegetative processes. Even the green stamens remind us of vegetative life…in the love-in-a-mist, the carpels grow together into one common ovary. A very strong influence from the moon manifests itself in this organ, which isolates itself uniformly from its surroundings and dominates the entire flower. **KRANICH**

SPIRITUAL PROPERTIES

The flower spirit of Nigella, also known as Love-in-a-Mist, reminds you to pause and breathe.

Close your eyes and slowly fill your lungs with cool, blue celestial light. Imagine the soft, hazy blue of the Nigella flower flowing into the crown of your head from above, filling first your stomach and then your lungs. **ECLARE**

PERSONALITY TRAITS

Love-in-a-mist, *Nigella damascena*, is one of the frothiest of plants. Mingling into surrounding greenery, it makes the planting float. Its relatively large flowers add to the impression as they hover above the fuzzy leaves.

CAROL KLEIN

RECIPES

GROUND SEED- Two grams daily for up to four weeks to improve immune system.

Do not use N. sativa, in any form, during pregnancy.

TINCTURE- Make a 1:5 tincture with freshly ground black cumin seeds in 60% alcohol. Use 10-30 drops as needed.

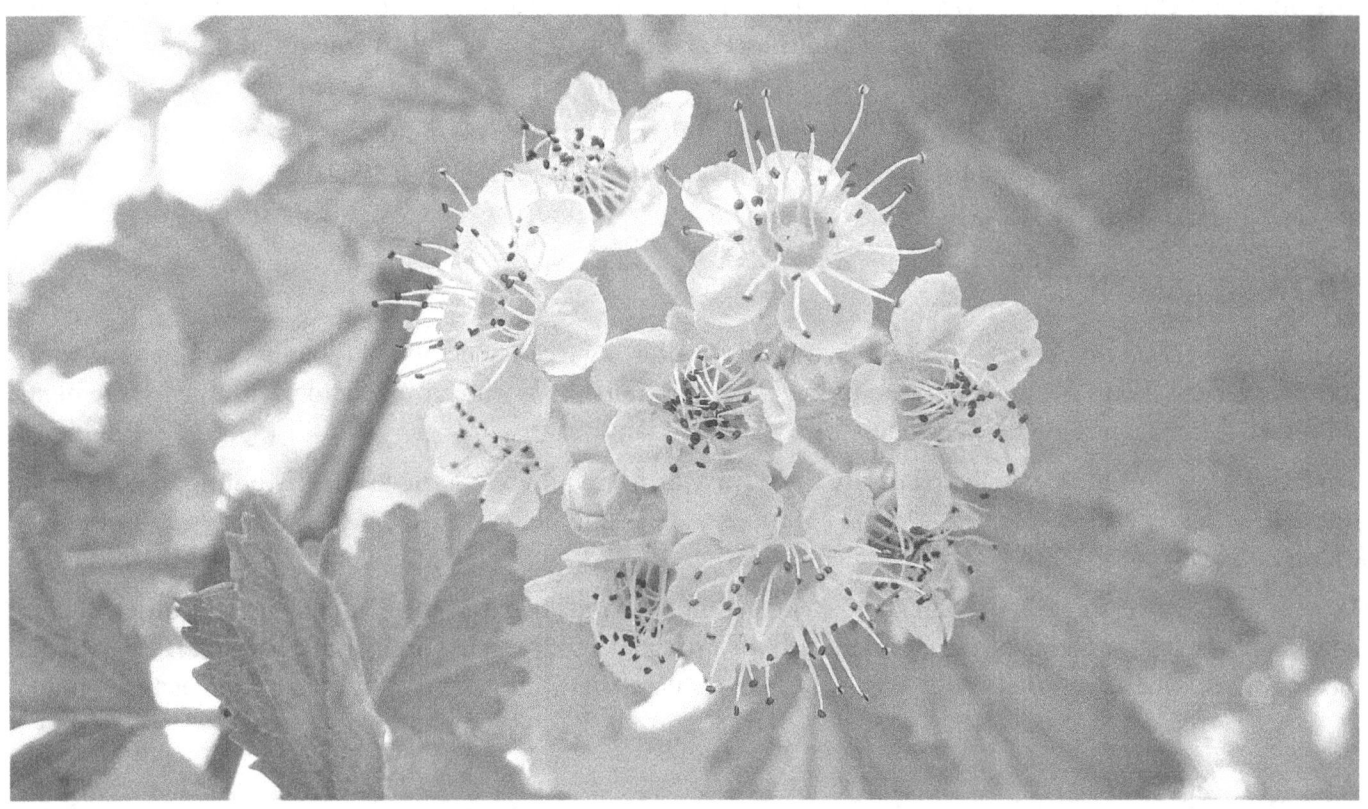

ATLANTIC NINEBARK

COMMON NINEBARK
(*Physocarpus opulifolius* [L.] Maxim.)
ATLANTIC NINEBARK
(*P. intermedius* [Rydb.] Schneid)
MALLOW NINEBARK
(*P. malvaceus* [Greene] Kuntze)
ROCKY MOUNTAIN NINEBARK
(*P. monogynus* [Torr.] J. M. Coult)
PACIFIC NINEBARK
(*P. capitatus* [Pursh] Kuntze)
PARTS USED- bark, flowers, seeds

Physocarpus means "bladder fruit", and refers to the inflated seedpods. Opulifolius means "leaves like opulus, and refers to likeness of the leaves to *Viburnum opulus* (Crampbark). It is related to the word opulent. Malvaceus means mallow.

Ninebark is believed to come from a time when plants were known for the number of medicinal cures they could affect. Ninebark is therefore, clearly better than Seven Bark (Wild Hydrangea). Hardly! Others believe it relates to nine layers of shedding bark. This is more likely.

Common Ninebark is an upright, spreading shrub or tree (2-3 meters) with creamy, white flowers, that later turn to an attractive red, dry fruit capsule.

It is not a very common shrub, in that is does not form groves, but is more solitary.

The bark is thin, and cinnamon brown, and layered in "nine" colored sheets as the given name suggests.

Mallow Ninebark was used by the southern Okanagan of Washington to make bows.

Rocky Mountain Ninebark grows on old dry, wooded slopes in the foothills and mountains down to New Mexico.

In autumn, the leaves turn orange and red.

The plant secretes a substance that does not allow other vegetation to grow near, so it is an ideal ground cover.

The Bella Coola of British Columbia made a decoction of the inner bark of *P. opulifolius* to be taken as an emetic by "persons dizzy with pain".

It was used for tuberculosis and gonorrhea internally; as well as a wash for the affected areas.

The Iroquois made a poultice of the plant, to be used when "women swell after copulation" or to counteract bad medicine.

Ninebark decoctions were taken by the Menominee, to help cleanse the female reproductive system, and enhance fertility.

Early settlers noticed this and for a woman who desires a baby and does not conceive, a bark decoction was prescribed.

The Carrier of the Arctic (?), according to Morice (1901), used the inner bark of willow with the outer bark of Ninebark for infected wounds and sores. They call it **SOES MAI TEON**, or Bearberry Stick or Bush.

"Cataract is easily discerned by the natives who treat it ...instead of birch bark other use for the same purpose a piece of calcined bone which, coming in contact with the waste tissue formed on the eye, seems to have the same drawing power as a magnet on a bit of iron. In either case, the eye is left sore and bloody. It is now carefully washed and as a final treatment, it is bathed in a cooled infusion of the inner bark of the bearberry bush to which a little woman's milk has been added. The former especially is reputed to be quite a specific against any soreness of the eyes, though its mordant properties render its application very trying at first."

Peter Smith, in *The Indian Doctor's Dispensatory* of 1812, wrote:

"Weaver quills are made of the pith. The Indians use a decoction of these roots for fomenting and poulticing... it removes the anguish and cures a burn beyond credibility; cases verging on mortification, felons, swellings, rising of a woman's breast, etc, yield to its application beyond anything else. To apply it boil the roots and make a strong decoction, then take the liquor and thick up a poultice with bran or Indian meal, this may be put into a little bag made of thin cloth and apply it as warm as can be born and then kept close while the case remains and so repeated".

Rafinesque considered "Ninebark has nearly the same properties as Hardhack (Spiraea), and is an equivalent."

According to Dr. Cook, the leaves are mildly astringent, tonic, a little demulcent and rather soothing in nature. They are used in sub-acute diarrhea where an astringent is needed.

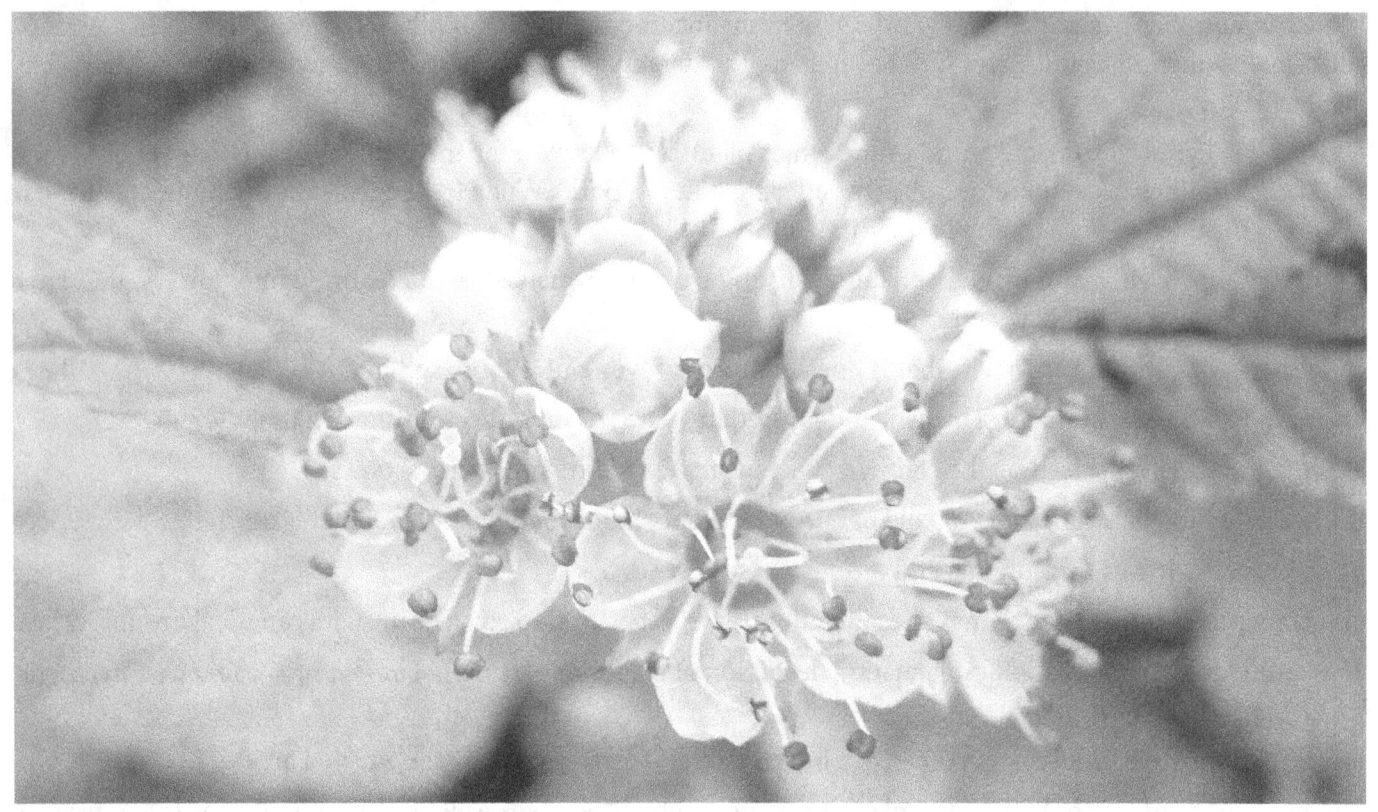

COMMON NINEBARK

Large doses of *P. opulifolius* are said to be toxic, due to varying levels of cyanide.

The seeds contain various cucurbitacins that exhibit antagonistic activity towards the steroid hormone found in Maral root and various Silene species, called ecdysterone.

Ninebark contains D-sorbitol, which has sweetening properties.

The Cowichan used Pacific Ninebark (*P. capitatus*) to make knitting needles, while the Nuu-chah-nulth made children's bows and other small items.

Pacific Ninebark root was decocted by the Kwatiutl for locomotor ataxia; while the boiled bark was taken to induce vomiting or relieve constipation.

The Nuxalk used a preparation for gonorrhea and scrofulous sores on the neck. The Karuk, further south, used the bark for stomach or intestinal ulcers and internal cancers including the throat. It is steeped in hot water and taken in small amounts at a time to avoid nausea and vomiting.

Mallow Ninebark was used as a good luck charm by Okanagan tribe to protect their hunting gear.

Several hybrids are available from prairie nurseries including Dart's Gold, Golden, and Tilden Parks. The latter is a low growing variety suited to groundcover.

MEDICINAL

CONSTITUENTS – *P. malvaceus* bark- cyanide compounds, cucurbitacin D & F, 3-epi-isocucurbitacin D.
P. intermedius- betulinic acid, ursolic acid, oleanolic acid, 3-O-caffeoyloleanolic acid, euscaphic acid (tormentic acid), 2 alpha-hydroxyursolic acid, maslinic acid.

Mallow Ninebark dried bark is decocted for relief of arthritis and rheumatism when added to a hot bath.

The infused bark tea is emetic and works quite quickly. The tinctured bark is a laxative but may cause stomach cramping if doses exceed 10-20 drops in hot water.

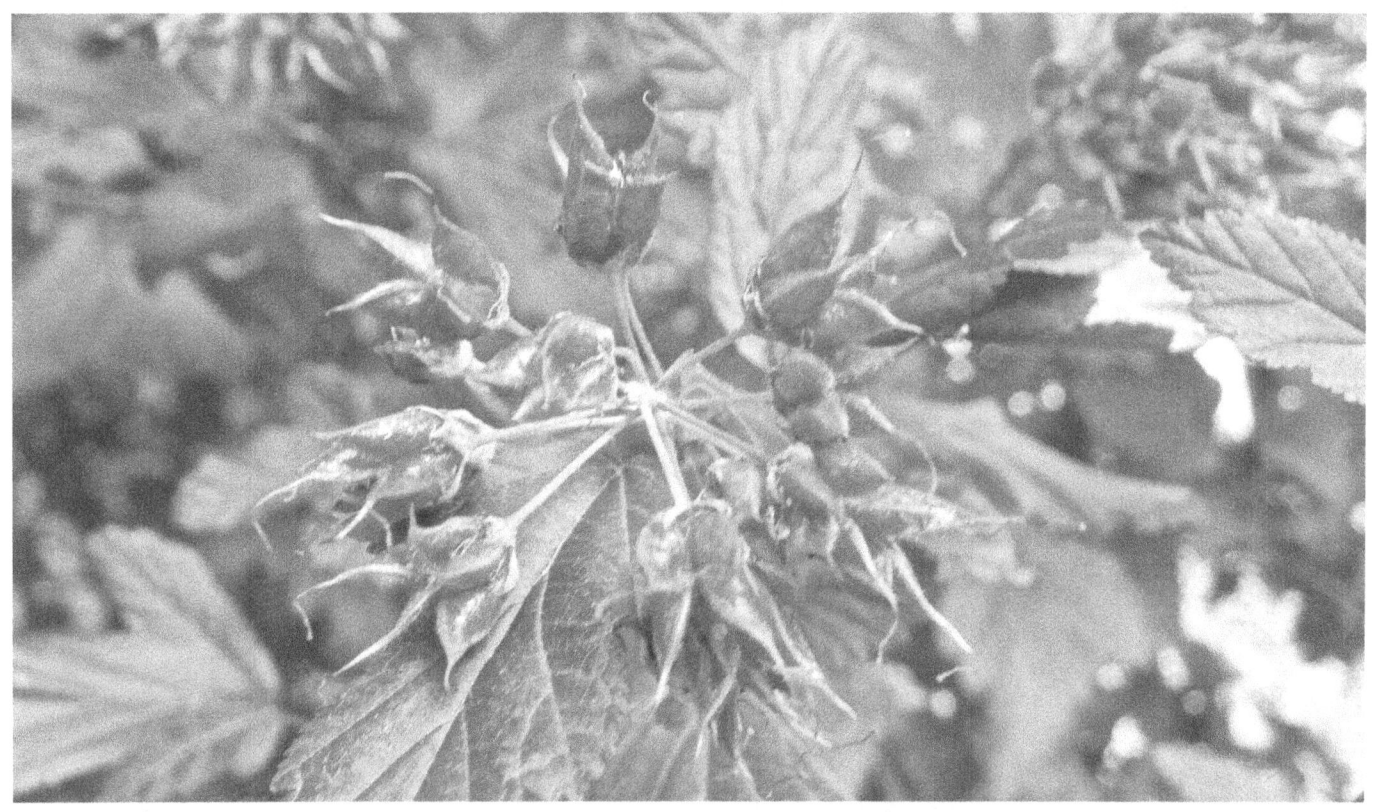

COMMON NINEBARK SEED PODS

The stem bark of the related *P. intermedius* has been found to contain active cytotoxicity against five human tumor cell lines, including non-small cell lung, ovary, melanoma, central nervous system and colon, *in vitro*. Kim YK et al, *Planta Medica* 2000 66(5): 485-6. Betulinic acid, derived from birchbark and other plants is a potent cytotoxic compound.

Ursolic acid shows significant anti-proliferative activity against liver and two lines of breast cancer cells. Wen L et al, *Food Chem Toxicol* 2017 100: 149-160.

Maslinic acid inhibits proliferation of renal cell carcinoma and suppresses angiogenesis of endothelial cells. Thakor P et al, *J Kidney Cancer VHL* 2017 4(1): 16-24.

Maslinic acid is an inhibitor of extracellular protease. It alleviated mild knee joint pain and promotes weight loss in the elderly in a randomized, double-blind, placebo controlled trial on twenty patients. Fukkumitsu S et al, *J Clin Biochem Nutr* 2016 59(3): 220-5.

Maslinic acid is able to stimulate NADPH production, through regulation of the two oxidative dehydrogenases of the pentose phosphate pathway. Rufino- Palmomares EE et al, *Comp Biochem Physiol C Toxicol Pharmacol* 2016 187:32-42.

Euscaphic acid may help prevent or treat atherosclerosis. Wang YL et al, *Mol Med Rep* 2016 14(4): 3559-64. It may be useful in the treatment of osteoarthritis. Yang Y et al, *Inflammation* 2016 39(3): 1151-9.

It may play a role in anti-proliferative activity on renal, prostate and melanoma cancer cell lines. It was more cytotoxic against ACHN cancer cells than vinblastine. Loizzo MR et al, *Anticancer Agents Med Chem* 2013 13(5): 768-76.

Other members of the rose family, including blackberries, agrimony and rose, contain euscaphic acid.

Pacific Ninebark contains cucurbitacins that cause actin aggregates and inhibit cell division. Maloney KN et al, *J Nat Prod* 2008 71(11): 1927-9.

FLOWER ESSENCES

Mallow Ninebark essence is the guardian of male fertility. **DARCY WILLIAMSON**

Ninebark (*P. capitatus*) is related to ancient wisdom that has been passed down and retained in our cellular memory and hearts. We may have long forgotten the context but need to tap into the message. The knowledge could be over many lifetimes. It may encourage us to seek out elders or family history to provide answers. It is also useful when feeling scattered, or when tying up loose ends. **NETTLES & MORE**

SPIRITUAL PROPERTIES

The number nine is one of our most mystical numbers, representing the trinity of trinities. The ancient Roman lunar week had nine nights in their method of tracking time.

In Norse mythology, the cosmos was a combination of nine worlds. Other nines include the nine-headed hydra, the nine lives of cats, and the Ninefold Goddess.

In Arabic numbers, every multiple of nine adds up to nine again, making for interesting mathematical calculations.

RECIPES

DECOCTION- prepare a 1:20 decoction of dried stems for 15 minutes.

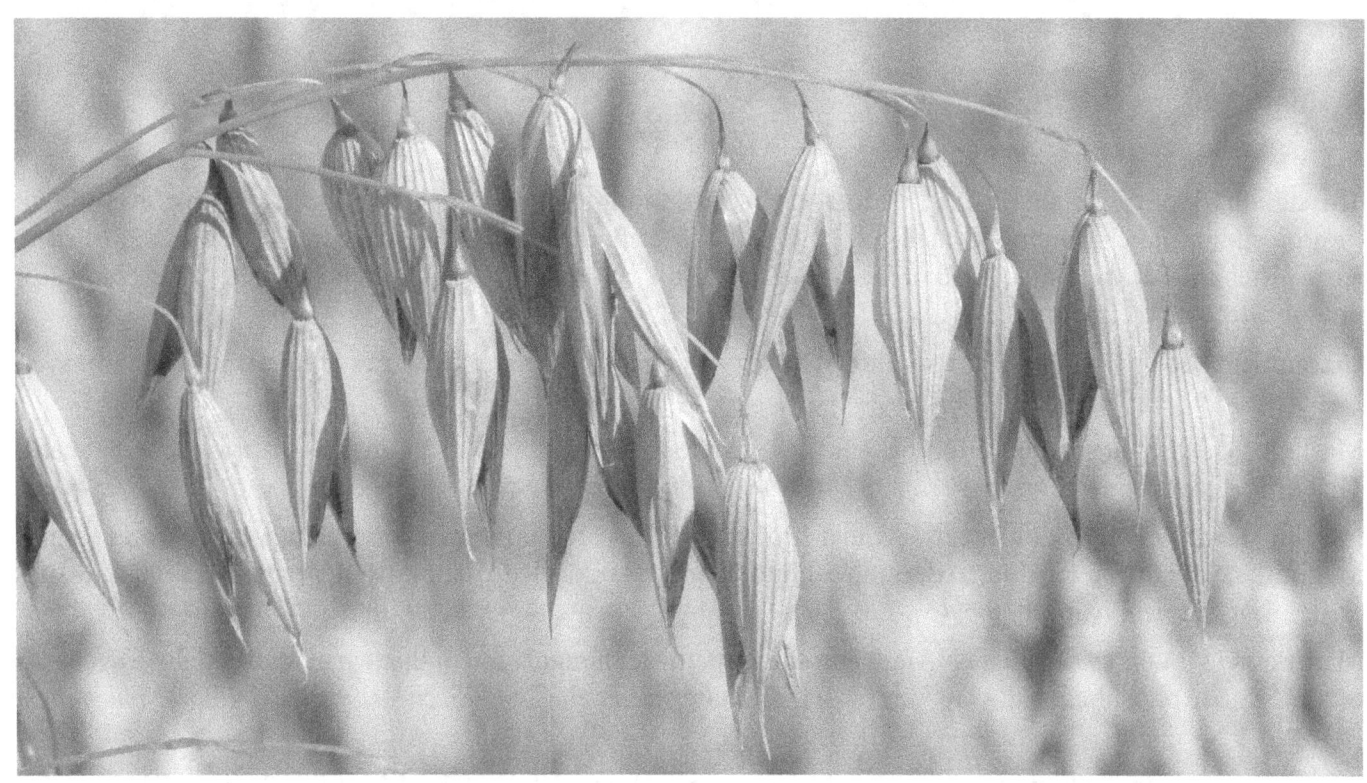

RIPE OATS

WILD OATS
(*Avena fatua* L.)
CULTIVATED OATS
HULL LESS OATS
(*A. sativa* L.)
PARTS USED–straw, milky stage seed, ripe grain, flower, sprouts.

That they may satisfy the foolish desires of certain light brains and wild oats, which are altogether given to new fangleness.

BERON 1542

Mares eat oats, and does eat oats, and little lambs eat ivy.

OLD SAYING

The young sow wild oats, the old grow sage.

WINSTON CHURCHILL

Most of us spend the first six days of each week sowing wild oats; then we go to church on Sunday and pray for a crop failure.

FRED ALLEN

Oat may stem from the Celtic or Anglo-Saxon **ATEN** or **ETAN** "to eat". This later became Oat. Avena means nourishment, and comes from the Latin **AVIDUS** for sought after. The Sanskrit word **AVASA** means nourishment.

Fatua means simple, or foolish; and sativum means, commonly grown as a crop.

Oats and all cereals are connected to the goddess Ceres, protector and benefactor of all agricultural crops. The grain was formerly used in ceremonies of prosperity, and the plant symbolizes music. Oats represent the birth date of August 5th.

It was cultivated much later than wheat, barley or rye, with early archeological evidence dating back to only the 2nd and 1st millennia BC.

Both wild and cultivated oats have contributed much to the earth's basic nutritional needs. The grain has nourished northern Europeans for centuries, while building a strong, robust constitution. Many of my former clients in their "eighties" started their day with a bowl of oat porridge. Wild oats are even better!

Hildegard de Bingen, the 12th century Benedictine Abbess, suggested that "Oats are a happy and healthy food for people who are well, furnishing them with a cheerful mind, and a pure, clear intellect."

Wild oats' beard was used at one time, as a hygrometer, to measure humidity.

Like wheat, oats contains a protein fraction called prolamin. In patients suffering celiac disease, they are told to avoid gluten. However, the oat prolamin, avenin, does not create inflammation and irritation in the manner of gliadin, from wheat.

Work by Kumar and Farthing in 1995 found that about 50 grams of oatmeal daily is safe for celiac patients.

Dr. Vogel, of Switzerland, says "oats have the highest content of iron, zinc and manganese of all grain species."

The Cree of Alberta called the introduced feed for horses, **MISTATIMOMECIWIN**.

Its sweet taste is nutritive, promoting growth in children, as well as strength and solidity.

In work by Holt et al, *Eur J Clin Nutr* 1995 49 oats were the third highest of 38 food tests for satiety. This phenomenon is mediated by increased secretion of gut hormones such as cholecystokinin, that enhance satiety and, in turn, weight loss.

Besides its nutritive qualities, oatmeal is used in beauty products for cleansing pores and toning the skin; as well as dermatosis, eczema and sunburn.

Norac, an Edmonton company specializing in supercritical fluid extraction, has extracted oat bran oil with great potential in health and cosmetics.

Ceapro, a biotech company in Edmonton, has standardized oat extracts, powders, and oils; as well as beta glucan for lowering cholesterol, and supporting immune function.

The gluten in oats has a soothing and moisturizing skin property, used in Dr. Redmond's Oat Shampoo, marketed to Japan, Australia, New Zealand, and Canada. They have 38 patents issued or pending on natural ingredients related to oat products. One, a dusting powder for surgical latex gloves, shows dramatic improvement over conventional dusting powders for total allergen uptake. Oat oil, which contains anti-oxidants, for skin health is another product with great cosmetic application, including neutralizing the oxidative effect of alpha hydroxy products.

They have developed AccuScreen, which uses an oat extract that allows early detection of Type 2 late onset diabetes.

Oat extracts are used in Aveeno Baby Wash and Shampoo and Salon Selectives Shampoo.

Oat powder is widely utilized by Aveeno and Cover Girl in various lotions, moisturizing bars, shave gels, and pressed powders. Johnsons Diaper Rash Cream with zinc oxide uses oat powder. Oat mucilage is used in a UK sunscreen product.

Avenanthramides are alkaloids found only in oats and possess strong skin soothing, anti-oxidant and anti-inflammatory properties. These compounds help restore the cutaneous barrier and relieve symptoms of atopic dermatitis. *Cutis* 2007 80:6 supplement.

Rhealba® is an oat plantlet extract that reduces facial inflammation and inhibits bacterial adhesion of *Propionibacterium acnes*. Fabbrocini G et al, *J Eur Acad Dermatol Venereol* 2014 28(suppl 6):1-6.

In 2002, ADL developed a new line of flavored beverages contains soluble fibre, with concentrated amounts of beta glucan. It should be noted that oat contains 1,4 beta glucans, unlike the 1,3 and 1,6 beta glucans in medicinal mushrooms. These linear compounds do not contain the high level of immune efficacy found in fungi fruiting bodies, but are still important and beneficial to for cholesterol and other cardiovascular risk.

Scientists at Ottawa's Eastern Cereal and Oilseed Research Centre have recently developed a new technology to derive components from crops like oats. It does not use anti-microbial agents or toxic solvents, but the equivalent of turbo charged vodka. The key is "designer" gels that can cheaply attract desired particles allowing for purification or fractionation of just about any component. The gels themselves are so benign they are edible.

Work by Drs. Thava Vasanthan and Feral Temelli at the University of Alberta developed a process to efficiently extract beta glucans from oats and barley.

A barley and oat-based Viscofiber, containing significant amounts of beta glucan is on the market and marketed by *Cevena Bioproducts*, a spin off company from the University of Alberta. It is 20-30 times more viscous than other beta glucan concentrates and contains up to 12 times more beta glucan than oat bran. It is GRAS and kosher certified and lends itself to functional foods and beverages. Visit www.cevena.com.

A recent pilot study of seven adults aged 25-35 who consumed 4 grams of Viscofiber daily for 16 weeks caused a significant loss of weight.

A study by Greenway et al, *J Med Food* 2007 10:4 found not only weight loss in obese patients, but also increased fasting levels of glucagen-like peptide-1 and peptide YY.

Researchers in Winnipeg are developing a test that allows plant breeders to quickly select oat and barley germplasm containing high levels of beta-glucans.

Both poultry and pig growth are negatively affected by beta glucans, suggesting different cultivars for different use. The removal of beta glucan may result in an increased feed energy value.

Researchers at the University of Saskatchewan, led by Pei Qiang Yu, have found a way to make oat hulls more digestible for cattle by removing ferulic acid. This was accomplished using *Aspergillus* ferulic acid esterase and *Trichoderma* xylanase. Considering that the hulls represent over one quarter of the oat seed weight, this leaves in excess of 100,000 metric tonnes of hulls available annually for other uses.

Herbalists, long ago, prescribed a solution of oats and wine for deficiencies of the nervous system.

Organic Oat Milk- made from whole oats and canola oil- is a new healthy alternative to soy, rice, or almond milk now on the market. At present it is processed in Sweden- why not here?

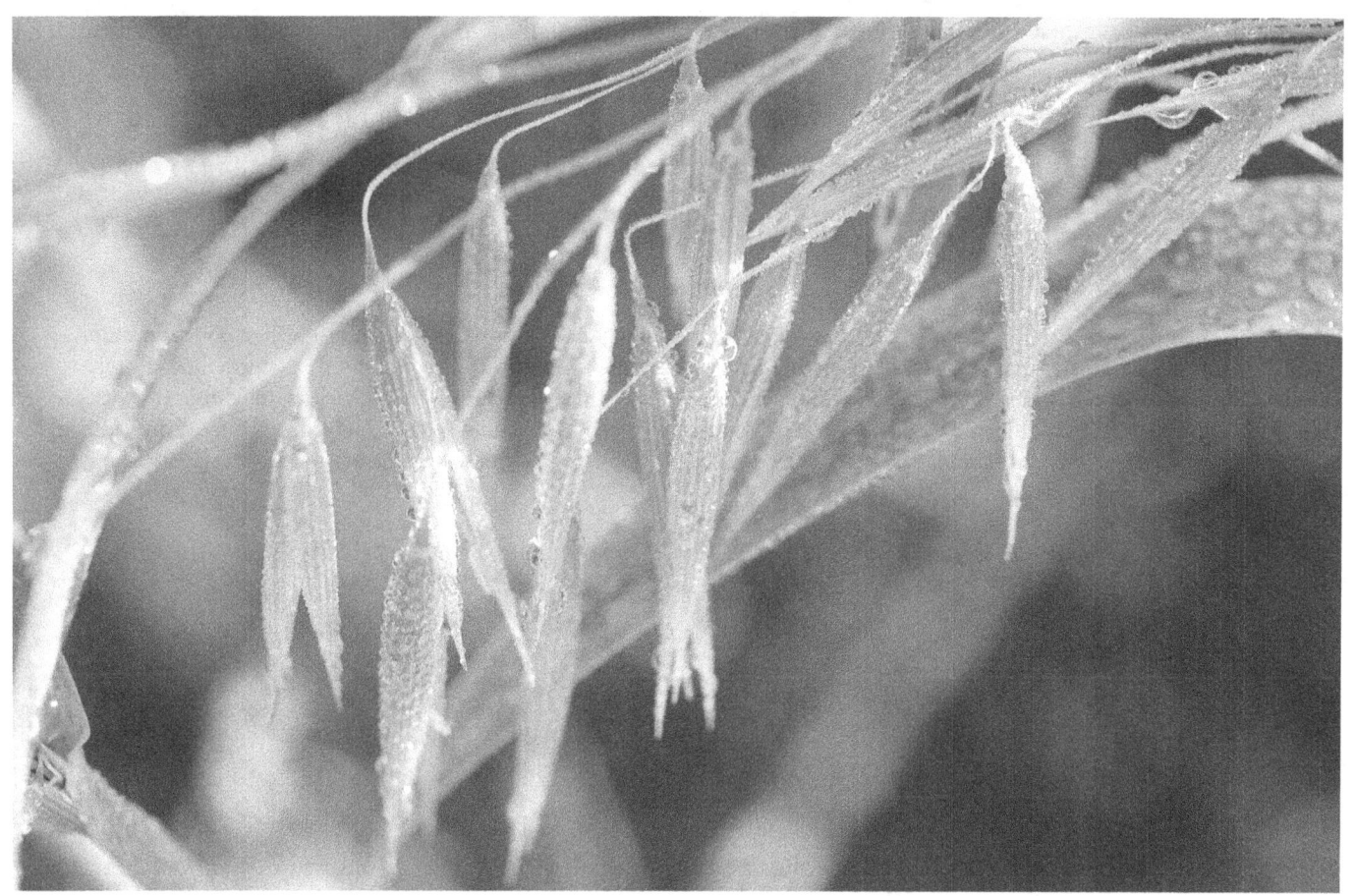

WILD OATS

Oat flour inhibits rancidity, and prolongs the shelf life of breads and other products.

Flowers of wild oats are an inexpensive alternative to fish flies used by trout fishermen.

Wild Oats are classified in the prairies as a noxious weed. However, the discovery of new genes in wild oats may lead to increased resistance to cold, as well as pathogens such as powdery mildew, crown and stem rust, cereal root nematode, and barley yellow dwarf virus; and other hybrid work.

Wild Oatmeal is marketed commercially, with the extra nutrition inherent in the wild cousin.

A soy-oat formula developed in Mexico is the nutritional equivalent of milk-based formulas, suitable for lactose intolerant infants.

Oat flour is the base of **FRESCAVENA**, a very popular South American beverage.

Rashbaum et al, have found a way to produce a commercial red dye based on fermentation using oats as a substrate.

Oat starch is a useful adhesive, a market presently dominated by wheat and corn.

Dr. Kevin Swallow with AAFRD is working at developing oat flour into pasta and noodles, creating new market opportunities.

Cultivated Oat plants (*A. sativa*) contain 0.21-1.18% aconitic acid. This has been shown by researchers to induce grass tetany or hypomagnaesasmia in lactating ruminants during grazing. Trans-aconitate is known to be a metabolic inhibitor of aconitase, thereby blocking the conversion of citric to iso-citric acid in the Kreb cycle.

Citrates and aconitates both form chelates with magnesium and calcium.

Oat seedlings can increase their scopoletin content by over 4000%, in response to environmental stressors. Oat sprouts increase vitamin B2 by 1450%, due to germination.

Hull-less Oats contain significantly higher amounts of six out of eight essential amino acids, compared to wheat.

Oats have been found as efficient as Indian Mustard in the bio-accumulation of zinc, according to a 1998 study out of Cornell.

MEDICINAL

CONSTITUENTS–seeds- zinc and other trace minerals including yttrium, carotene, folliculin-like hormones, gramine (an indole alkaloid), avenine (alkaloid), an unusual amino acid, avenacosides A and B (steroid saponins), hordenine, acetyl cysteine, betaine, aconitic acid, trigonelline, ergothioneine, flavonoids, soluble oligo and polysaccharides, including (1,3), (1,4) beta-d-glucan (2-4%) and saponins. These include steroid saponin avenacosides A and B, whose aglycone is nuatigenin from leaves and seeds. Also contains avenanthramides which show higher anti-oxidant levels that ferulic, gentisic, p-hydroxybenzoic, proto-catechuic, syringic, vanillic, and phytic acid.
A new galactolipid comprising 0.5-0.6 mg per gram has been found in oat seed; and named avenoleic acid.
root- avenin, avenacins, avenic acid, graminine
petiole- tartaric acid, methoxy-malic acid, glutaric acid, dimethoxy-butyl benzene.
flower- flavones
leaves- triterpenoid saponins of the furostanol type-avenacosides 1-3mg/g when fresh; carotenoids and chlorophyll.
straw- up to 2% esters of silicic acid. The leaves contain high concentrations of vitexin (over 2%).

Richer in zinc than any other plant, Oats soothe an exhausted nervous system. Green flowering oats are thymoleptic, especially associated with relieving depressive mental states.

Depression is a complex condition, and some differentiation may help direct the beginner.

For depression with restlessness, look to Scullcap and California Poppy. For caffeine abuse and addiction, try German Chamomile or Pineapple Weed. For depression during pregnancy, try Raspberry leaf, while young children suffering bedwetting may benefit from Licorice root. The weekend alcoholic may benefit from Ginseng, while the older gentleman with prostate enlargement, may find Pulsatilla helps lift depression.

Avenine, one of the alkaloids, stimulates the central nervous system, and is a wonderful cerebral restorative. Gramine, an indole alkaloid in the flowering tops, has a mildly sedative and hypnotic property. It combines well with Valerian or Scullcap for those individuals attempting withdrawal from addictions; or taken alone for convalescence after flu or viral infections, with nervous insomnia and exhaustion.

It also combines well with Marsh or Wood Betony for nerve weakness, and/or with Scullcap to minimize attacks of petit mal epilepsy and other convulsive states. It does not seem to combine well with Lady's Slipper.

It combines well, three parts, with Calamus root, one part, in cases of various drug withdrawal programs.

Patients with multiple sclerosis report less nerve pain and fatigue, with a greater sense of wellbeing, but no definitive studies have been conducted.

It should be noted that the herb works best for normally strong individuals with above indications, rather than for chronically deficient patients.

It should be included in diets for hyperacidity and a number of related disorders like jaundice, gall bladder, rheumatic pain, eczema and diabetes.

Although much credit is given to the power of oat straw, the entire above ground herb should be recognized for its healing properties.

Like horsetail, oats are a good source of organic silica that the body converts into usable calcium. It helps treat osteoporosis, not only as re-mineralizer, but as hormone regulator.

Oat straw baths, however, are perfectly suited and still recommended by medical doctors for acute itchy dermatitis, like dry eczema and psoriasis. It is a useful, soothing bath for children with chicken pox and the like. Oat straw footbaths are useful for excessive foot perspiration, hardened skin, blisters and ingrown toenails.

For persistent vomiting take one part of oats to four parts of boiling water. Drink as often as needed for relief. Oat straw decoctions used in the form of hot fomentations can be applied to kidney pain or tenderness.

Fresh oat grass tea is used to balance the menstrual cycle and relieve dysmenorrhea, and is recommended for osteoporosis and urinary tract infections.

Animal studies on oats show it stimulates the release of luteinizing hormone from the pituitary gland, suggesting a role in reproductive health.

Soluble fibre, as found in oats, lower serum cholesterol levels in several ways. It will bind bile acids in the intestine and increase amount of cholesterol excreted in stool.

Intestinal bacteria ferment soluble fibre into short chain fatty acids that help decrease cholesterol production by the liver. These fatty acids may play a role in lowering serum cholesterol.

Oats reduce blood pressure, and in one study were found to help patients eliminate medications. Pins et al, *J Fam Prac* 2002 51.

A randomized, controlled study by Saltzman et al, *J Nutrition* 2001 131:5 looked at 43 adults for 8 weeks on a low calorie and oat diet. Improved lipid and blood pressure levels were noted.

Oats not only lower cholesterol levels, but also support the heart muscle and circulatory vessels. This includes tightening and rebuilding the veins, making it useful for hemorrhoids and reducing varicosities. Saponins in oats help to bind bile acids and reduce the amount that can be transformed into toxic secondary bile acids.

These can damage the intestinal walls and lead to cancer risk. Acetyl cysteine, from oats, has been found to inhibit colon tumours.

Oats and green flowering oats are both useful in regulating blood sugar swings. Mild diabetic tendencies are greatly improved by simply including oatmeal in the diet. It is used for asthenia and weight loss in the diabetic, and the alkaloid, trigonelline, helps lower post-prandial blood sugar levels.

Recent studies have indicated that oats contain acid stable lipase, explaining their usefulness in diabetes. Lipase is a superior lymphatic decongestant and anti-inflammatory where congested conditions are improved by heat. As a plant enzyme it should be taken between meals for optimal lymphatic decongesting results.

Extracts made from green oats or the milky stage, are useful for several reasons, and may be purchased commercially or made in your own kitchen.

Green oat extract, combined with calamus root, licorice root and scullcap is a specific for helping withdrawal from addictions of tobacco, alcohol and cocaine.

In one placebo-controlled clinical trial of 28 days, fresh green oat extracts resulted in tobacco smoking diminishment from 19.5 to 5.7 per day as compared to the placebo (16.5 to 16.7). Anand, *Nature* 1971 233; Jack et al, *Brit Med Journal* 1971 4:48.

The same author investigated green flowering oat extracts for treatment of opium addiction. On the patient's own initiative, six gave up opium completely, 2 had reduced intake, and 2 showed no change. No serious withdrawal symptoms or side effects were noted. Connor et al, 1975. As reported in the *British Medical Journal*, 10 chronic opium addicts with an average of over ten years dependence were given 2 ml doses of green flowering oats three times daily.

Children who exhibit nervous symptoms such as bedwetting, colic, allergies and hyperactivity all greatly benefit from green oat tincture. I have personally used Green flowering Oats with good success in treating children diagnosed with ADD or ADHD spectrum disorder.

It helps reduce symptoms of withdrawal from Ritalin. It combines well with hawthorn berry for this purpose, especially individuals with low-level allergies.

Work by Schellekens et al, *Phytother Res* March 25 2009 found green wild oats improved rat behavior under a number of stressful situations.

Oat extracts have an antispasmodic action that relieves bladder spasms and pain. It combines well with willow bark, and nettle root for prostate pain and inflammation.

Green Oats also help in the treatment of wasting disease related to nerve paralysis, according to Dr. Bastyr.

Many years ago, a rancher mentioned to me that expressions like "feeling your oats" and even "sowing your wild oats" have a basis in fact. It seems that older bulls or stallions, whose fertility rates are in decline are fed sprouted oats. They became friskier and are once again able to perform their job.

As the story goes, a Chinese carp farmer harvested a small field of oats, but was too green to mix with other feed.

He dumped his load of green oats into his carp pond, which increased the mating behavior of his fish dramatically. It's just a fish story. Fish don't really mate.

More recently, a product from Switzerland contains green oats, nettles and sea buckthorn for human purposes. It frees the bioavailability of free testosterone, increasing the sex drive.

Researchers have found women have more receptors for testosterone in the female brain than the male, suggesting its usefulness for both sexes.

A study conducted at the Northeastern Ohio College of Medicine, evaluated this herbal product on men diagnosed with erectile dysfunction. Definite beneficial effects on sexual functioning were found.

Studies in Japan reveal avenine can be extracted from oats and used to obtain a substance with luteinizing hormone releasing activity. It has been shown to increase plasma follicle stimulating hormone (FSH) without increasing prolactin levels.

Wild Oats are a thyroid stimulant, helpful in treating sexual organ functions of impotence, luteal insufficiency and infertility.

In lay terms, the possibilities with regard to male virility and female fertility are confirmed. Further studies in Hungary have shown this herbal combination capable of increasing muscle strength and mental equilibrium.

The continual release of LH may, however, interfere with normal production of testosterone in men over fifty, if used for a period of time. I have found combining oats with puncture vine prevents any such problem.

Green flowering oats help lower blood uric acid levels, making it a good addition to arthritis and rheumatism therapy.

Add to this the fact that oats contain 24 compounds with anti-oxidant activity, helping reduce the aging factors attributed to free radicals. Structurally, both caffeic and ferulic acid are closely related to the common commercial anti-oxidants BHT and BHA. Health concerns will lead to restricted use of these widespread synthetics in near future.

Oat juice, from the fresh plant is recommended in cases of exhaustion, loss of appetite and building up the body after illness.

In cases of overwork and for sleep it combines well with skullcap. It is a useful detoxifier in addiction withdrawal programs.

Green oats combines well with Mugwort for depression, with Prickly Ash for stimulation, with Gravel root, Nettle root or Goldenrod for urinary deficiency and prostate inflammation.

Frutarom selected optimal accessions of *Avena sativa* to produce an extract called EFLA955 Wild Green Oat Neuravena® Special Extract.

In the process of research, they used a CNS system to test for cognitive function, stress/burnout and chronic fatigue. This sets the bar a little higher for green oat extracts.

Two enzymes, closely related to mental health, have been identified and stabilized in this green oat product. They inhibit MAO-B and phospho-diesterase 4, associated with anti-depressant and cognitive enhancement capabilities.

MAO-B is responsible for metabolizing dopamine, and levels in the brain are important for mental health and cognitive function. Inhibitors of MAO-B are used to treat neurodegenerative conditions such as Alzheimer's and Parkinson's disease.

Inhibition is associated with mood enhancing, stimulating and neuro-protective properties. Riederer P et al, *Curr Med Clin* 2004 11.

PDE 4 is responsible for the degradation of the key second messenger molecule cAMP, which is used for intracellular signal transduction, such as transferring the effects of neurotransmitters like noradrenaline.

PDE 4 inhibitors increase cAMP levels in the brain, acting as signal enhancers. They are used in the treatment of depression and enhancing cognitive enhancement.

A recent study found 1600 milligrams daily of Neuravena® acutely improved attention and concentration and the ability to maintain task focus. Berry NM et al, *J Altern Compl Med* 2011 17(7): 635-7.

Neuravena® improved cognitive function in a double blind, placebo-controlled, counter-balanced cross-over study of healthy adults aged 40-65 years of age. The optimal dose for confirmed acute cognitive benefit is around 800 mg. Kennedy DO et al, *Nutr Neurosci* 2017 20(2): 135-51. A follow-up study found supplementation to 37 adults averaging 67 years old does not translate the cognitive benefit of acute use to chronic treatment in older adults with normal cognition. Wong RH et al, *Nutrients* 2012 4(5): 331-42.

But it does improve vasodilator function in systemic and cerebral arteries in adults over 60 years of age. A 24 week randomized, double-blind, placebo-controlled two-way crossover studied involved 1500 mg daily of wild green oat extract or placebo, on 37 seniors. Wong RH et al, *J Hypertension* 2013 31(1): 192-200.

Studies on various saponins, including discovery of Avinocoside-A from *Avena sativa* in India in 1992, have shown promising anti-fungal activity that may be useful in controlling plant disease under field conditions.

A water extract of roots shows activity against mycobacterium. Traditionally, the roots were powdered and mixed with vinegar and wine for diaphoretic purpose during the plague.

Oat hulls contain a factor with cariostatic activity, according to studies by Constant et al, 1952. Ethanol extracts have been found to inhibit not only dental caries, but the growth of cariogenic micro-organisms. Chewing gum containing oat extracts has been developed experimentally, but has not yet found its way to market.

Oat hull pentosans can be used for the production of sweetener xylitol; and anti-skid compounds, Boyle, 1952; brewery filter aid, Myasnikova 1969; a hydrogen peroxide explosive component, Baker, 1962; linoleum, Kent 1966; and as a component of plywood glue extenders, Stone and Robitschek 1978.

And of course, oat bran has recently been approved as a health claim for reducing cholesterol, but this is such a small part of the story. The USDA now permits food manufacturers to make health claims on products containing a minimum of 0.75 grams of soluble fibre per serving.

Sulphated beta glucan, derived from oat bran, has been found to exhibit anti-HIV activity, even post-infection, and may have application as a vaginal microbicide. Wang et al, *J Ag Food Chem* 2008 56:8.

Oat extract, a filtered product from oat groats, is a hypoallergenic sweetener, suitable for breads, muffins, bars, cereals, dairy products and puddings. It is a rich, sweet oat flavour with a light red brown colour.

Oat Milk was tested in a randomized, double-blind study for five weeks on 65 men with moderate hypercholesterolemia.

Intake of oat milk resulted in significantly lower serum total cholesterol and LDL cholesterol levels. Both HDL and triglycerides did not change significantly.

What is significant is that the oat milk was screened for soluble fibre, and thus some other factor like beta-glucan is involved. Onning et al, *Annals of Nutrition and Metabolism* 1999 43:5.

In another study from Australia, athletes placed on an oat-based diet for three weeks showed a 4% increase in stamina. It is thought that oats help maintain muscle function during training and exercise.

Oats contain the trace mineral yttrium. It has been largely dismissed, and yet it is one of only three stop codon triggers in amino acid production.

Hydrogen and sulfur are the other two, and plentiful in nature. Yttrium is not on lists of required minerals for life and yet is governs the third termination point of protein production. One genus of bacteria, *Bifidobacterium longum* and *B. bifidum* specifically, are the most important intestinal bacteria. Oats and cranberries are organic sources. Aluminum interferes with yttrium absorption, explaining in part, its widespread deficiency.

Selenium can substitute in the termination point when deficient, explaining the importance of selenium in prevention of disease. Yttrium, like selenium, may invoke tumor suppressing proteins into action, the most notable being p53.

Beta glucans, from yeasts and medicinal mushrooms, have been shown to potentiate immune functions, and contain a (1,3)-(1,6) linkage that is largely water insoluble.

Beta 1,3 1,4 glucan, derived from oats shows this ability both *in vivo* and *in vitro*. Estrada et al, *Microbiology and Immunology* 1997 41:12.

A study by Queenan et al, *FASEB J* 2005 19 involved 54% beta glucan tested against placebo in 90 modestly hyperlipidemic men and women. After six weeks the oat group exhibited LDL decline of 9%. Total cholesterol changes were not significant, however, and no difference was found in HDL, fasting glucose or insulin, homocysteine or C-reactive protein. This suggests that more definitive tests are required to validate some of the present claims.

A randomized, controlled study of 12 non-insulin dependent diabetics in Finland, showed that eating higher beta glucan oak snacks produced lower glucose fasting and load tolerance levels compared to control. Tapola et al, *Nutr Metab Cardiovas Disease* 2005 15:4.

A study by Smith et al, in the above journal looked at a small study of subjects exposed to six grams of beta glucan. The diet produced marked pro-inflammatory response, suggesting the need to research immune response to oat derived beta glucan.

Norwegian salmon farms use beta glucan in their fishmeal instead of antibiotics.

Hopefully, this trend will catch on in British Columbia's fishery, and then, of course, spread to the poultry and beef/milk cow industry.

Rhealba® is an oat plantlet extract that has removed protein. Studies have found it anti-inflammatory and immune regulatory. Mandeau et al, *Planta Medica* 77:9 900-906.

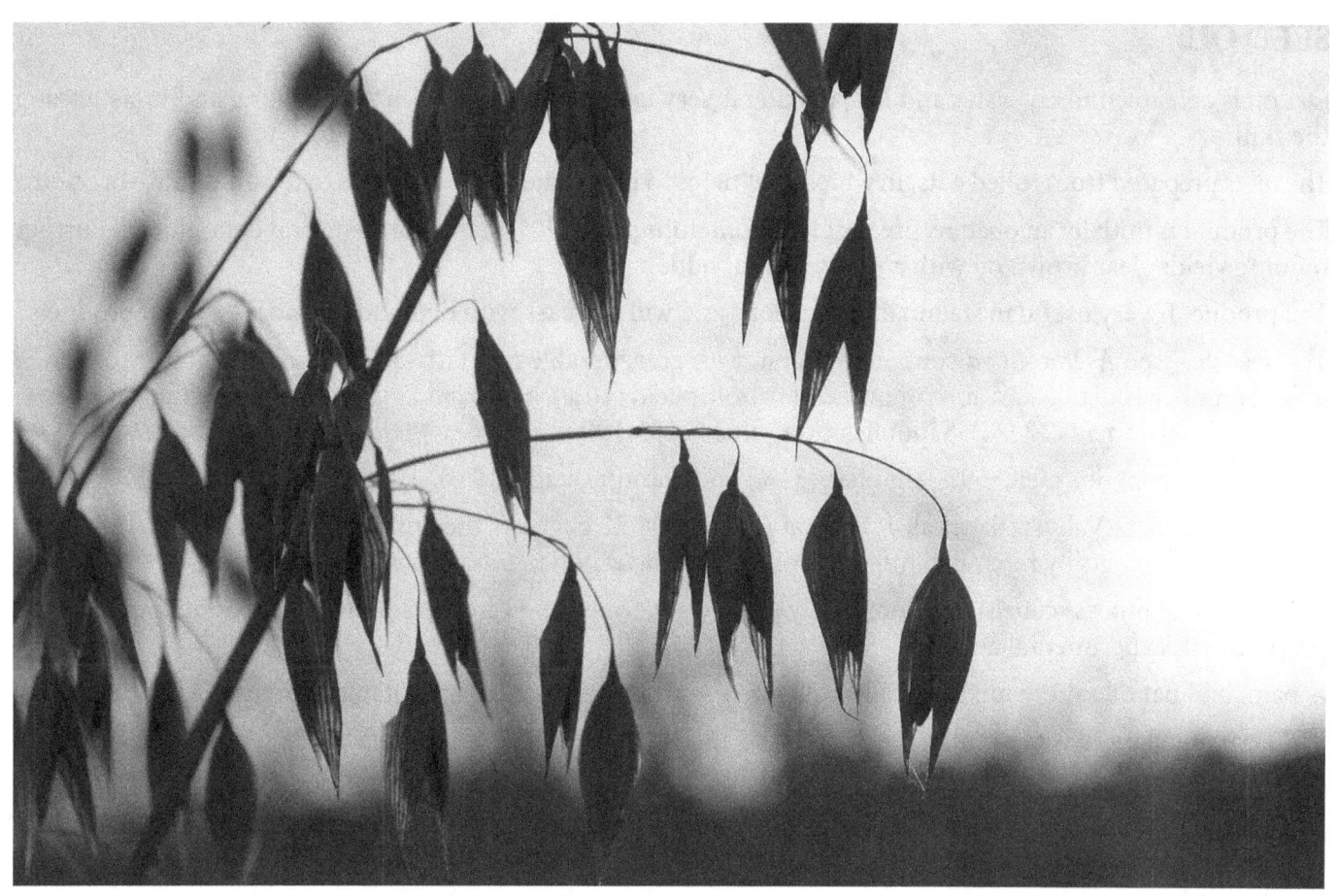

OATS

Strategic alliances between various nutraceutical concerns on the prairies could lead to significant overseas markets.

Wild Oats (*A. fatua*) is used in TCM, and known as **YAN MAI CAO**. It is used to supplement vacuity detriment and to treat vomiting of blood, vacuity sweating and menstrual flooding.

A review of Oats potential as a neutraceutical by Singh R et al, cites a number of relevant studies. *Crit Rev Food Sci Nutr* 2013 53(2): 126-44.

HOMEOPATHY

Avena sativa has been used by homeopaths for much of the above mentioned. In addition it soothes nervous headaches during menstruation, with burning on the top of the head. It seems to ease irregular or painful periods, as well as improving the sperm count in males. As a general tonic it combines well with alfalfa.

Patients does not sleep well, sleep is light, easily awakened, troubled dreams of blood, chilly when she moves, has cold crawls all day. Indicated in those who do mental work, teachers, and women who have become exhausted and anemic, due to worry and acute disease.

Disposition to masturbation is found in teenage males (Really?). Numbness of limbs.

Dose- Ten to twenty drops in hot water when needed. Mother tincture is made from the fresh plant in flower. Clinical trials have shown the 1X potency superior to the mother tincture. Clinical observations with use of tincture in 10-20 drop doses in hot water, in Boericke. Proving, by Swan with one female CM in 1886.

SEED OIL

Oat oil is able to emulsify water and fats, making it very useful for cosmetics, and hydrating and moisturizing the skin.

The oil is prepared from rolled oats, in which heat helps to inactivate lipase enzymes that would cause rancidity.

The product is initially an opaque, green colour containing up to 20% starch, protein, and beta-glucan. Further refining yields clear brown oil with a nutty, natural odour.

The product is very useful in stabilizing emulsions and will increase with demand for more "natural products".

The seeds of ripe *Avena sativa* contain 3-5% oil, with considerable free fatty acids, a specific gravity of 0.925, iodine number 100-114, and are composed of palmitic acid (10%), oleic acid (58.5), alpha linoleic acid (17.2%), and beta-linoleic acid (13.9%). Saponification value is 185-199.

Oat germ oil contains oleic (59%), linoleic (31%) and palmitic acids (10%).

Work by Marjatta Vahvaselka et al, *J Ag Food Chem* 2004 52 suggests the enrichment of CLA, or conjugated linolenic acid in oats by microbial influence of *Propionbacterium freudenreichii* ssp. *shermanii*.

This microbial process consists predominately of the cis-9, trans-11-11 isomers shown to have anti-carcinogenic properties in experimental animals.

A palm and oat oil satiety mixture, called Olibra, is marketed by Lipid Technologies Provider AB, of Sweden.

Wild oats seed oil is very similar, yielding 9.6%, and composed of42.9% oleic acid, 36.5% linoleic acid, and 15.6% palmitic acid.

In general, wild oats tend to have higher oil content and 18:1 fatty acids and lower amounts of 18:2 and 18:3 fatty acids compared to cultivated oats. Leonova et al, *J Ag Food Chem* 2008 56.

FLOWER ESSENCES

WILD OAT (*Avena fatua*)

Wild oat is about the soul qualities of reservation. At times, it is more appropriate to curb impulsiveness and spontaneity; and look at the larger picture. While it is true that many of us, especially adults have lost spontaneous reactions; for others it acts as impulsiveness that leads to restlessness and despair. Wild Oat flower essence can help restore a sense of fun and appropriateness to one's life.   **PRAIRIE DEVA**

NOTE: The Wild Oat essence developed by Dr. Bach, was prepared from Bromegrass.

Wild Oats essence enhances and develops a sense of humor. We can let go and laugh our way past inhibitions holding back our natural growth.   **PETITE FLEUR**

PERSONALITY TRAITS

Oat personalities are athletic, sports minded people and rugged manual laborers. Resistance and strength must be built up to perform their daily tasks.

As these people grow older, the muscles begin to lose tone. There is often an accompanied fatigue, and sudden exertion is a strain on the heart. Oats will help these people keep their tone; preventing previously hard-worked muscles from atrophying.

Many athletes run on adrenaline and have a hard time unwinding afterwards. Green oat tincture will ensure they have a relaxing, unwinding sleep.

The oat person needs to keep active, especially in old age. The oats eaten for breakfast, or the tincture taken to ensure good rest at night, both benefit this individual.   **HALL**

When Oat plants get knocked over, they have a way of righting themselves and growing vertically again. The plant produces a messenger chemical, inositol triphosphate that announces within the plant that it is flat out and needs to straighten up. After a while, cells begin to elongate on the underside of the pulvinus- a swollen joint on the stem where leaves are produced. This one-sided elongation bends the stem upward to resume normal growth.

It doesn't lie there and give up, nor does it wait for external remedies. The oat contains within itself the resources to evaluate and change the situation.

If you've been knocked down by disappointment or failure, it is important to realize that you can recover and continue to grow. Give yourself time to assess the situation. Avoid blaming others. Then galvanize the special abilities that you have been blessed with to aright yourself- you'll find that you have the resources for just such times.
G. MOHAMMED

Oat Straw's keyword is communication. It encourages clarity of thoughts and certainty of communication and helps to initiate action. Oat Straw helps anyone setting out on an endeavor or setting an intention.
EVELYN MULDERS

MYTHS AND LEGENDS

When god named and distributed plants, the devil complained and whined. God took pity and said, "remember this name- oats. Go to the Great Recorder and put down that I have made you in charge of oats". The devil set off, repeating "oats, oats, oats" to himself. As he passed a forest, the birds were singing "koukil, koukil, koukil."

The devil forgot the original name and began repeating koukil over and over. When he came to the Great Recorder, he said this word and instead of being put in charge of oats, he was given charge of koukil, the flower-like fungus that grows on oats.
UKRAINIAN LEGEND

Norse myths link Loki, the often malevolent trickster, with oats— "oats of the devil", they are called in myths, or Loki's oats." Loki is a complex figure – basically a trickster, but often an adversary to the gods as well. In one legend the earth mother put werewolves at the corners of the grainfields to scare off predators, but Loki sneaked past them and scattered his oat seeds. The myth fostered a connection between oats and naughtiness.

People in Germany and neighboring countries typically personified the last sheaf of oats as a horse, a cow, a wolf, or a goat. All of these animals represented not only the last sheaf but the spirit of the growing oats.
TAMRA ANDREWS

BOTANICA POETICA

Did you eat your oats today?
Your colon would approve
You'd also feed the nervous system
Tensions you could soothe
Exhaustion you can turn around
Insomnia relieve
It's good for debility
A tonic when you need
Put the straw in the bath
For itch and inflammation
Or drink a little tincture
To boost your urination
For itchy skin, think of this plant
That you can apply
For a daily nervine tonic
It's also worth a try!

SYLVIA CHATROUX

RECIPES

TINCTURE- Fill a glass jar with one part milky stage green oats. Pour and cover with five parts vodka or other grain alcohol (60% ideal). Shake daily for two weeks and strain. One tsp three times daily. Put in hot water during day and in cold water before bedtime.

FRESH JUICE EXTRACT- Fill a blender with cultivated oat seed heads that are in the milky stage. Cover with water and blend. Strain and drink one to two ounces daily. Fresh juice is also available commercially.

DECOCTION–Although oat straw is above ground it requires vigorous boiling to extract the rich organic minerals like silica. Take two heaping tablespoons of dried oat straw to one pint of water. Simmer for 30 minutes and strain. Drink one to two cups daily.

Use 100 grams in three litres of water for twenty minutes. This can be used as a footbath, or strained and added to whole body bath.

CAUTION- Jeremy Ross suggests green oats is inadvisable for Spleen deficiency with stagnation and dampness. Thomas Bartram suggests the herb does not combine well with Passionflower or Lady's Slipper (*Cypripedium*). It seems that way.

CURLED PARSLEY
(*Petroselinum crispum* [Mill.] Fuss)
(*P. hortense* Hoffm.) not accepted
(*P. sativum* Hoffm.) not accepted
(*Carum petroselinum* [L.] Benth. & Hook. f.)
ITALIAN PARSLEY
(*P. crispum* [Mill] Fuss. **var.** *neapolitanum* Danert (nom inval))
(*P. horstense* **var.** *filicinum*)
HAMBURG PARSLEY
DUTCH PARSLEY
(*P. crispum* **var.** *tuberosum* [Bernh.] Mart. Crov.)
PARTS USED- leaf, seed, root

It produces seriousness in the mind of a person.   **HILDEGARD VON BINGEN**

The tender tops of Parsley next he culls,
Then the old rue bush shudders as he pulls.   **THE SALAD**

The often use of parsley taketh away the stinking of breath, especially from such as have drunk much wine or eaten garlike.   **RICHARD SURFLET 1600**

At Sparta's palace twenty beauteous maids
The pride of Greece, fresh garlands crowned their heads
With hyacinths and twining parsley drest
Grace joyful Menelaus' marriage feast.   **THEOCRETUS**

Where the mistress is the master
The parsley grows the faster.   **OLD ENGLISH**

In Greek, the word parsley means stone- breaker in reference to kidney stones. The genus *Petroselinum* or rock parsley is believed to come from Dioscorides, the Greek herbalist. He wanted to differentiate celery and parsley, both called Selinon. Celery was called Heleioselinon, or Marsh Selinon, and Parsley was Petroselionon, or Rock Selinon.

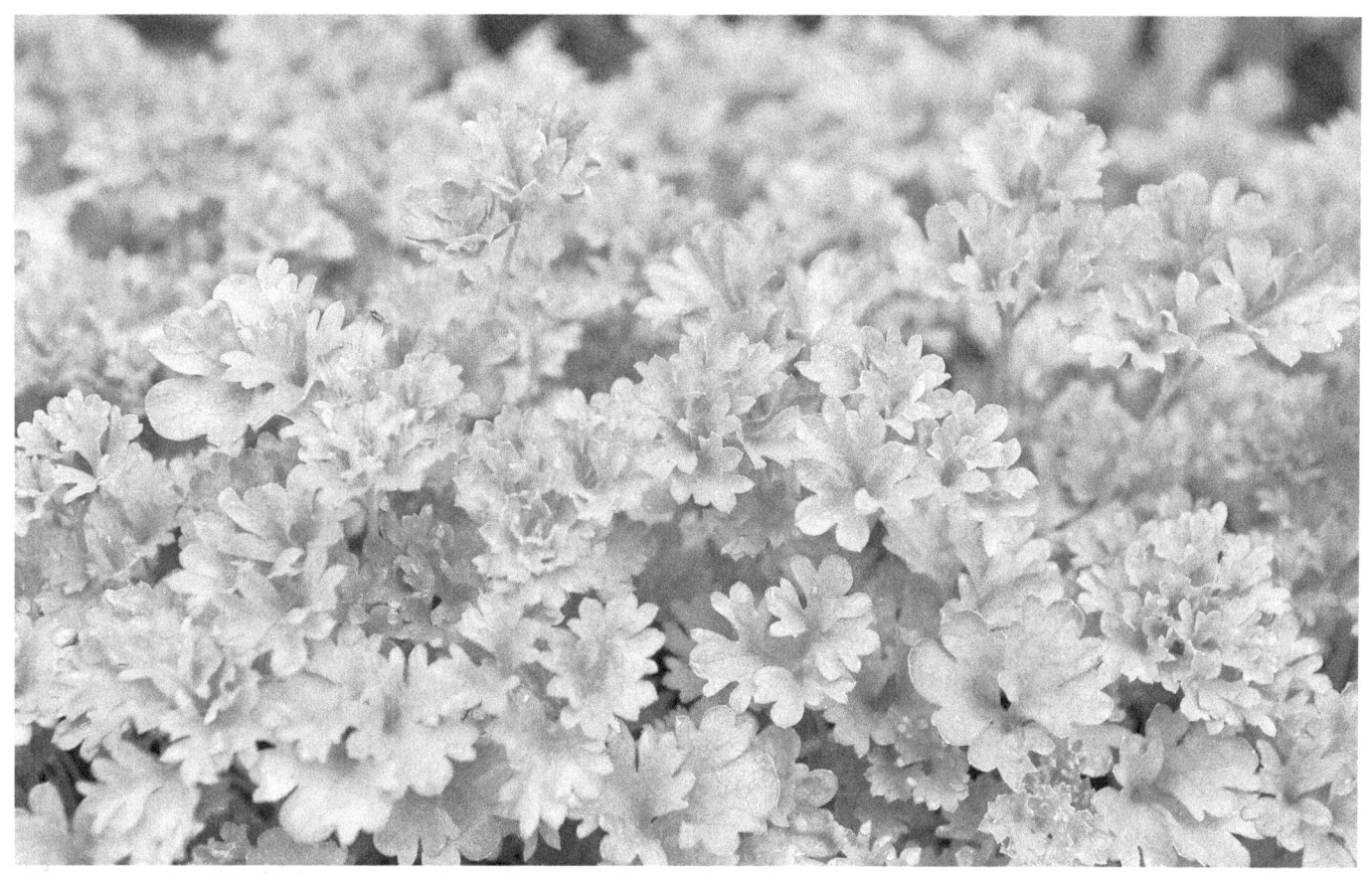

CURLED PARSLEY

Petroselinon evolved over time into the medieval petrocilium, petersylinge, and persele into the French **PERSIL**, and finally Parsley. In Russia, petroselinum became Petrosila meaning Peter's strength.

The origin of Selinon is obscure, perhaps referring to Selene, goddess of the moon.

Parsley is probably native to southern Europe, Sardinia, Turkey or Lebanon. Until recently, Sardinia coins were imprinted with parsley.

Parsley seed is credited with magic powers both supernatural strength and invisibility.

The Greeks said that Hercules chose parsley for his garlands, and wove it into the crowns presented at athletic games. They fed it to their horses, before races, to help them run faster. They even used the herb at their orgiastic banquets, to absorb wine fumes and help retain a modicum of sobriety.

They associated it with Persephone, goddess of the underworld, and Charon, the ferryman of dead souls over the river Styx. It was associated with, and sprang from the blood of Archemorus ("harbinger of doom"), the old fertility king and Herald of Death. They decorated their tombs with the herb.

Another version says that parsley sprang from the blood of Opheltes, the infant of King Lycurgus of Nemea, who was killed by a serpent while the nanny was directing thirsty soldiers to a source of water. For some 500 years, Crowns of parsley were given to victors at the Nemean Games, identifying the herb with the hero cult. In June 1996, the Nemean Games were re-instated in Greece, and participants again used wild parsley to crown the winners.

Parsley has come to symbolize feasting, and relates to the birth date of December 22nd.

They associated parsley with death, and rebirth, planting it around graves, to soothe restless spirits. Someone in need of parsley meant they were close to death. Parsley is said to most powerful when picked on Friday, to coincide with Venus, during waxing of the moon.

Parsley and Rue were used to border Greek gardens, and from this arose the idiom of an undertaking spoken of, but not yet begun. "Oh, we are only at the Parsley and Rue".

This legend led to the expression, "in need of parsley"; which means you are seriously ill.

The Hebrew celebrate it as a symbol of new beginnings, in the Passover meal, Seder.

I love lots of parsley in tabouli, a mixture of bulgur wheat, or quinoa with garlic, lemon, mint and olive oil.

Parsley is part of Baba ghanoush, gremolata from Italy, and in sofrito, a Cuban hot sauce that needs to mellow. In Argentina, it is part of a green sauce called chimichurri for grilled meats. In Peru, a variation of this was a delicious condiment I enjoyed with grilled guinea pig.

The Christian tradition says that parsley can only be planted on Good Friday, the day of death for Jesus, Attis and Adonis. They consecrated the herb to Saint Peter, the guardian of the gates of heaven.

Galen pronounced parsley "sweet and beneficial to the stomach", and to "take away stoppings and provoke urine".

He noted that the seeds "waste away wind, are good for suche as have dropsie, draw down the menses, bring away the afterbirth; they be commended also against the cough."

Pliny thought parsley, or apium should be in every sauce. He even recommended the leaves be strewn on villa stew ponds to cure sick fish. Turner reiterated this.

In the Middle Ages, parsley root was used for urinary infections, intestinal gas, and menstrual difficulties, just as today. Hildegard de Bingen recommended poultices for arthritis, and boiled in wine, honey and vinegar for chest and cardiac pain. "One who is in pain from a stone should take parsley and add a third part saxifrage. He should cook this in wine... and drink it in a sauna."

Witches mixed the root into flying ointments, intended to induce erotic dreams. Apiol is irritating to the urogenital tract, and may be sexually stimulating as well.

Parkinson noted that "the rootes boiled into broth help open obstruction of the liver, veines, and other parts... boiled with leg of mutton...will have their operation to cause urine." Various clinical physicians, over the past century, have noted benefit in cases of liver disease.

This fits in well with an old English belief that Parsley seed is taken to prevent drunkenness, as it "helpth men that have weak brains to drink better."

An old English adage is "fried parsley will bring a man to his saddle, and a woman to her grave". Whatever that means!

In parts of England, parsley wine is esteemed as an aphrodisiac. Virgins feared planting it lest they become impregnated by Satan. Many stories abound related to sex, fertility, pregnancy and babies found in parsley patches over much of Europe.

A Russian product, Supetin, containing about 85% parsley juice, is used to stimulate uterine contractions during labor.

The leaves were used for eye inflammation and conjunctivitis. Romanian gypsies apply parsley leaves as a poultice to bruises, repeating the applications until cleared.

In Spain, parsley is fed to sheep and goats to keep them healthy, and free from foot rot; or to bring them into heat at any time of the year.

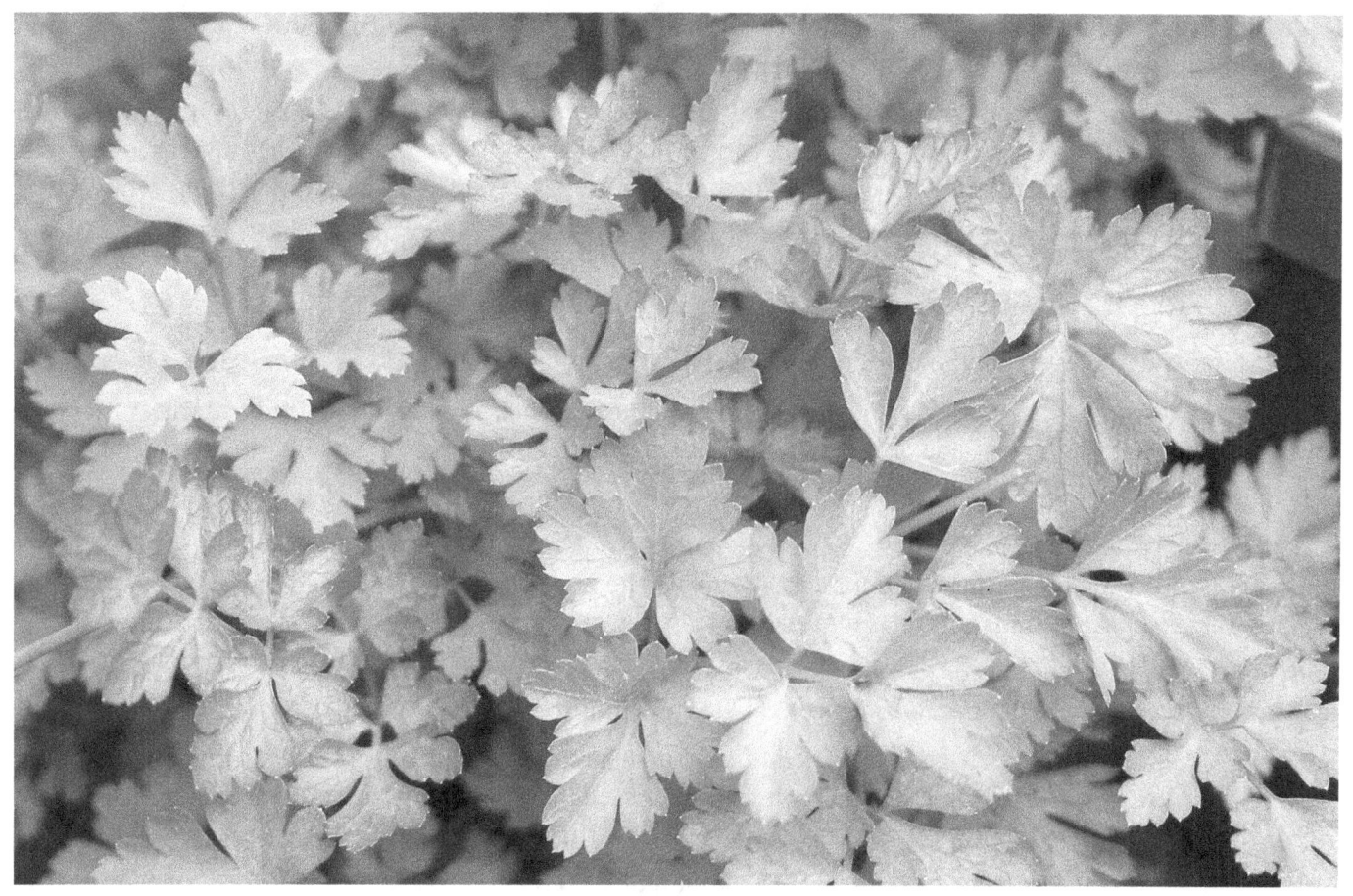

ITALIAN PARSLEY

In France, it was fed to horses, to increase stamina, while in Ireland it was given to quiet vicious horses. Parsley root is useful for animals suffering arthritis that is aggravated by uric acid buildup in the joints.

Even Peter Rabbit knew that when he was "feeling rather sick, he went to look for some parsley."

Parsley was brought to Newfoundland before 1620, by the British sea captain, John Mason.

Parsley has a folk reputation as a cancer preventative, and has been used for tumours of the bladder, breast, eyes, liver, throat and mouth.

Sauer, in his Compendious Herbal, mentioned using parsley greens boiled in lye water with southernwood and willow leaves, as a hair wash to prevent falling out.

During WWI, the herb was used to prevent kidney complications associated with dysentery.

After its introduction by settlers, the Cree incorporated the plant into their own Materia Medica. They named the plant, **OHPIKECIKANA** or **KISTIKANIS**, or sometimes **WEHIMAK OHPIKECI-KANA**, meaning herb with aromatic leaves.

The Micmac were quick to add parsley to their medicinal repertory, as a remedy for cold in the bladder. Further south, the Cherokee infused both the root and tops of *P. crispum* as an abortive, when discharges were too scanty, and for dropsy, kidney and bladder complaints.

In Central and South America, the herb is used as an aphrodisiac, and to treat kidney infection, and hypertension. In Turkey, the herb is used to help lower blood sugar levels in diabetics. I'm sure it is used medicinally in Japan, where they lightly batter and deep-fry it as a vegetable tempura.

It is a biennial, growing up to 8 inches in the first summer. The plant is only hardy to zone 6, where the second year it will grow to 3 feet, flower and then form seed.

Curled Parsley is the most commonly grown variety, produced commercially for the restaurant trade, and dried product. Parsley and watercress are rarely sprayed, and are good "organic greens" without being advertised that way. Parsley is often overlooked in cooking. The stems do not color green, and make a fine addition to any white sauce.

California is the major US producer of parsley with an estimated 1360 tons of leaves dehydrated in 1990, and more than a million tons of fresh plant produced annually.

Italian Parsley has flat leaves that resemble celery, and is hardier, but also stronger in taste. This is better for soups, stews and sauces where the more pronounced flavor is sought after.

Hamburg or Turnip Root Parsley is grown for its thick edible taproots; and only available in specialty markets. The roots can be grated into salads or borscht soup, or simply cooked like small parsnip.

When growing parsley from seed, at least 3-6 weeks are needed for germination. Planting a few radishes will help mark the rows for early weeding.

It can withstand a frost. Freezing seeds for a week can also help germination if followed by a warm 24-72 hour soak in warm water. Germination rates increase up to 70% if stratified for one week or soaked as above.

Thin to 8-10 inches in raised beds two feet apart; with soil pH of 5.3-7.3, and good drainage. Fresh parsley leaves will store at freezing temperature for 6-8 weeks at 90-95% humidity.

Parsley contains a water-soluble germination inhibitor, heraclenol, which greatly affects germination. Priming seeds, which involves the controlled osmotic injecting of seeds with moisture has enhanced germination by 78%. Or soak them for three days at 25 degrees Celsius water slightly aerated.

Osmotic priming is the immersion of seeds in a solution of PEG 8000 or polyethylene glycol, for four days at 77 degrees Fahrenheit. This would preclude an organic certification.

Parsley: A Production Guide by Simon el al, produced by Purdue University is very helpful book for the serious grower.

Work by Atta et al, *Scientia Hort* 1999 82:1-2 found low levels of nickel solution, strongly improves parsley leaf yield and quality, and reduces both nitrate and ammonium content, making it safer for human consumption.

An old German recipe says that mixing the ashes of faba bean straw in soil will help parsley seeds germinate more quickly. To deter the devil, boiling water was poured on the ground before sowing parsley seed. This probably worked, by warming the soil to encourage germination.

Twelve pounds of fresh parsley will produce about one pound dried leaf. Chewing either the fresh leaf, or dried seeds makes a good breath freshener. The seeds were at one time added to flavor cheese.

In Spain, parsley is fed to sheep, to bring them into heat at any time of the year. The whole plant can be fed fresh to horses for relief of arthritis. Dogs and cats will benefit from a strong tea, or juice, one tsp of the latter for each twenty pounds of weight.

Grieve, in Modern Herbal, mentions that rabbits love parsley, but that it kills small birds. I'm not certain of that, but it does repel the asparagus beetle when companion planted. Fresh parsley juice is also an effective non-toxic insect repellant. Parsley mixed with carrot seed helps repel carrot flies with masking odor. It also protects roses against rose beetle, and adds vigor to tomatoes and asparagus. And it is active against *Rhizoctonia solani*. Tiina Ojala et al, *J Ethnopharm* 73 299-305.

Parsley seed decoction rinses have been used traditionally to treat hair lice. Pour over the head and then wrap head in towel for half hour, and dry naturally.

Parsley is according to John Heinerman, a mild aphrodisiac for couples with sexual frigidity of any kind.

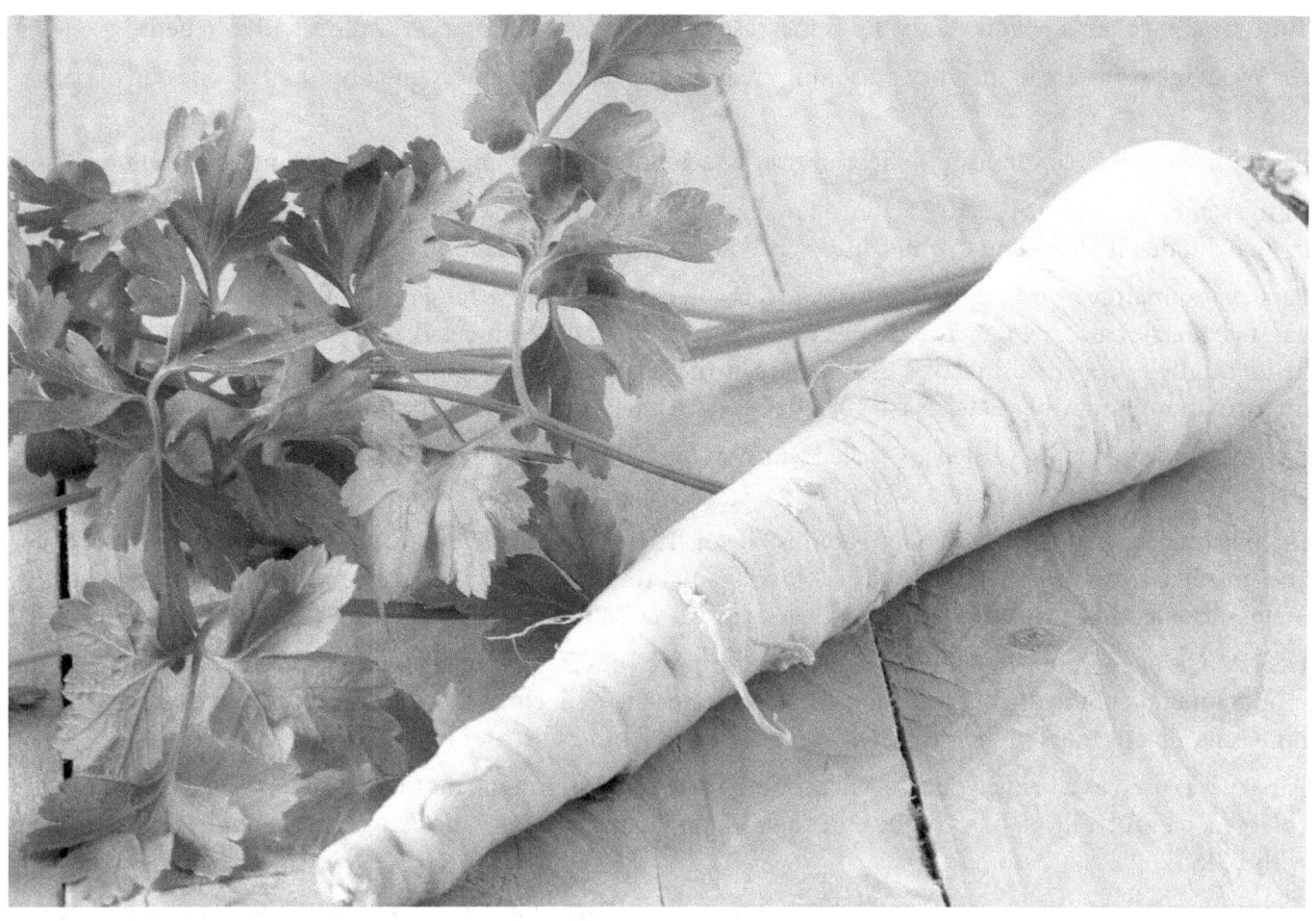

HAMBURG PARSLEY ROOT

MEDICINAL

CONSTITUENTS- seed- 22% protein, apiin (glucoside); alkaloids, inositol, sulphur, vitamins C and K, B12, carotene, essential oils (2-7%), apiol, myristicin, various furanocoumarins like below, and fatty acids, mainly petroselic acid.
leaf-20-22% protein, vitamins A (22,550 I.U/oz), and C (165mg/100 g), calcium, iron (5X spinach), copper, manganese, vanadium (1.8 mcg/g), magnesium, B1,B2,B3, potassium (1%), phosphorus, volatile oils (0.3%), apiole, myristicin, 1-allyl-2,3,4,5-tetrameth-oxybenzole, furano-coumarins including bergapten (21-2000 ppm) oxy-peucedanin, isopimpinellin (79 ppm), psoralen, xanthotoxin (3-289 ppm), and imperatorin; flavonoids (1.9-5.6%) including apiin, 6"-acetylapiin, luteolin, crisoeriol, apigenin, cosmosiin, and petroside (monoterpene glucoside); para-1,3,8-menthatriene, alpha pinene (31,080 ppm), beta pinene (26,460 ppm); sesquiterpenes such as siol angelate and lasidiol angelate; and a novel phenylpropanoid, apional.
root- volatile oils (0.1%), phthalides including ligustilide, senkyunolide, and 3-butyl-5,6-dihydro-4H-isobenzfurane-1-one; various furanocoumarins like leaf; apiin, and polyynes like falcarinol and falcarindiol, flavonoids mainly apiin (0.2-1.3%).
Ratio of apiole to myristicin is 1:1 in roots and 3:1 in leaf of *P. crispum*.

Both the leaves and seeds have been used medicinally as a diuretic, stomachic, carminative, anti-spasmodic, expectorant and emmenagogue.

Traditionally, the Europeans have used parsley seed for its diuretic effect, in the form of a cold infusion. This is probably due in part to parsley directly inhibiting salt re-absorption by various body tissues. Early work by Kaczmarek et al, *Biuletyn Instit Roslin Leczniczych* 1962 8 showed parsley to possess both diuretic and spasmolytic activity.

Both sodium and potassium re-absorption mechanisms appear involved in diuresis. Kreydiyyeh et al, *J Ethnopharm* 2002 79.

This pump mechanism works not only to increase urine output, but increases mild laxative benefit.

Dr. Weiss relates a case of mercury poisoning creating total anuria that was quickly cured by one cup of parsley seed tea.

Parsley has a warming, stimulating effect on gastric secretions, helping improve digestion and assimilation of food.

At the same time, its carminative action allays flatulence and intestinal colic, relieving spasms and pain. It may irritate duodenal ulcers and Crohn's disease in some individuals so caution is advised.

Parsley leaf mainly nourishes and restores, helping in cases of anemia, fatigue, delayed menstruation and even hair loss. Parsley also helps relieve the flushing of menopause and the bloated, water retentive condition of PMS, being mildly estrogenic. It relaxes the muscles of the heart and uterus, and helps to normalize a slow, clotty menstruation. It may be useful as part of a daily tea to relieve menopausal symptoms.

Leaf tea helps attenuate glycation associated with development of diabetic complications. Tupe RS et al, *Pharm Biol* 2017 55(1): 68-75.

Ketohexokinase-C is the key enzyme responsible for fructose metabolism that drives its adverse effect. Parsley and angelica extracts show inhibitory activity against this enzyme, suggesting efficacy in blunting negative metabolic effects of fructose-containing added sugars. Le MT et al, *PLoS One* 2016 11(6): e0157458.

Dr. J. V. Cerney wrote. "In addition to being a kidney cleanser, parsley supplies properties that maintain the proper function of the thyroid and adrenals. It maintains the wellbeing of the smaller blood vessels. Of particular note is its effectiveness in the treatment of weak eyes and other diseases of the eyes."

Parsley leaf used as a breast poultice will arrest the milk flow of nursing mothers; relieving swollen breasts and enlarged, painful milk glands. On the other hand, a poultice may relieve the pain of breast tenderness associated with PMS.

The fresh juice restores appetite, and relieves slow painful digestion, or cases of gastritis. Its antiseptic action helps neutralize acute halitosis, associated with poor digestion, or the forming of sulphur compounds. It contains a laxative compound that assists in constipation.

Recent studies indicate parsley decoctions help inhibit adhesion of *Helicobacter pylori* to stomach walls. This bacterium is associated with gastric and duodenal ulcer formation. O'Mahony R, *World J Gastroenterol* 2005 11:47. Another study in *Am J Chin Med* found the herb prevents experimental-induced stomach ulcers.

The juice or tincture helps tone the arteries, capillaries and smaller arterioles.

A study in *The Journal of Ethnopharmacology* concludes, "the dietary intake of parsley may benefit…the nutritional prevention of cardiovascular disease."

Crusty eyelids benefit from a fresh parsley juice application. Topical application may help reduce severity of epidermal melasma. Khosravan S et al, *Holist Nurs Pract* 2017 31(1): 16-20.

Parsley is rich in apigenin, a flavonoid that helps reduce allergic reactions, and is an effective anti-oxidant.

One study at Harvard Medical School analyzed the flavonoid content of diet of 1140 women with ovarian cancer and 1180 without the disease. They found that apigenin intake was linked to a 21% decrease in this difficult cancer.

Apigenin has been found to inhibit breast cancer cells from multiplying and growing, by inhibiting blood vessel formation. Salman Hyder et al, *Cancer Prev Res* 2011, May 11. Apigenin does all of above as well as oppose chemokine signaling pathways that direct metastasis, including gastrointestinal cancers. Lefort et al, *Mol Nutr Food Res* 2013 57:1.

The compound down-regulates TNFalpha mediated release of chemokines from human triple negative breast cancer cells (MDA-MB-231). Bauer D et al, *PLoS One* 2017 12(4).

Parsley leaf and stem extracts inhibit the proliferation and migration of breast cancer cells MCF-7. This suggests protection against metastasis. Tang EL et al, *J Sci Food Agric* 2015 95(13): 2763-71.

Parsley seed extracts exhibit cytoactivity against MCF-7 breast cancer cells, and induce programmed cell death. Farshori NN et al, *Asian Pac J Cancer Prev* 2013 14(10): 5719-23. Parsley leaf extract is cytotoxic and induces apoptosis in A375 melanoma cells. Dorman HJ et al, *Food Funct* 2011 2(6): 328-37.

Apigenin promotes cancer cell cycle arrest and induces apoptosis through the well-known p53 related pathway. It also induces autophagy in several human cancer cell lines. Sung B et al, *J Cancer Prev* 2016 21(4): 216-26. Beside parsley, apigenin is abundant in German chamomile flowers.

A mouse model found apigenin alleviates *Staphylococcus aureus* pneumonia by inhibiting the production of alpha-hemolysin, and alleviated injury of lung tissue. Dong J et al, *FEMS Microbiol Lett* 2013 338(2): 124-31.

The epithelium of the gastrointestinal tract is exposed to higher concentrations of apigenin, accounting for its ability to halt cancers progressing and spreading. Apigenin inhibits cell growth, sensitizes cell to apoptosis, and hinders blood vessels from feeding a growing tumor. It also reduces cancer cell glucose uptake, and opposes chemokine signaling pathways that direct course to other location. Lefort EC et al, *Mol Nutr Food Res* 2013 57(1): 126-44.

Genins are aglycone flavonoids without a sugar group. Genins in parsley display a potent anti-platelet activity, suggesting benefit in thrombosis and cardiovascular disease. Gadi D et al, *J Complement Integr Med* 2012 9:9.

The herb inhibits the body's release of histamines, making it a useful addition to allergy, cold and congestive lung formulas. This is due, in part, to the vitamin C content, four times that of oranges, by weight.

Human studies by Nielson et al, in Denmark showed increased levels of SOD, or superoxide dimutase, and glutathione reductase from parsley ingestion. Both of these compounds are powerful anti-carcinogens.

Ogino et al, *Journal Jap Soc Nut Food Science* 1997 50:1 found butanol and water extracts of parsley to possess effective anti-tumor activity.

Parsley is considered by some herbalists a biocatalyst, or agent that helps change metabolic function in the body.

Parsley was traditionally considered very therapeutic for the optic nerve, and the brain in general. Apiin, present in both the leaf and seed, is a potent inhibitor of lens aldose reductase, promoting eye health. It contains nearly ten times the vitamin A of carrots, and is a rich source of thiamine.

Combined with red raspberry leaf, the two herbs help flush excessive mucous from the body via the kidneys. This is an excellent combination for first stages of cold and flu, helping relieve congestion.

Be careful, however, as parsley will attempt to remove toxins too quickly, if taken in excess; and may cause skin rashes, or kidney pain. Parsley leaf, added to urinary herb formulas, relieves prostate pressure and inflammation, as well as cystitis and scanty urination.

Parsley contains psoralen, a coumarin that may cause light sensitivity. Fresh parsley juice may be applied to psoriasis lesions, followed by exposing the area to sunlight, repeating as needed.

The herb may play a role in prevention of cancers, as shown by several studies on coumarins in general. Various polyacetylenes, for example, have been found to neutralize the carcinogenic benzopyrene.

The root is similar, but has the added activity of cleansing, clearing toxins and relieving toxic conditions. Its activity is still centered on the kidney system, but is more useful in cases of uric acid, urinary stones, gallstones, and water retention.

A rat study found water extracts of leaf and root reduce the number of calcium oxalate stone deposits. Saeidi J et al, *Urol J* 2012 9(1): 361-6.

Twenty humans were divided into two groups. One drank 1.2 liters of parsley leaf tea daily for two weeks, and the other groups similar amount of bottled water. A two week washout was used and then the two groups crossed over for two weeks. No difference in a variety of parameters was noted. Alyami FA et al, *Saudi J Kidney Dis Transpl* 2011 22(3): 511-4.

It may only be useful when stone formation is already present.

It works better in acute, and even sub-acute conditions, and may be given even in inflamed conditions of the latter. It is a forceful diuretic that must be used with care.

For gout, combine parsley root with dandelion root, cleavers, gravel root, and celery seed. For gravel and kidney stones combine the root with hydrangea, gravel root and marshmallow. The fresh root can simply be chewed for medicinal benefit.

Or combine parsley herb with celery stalks in 1:4 ratio as a juice, eight ounces twice daily. Both leaf and root show good activity against oxidative stress. Popovic et al, *Phytother Res* 2007 21:8.

Parsley root promotes tissue repair including fractures, due in part to its content of vitamin K and trace minerals, like boron and fluoride. Fresh root juice helps reduce swelling and heal skin wounds.

Parsley root extract shows anti-proliferative effect on MCF-7 and MCF-12A breast cells. Schroder L et al, *Anticancer Res* 2017 37(1): 95-102.

Parsley seed is much richer in essential oils, and thus is more stimulating, as well as anti-spasmodic and antiseptic in activity. The seed is approximately five times more powerful than the root.

Its main action is on the kidney and uro-genital system, helping to clear infections and relieve spasms. Anti-spasmodic activity also reduces contractibility in other body tissue and blood vessels, leading to its use in migraines, asthma, tension or weakness of the bladder, as well as intestinal hyperactivity.

Ethanol extract appear to exert more anti-spasmodic activity than water extracts, on ileum tissue. Brankovic S et al, *Med Pregl* 2010 63(7-8): 475-8.

Although recommended by some herbalists for treating nephritis, I would be careful and include an herb like goldenrod, and perhaps marshmallow root to prevent aggravation of kidney tissue.

Parsley seed promotes menstruation, and may be used for delayed or clotted conditions, but not during pregnancy for obvious reasons. It combines well with Cramp bark (*Viburnum spp.*) for painful cramps aggravated by delayed periods.

It will help expel the placenta afterbirth, if this is a problem. As with other emmenagogues, parsley will initially promote milk production, and help ensure normal involution of the womb.

Carotenes are fat soluble, and vital for the proper development of the luteal phase of the reproductive cycle. Vitamin A supplements do not satisfy the need of the ovary for carotene. The corpus luteum has carotene cleaving ability, which at mid-ovulation is twice that of intestinal levels. This un-esterfied retinol will help ensure normal ovulation and regular cycles.

William Fernie in his publication of 1914 wrote, [it is] "beneficial for women who are irregular as to their monthly courses due to ovarian debility." He was right!

Parsley is one of the few green land plants containing B12, the other being comfrey. Water extracts contain, however, an anti-thiamine or B1 substance, unaffected by temperature or gastric juices.

Note that parsley seed can both relax uterine tone as well as stimulate the uterus. The root can nourish and restore uterine blood, as well as stimulate. The differences are subtle, but of course, important when looking at the underlying disharmony associated with individual cases of amenorrhea.

For enlarged prostate with painful dribbling urine, it combines well with black cohosh and stinging nettle root.

For urinary stones, combine parsley root, gravel root, and half parts marshmallow root and corn silk.

For rheumatic pain, combine parsley seed with buckbean, juniper berries, and dandelion root.

It is far more antiseptic than carrot seed, and in work by Marczal et al, *Acta Agron Acad Sci Hung* 1977 26, mild anti-bacterial and anti-fungal activity was noted, in test tube studies.

Ohyama et al, in *Mutation Research* 1987 182:1 studied parsley's ability to inhibit the mutagenic elements in the urine of cigarette smokers. This Japanese study, only on three men, showed a reduction of over 50% of cancer causing compounds in urine, after eating charcoaled salmon. Histidine, an amino acid, in parsley, was found in *Mutation Research* 77 to strongly inhibit tumor development in the body.

Another good reason to eat the lemon (limonene) and parsley with your plate of fried fish!

Parsley seed is considered a good constitutional remedy for the Wood element in TCM, with a special reputation for reducing hypertension associated in this bilious migraine type person.

Work by Gadi et al, *J Ethnopharm* 2009 May 23 found parsley normalizes platelet hyperactivity and is a good nutritive prevention of cardiovascular disease.

Myristicin is present in nutmeg, and during the 1960', both products were smoked for their psychotropic nature.

The compound exhibits an MAO-like action, promotes platelet aggregation, and is spasmolytic. Myristicin is believed converted in the body to amphetamine, to which it is structurally similar. It is also found in basil, carrots and cinnamon.

Researchers in Minneapolis looked at myristicin. They found in studies with mice, that it induced the powerful protective detoxifying enzyme glutathione S-transferase. When given cancer causing chemicals, they developed significantly less lung cancer than controls. It inhibits formation of benzo(a)pyrene formed by cooking meat over high heat. Ahmad et al, *Biochem Biophys Res Commun* 1997 236:3; Zheng et al *Carcinogenesis* 1992 13:10.

Myristicin appears to protect and enhance cell viability in hypoxia-induced neurons via inhbition of the endoplasmic reticulum stress pathway. Zhao Q et al, *Mol Med Rep* 2017 15(4): 2280-88.

Luteolin, a flavonoid in parsley, celery and perilla, inhibits DNA oxidative damage. In a study against 27 citrus flavonoids, luteolin showed the second most anti-proliferative effects against various cell colonies. It reduces excess levels of interleukin-6 and interleukin-1β.

Hydroquinones, found in members of the Vaccinium genus, are present in parsley and display anti-bacterial, hypotensive and anti-oxidative properties. Petkov, *Am J of Chinese Medicine* 1979 7:3 showed parsley possesses both coronary relaxing and hypotensive activity. In fact, angelica, carrot, celery, parsnip and parsley all contain calcium channel blocking phytochemicals; and all are good for the heart.

An 80% ethanol extract of the seed, for example, relaxed ileum contractions in one study by blocking calcium channels. Moazedi et al, *Pak J Biol Sci* 2007 10:22.

In addition, apiin, apigenin, as well as organic magnesium and potassium are anti-arrhythmic compounds that help maintain heart health.

Cold infusions of the seed, combined with goldenrod are good for anuria, nephritis and inflamed kidney disorders.

Ziyyat et al, *J of Ethnopharmacology* 1997 58 looked at parsley for its role in treating hypertension and diabetes.

Aqueous extracts of the leaf normalize platelet hyperactivity and help restore cardiovascular health. Gadi et al, *J Ethnopharm* 2009 125:1. Both cosmosiin and apigenin interfere on haemostasis inhibiting platelet aggregation. Chaves DS et al, *Nat Prod Commun* 2011 6(7): 961-4.

In the same journal, issue 104:1-2, Ozsoy-Sacan et al found parsley protected against hepatoxicity caused by diabetes, in a manner similar to glibornuride. Bolkent et al, *Phytother Res* 18:12, found parsley leaf lowers blood sugar levels.

Pretty good for a garnish!

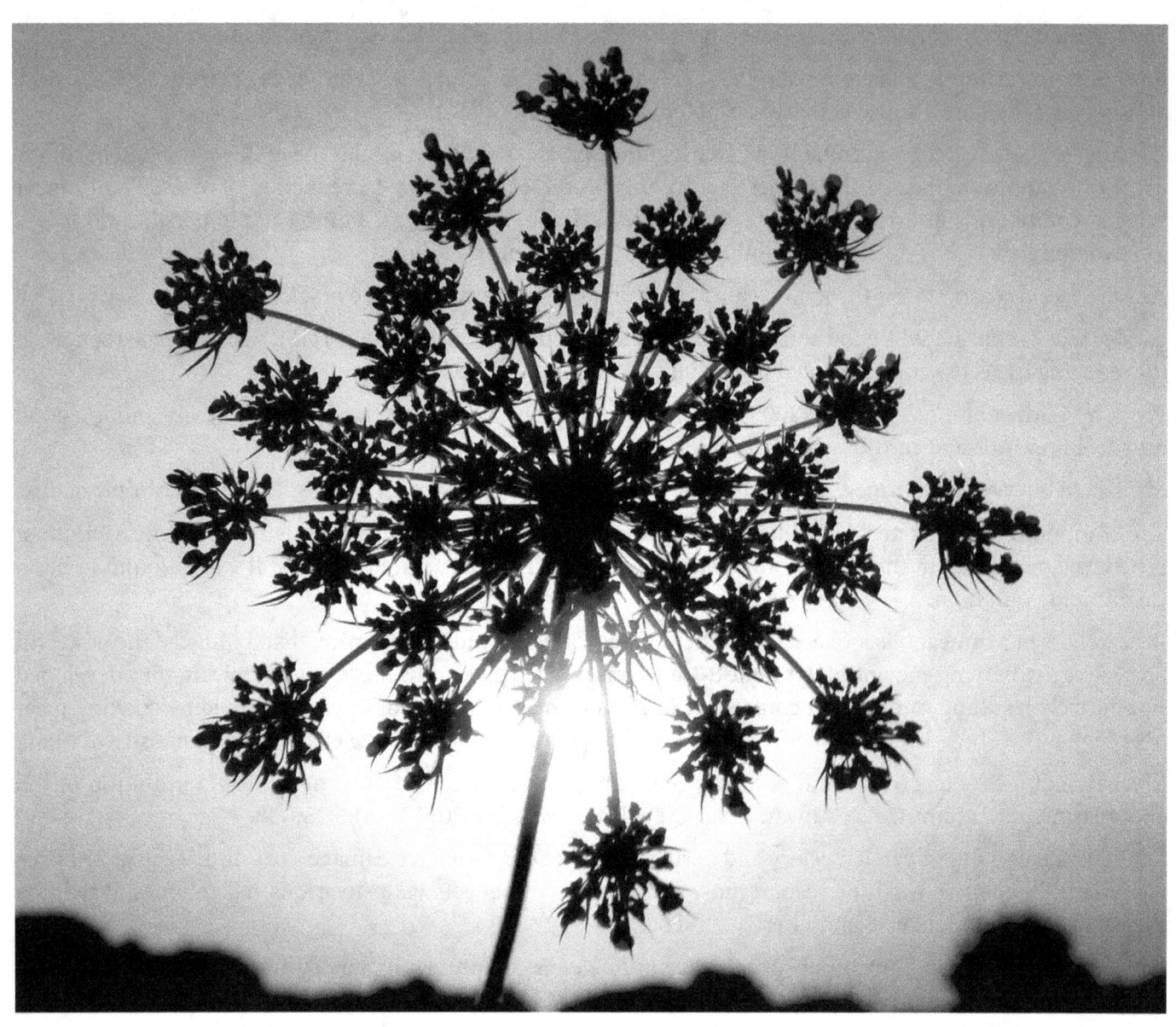

PARSLEY SEED

HOMEOPATHY

Parsley (Petroselinum) is used for urinary symptoms including burning, tingling or sudden urge to urinate. There may be intense biting, itching pain deep in the urethra, and a milky discharge.

The patient may be thirsty and hungry, but this fails at the beginning of food or drink.

There may also be hemorrhoids with much itching. Bubbling in muscles of back and arms are noted.

There may be shrill sounds in the ears, like a bell out of tune.

The itching in the urethra may cause impotence owing to a persistent disorder resulting from the impregnation effects of re-toxic treatment of gonorrhea.

This would be a milky, yellow discharge from urethra with opening glued. It is usually worse after alcohol or spicy food. Urination feels crawling and burning.

DOSE- First to third potency. The mother tincture is prepared from the whole fresh plant, when coming into flower. Apiol, the active principle of parsley, is used in dysmenorrhea.

ESSENTIAL OIL

CONSTITUENTS- seed- apiol, myristicin (ether oxides) ; alpha pinene. Yields of up to 7% can be expected.
leaf- apiol 50%, bergapten, alpha and beta pinene (2.8-22%), beta myrcene (3.5-5%), beta phellandrene (4-30%), terpiniol (3-4.5%), p-methatriene-1,3,8 (28-50%), beta caryophyllene (1.2%), linalol (5.8%) carotol, myristicin (5-17%), p-mentha- triene-1,4-al-7, p-methylaceto-phenone, 4-isopropyyl-1-methylbenzene (4%), kryptone (6%), beta bisbolene. The most characteristic note of parsley leaf oil is mentha-1, 3, 8-triene.
Leaf essential oil yield is only 0.04 to 1.15%.
root- 50-77% apiole, 3-30% myristicin, beta pinene. The root is predominantly polyacetylenes such as falcarinol and falcarindiol.

Parsley leaf oil is pale yellow to greenish yellow, with a peculiar warm spicy, heavy leafy fresh herb odour.

It is very representative of the fresh herb, with a bit of a burning, bitter edge.

Apiol, known as parsley camphor, and myristicin are the main components of the oils, comprising from 50-80% of the content. The familiar odor of parsley is the para-1,3,8-methatriene that is present from 6-65%, while beta phellandrene gives the nutmeg, celery, and spearmint type scent.

It has an antiseptic activity on the urinary tract, as well as a stimulating effect on uterine tissue.

Parsley leaf oil is, of course diuretic, and useful in insufficient urination. It is anti-spasmodic and anti-epileptic, making it useful in relieving the pain of spasmodic enter-colitis and tendency to epileptic seizure associated with nervous disorders.

Parsley oil suppresses both cellular and humoral immune response, decreases NO production and function of macrophages in test tube work. Yousofi et al, *Immunopharm Immunotoxicol* 2012 34(2): 303-8. This suggests it may be useful in various allergic, autoimmune or chronic inflammatory conditions.

Parsley oil may be useful in ameliorating the liver and cardiac toxicity associated with cisplatin. Abdellatief SA et al, *Biomed Pharmacother* 2017 86: 482-91.

The leaf oil shows anti-bacterial activity against *Staphylococcus aureus*, *Listeria monocytogenes* and *Salmonella enterica*, as well as anti-fungal activity against *Penicillin ochrochloron* and *Trichoderma viride*. Linde GA et al, *Genet Mol Res* 2016 15(3).

It may be useful, when mixed with water and liquid soap, for organic gardens overrun by army worms. Sousa RM et al, *J Agric Food Chem* 2013 61(32): 7661-72.

The leaf oil is not used in perfume work, but is often used in pickles, and other spice work, including alcohol and soft drinks.

Both leaf and seed oils are used to flavor canned or cured meats, sauces, baked goods and soups.

The seed oil is more nervine, helping both mental fatigue and overexcitement.

It works well for urinary and genital tract infections, as well as menstrual difficulties such as amenorrhea. Work by Abdullin in *Uch Zap Kazansk Vet Institute* 1962 84 found parsley essential oil possesses bactericidal activity. This extends to uro-genital infections including urethritis, and in small amounts for leucorrhea.

The seed oil is somewhat anti-catarrhal, and can be used in adult asthma.

It can be diluted and used externally in cases of arthritis, rheumatism, cellulitis, and sciatica pain.

This oil is neurotoxic and abortive in strong doses so be careful. Ciganda et al, *J Tox Clin Tox* 2003 41:3.

Parsley seed oil is often produced from seeds that no longer are useful for seeding. The spent seed meal is sold as cattle feed.

Parsley seed oil is not reminiscent of parsley herb, and although rich and warm and spicy, it has a bitter tone.

In perfume work, this must be accounted for with sweeter oils. It is more spicy and aromatic and less fatty-woody than carrot seed oil.

It is often used in modern fantasy perfumes, and men's fragrances; as well as soaps, creams, and dry hair conditioners.

The oil is used in food flavouring and even tobacco mixtures.

Parsley seed oil has a specific gravity very close to water, and separation can be difficult. The use of two separators in series can be most useful.

Parsley oil is available off the shelf in a popular herbal halitosis breath freshener capsule. No warning for pregnant women is present, and probably should be.

One case of nerve damage and paralysis following the use of apiol to induce abortions, was determined to be caused not by apiol, but by tri-ortho-cresyl phosphate.

Essential oil from parsley seed and leaf had an estimated value of just under one million US dollars in 1993.

Two to three drops of the leaf oil, twice daily, may be used instead of parsley root in diuretic conditions.

A 10-25% increase in the content of p-menthatriene is realized when nickel content of the soil is higher than 25 mg/kg.

Parsley seed essential oil is synergistic with pyrethrins, for use on organic crops. Joffe T et al, *Pest Manag Sci* 2012 68(2): 178-84.

Parsley seed oil, high in myristicin, is used in the illegal manufacture of MDA or MDMA type psychoactive drugs.

SEED OIL

Parsley seeds contain fatty oils composed mainly of petroselinic acid, as well as oleic, linoleic and palmitic acids.

Parsley seed oleoresin (12-14%) is widely used in the flavouring industry.

Work by Gershbein, *Food Cosmet Tox* 1977 15 found parsley seed oil to stimulate hepatic regeneration.

The root was traditionally slowly cooked in lard to produce an ointment for inflammation, erysipelas, etc.

HYDROSOLS

"The water distilled from parsley greens and root at the beginning of spring will open blockages of the liver, purify the kidneys and bladder, carry off sand and stones, and force down trapped urine. Drink half a gill in the morning before breakfast."
SAUER

Parsley water distilled from the herb and roots is good for breaking and removing gravel from the bladder and kidney, causing increased urination, or decreasing the pain of passage; helping the liver to improve digestion and helping replace hair on bald patches of the head.
BRUNSCHWIG

The distilled water of Parsley is a familiar medicine with nurses to give their children when they are troubled with wind in the stomach or belly which they call the frets.
CULPEPPER

Viaud found parsley water to be anti-cancerous, litholytic to the kidneys, and a red cell regenerator. Parsley leaf hydrosol is readily available.

FLOWER ESSENCE

Parsley flower essence helps relieve thoughts and concepts continually buzzing around the mind.
BRYNAHERB

PERSONALITY TRAITS

Parsley's keyword is circumspect. It is useful for those who are overly enthusiastic and can get carried away. It will help these people to gather in their energy and become more circumspect and contemplative. Parsley's attitude is like a shy smile under a big hat.
EVELYN MULDERS

MYTHS AND LEGENDS

In Greek mythology, parsley sprang from the ground where the blood of the hero Archmorus (forerunner of death) was spilled as he was devoured by serpents. In general, the Greeks associated parsley with death and oblivion…Yet it was also associated with the heroic Hercules and garlands of parsley were given to the winners of athletic competition.

FOSTER

In a Greek myth, seven warriors known as the Seven Against Thebes stopped in Nemea on their way to battle. There they met a slave girl named Hypsipyle, who held the infant Opheltes, son of Lycurgus, the king, in her arms. When the warriors asked Hypsipyle to lead them to water, she put the infant down on the ground by a spring for a moment, and the guardian serpent of the stream struck the infant and killed him. Parsley grew from the ground by the stream, from the infant's blood. Amphiarius, one of the seven men, was a great seer as well as a courageous warrior, and he knew that the infant's death foretold disaster for their mission and the death for their chiefs. He renamed the infant Archemorus, which meant the "beginner of doom". They gave an elaborate funeral and found the Nemean Games in his honor, and used the parsley to crown the winners.

TAMRA ANDREWS

When St. Peter became the Christian guide of the souls of the dead, parsley became his symbolic herb.

SMALL

BOTANICA POETICA

Parsley used to decorate
Little sprig upon your plate
It's got herbal qualities
And a taste that's sure to please
Vitamin C, it has in wealth
It's a tonic for the health
It can help you urinate
Your menstruation stimulate
Avoid its use in pregnancy
Or if the kidneys have disease
A nibble here or there won't harm
But in full dose would cause alarm
Apply it to your itchy skin
As a soothing medicine
This diuretic herb and root
Is an expectorant to boot
Petroselinum Crispum, you'll agree
Is more than it appears to be!

SYLVIA CHATROUX

RECIPES

LEAF INFUSION- One tsp. of fresh or dried parsley to one cup. Simmer slowly. Take one cup three times daily. Many of parsley's compounds of benefit are not water-soluble, suggesting tinctures for maximum benefit. A small amount of butter, coconut oil or ghee in a tea will also help absorb fat-soluble nutrients.

ROOT DECOCTION- One tablespoon of dried root to each cup. Simmer for 15-20 minutes. Take one-half cup as needed.

TINCTURE (ROOT OR SEED) 40-50 drops in water. Fresh root tincture is made 1:5 at 60% alcohol; leaf at 40%.

FRESH JUICE- 1-2 teaspoons as needed; but diluted in ten parts water.

ROBERT'S KIDNEY TONIC- Combine equal parts parsley root, carrot tops, juniper berries, cleavers and flax seed by weight. Simmer twenty minutes in four times the volume of water. Cool and drink one cup four times daily.

CAUTION- Large amounts of parsley juice may decrease cytochrome P450 detoxification of liver, resulting in increased activity of analgesic and hypnotic drugs. Parsley in therapeutic doses should be avoided during pregnancy. Myristicin is reported to cross the placenta, causing fetal tachycardia. Avoid large amounts if sensitive to sunlight or fair skinned. Limit fresh juice use if kidneys are inflamed or you are taking blood thinners. Parsley in large amounts can cause intestinal spasms and may irritate duodenal ulcers and Crohn's disease. Avoid during menorrhagia or dry cough.

Ethanol extracts of leaf show liver and kidney toxicity at continued doses of 1000 mg/kg in a rat study. Lower doses caused no pathology. Awe EO et al, *BMC Complement Altern Med* 2013 13:75.

From TCM perspective, do not use alone or for considerable period of time in yin deficiency with heat, or liver yang rising.

The chronic and excessive consumption of fresh parsley for thirty years has been associated with itching and pigmentation of lower legs in a 70 year-old woman. Do not take parsley in excessive amounts for more than thirty years!

Parsley tea consumed on a daily basis for a long period of time is a concern. Alajlouni AM et al, *J Agric Food Chem* 2016 64(45): 8640-6.

PARSNIP
WILD PARSNIP
(*Pastinaca sativa* L.)
PARTS USED- root, seeds.

If you want a parsnip good and sweet,
Sow it when you sow the wheat.   **LEATHER**

Parsnip comes from the Latin *PASTINARE* meaning "to dig up or trench", or **PASTUS** "pasture"; pertaining to where to grow or find the valuable long, fleshy, edible roots.

Pliny, the Elder, described Pastinaca, in his 1st century AD, *Naturalis Historia*. This became the French **PASNAIE**, and then corrupted into Old English **PASNEPE**, from pasnaie and **NAPUS**, meaning turnip. The Russian surname Pasternak is from the same root.

Parsnips are grown for their white, fleshy roots that become sweet overwinter. This is because the starches transform into simpler sugars. They are a favorite of my wife, Laurie, and myself.

Parsnips exceed almost all vegetables, save potato, in terms of food value.

The next year, as the biennial begins to develop a flowering stalk, the root becomes woody.

It can still be eaten raw, grated, chopped or cooked and becomes less fibrous by using a food processor. As the plant goes to seed, however, the root becomes rank, acrid and somewhat poisonous. It can cause inflammation of the alimentary tract, followed by colic and diuresis. In medieval England, the long in ground root was called Madnip, and said to cause insanity.

The seeds may be used in salads, soups and sauerkraut, in place of juniper berries.

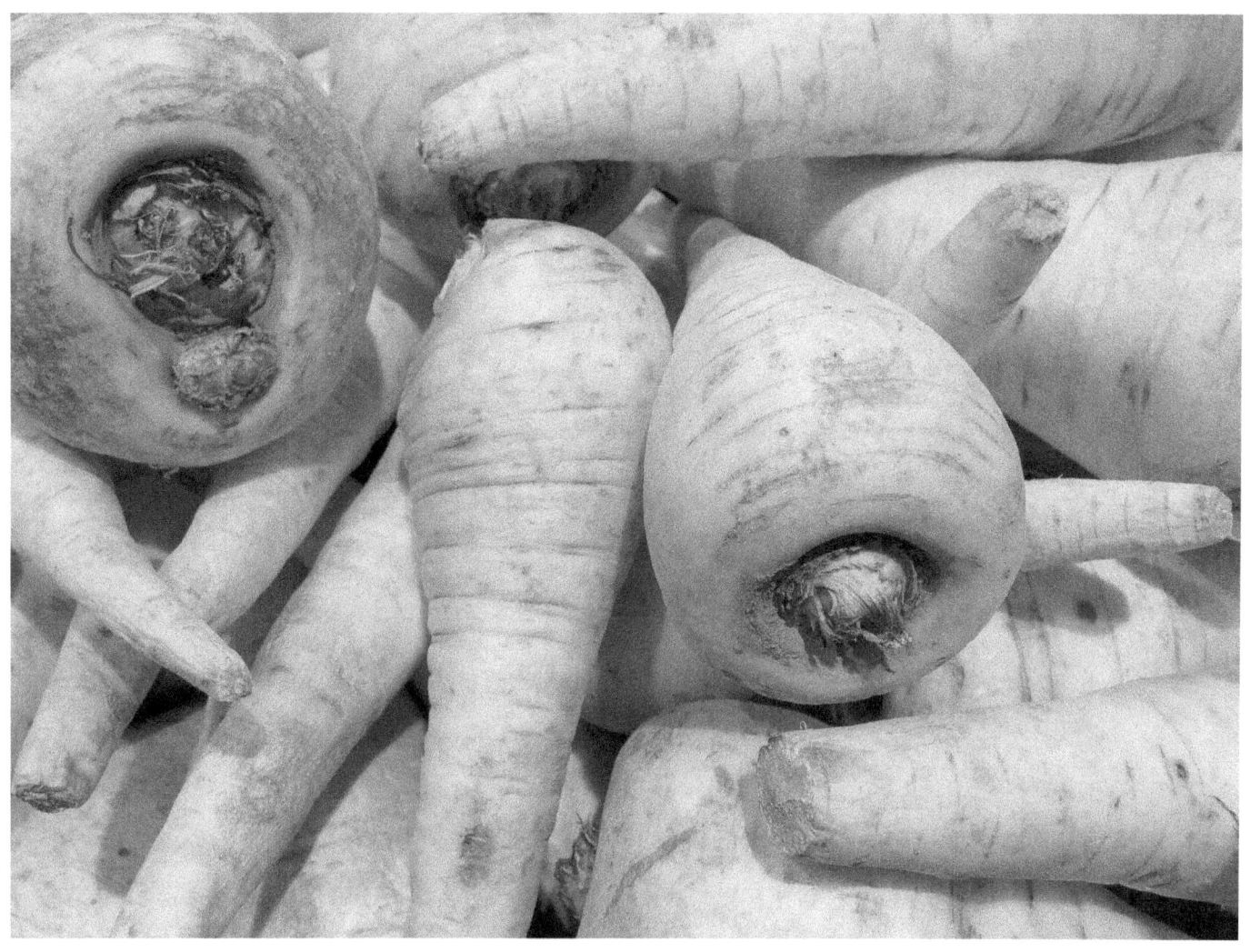

PARSNIPS

The seeds have been used traditionally in stomach and intestinal problems, agues, dropsy, kidney and bladder complaints and intermittent fevers.

In Gerard's time, Parsnip roots were called **MYPES** and made into Marmalade. They were used to improve appetite, and as a restorative to those recently ill.

In parts of England, the cold, previously boiled young roots are called Poor Man's Lobster Salad.

John Wesley, in Primitive Physic wrote, "wild parsnips both leaves and stalkes bruised seem to have been a favorite application; and a very popular internal remedy for cancer, asthma, consumption and similar diseases".

Parsnips are great in soup and stews, a fact not lost on the Cree of Alberta. They named the introduced plant, **WAPISKI OSKATASK**, or white carrot.

The soup is a very nutritious and easily digested restorative for the elderly. The roots also have diuretic and emmenagogue properties.

Early Ukrainian settlers made a decoction of parsnip root and spruce gum for heart problems.

Early German settlers made use of the parsnip, and the fact it can be left in the ground in winter and harvested as needed. Not just for food, as parsnips were one the few medicines available to help new mothers produce more breast milk.

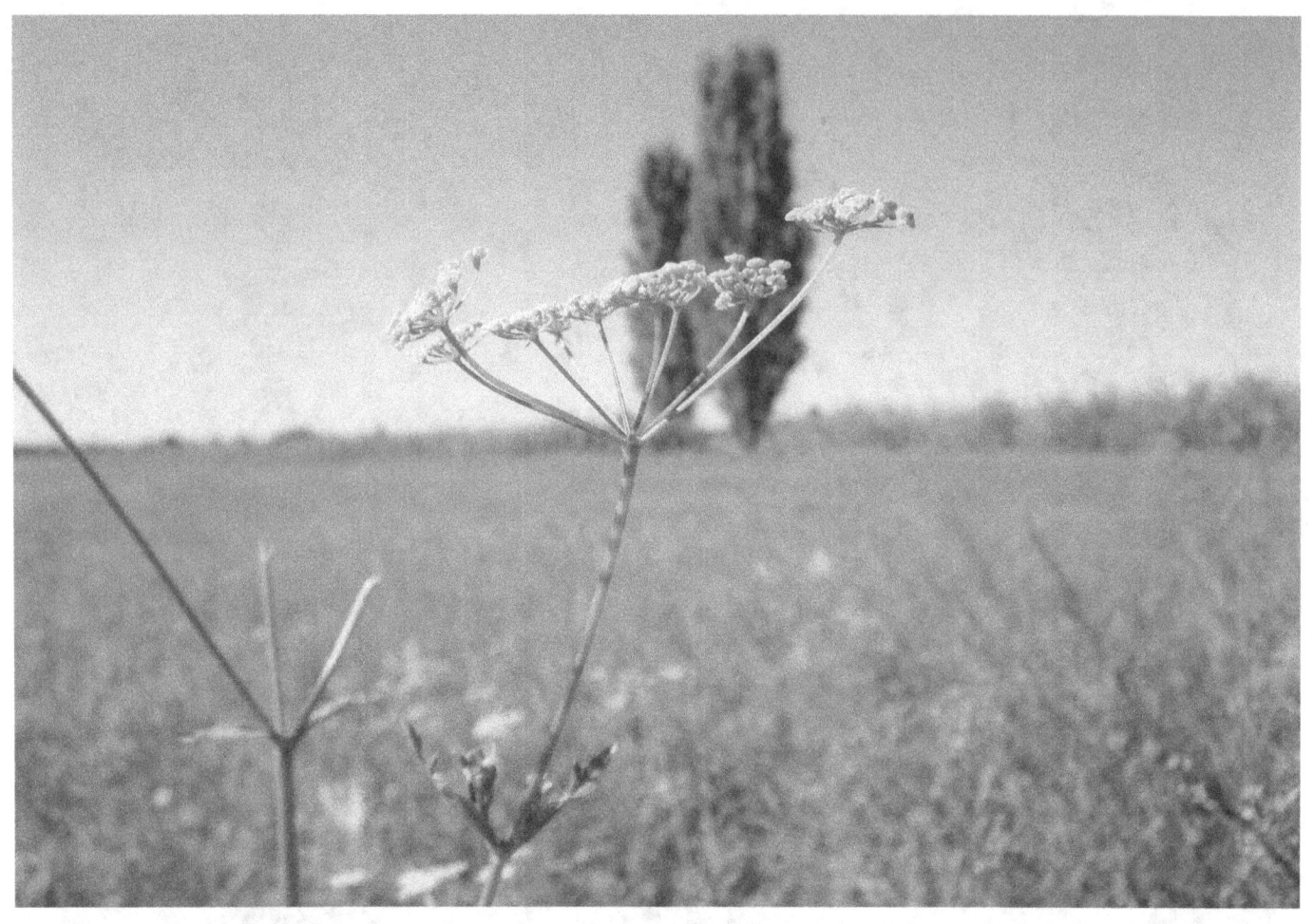

WILD PARSNIP IN FLOWER

The second year roots, or those of the so-called Wild Parsnip, are a different matter.

The Cherokee took small pieces of the root for sharp pains, while the Iroquois used a compound decoction containing wild parsnip root or a poultice for reducing chancres or lumps on the penis.

The Ojibwa compounded infusions of small pieces of wild parsnip root for female troubles. They considered small pieces of root a powerful medicine, and large amounts poisonous.

The Potawatomi tribe applied root poultices to inflammation and sores, but considered internal use too dangerous.

This may be a case of plant misidentification, as there is no proof the wild parsnip is poisonous. Likely suspects include Conium and Cicuta species, or the water parsnip, *Sium latifolium*.

Early work by Dr. Power failed to detect any toxic or poisonous principles in the true wild parsnip.

The young shoots can be eaten raw, the older stalks are better steamed. The fruits contain an essential oil, that have a smell like the fruit of cow parsnip.

The fresh leaves and root surfaces contain furanocoumarins that can irritate the skin of those who are photo-sensitive. The parsnip webworm (*Depressaria pastinacella*) takes advantage of this by ingesting these furanocoumarins and sequestering them in their silk glands, and ultimately into the silk they use to web the flowers they live in.

Because webworms are very sensitive to ultraviolet light, the presence of UV absorbing furanocoumarins in their silk houses is very adaptive. These phytochemicals are anti-microbial against both bacteria and fungi, and provide protection.

Improperly stored parsnips may dramatically increase in furocoumarin content, leading to photo toxicity in susceptible individuals.

In the north of Ireland a kind of beer is made by brewing the roots with malt instead of hops, and a good wine is also made from them. This is distilled, and a product similar to a sorghum alcohol is produced.

In Germany, of course, the root extracts are used to flavour schnapps.

The roots contain up to 200 ppm of myristin, which is synergistic with pyrethrum, in creating a stronger natural insecticide.

Wild Parsnip hosts a fungus that attacks Celery, so be aware.

They are considered better for fattening pigs than carrots.

MEDICINAL

CONSTITUENTS- roots- starches, resins, furocoumarins [15 mcg/g] (see leaf), 5-alpha-androst-16-en-3-alpha-ol, apterin, boron (25 ppm), limonene, p-cymene, spondin, zinc (70 ppm). Xanthotoxin may be present in levels of 8.5 mcg/gram. Significant levels of folic acid, potassium, myristicin, and falcarinol.
leaf- furocoumarins including angelicin, bergapten, xanthotoxin, imperatorin, 5 and 8-methoxypsoralens.
seed- rutin, volatile oils, fatty oils, furanocoumarins, bergapten, imperatorin, petroselinic acid (132,000 ppm),

Parsnips contain both soluble and insoluble fibre, in fairly substantial amounts. The insoluble fiber, of course, helps absorb fats, dilute bile acids inthe intestine and form a gel like mass to ease the passage of stool. Soluble fibre speeds up the rate at which stools pass the intestine.

This helps prevent hemorrhoids, as well as regulate blood sugar swings.

They are rich in folates, fibre and phenolic acids, all of which have shown in lab studies to help block cancer.

Parsnip root is used medicinally in cases of kidney complaints, and fevers. It is also an effective analgesic and diuretic.

The root is indicated whenever potassium and silica are needed, such as falling hair, neurasthenia, ulcerations and nervous dyspepsia.

The fresh root is considered stimulating in small doses, but a nervous sedative in larger amounts.

Parsnip contains enough sulphur to be useful as a natural antiseptic.

The leaf is used in kidney and gastrointestinal complaints and digestive problems.

Like carrots, and angelica, the root contains compounds that act in the body as calcium channel blockers, for preventing and regulating angina pain.

They contain phenolic acids that attach themselves to potential cancer causing agents in the body. This creates a larger molecule that cannot be absorbed.

When juiced and combined with carrot juice, parsnip appears useful in helping to encourage healthy hair, skin and nails. Over time, parsnip juice will help to break down and crush small kidney stone formation, so they can be expelled.

Work by Bunger et al, *Aktuelle-Ernahrungsmedizin* 1996 21:5 found that multiple sclerosis patients taking psoralen rich teas and vegetables showed improvement in functional deficits in a three week study. No follow up has been done.

Pure 5-methoxypsoralen is a synthetic potassium channel blocker drug. The psoralen-rich diet produced improvements consistent with the known actions of the drug.

Xanthotoxin (8-methoxypsoralen) was found synergistic with several anti-convulsant drugs, oxcarbazepine and topiramate. Zagaja M et al, *Fitoterapia* 2016 115: 86-91.

Xanthotoxin and bergapten inhibit CYP2A6, slowing the metabolism of nicotine, prolonging the anti-depressive and cognitive ability of the drug. This may offer a new approach to nicotine addiction. Maybe. Budzynska B et al, *Psychopharmacology* (Berlin) 2016 233(12): 2289-300.

The parsnip seed is an effective diuretic, similar in most ways to carrot seed.

Ethanol extracts of the seeds have been found to induce apoptosis in various human leukemia cell lines. Bogucka-Kocka et al, *Fitoterapia* 2008 79 487-97.

Bergapten may help inhibit diabetes-related osteoporosis via various signaling pathways. Li XJ et al, *Int J Mol Med* 2016 38(6): 1661-72.

Parsnip root is rich in potassium and should be used with caution by those on dialysis and kidney disease.

Myristicin is found in large amounts in parsnip root. Myristicin can be converted into MMDA using the reaction used for converting safrole into MDMA.

It can induce active psychoactive states with visual distortions and the dosage is widely variable person to person. Be careful.

The real role of myristicin is as anti-feedant for insects.

HOMEOPATHY

Parsnip roots are cooked in water, or as a salad for consumption, and kidney stones. It is for loquacity, delirium tremens, intolerance of milk, and illusions of vision. Dilated pupils, vertigo, difficult breathing, and a weak, slow pulse.

Patients stared and grasped at imaginary objects in air and two of them used inarticulate sounds.

A child of two years eating parsnip vomited milk in large, hard curds, and the skin was red, hot and swollen, with blebs and blisters on hands and fingers from handling the roots externally.

DOSE- Mother tincture as needed.

The mother tincture is made from the roots of second year growth, or those from the wild. The resulting tincture is almost colorless, being slightly yellow, very gummy, with a peculiar honey-like odor, sweet taste and acid reaction.

Symptoms were observed in seven children by Pupcke in 1848 and reported in Allen. A report in *Hom Physician* in 1889 is included.

See Vermeulen & Johnston *Plants* vol 1 page 321 for case history.

SEED OIL

Parsnip seed oil is composed of petroselinic acid (46%), oleic acid (32%), linoleic acid (21%), and traces of palmitic acid.

CROSS SECTION OF PARSNIP ROOT

ESSENTIAL OILS

CONSTITUENTS- seed-terpinolene (40-70%), myristicine (17-40%), and furocoumarins; aliphatic esters butyl-, hexyl-, and decyl butryate, decyl acetate; hexanol, decanol, octenol, acetic-,butyric- and caproic acid esters, etc.
leaf- cis beta and trans-B-ocimene, terpinolene (64%) trans-B-farescene, y-palmitolactone, myristicine (23.6%) as well as mono and sesquiterpene hydrocarbons; mycrene, pinene, and limonene.
root- terpinolene, vanillin and myristicine (80-88%), as well as minor amounts of mono and sesquiterpene hydrocarbons.

From parsnip seeds, an essential oil is steam distilled. It is a powerful antispasmodic, with particular affinity for the gastro-intestinal region and used for spastic colon, irritable bowel, Crohn's and colitis.

It is used in cases of glaucoma, and various opacities of the sclera of the eye.

It should be used dermally and not put anywhere near the eyes.

It is of some interest that the so-called boar pheromone has been identified and present in parsnip at a concentration of 8 ng/gram of the plant. The chemical configuration for this sex hormone is 5 alpha-androst-16-en-3-one.

Their odour for humans has been qualified as a primary odour on the basis of specific anosmia distribution. The existence of a specific androstenone receptor has been postulated, by numerous researchers.

The pheromone 3alpha-androstenol is produced in a male boar's saliva, and the odour advances puberty in juvenile female pigs by a least a moth.

Confined pigs may suffer delayed puberty, especially in confined pens, and priming pheromones are an inexpensive, labor saving and hormone sparing approach to livestock production.

Much of the musky odor associated with male underarm is caused by 3alpha androstenol, and 5alpha androstenone; with men producing up to 50 times more of the latter than women. The latter is found in truffles, a gourmet fungi, rooted out from the base of oak trees, by trained pigs and dogs.

The 19th century chef Brillat Savarin suggested that truffles are not a true aphrodisiac but "it can make women more affectionate and men more attentive."

The chemical is present in the root and the essential oil, and definitely acts to stimulate sexual arousal in a number of female species, including human. Celery is similar in effect.

An essential oil steam distilled from the root is quite aromatic, with the suggestion of vetiver. It is occasionally used in spicy, herb-like perfumes.

The umbels, without seeds, produce an essential oil similar to ambrette seeds, and valuable indeed.

Essential oil from the whole plant is about 30% effective against the pine wood nematode in work by Kim et al, *J Ag Food Chem* 2008 56.

RECIPES

FRESH ROOT- Take one teaspoon of the freshly, grated root three times daily

DECOCTION- Take one teaspoon of the dried leaf to one litre of water and simmer for ten minutes. For the first 8 days, drink 4 ounces three times daily, during the second week drink 8 ounces, increasing up to two litres daily as needed for 4-6 weeks.

Furocoumarins, like those in grapefruit juice, can act as highly potent inhibitors of cytochrome P450 and affect drug metabolism. Be aware if taking meds!

PEARLY EVERLASTING
(*Anaphalis margaritacea* [L.] Benth & Hook.)
(*A. occidentalis* [Greene] A. Heller) not accepted
WESTERN MARSH CUDWEED
(*Gnaphalium palustre* Nutt.)
SLENDER CUDWEED
WRIGHT'S CUDWEED
WHITE EVERLASTING
(*Pseudognaphalium microcephalum* [Nutt.] Anderb.)
(*G. microcephalum* Nutt.) not accepted
(*G. thermale* E. E. Nelson) not accepted
(*P. thermale* [E. E. Nelson] G. L. Nesom)
LOW CUDWEED
COTTONWEED
GOLDEN MOTHWORT
LIFE EVERLASTING
MARSH EVERLASTING
(*G. uliginosum* L.)
(*Filaginella uliginosa* [L.] Opiz) not accepted
COMMON CUDWEED
SWEET EVERLASTING
RABBIT TOBACCO
(*Pseudognaphalium obtusifolium* [L.]
        Hilliard & B.L. Burtt)
(*G. obtusifolium* L.) not accepted
CLAMMY EVERLASTING
WINGED CUDWEED
MACOUN'S CUDWEED
(*P. viscosum* auct. non[Kunth] W. A. Weber)
(*P. macounii* [Greene] Kartesz)

ROSY EVERLASTING
PINK PUSSY TOES
(*Antennaria rosea* Greene)
PLANTAIN LEAF EVERLASTING
WOMAN'S TOBACCO
(*A. plantaginifolia* [L.] Richards.)
SMALL FLOWERING PUSSYTOES
(*A. microphylla* Rydb.)
(*A. rosea* var. *nitida* [Greene] Breitung) not accepted
LOW EVERLASTING
SMALL LEAF PUSSYTOES
(*A. parvifolia* Nutt.)
LESSER CAT'S FOOT
FIELD PUSSYTOES
FIELD CAT'S FOOT
PRAIRIE EVERLASTING
(*A. neglecta* Greene)
HOWELL'S PUSSYTOES
(*A. howellii* var. *athabascensis* [Greene] Boivin)
        not accepted
(*A. howellii* var. *campestris* [Rydb.] Boivin)
        not accepted
(*A. howellii* ssp. *neodioica* [Greene.] Bayer)
ALPINE PUSSYTOES
ROCKY MOUNTAIN PUSSYTOES
(*A. media* Greene)
(*A. alpina* [L.] Gaertn.)
PARTS USED-leaves and flowers

Look at those cats, all in rows
Lying on their backs, showing their toes.
With the sun burning bright, that's bad because
Cats on their back will get sunburned paws.

JACK SANDERS

Antennaria is derived from the antennae- originally from the Latin **ANTENNA**, literally the yard of a sailing ship.

To me, it looks like a cat's paw, and hence the other common name.

Margarites is from the Greek **MARGARON** for "pearl", while Gnapalium or Gnaphalis is from the Greek **GNAPHALLON** meaning, a lock of wool, or **GNAPHALION**, a downy plant with soft white leaves used for stuffing cushions. Note how anaphalis is an anagram of gnaphalium. Well, sort of!

Cudweed is derived from the word Cud, in turn derived from the Anglo-Saxon and Dutch words for vulva. Related species were used in Europe to prevent or relieve chafing. Other sources claim it was given to cattle that had lost their ruminating (cud) ability. Uliginosum means, "of marshy places".

There is some taxonomic confusion over the naming of these beautiful plants. For example, some authors believe that *A. rosea* was changed to *A. microphylla* in 1973. It can be confusing, but fortunately they all have similar benefits.

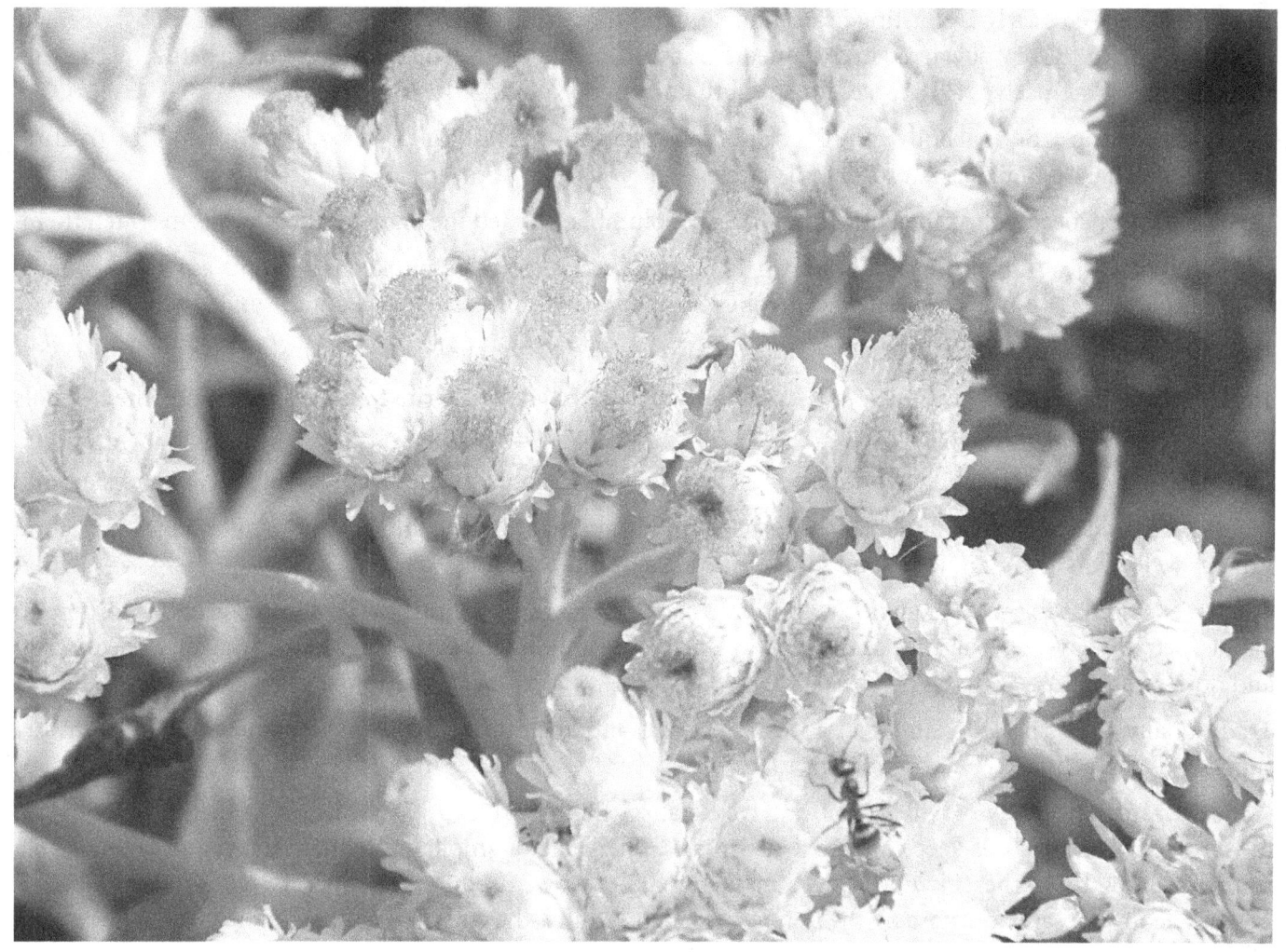

PEARLY EVERLASTING

The Antennaria are examples of so-called incomplete flowers, having only female components. As there is no male, there is no pollen. Instead the ovules fertilize themselves and produce seeds that in turn produce identical clones. To add confusion, they will on rare occasion produce male colonies!

Pearly, or life everlasting is also a perennial that produces both sexes. As the name connotes, the herb has long been associated with longevity and healing. It was traditionally used in spells to ward off aging and restoring youth. Everlasting also refers to the dried flower heads keeping their shape and color indefinitely.

Under a microscope, the flowers resemble miniature blossoms of the pond lily.

An old English cure was a cup of everlasting tea accompanied with this verse.

> "Chill and ill, pains and banes,
> Do your fasting with life everlasting".

The dry plant infusion is a pale yellow green, slightly bitter, but significantly salty, with a warm aromatic, relaxing quality.

It is a pleasant freshener of linens and chest of drawers. Early pioneers, as well as the Thompson and other indigenous healers filled pillows with the pungent plant to guard against tuberculosis. It smells a bit like acorns.

The Chippewa smudged pearly everlasting flowers, known as **WA'BIGWUN** in ritual sweats for rheumatism and combined it with mint for treating paralysis.

The Cherokee used pearly everlasting in steam treatments for curing headaches or blindness caused by excessive sun. They carried the dry powdered herb in medicine bundles, and protected themselves before battle, by chewing and spitting on themselves and horses for strength and energy.

The Mohawk and Iroquois both combined mullein root and everlasting flowers as an infusion for treating asthma; the Nlaka'pamux used it for flu mixtures.

Various native tribes, such as the Ditidaht of British Columbia, rubbed the plant on their hands to soften them.

The leaves of Ladies' Tobacco, as it was known, and Rosy Everlasting were smoked for asthma as well as coughs, colds and fevers. A gum from the stems was chewed and said to make the user want to sing!

The Karok tribe used cold infusions of Slender Cudweed (*G. microcephalum*) to wash sore eyes.

The introduced Marsh or Low Cudweed (*G. uliginsoum*) makes a good hair rinse for lice infestation. The Iroquois used the plant for bruises, and as part of a compound infusion for asthma.

In Russia, it is used for treating hypertension. It is thought to be both an anti-depressant and aphrodisiac.

Marsh Cudweed has a warm and dry nature, used traditionally in Europe for killing worms, congestion of the liver, as well as dissolving mucous and sand in the kidney and bladder.

The Greeks used it for swollen glands with mumps, applying a dipped cloth to the affected area. According to Culpepper, Pliny wrote, "the juice of the herb taken in wine and milk is a sovereign remedy against the mumps and quinsy."

Traditionally, it was boiled with lye as a wash for mites and lice of the scalp. As the name Golden Mothwort suggests, it can be placed among woolens to keep away moths and other insects.

Gerard wrote "*Gnaphalium* boiled in strong lye, cleanses the hair from nits and lice: also the herb being laid in ward-robes and presses keeps apparel from moths. The fume or smoke of the herb dried and taken with a funnel, being burned therein and received in such manner as we used to take tobacco that is with a crooked pipe made for the same purpose by the potter, prevaileth against the cough of the lungs, the great ache or pain of the head and cleanses the breast and inward parts".

When dried and smoked like tobacco, it is good for toothaches and draining the sinus cavities of the head.

Both *G. ulignosum* and *G. palustre* look similar. The former is introduced, likes moist environments, has been found around Fort Chipewyan, and has green to brown tips. The latter is more widespread around southern Alberta, and usually has white tips. It is unfortunate they have the same common name, but are so similar in appearance and constituents that they can be used interchangeably.

Marsh Cudweed is used in Kentucky and Georgia for treating asthma. In South Carolina, "life everlasting tea is considered to be the most popular native cold remedy."

Tommy Bass, a famous southeastern American herbalist, says that the plant is excellent for asthma and sinus trouble, and that "one man and his wife put the plants in a stewer and set it on a heater in the room, and they slept so good they almost didn't get up the next morning."

He used the herb for migraine headaches, and as a cough syrup that doesn't upset the stomach.

Common Cudweed (*P. obtusifolium*) is found as far west as Manitoba. It is also known as White Balsam and Poverty Weed.

It has the nicest scent of any members of this family.

Rosy Everlasting, also known as Pink Pussytoes, root was used by the Okanagan as part of a winter dance ceremony. The smoke from a smudge was said to drive away bad spirits and revive tired dancers.

The fresh leaves were chewed to improve male potency. The closely related *A. luzuloides* was used for similar purpose.

The neighboring Nlaka'pmx, chewed the stems and leaves as a cough and cold medicine.

The fresh juice enjoyed early reputation as an aphrodisiac. It was soaked in wine for removing intestinal worms in various cultures around the globe. In Quebec, the plant is infused for treating burns.

Smaller or Lesser Cat's Foot (*A. howellii ssp. neodioica*) is a common mat forming perennial of the open woods and grasslands of the prairies. The Fox tribe used the whole plant infusion for preventing hemorrhage during childbirth. The

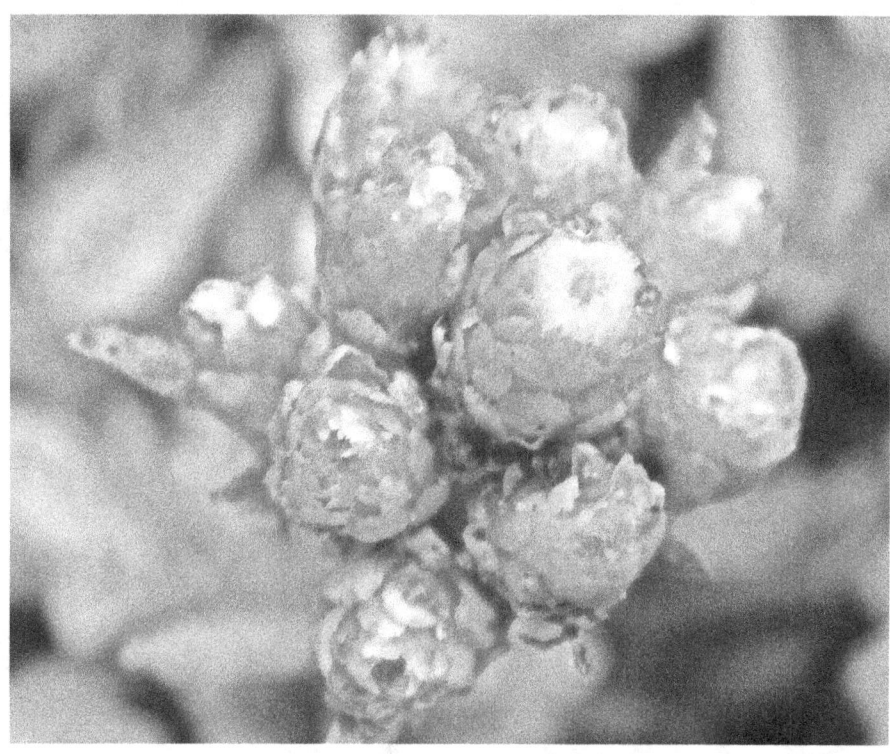

PINK PUSSYTOES

Flambeau, another member of the Ojibwa confederacy, also used the whole herb, called **GAGIGE'BUG** after birth.

The Navaho Ramah used *A. parvifolia* ceremonially to treat mad coyote bites, or drank cold infusions as protection against witches. The neighboring Navaho Kayenta chewed the plant with deer or sheep fat as a blood purifier.

Lesser Cat's Foot (*A. neglecta*) leaf was decocted, by the Bella Coola for pain in the body, but not the limbs. The Ojibwa gave infusions after childbirth to remove the placenta and help heal. Several groups chewed the plant for coughs and colds. The plant is found in British Columbia and on the dry prairies.

Gnaphalium viscosum shows a range of anti-bacterial activity. Villagomez-Ibarra JR et al, *Fitoterapia* 2001 72(6): 692-4.

Clammy Everlasting is an annual/biennial that looks somewhat like Pearly but has a white centre on the flowers, instead of yellow. It is rare but can be used in a similar manner.

The Cherokee call it **KÂSD'ÚTA** or stimulating ashes, due to appearance of leaves. Decoctions are taken for colds and used in sweat baths.

Plantain-leaved Everlasting is found in southeastern Manitoba, but no further west.

The leaf tea was used, by the Meskwaki every day for two weeks before childbirth, to prevent sickness in mother. Eclectic physicians have used the plants volatile oils as a soothing expectorant. Natives of Quebec used it for coughs, colds and pulmonary inflammations. Early German settlers used the plant for dysentery.

In India, the related *G. polycephalum* is widely used for the anti-malarial and anti-febrile action. The Chinese use the same plant for driving away insects and moths.

This plant is found down east and was reported by Smith to be used by the Meskwaki as a smudge for bringing back loss of mind, or to revive consciousness.

Anaphalis contorta, another closely related plant from the Himalayas, is used to stimulate appetite and is a general tonic.

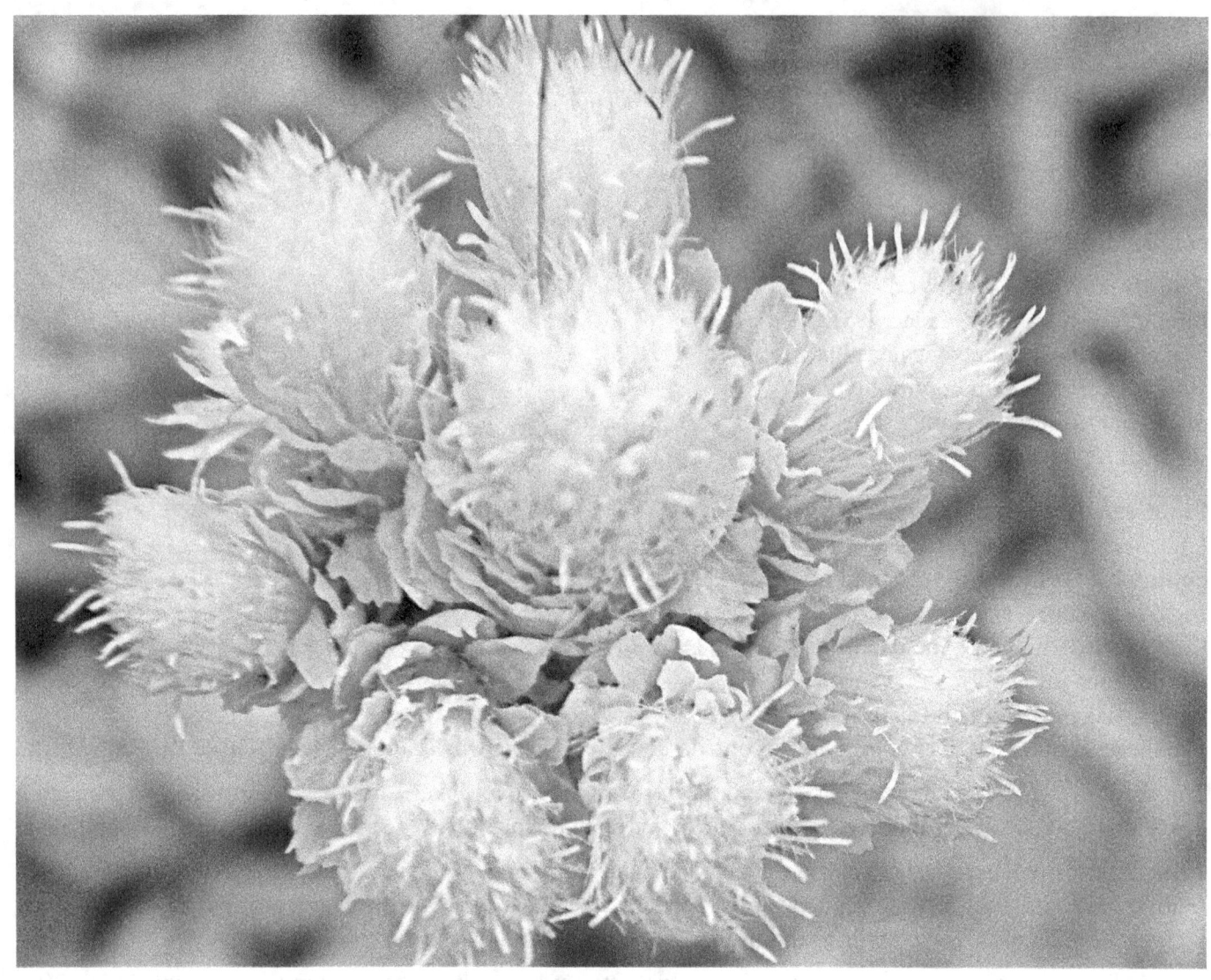

WOOLLY PUSSYTOES (*A. lanata*)

MEDICINAL

CONSTITUENTS- all of the above plants contain in the leaves and flowers bitter principles, monoterpenes anaphalin, the flavone gnaphaliin; flavonoid aglycones including the rare 3,5-dihydroxy-6, 7, 8-trimethoxyflavone, quercitin, luteolin, and essential oils.

A. margaritacea roots- tridecapentainen, trans-dehydromatricaria ester, and 5-chlor-2 [octatriin-(2,4,6)-yliden]-5,6-dihydro-2H-pyram.

aerial- 2 hydroxylactones, apigenin, quercitin, spiraein, tiliroside, ursolic acid, polnolic acid.

P. microcephalum- obtusifoline, and 3,5-dihydroxy-6,7,8-trimethoxyflavones.

G. uliginosum- various carotenoids including gamma, beta and alpha carotene as well as lycopene in the lipid fraction of the plant, resins, essential oils, tannic acid; gnaphalin, quercitin, phytosterols, 6-hydroxyluteolin-7-O-beta-D-glucopyranoside, 6-methoxyluteolin, scutellarein 7-O-beta-D-glucopyranoside.

Pearly everlasting and cudweed are principally astringent pain relievers. Hot decoctions will greatly benefit lung congestion, as well as sore throats and mumps. The flowers are cooling and drying in nature.

Warm infusions of the leaves and flowers help resolve fevers if caught in the early stage. It is a weak anti-histamine that helps reduce mucous membrane congestion. The tongue is red-tipped and moist, when examined.

Cold infusions, or retention enemas on the other hand, are useful for diarrhea, irritable and bleeding bowels. This is due to the relaxing quality, as well as soothing and strengthening the mucous membranes. Gently warmed, the infusion is a mild, but effective douche for vaginal discharge and itching.

The flowers and leaves may be chewed, fresh or dried and the juice swallowed for mouth and throat ulcerations. It may also be smoked to cool the mucous membranes of the lungs, decrease inflammation and act as a mild expectorant. A flower tea helps promote restful sleep.

A poultice of fresh flowers relieves insect bites, burns, sores and joint pain as a topical foray first aid.

The tincture combines well with yellow dock, Oregon grape root or burdock root for psoriasis.

Externally, both pearly everlasting and cudweed make a good poultice or fomentation for sprains, bruises, boils, sunburns and other painful swellings; due to their mild pain-relieving and anti-inflammatory properties. The roots contain constituents similar to pineapple weed and yarrow.

The flowers, leaves, root and stems of *A. margaritacea* have been extracted in both alcohol and water and show activity against both gram positive and negative bacteria. Work by Borchardt et al, *J Med Plants Res* 2008 2:5 found leaf extract inhibited *S. aureus* significantly.

Two dipterpenes from the flowering aerial parts show activity against *Bacillus cereus, Pseudomonas aeruginosa* and *E. coli*. Ahmed et al, *Phytochem* 2004 65.

Both pearly everlasting and cudweed aerial parts contain the anti-oxidant and anti-inflammatory compounds tiliroside and gnaphaliin. The latter compound shows relaxant effect on tracheal smooth muscle. Rodriquez-Ramos F et al, *J Nat Prod* 2009 72(6): 1061-4. The compounds bind to the same sites as sildenafil.

Cudweed (*G. uliginosum*) has been an official medicinal plant in Russia since the 1930s. The herb is cool and drying. Internally, infusions are used to relieve early symptoms of hypertension, heart palpitations and stenocardia. It helps reduce arterial pressure, and dilate blood vessels. Footbaths made from decoctions are complimentary.

It is used for a condition known as "hypotonia", which is, according to Zevin, "muscular tension of the arteries relaxes, which can impair the flow of blood into the heart". It is reminiscent of passive venous congestion at first observation.

He suggests one part of this herb, two parts horsetail, one part *Vinca minor* and one part yarrow for hypotonia.

For thrombophlebitis, he suggests four parts of the herb with two parts birch leaves, two parts chamomile flowers and one part yarrow flower.

Work by Turova et al, *Med Plants of USSR* Moscow 1989 showed benefit in the treatment of thrombophlebitis.

It is a weak diaphoretic and anti-tussive, useful as a hot tea in coughs, fevers, bronchitis, whooping cough, and respiratory bleeding.

Infusions are used for treating headaches, insomnia, depression, nervousness, asthma, and diabetes. It makes an excellent gargle for sore throat, tonsillitis, pharyngitis, nasal congestion and inflammation of the parotid glands (mumps).

Studies by Loukova et al, in 1996 showed Marsh Cudweed concentrates chromium in doses higher than usual for plants, and hence, possibly of benefit for type two diabetes.

The herb is often used in smoking mixtures. For excessive phlegm, or head colds combine and smoke Marsh Cudweed with goldenrod bud tops or elderflowers. For tonsillitis, combine with cleavers and echinacea.

It is widely used by Russian herbalists for its anti-depressive, aphrodisiac and hypotensive activity.

The herb tea has been used as a hair wash for lice.

The various Antennaria Pussy-toes and everlastings have mild choleretic action, and promote the flow of bile. This makes them excellent for liver inflammations and mild recurrences of old hepatitis symptoms. They all possess soothing, demulcent properties for intestinal irritations above the ileocecal valve, like fireweed, but without anti-fungal activity.

Action on the large intestine is minimal with ingestion, but like pearly everlasting, good results can arise from retention enemas.

Antennaria has the added bonus of raising blood pressure in those suffering from chronic low circulation of blood.

Rosy Everlasting has not been well studied. What is known, however, is that it contains ordinary flavonoids, stimulates phagocytosis by the reticulo-endothelial system (immune stimulating), and is anti-tussive.

It is a useful herb for liver inflammation and recurrent symptoms of hepatitis, according to Michael Moore. He suggests using the herb as a non-irritating astringent for intestinal irritation above the ileo-cecal valve. Also, the herb can be used as a gargle for sore throat, and as a douche for vaginitis.

The pleasant taste makes it suitable for children with hot, febrile conditions associated with "poorly organized fruitless expectoration."

A study of the entire plant showed the expressed juice inhibiting gram positive bacteria.

Small flowering pussytoes activate pancreas function in cases of diabetes. This was shared with me, by Greg Brandenburg, an accomplished Alberta herbalist.

Diana Beresford-Kroeger suggests the plant carries anti-venin biochemicals.

Clammy Everlasting (*G. macounii*) alcohol extracts show activity against *Staphylococcus aureus*. Bishop and MacDonald, *Can J Botany* 29.

HOMEOPATHY

Gnaphalium polycephalum (Rabbit Tobacco) is the remedy of unquestioned benefit in sciatica; especially when there is pain associated with numbness. There may be neuralgic face pain, or affections in various parts of the abdomen, particularly menstrual or prostatic.

There is often chronic lower backache in the lumbar region that feels better by resting on the back. Lumbago with numbness in the lower back, with radiating pain down the legs also calls for this remedy.

The calves and feet may cramp at night, but the biggest indicator is intense sciatic nerve pain. Relief may also come for gouty pains of the big toe, or chronic rheumatic pain in the back or neck.

If there are joints that feel lacking in lubrication, this remedy should be considered.

DOSE- Third to 30th potency. The mother tincture is prepared from the fresh plant in flower. Rabbit Tobacco is now recognized by its official binomial *Pseudognaphalium obtusifolium*.

ESSENTIAL OIL

CONSTITUENTS- *A. margaritacea* contains various esters including hexyl, phenethyl, and heptyl-2-methyl butyrates.

Distilled in China, pearly everlasting produces Shanqiu Oil; a long lasting aroma used as a perfume raw material. This is a fresh, green honey rose-like fragrance with sweet wine undertones. From the dried flower, a yield of 0.1-.25% can be expected; and from the whole plant up to .28%.

The related *Anaphalis contorta* produces an essential oil from the leaves that is an inhibitor in vitro against five human pathogenic bacteria and three fungi.

The pure oil has greater inhibitory activity in vitro than 1000 ppm griseofulvin as a control.

It contains alpha thujene 14.8%, alpha thujol 10%, nerol 8.7%, linalyl acetate 8.2%, p-cymene 5.8%, linalool 5.4% and alpha pinene 5.3%.

HYDROSOL

Pearly Everlasting hydrosol is useful for an after workout or sport rub due to anti-inflammatory and analgesic properties. It is helpful for after surgery to speed healing of incisions and needle wounds while reducing swelling and bruising. It can be used to clean and heal tattoos or body piercing and help to heal scar tissue.

It is good splash for congested, sensitive or mature skin and for men as an aftershave to prevent ingrown hairs.

FLOWER OIL

Sun infused oils of cudweed are useful additions to blends for healing old wounds, chemical or thermal burns, ulcers, fungal skin problems, and wet eczemas. It can be combined with nettle oil for preventing balding, by rubbing it into the scalp.

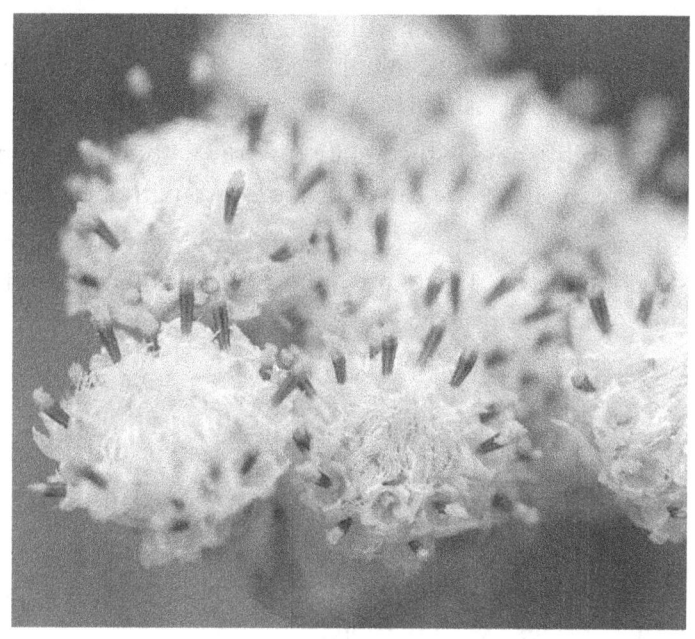

ANTENNARIA PLANTAGINIFOLIA
(Courtesy of southeasternflora.com)

FLOWER ESSENCES

Pussytoes (*A. rosea*)–The key words with this flower essence are reversing judgement. There is an increase and understanding of compassion. In meditation, the essence can be used to become at one with people, plants, animals, or even places.
GURUDAS

Small leaf pussytoes flower essence is for looking at all the angles and finding the simplest, and quickest solutions to problems, motivation.
ROCKY MTN

Pearly everlasting flower essence is useful for those who have suffered amnesia, due to injury. It will help bring back the loss of mind and memory, particularly long-term associations.

It can also be useful whenever the death of a loved one creates disturbed dreams or nightmares. Often times, the unconscious mind is manifesting feelings of guilt or remorse that result from the unresolved. Pearly everlasting, or immortelle, as it is sometimes known, helps connect us with the reassurance of the continuity of the soul.
PRAIRIE DEVA

Pearly Everlasting (*A. margaritacea*) flower essence helps us to deepen our connection with the other. The purifying fire of anger becomes a powerful ally, which can be used to create transformation. This remedy can be especially helpful to those who feel unwilling and/or unable to make a deep and lasting commitment in relationship.
PACIFIC

Woolly Everlasting essence helps address issues involving money.
ROCKY MTN

Pussy-Toes Everlasting essence helps deepen one's connection with others. Everlasting connects between the spirit world and the physical world.
WILD ROSE

SPIRITUAL PROPERTIES

The Everlasting flowers have a gentle persistence that can be transferred in herbal form to people. It gives extra patience and a willingness to stick to it for longer. The flower helps set up an inner balance so that new approaches and points of view can come forward.

Often, there is an inner willingness to let go of what no longer fits the picture. In spiritual growth and wisdom, there is often the need to hold two separate ideas simultaneously. This can lead to great restlessness that is eased with using everlasting.

Psychically, there is the ability to grow without worry of the past; with great acceptance and more energy to explore the new. The throat chakra is strengthened. There is a great opening that takes place in the heart.

The positive aspects of Neptune are explored; the slowing down, and willingness to go into the deeper intuitive side of the soul. Those individuals with positive ascending of Neptune in their astrological charts will receive the energy of this herb more readily.   **GURUDAS**

RECIPES

INFUSION- hot or cold- One tsp of fresh or dried herb one pint of water. Drink cool up to three times daily.

DECOCTION- One ounce of herb to three cups of water. Simmer slowly, down to two cups. Drink cool, two ounces every two hours.

TINCTURE- 10-15 drops 3x daily. Fresh tincture of Marsh Everlasting is produced at 1:4 and 50% alcohol. Other species use similar preparations.

ESSENTIAL OIL- when available- use externally, in 3% dilution for massage, or in diffusor for psychological benefit.

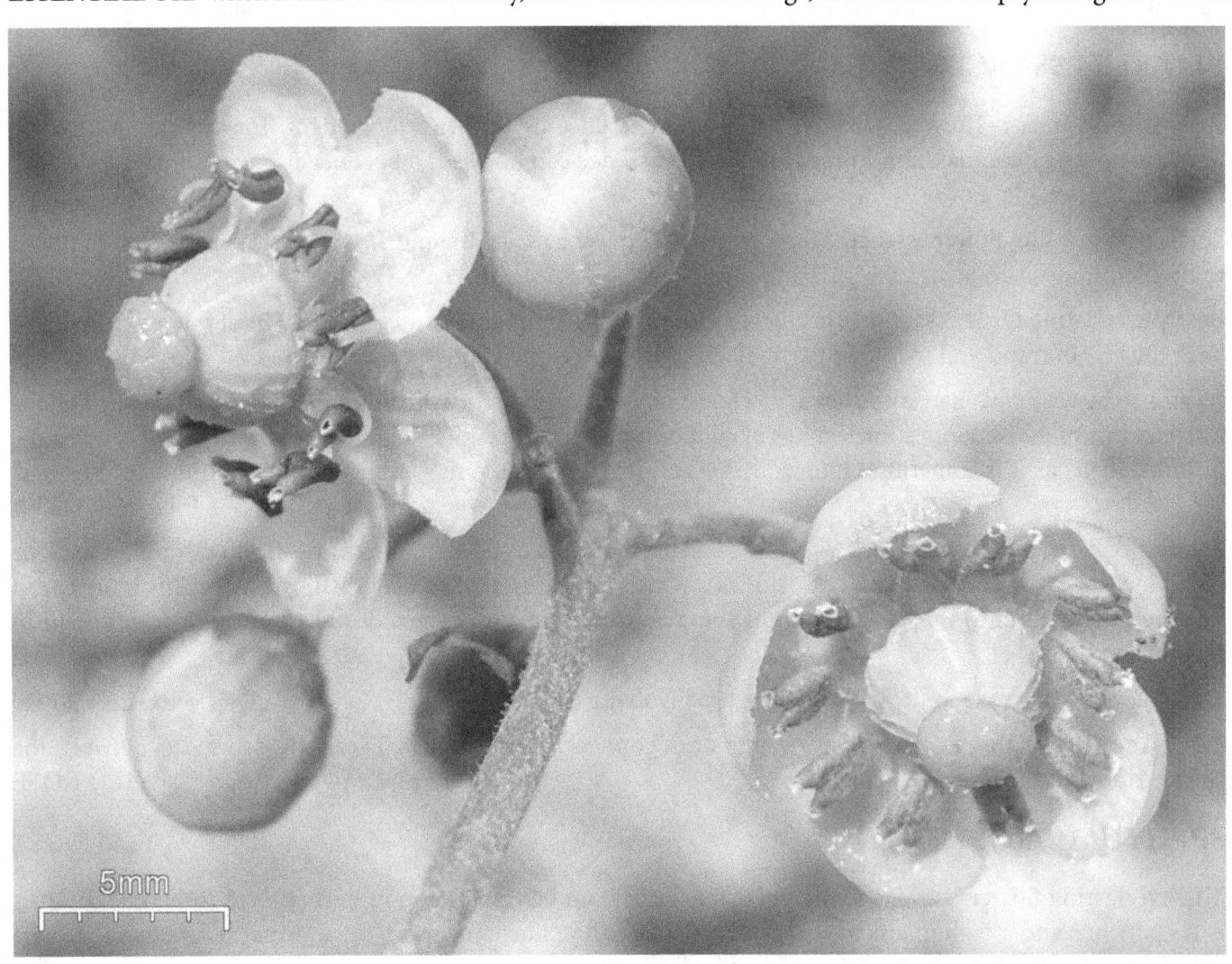

PRINCE'S PINE FLOWER- CLOSE UP

PIPSISSEWA
PRINCE'S PINE
(*Chimaphila umbellata* [L.] Nutt.) not accepted
(*C. umbellata* [L.] W. Barton)
(*Pyrola corymbosa* [Pursh] Bertol.) not accepted
(*Pyrola umbellata* L.) not accepted
PARTS USED- root, leaves, flowers

Pipsissewa is from the Cree **PIPISISKWEU** meaning, "it breaks it into small pieces", and refers to the leaves containing a substance that breaks down kidney stones.

It is one of my favourite examples of herbal onomatopoeia, which refers to the word describing the act of urination. The Abenaki name is **KPI PSKW AHSAWE** means flower of the woods.

Chimaphila is derived from the Greek **CHEIMA** meaning winter, and **PHILOS** meaning, love, in reference to the evergreen leaves. Umbellata describes the flower cluster or umbel.

Pipsissewa is common throughout the pine forests of the Rockies and in the Cypress Hills of southern Alberta. Native people of the province used the plant for a variety of problems involving inflammation of the skin, kidneys and menstrual cycle.

The Cree of northern Saskatchewan call it **AMISKWATHOWIPAK**, meaning beaver tail leaf. Decoctions of the whole plant were used for stabbing pains in the chest (angina pectoris), backache, coughing up of blood, and various fever and pain states.

The Blackfeet dried the leaves of **O-MAKSI-KA-KA-SIN**, and used them as part of smoking mixtures; while the Chippewa decocted the root and used the water to soothe sore eyes; or part of a combination to treat gonorrhea. The Anishinaabemowin names are **GAAGIGEBAG** meaning everlasting leaf, and **MAKOONSOMIN** for pipsissewa berry.

The Catawba called it Fire Flower, and used it for backaches.

The Karuk name **XUNYEEPSIIURUK IIITIHAN** means, "one who is under tan oak trees", which is true in that part of the world. The leaves and stems were steeped into a tea for bladder complaints.

Sam Hill, Onondaga herbalist from the Six Nations Reserve, had this to say about the herb in 1912.

"When a pregnant women feels feverish and drowsy, she is not sick, her baby is. Make a small bundle of pipsissewa about one inch thick using the whole plant. Put this in one half quart of water to steep. Take a cupful four times a day until it is used up."

The Wasco of Oregon decocted whole plant to treat tuberculosis.

It was used with wild sarsaparilla as part of traditional recipes for root beer.

The raw leaves can even be eaten, although somewhat stringy and fibrous. In parts of Appalachia, the leaves are chewed to relieve heartburn.

The fresh leaves were bruised and applied to rheumatic pains, and scrofula. A reddening and blistering of the skin can result, however, from prolonged application.

The leaf and root decoctions are red brown with a clean bitter taste that changes to sort of sweet taste, with no sign of wintergreen flavour.

Samuel Thomson used it as a tonic for kidneys and urinary tract, while Dr. Cook used it for vaginal and uterine weakness.

Felter used it for elder people with "chronic cystitis with a pinkish or reddish sediment of mucus, pus, blood and brick dust in the urine", and prostatitis.

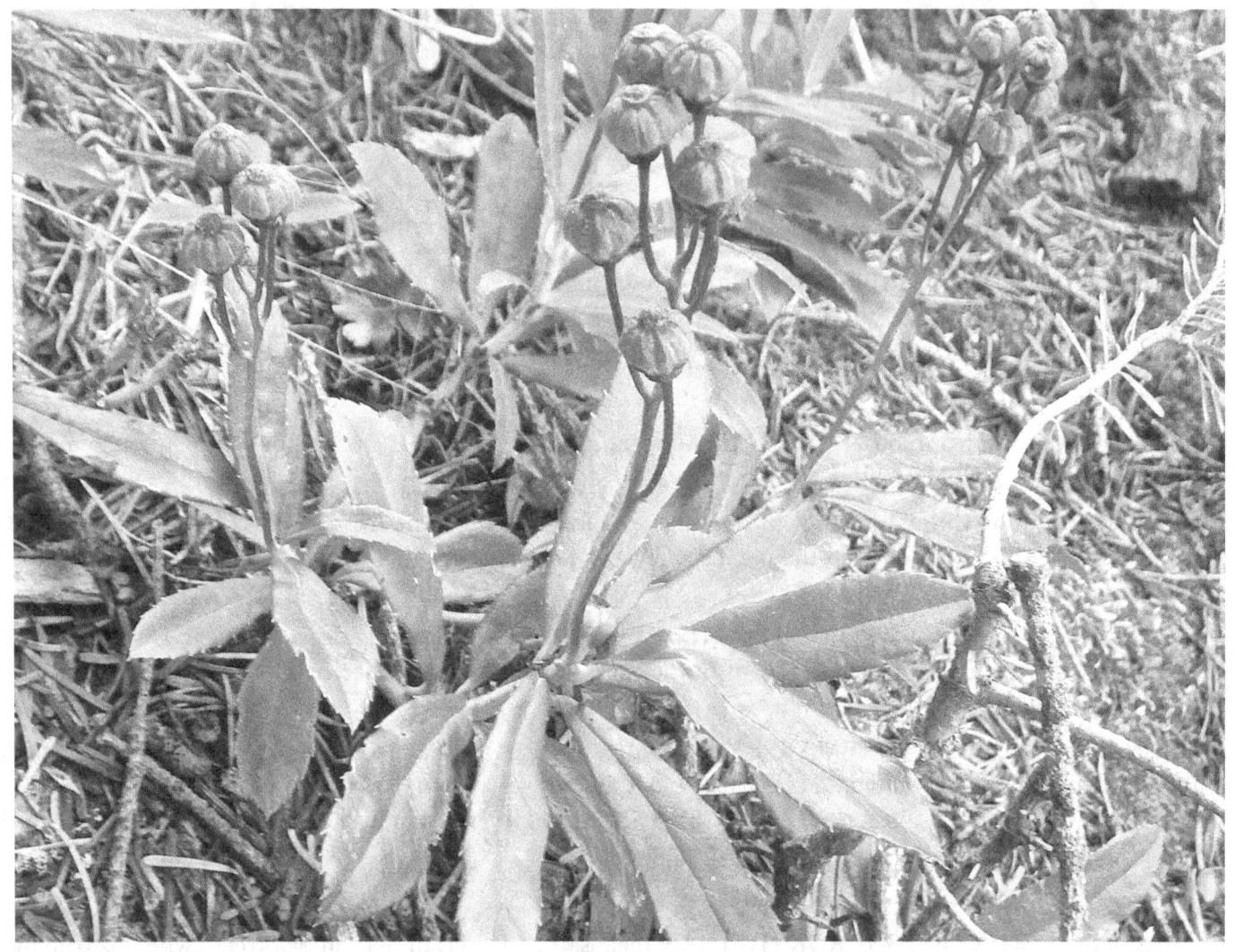

PIPSISSEWA PLANTS IN SEED- NOTE THE EVERGREEN LEAVES

Dr. Eli Jones suggested its use for breast cancer in large breasted women, where the lymphatic glands are involved. Other Eclectic physicians used it as part of formulas for prostate and bladder cancer.

Various tribes ate the berries as stomachics, or digestive tonics.

Pipsissewa extracts are used as "secret" flavour components today for root beer and sarsaparilla soft drinks, as well as candy, frozen dairy, baked goods (290 ppm), gelatins, puddings and sweet sauces (365 ppm). It is wild-crafted extensively, and rapidly disappearing from the Pacific Northwest.

Pipsissewa was carried traditionally to attract money. When crushed and combined with rosehips and violet flowers, and burned, it was said to draw good spirits for magical aid.

The herb is used in traditional Chinese Medicine, as a diuretic, anti-fungal and to relieve stomach, tooth and after birth pains. It is called **MEI LI CAO.**

The closely related *P. maculata* is European, but nearly identical in composition. It is commonly found throughout the Appalachians.

In Germany it was called **HARNKRAUT**, meaning Urine Weed; alluding to the plant's urinary activity.

Paracelsus wrote of the plant "for wounds, for old weeping injuries...to stop abdominal fluxes...and for fresh wounds, there is hardly a remedy in greater repute for healing these."

MEDICINAL

CONSTITUENTS- flavonoids including hyperoside, quercitin, and avicularin; arbutin (7.5%), isohomo-arbutin, homoarbutin, hyperin, avicularin, kaempferol, chinic acid, urson, ericolin; taraxasterin, sitosterin, renifolin, hentriacontane, nonacosane (C29H60), ursolic acid, toluquinol, silicic acid, sufphuric acid, epicatechin gallate, methyl salicylate, kaempferol, quercitin, naphthoquinones such as chimphilin (2%) and 3-chloro-chimaphilin; tannins, including epicatechol gallate (4%), beta amyrin, pectin, gums and bitters.

Pipsissewa is a valuable cool and dry herb for scanty urine and urinary infections. It is somewhat less astringent than bearberry, but a stronger diuretic with less stomach irritation due to less tannin. It does, however, remove gravel and uric acid, and relieves chronic prostate irritation in the manner of bearberry.

It was considered at one time to be a specific for men over fifty, suffering from chronic bladder irritation.

Various Eclectic physicians, including Felter, Ellingwood and Lloyd prescribed pipsissewa for burning urination associated with chronic cystitis and prostate congestion.

For chronic nephritis, combine pipsissewa with goldenrod; while lymphatic congestion of the breast calls for the addition of cleavers and red root.

It may be used over the long term for benign prostatic hyperplasia, or enlargement of the prostate, general kidney weakness and mild nephritis. It is used for chronic low-grade infections of bacterial vaginosis and chlamydia, with enlarged lymph glands in the groin.

It may be used concurrently with antibiotics to treat gonorrhea.

Many of the bactericide constituents are excreted as disinfectant substances, making it a valuable plant for chronically suppressed skin eruptions.

For swollen and congested lymphatic glands, ovarian cysts, and lipomas (congested fat lumps under the skin), it can be used internally as a cool decoction and externally as a poultice or wash for ulcerous sores, tumours, blisters and swelling. Inflammation of the cervical lymph plexus is relieved.

Michael Moore suggested "it is an effective alterative for lingering skin conditions characterized by dry, flaky inflammation, vague aching in the joints, and frequent urination at night."

Matthew Wood added. "Pipsissewa is a great 'eliminator of kapha', if I may coin a phrase. It warms and activates the lymphatics and kidneys, the carriers and dispersers of water in the body...It is indicated in the sluggishness, water retention, and weight gain of middle age. It is indicated when the tongue is swollen and coated white in the middle. This might be an indication of 'spleen yang deficiency' in traditional Chinese medicine, a category similar to 'scrofula' in old-time Western medicine."

Ursolic acid inhibits COX-2, thereby alleviating pain and inflammation. Dr. Hale, an Eclectic physician wrote. "It is chiefly in chronic rheumatism that its curative powers have most observed".

Laboratory studies have confirmed pipsissewa's benefit in hypoglycemia, and its tonic effect in late-onset diabetes. Arbutin is not only anti-bacterial and anti-tussive, but inhibits insulin degradation.

It relieves rheumatoid aliments, and restores mobility in rundown and debilitated individuals.

As a hot infusion, it helps reduce fevers due to infection, especially if caught early. Cystitis, including interstitial, urethritis, prostatitis, and nephritis all respond better to infusions at body temperature.

Beta-sitosterin, for example, has been found to reduce growth of the prostate. Kassen A, *Krankenpfl J* 1999 37(7-8): 286.

Early work found sitosterin, as adjuvant medication, reduced prostatic hyperplasia and prostatitis. Bauer HW & Bach D, *Urol Int* 1986 41(2): 139-44. Sitosterin capsules for prostatic adenoma and prostatitis showed therapeutic efficacy. Dorner G & Fritsche C, ZFA (Stuttgart) 1982 58(3): 167-9.

Sitosterin also showed efficacy in chronic polyarthritis and rheumatism. Zorn J, *Med Welt* 1981 32(4): 135-8.

Tannic astringency in the herb is of benefit in diarrhea, and internal bleeding such as stomach ulcers, birthing and peridontal disease. Long decoctions create more astringency.

Due to methyl salicylate content and its pain relieving property, the plant is useful for urinary tract infections associated with pain, and postpartum hemorrhage.

Chimaphilin stimulates phagocytes, one of our non-specific immune cells, at low doses. Harbourne et al, 1993.

It was first isolated in 1860 by Samuel Fairbanks, upon distillation. Its structure is similar to vitamin K, and several studies confirm reduction of clotting time.

Chimaphilin shows greatest activity against *Staphylococcus aureus*, moderate benefit against *E. coli* and *Candida albicans*, and some activity against *Shigella sonnei*, Ambrogi et al, *British J Pharmacy* 1970 40.

Anti-fungal activity was noted by Steffen and Peschel, *Planta Medica* 1975 27.

Work by Towers et al, at the U of British Columbia found aerial parts active against all nine fungal species tested. Ethanol extracts of the whole plant show activity against *Candida albicans*. Jones et al, *J Ethnopharm* 2000 73.

Chimaphilin is a powerful anti-fungal with significant activity against organisms responsible for dandruff. Galván et al, *Phytochem* 2007 Oct 23.

Chimaphilin, *in vitro*, inhibits platelet aggregation induced by collagen and ADP, and is active on atrial tissue from guinea pigs.

Bishop & MacDonald *Can J Botany* 1951 29 tested 209 plant species, and found *C. umbellata* ether extracts one of the most effective against *S. aureus* of all plants they tested. Only Sweet Gale (*Myrica gale*) in alcohol showed more inhibition.

Moving ahead to 2015, a recent study looked at a few northern plants and found pipsissewa exhibits anti-microbial effects. Vandal J et al, *Pharm Biol* 2015 53(6): 800-6. Inhibition of *E. coli*, *Staphylcoccus aureus*, *Pseudomonas aeruginosa* and *Candida albicans* was noted.

Some Eastern Native healers combine the leaves, with mint as a tea for stomach cancer.

Work by Oka et al, *Phytomed* June 20 2007 found a combination of Pipsissewa, Aspen Poplar, *Pulsatilla pratensis*, Horsetail and wheat germ oil reduced benign prostatic hypertrophy. The individual constituents did not show any effect, and yet the combination showed significant improvement.

The proprietary compound Eviprostat® is used in Japan and Europe for treatment of BPH, or benign prostatic hyperplasia.

A newly isolated naphthalene glycoside with acronym DMDHNG has been isolated from the stem and leaves. It appears to inhibit the receptor activator of nuclear factor-KB lignan-stimulated osteoclast differentiation. This suggests possible use for bone health. Shin BK et al, *Arch Pharm Res* 2015 38(11): 2059-65.

The fresh leaves are good counter-irritant, if poulticed and left for at least 30 minutes. Use for arthritis, rheumatism and associated congestions, but caution against blistering of skin is advised.

Some herbals suggest you can substitute *Uva ursi* for this herb. In terms of astringency, this is true, but it lacks the analgesic effect of methyl salicylate. In this case use two parts bearberry and one part birch twigs as a substitute.

Like Uva ursi, the content of arbutin is from 17-22%. Arbutin, of course, converts to hydroquinone after metabolic or bacterial conversion, and is anti-bacterial.

The flavonoids and their glycosides show anti-inflammatory activity, as does beta sitosterol. The latter, however, is insoluble in water and minimally soluble in alcohol.

The whole plant suppressed oxidative stress in rats with surgically induced bladder outlet obstruction. Oka et al, *The Journal of Urology* 2009 182 382-90.

Watkins, in the *Eclectic Med Journal* 1902 62 found the fluid extract more active after sitting for 6-12 months. With time, the liquid becomes more gelatinized, with patients reporting better results from the aged product. Not sure why.

HOMEOPATHY

Pipsissewa acts principally on the uro-genital tract, and lymphatic glands. For bladder infections with notable mucous in both acute and chronic conditions, it is very useful. There may be scanty urine, with lots of ropy, mucous sediment. The prostate may be inflamed, leading to scanty and burning urine, with high sugar content possible.

The female labia may be inflamed and swollen, with or without vaginal pain. The breast may have painful tumours, with unexplained milk secretion; and more common in women with large, cystic, painful breasts.

In males, there may be prostatic enlargement with loss of seminal fluid.

Incipient and progressive eye cataracts may be arrested in their growth.

Blue rings around eyes, pain around teeth and jaw. Tongue sore and full of little vesicles.

The symptoms are worse on the left side of the body, in damp weather, and from sitting on cold.

DOSE- Tincture to third potency. Mother tincture is prepared from the whole fresh plant in flower. Provings by Jeanes in 1840 and Bute in 1856. Clinical observations by Hering and Stauffer.

FLOWER ESSENCE

Pipsissewa is the flower essence for clearing ambivalence. It is a decision maker, helping us choose as a responsible act. It also helps resolve the frustration around having made a choice which seems not to turn out the way we thought it would. Instead of wasting energy bewailing where we find ourselves, the essence will help move us to the point of power in the present where we can make a new choice.

Physically, it impacts upon the brain and awakens that area involved in choice. It affects the throat and solar plexus chakras.   **PACIFIC**

SPIRITUAL PROPERTIES

Pipsissewa is a powerful healer for deep release. It creates a spiral of energy in the abdomen that is ongoing. Blockages of spiritual growth such as fear and guilt are released. The cleansing is from the heart down, and negative thought forms are released. It does not, however, have the energetics to release past life patterns.

If in an intimate relationship, both of you may take pipsissewa to release negative energy and help develop greater love. There may be initial irritation, but then an emotional cleansing takes place.

The whorl pattern of the leaves is representative of spiral energy. The etheric body is cleansed and a few hours after taking the tea, the etheric is strengthened.

Mars, and its negative effect when in opposition or squared are eased.   **GURUDAS**

Pipsissewa's key word is awareness; both self-awareness and environmental awareness. It enhances the awareness of every piece of information, of every stimulus, in every sense.   **MULDERS**

PERSONALITY TRAITS

As a child, the pipsissewa type suffers from chronic lymphatic congestion. The tonsils and/or appendix have been removed, or as a teenager, mononucleosis has affected the spleen.

Later in life there is poor skin with lymphatic congestion and sluggishness. The kidneys are weak, and there may be prostate inflammation in the male.

On the negative side, the pipsissewa person is prone to fears and lack of self-esteem. They may rely on others for approval, and choose careers or marriage partners that reflect that internal imbalance.

On the positive side, the pipsissewa person learns at an early age to care for themselves. They may be overly sensitive as children, and as adults learn to not take things personally.

They also recognize the symptoms of congestion that lead to stagnation on a physical and emotional plane.

PRAIRIE DEVA

BOTANICA POETICA

Pipsissewa, an Evergreen
Helps to keep the urine clean
With its tannins, it's astringent
Salicylates and quinones in it
For urinary disinfection
Also calms the inflammation
And if the prostate's oversized
Give Pipsissewa a try
A bitter tonic, diuretic
Use the leaf for joints arthritic
Chimaphila Umbellata
Cleanse the blood and the liver
Take this herb for UTI
Also known as Prince's Pine
It's endangered so make haste
Don't overuse and create waste
Truth be known to all who care
Though it smells rather fair
The infusion as my tea
Did not taste so good to me!

SYLVIA CHATROUX MD

RECIPES

DECOCTION- Take one heaping tablespoon of dried leaf to one pint of hot water. Simmer twenty minutes. Drink at body temperature for skin or urogenital infections, cold for lymphatic, lipomas and breast affections, and hot for fever-like conditions. Four to eight ounces 3 times daily. The fresh leaf tea is irritating to the kidneys.

POWDER- 30-90 grains daily

TINCTURE- fresh preferred- 15-60 drops in divided doses daily in water. For a dry plant tincture use a 1:5 ratio with 50% alcohol. For fresh tincture, my own preference, use a 1:2 ratio of 60%. For bladder cancer use ten drops in large amount of water up to three times a day.

In general, only use for ten days, take a five-day break and repeat. For urinary tract infections, combine with equal parts of uva-ursi and usnea/lomatium- 90 drops 4x daily in warm water with pinch of baking soda.

For kidney stones take two tsp twice daily in cool water. For pulmonary edema, use 10ml of fresh leaf tincture per liter of water. Drink in divided doses daily until improvement.

CAUTION- urine may have a green tone, it is harmless. Do not use during pregnancy or lactation.

FLUID EXTRACT- One tsp three times daily.

A method for determining chimaphilin content can be found in *Pharmazie* 1997 52:2 based on work of Michelitsch.

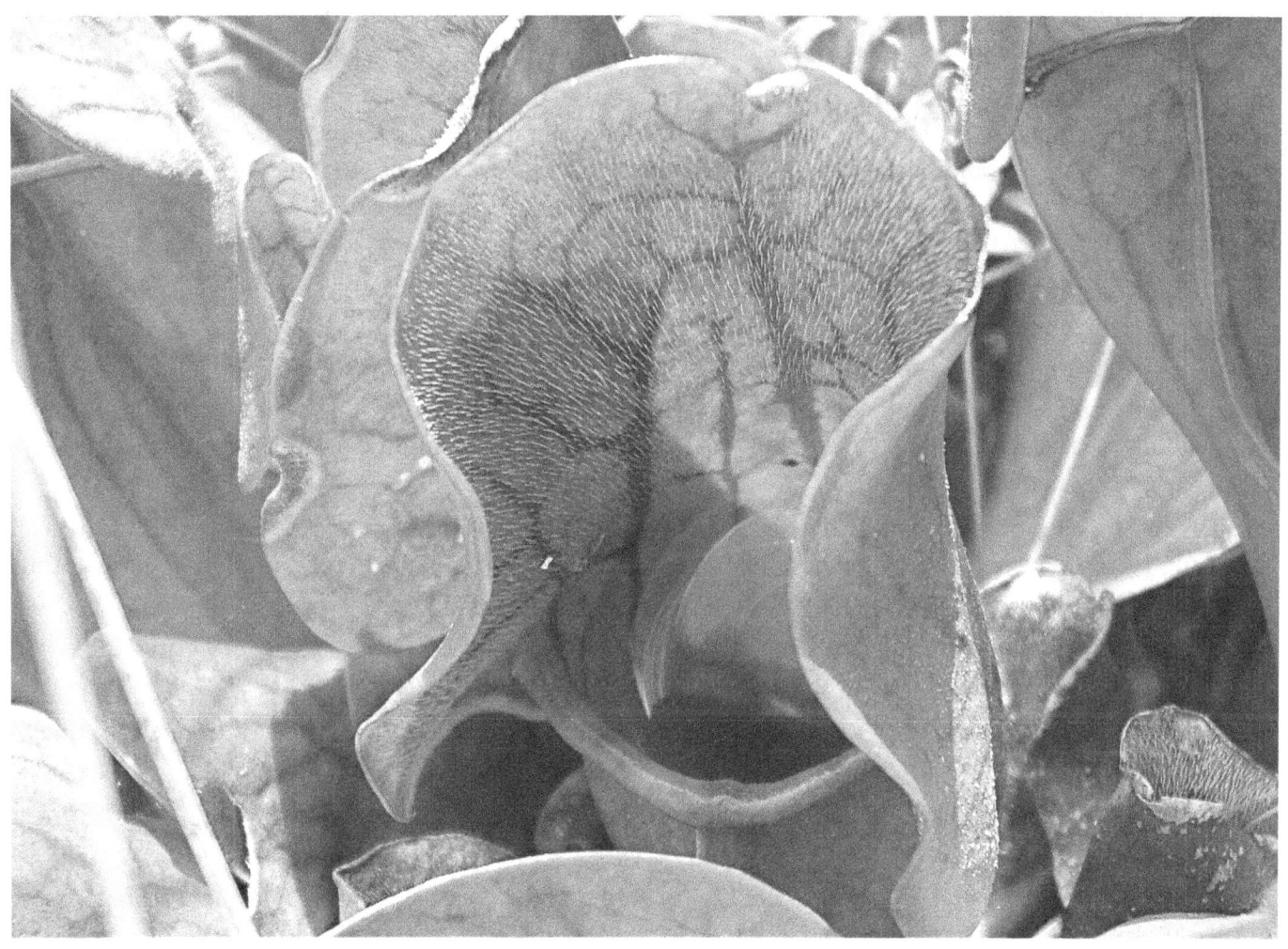

PITCHER PLANT

PITCHER PLANT
(*Sarracenia purpurea* L.)
(*S. purpurea* **f.** *purpurea* L.)
(*S. purpurea ssp. venosa* [Raf.] Wherry)
PARTS USED- root, leaves.

Hovering over a pool on a long and delicate pink stalk is a flower of magnificient proportions, arising like a red lantern in a sea of green.   **BERESFORD-KROEGER**

Sarracenia is named after Dr. Michel Sarrasin de l'Etang, Canada's first professional botanist, who came to Quebec in 1685.

He wrote *L' Histoire des Plantes de Canada*, a botanical first for the new country. He received information on this plant as a remedy for smallpox from the Quebec natives. Linnaeus honored him by naming the plant after him.

Today, the Prix Michel-Sarrazin is awarded annually to a Quebecois scientist that makes contribution to biomedical research.

Purpurea means purple, referring to the leaves and flowers.

Pitcher Plant is the floral emblem of Newfoundland, but is found plentifully in northern peat bogs and muskegs; and all the way south to the swamps of Louisiana.

It is quite common in the boreal forests of Saskatchewan, but in Alberta is found only on the Athabasca River up to Fort Chipewyan, and near Lesser Slave Lake.

The plant is most unusual, reminding me of the extra-terrestrial plant in the play "Little Shop of Horrors", about a plant that grows larger on human blood. An older name Dumb watches, in the New Jersey Pine Barrens, comes from the expanded style and sepals remaining after flower. They were thought to look like older style pocket watch, whose cover opened in a star-shaped pattern. No hands to tell time makes it mute.

One small mosquito larvae, *Wyeomyia smithii* lives solely, in the leaf water. For other insects, it is a final resting spot. One study found 14 orders and 150 families of insects in the pitchers, as well as slugs and snails.

Pitcher Plant, like the Sundew, requires nitrogen that is not easily available in the acidic, northern bogs. It has developed an elaborate system of trapping insects in its leaf tubes, with the inner hairs pointing downward. This makes it nearly impossible for an insect to crawl back up and out to freedom. Young plants trap the majority of prey, with new leaves trapping up to 82% of plant's total prey. The compound sarracenin is a volatile that helps attract insects to pitcher plants.

The hairs at the base of the tube probably act as absorbents of nitrogenous matter decaying within the leaf. Millspaugh wrote, "some acute observers claim that at the end of each hair there is a minute opening, thus allowing the nitrogenous fluid to pass directly into the apical cell of the hair.

This does not seem to be the case, but instead, the wall surrounding the entire cell is very thin. Unlike the tentacles of Sundew, in no case do the spiral bundles enter their tissue."

Later, when the leaf has nearly stopped absorbing fluid from the tube, it still acts as an insect trap. At this time it gives off the strong odor of rotting insects. When these leaves decay, they act as fertilizer around the plant roots.

The raw-meat coloring, and red-purple veins are lessened when the plant is exposed to full light. The green color then dominates, but it is still beautiful.

Work by Chapin and Pastor, *Can J Botany* 1995 73 showed that the amount of nitrogen from captured insects is still only 10% of the plants annual requirement.

The first recorded use of this plant was among the Native people of Canada. Smallpox, carried from Europe, caused widespread epidemic among the previously unexposed native population. With no natural immunity, the death rate was alarmingly high.

The Woods Cree of Saskatchewan know the plant as **ATHIKACAS**, meaning "little frog pants". In Alberta it is a very similar, **AYIKITAS**, meaning "frog pants".

Russell Willier, noted Cree healer, uses the plant in combinations for menstrual problems, coughing and back problems due to kidney weakness. It is an effective diuretic.

The Chipewyan of northern Alberta call the plant **TS'ELI TILI**, or "frog pail".

The Cree know the plant as Frog's Legs, and used it for those who were very sick. In the new Cree dictionary, Pitcher Plant is known as **ASKIHKOSIHK KOHPIKIHCIKESIHK**.

Cree healers use it for respiratory and heart ailments, often in combinations.

The root was decocted and given to a woman to prevent sickness after childbirth; and combined with other plants in decoction to expel the afterbirth. It was also used for kidney problems and associated back pain.

The Fox used the root tea when labour was imminent.

The root decoction was used in attempts to cure venereal disease.

The Iroquois combined the plant's leaves with Giant Bur reed as an infusion for chills. They call the plant Turtle Socks, or Turtle Shoes.

The boiled root is one of our mildest laxatives, for both children and adults.

The leaf was infused or decocted was given to women suffering from amenorrhea, or lack of periods.

The Iroquois used the plant as a medicine for thirst. They infused the dried leaves for high fevers, and shakiness; the root was infused for liver maladies. Cold decoctions of the whole plant were used in whooping cough and pneumonia.

The powdered root was sprinkled on a person as a love or lacrosse medicine, while the pitchers were considered a specific love medicine.

The whole plant was used with other unspecified plants in a combination for lower back pain. The children used the leaf as toy kettles.

The leaf tube was also used as a leaf wrap for meat cooked over open fires.

Pitcher Plant root was used as a specific by a number of Native tribes for treating smallpox, with varying success.

The Mi'kmaq of Nova Scotia used root decoctions for a variety of respiratory ailments, including sore throats, spitting blood and tuberculosis.

Various tribes used the leaves for kidney problems, taken as an infused tea.

Pitcher Plant was used traditionally in the southern United States as a cure for dyspepsia.

Pitcher Plant is protected by CITES (*Convention in International Trade in Endangered Species of Wild Fauna and Flora*, to save it from extinction. It is common in parts of the boreal forest and Atlantic Canada.

MEDICINAL

CONSTITUENTS- Sarracenin (volatile monoterpene with diacetyl group), acrylic acid, sarracenic acid, flavonoids (quercitin, rhamnetin, hyperoside), tannins, resins, triterpenes such as betulin, amyrins and lupeol, as well as piperidine alkaloids such as coniine, histamine, erucamide, and bitters.
Anthocyanidins are present in the flowers and leaf, including cyanidin, delphinidin, pelargonidin, peonidin, petunidin, and malvidin.
Water- *Mycobacterium sarraceniae* sp. nov and *M. helvum* sp. nov.

The acidity of the water, after sitting in a leaf tube for some time, is due to malic acid, citric acid, and gamma conicein. Nitrogen-fixing bacteria live in the pitcher.

The plant is too rare to use except in homeopathic form. This means that not only does a small amount go a long way, but it keeps the plant protected and allowed to flourish.

It is worth noting that Dr. Cigliano, in experiments with the root tincture, showed that it produces "eruptions similar to *crusta lactea* on the forehead and hands papular eruptions, changing to vesicular with the depression, as with smallpox, lasting from 7-8 days."

This appears to confirm native use of the plant.

Coniine is a piperidine alkaloid present in much higher amounts in poison hemlock. In this plant, it appears to be the insect-paralyzing principle. A dose as little as 100 nanograms caused partial paralysis in ants in less than thirty seconds.

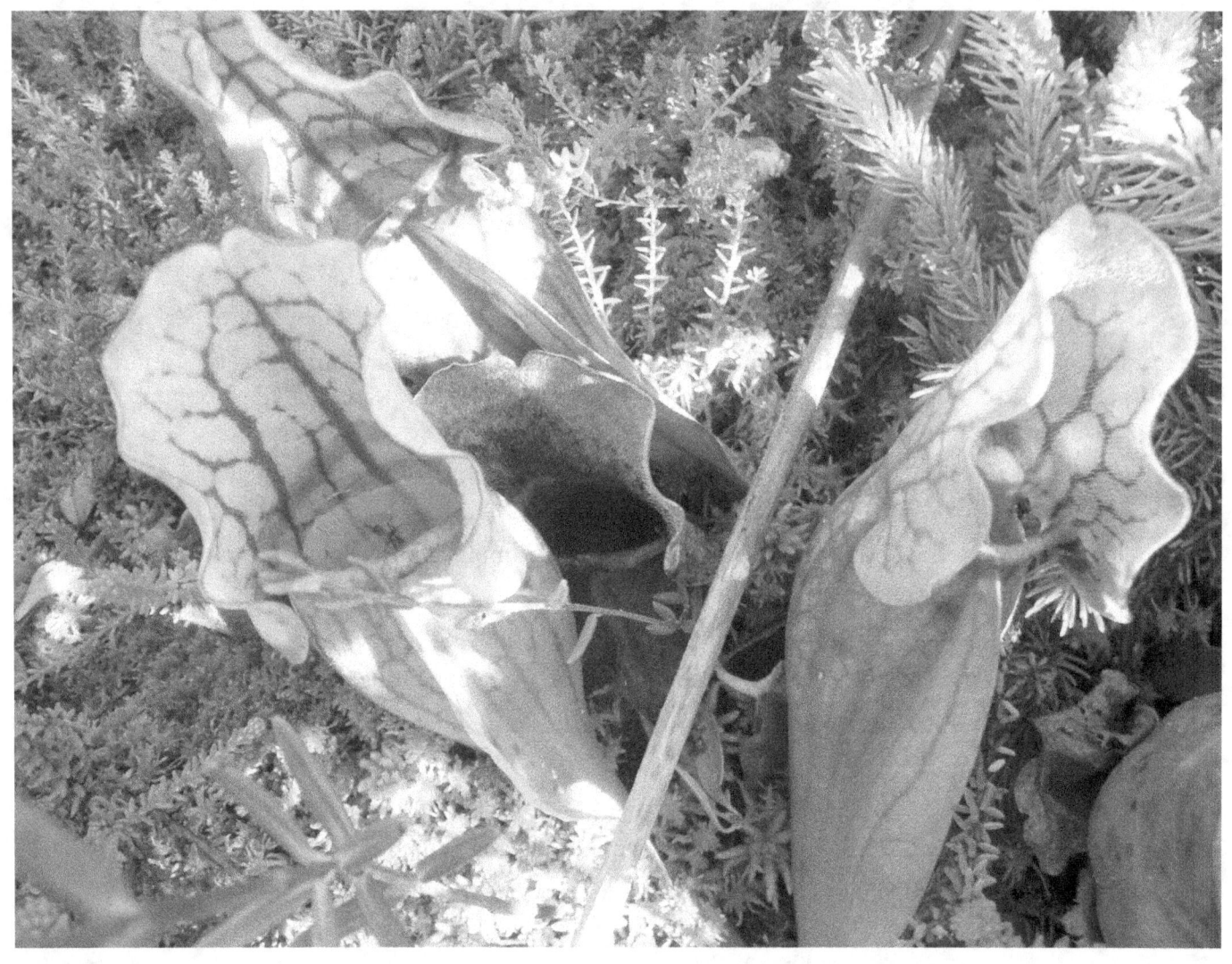

PITCHER PLANT- LATER IN SEASON

Coniine exerts inhibitory effects on nicotinic receptor-mediated nitrergic and noradrenergic transmitter response. Erkent U et al, *Z Naturforsch C* 2016 71(5-6): 115-20. Nitrergic neurons are nerve cells mediated by nitric oxide.

Sarracenin is similar to veratrin, found in false hellebore. It is an insect attractant, and synthetically is employed as a flavoring agent for microwave popcorn, to give it a buttery taste.

Note that a number of cases of *bronchiolitis obliterans* have been found in popcorn-flavoring plant workers. This is a rare, and potentially fatal obstructive lung disease that causes victims to slowly suffocate, with inflammation and scarring of lungs, dry cough, shortness of breath and diminished breathing capacity.

Erucamide is a fatty acid amide, similar to the endocannabinoid analogue oleoylethanolamide.

Given orally to mice, it alleviates depression and anxiety, possibly due to regulation of the HPAA, or hypothalamic-pituitary-adrenal axis. This suggests an adaptogenic influence that should be further explored.

The closely related *S. flava* has been examined for constituents in the root and leaves. Besides the ever-present beta-sitosterol and alpha amyrin, the plant contains lupeol, betulin and betulinic acid. The leaf and root extracts show anti-tumor activity against both naso-pharynx carcinoma and lymphocytic leukemia P-388. Miles and Kokpol, *J of Pharmaceutical Sciences* 1974 63:4 and 1976 65:2.

A proprietary liquid extract of *S. purpurea* powdered root, called Sarapin, has been locally injected, by physicians treating neuralgia. An undetermined compound may be responsible. Bates, *Am J Surgery* 1943 59:83.

Manufacturers of the product list painful syndromes relieved by Sarapin as sciatic pain, intercostal neuralgia, alcoholic neuritis, occipital neuralgia, brachial plexus neuralgia, meralgia [thigh] paraesthetica, lumbar neuralgia and trigeminal neuralgia. These are pinched or trapped nerves, reminiscent of the entrapment strategy of pitcher plant.

See www.saparin.com.

Like sundew and stinging nettles, the fresh plant contains histamine that is anti-inflammatory, vaso-dilating and broncho-constricting. It can be used topically to relieve chilblains, and internally to promote gastric pepsin secretion.

Work by Spoor et al, *Can J Physiol Pharmacol* 2006 84 examined eight indigenous plants of Quebec used traditionally for diabetic-like symptoms.

Pitcher Plant (*S. purpurea*) extracts appear to possess insulino mimetic activity, as supported by a rapid and insulin independent effect on uptake in muscle and fat cells.

The effect was quantitatively greater than 400 micromol/L of metformin. It showed protection under both cytotoxic conditions tested.

Work by Tam et al, *Can J Physio Pharmacol* 2011 89:1 found the plant inhibits CYP3A4 cytochrome liver enzyme system, at least in vitro. This suggests a reduction in the speed of breakdown associated with drugs and other herbs by the liver. Caution is advised, at least theoretically.

Two mycobacterium living in pitcher plant waters have been studied. One strain was positive for arylsulfatase production. Tran PM et al, *Int J Syst Evol Microbiol* 2016 66(11): 4480-5.

The genetic disorder Maroteaux-Lamy syndrome manifests in skeletal abnormalities and short stature, based on mucopoysaccharidosis, due to deficient activity of arylsulfatase B; also known as N-acetylgalactosamine-4-sulfatase.

Pseudomonas bacterium are a sulfatase producing organism, often resulting in respiratory infections in patients with cystic fibrosis (CF). Diminished activity of arylsulfatase B is noted in lymphoid cells of patients with CF compared to normal subjects.

The genome of *Mycobacterium tuberculosis* encodes nine putative sulfatases. Sulphatase enzymes hydrolyse the sulphate ester, found on the surface of pathogens, and playing a key role for host-pathogen interaction. Arylsulfatase B can degrade chondroitin sulfate and dermatan sulfate. Tobacman JK et al, Chest 2003 123(6): 2130-9.

It is purely speculation, but could it be that the arylsulfatase developed by mycobacterium in pitcher plant water, somehow interferes with mediating or regulating host-pathogen interactions. This would explain, in part, the traditional use in various respiratory conditions.

Arylsulfatase was used to differentiate between human and bovine tuberculosis at one time.

HOMEOPATHY

Pitcher Plant is used for a variety of visual disorders, including photophobia, sore and swollen eyes, and pain in the eye orbits. Black objects appear to move with the eye.

There may be congestion in the head, or a sick headache, with throbbing in the neck, shoulders and head that feels like bursting.

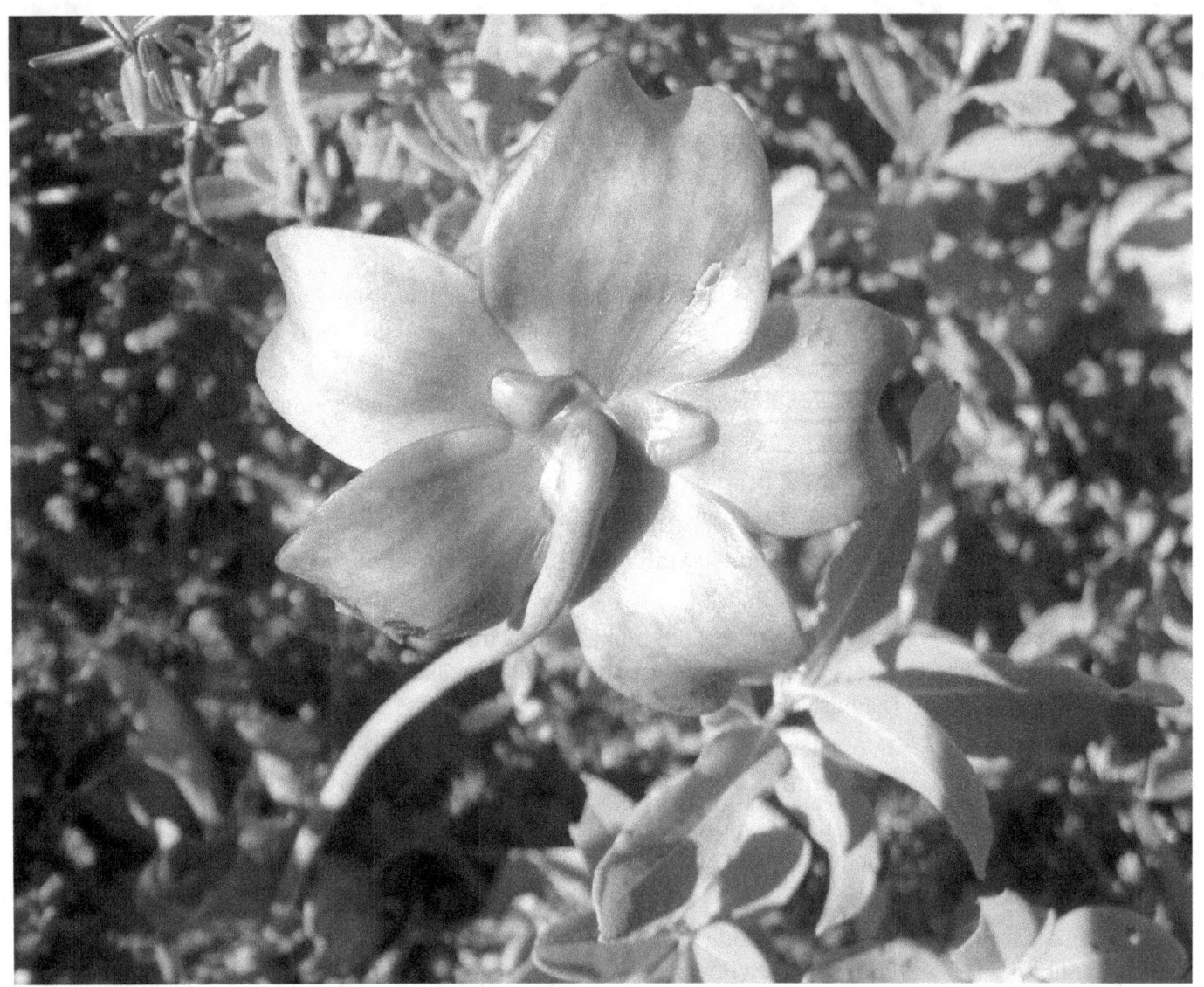

PITCHER PLANT FLOWER

The stomach feels hungry all the time, even after meals. Patient may be sleepy during meals, or have copious, and painful vomiting.

There may be shooting pain in a zigzag course from the lumbar region to the middle of the scapula.

There may be an irregular heartbeat, weak limbs, bruised feelings in the knees and joints. The bones in the arms feel weak, as well as between the shoulders.

It was formerly considered a remedy for smallpox (variola) helping abort the disease and arrest pustulation.

DOSE- Third to sixth potency. The mother tincture is produced from the whole, fresh root. Porcher self experimented with sixty pills, three grains each of the dried root in 1848. Proving by Ducan with infusion, decoction and tincture in 1866. Effects in cases of smallpox, Cigliano 1871; McFarlan 2M in 1893.

FLOWER ESSENCE

Pitcher Plant flower essence is for helping those who are in transition towards a vegetarian diet. It helps to release people from the karmic burden of discharging negative thought forms into the bodies of insects.

PEGASUS

SPIRITUAL PROPERTIES

The pitcher plant is considered by the medicine men and women of the North American aboriginal world to hold the most powerful medicines. The complex medicine of this plant has been used for witchcraft, lovesickness, fevers, kidney disease, and migraines. It has been used as an oxytoxic childbirth medicine and to regulate menses. It is a cardio and capillary tonic and it is thought to have anti-leukemia properties. The beast of the Boreal may well turn into a beauty after all.
BERESFORD-KROEGER

RECIPES

DRY POWDER- 10-30 grains

TINCTURE- The fresh root is gathered after fruiting; or the whole fresh plant when budding to blossom (before the leaves are fully expanded) are chopped into a pulp. For every part of root by weight, add two parts of 76% grain alcohol. Shake thoroughly each day for two weeks.

The resulting tincture after filtering is a deep, brown red; with a taste that is first sour, then bitter and slightly astringent, and strongly acidic.

DOSE- 10 drops as needed.

POISON HEMLOCK
(***Conium maculatum*** L.)
WATER HEMLOCK
SPOTTED WATER HEMLOCK
(***Cicuta maculata*** L.)
(***C. maculata var. angustifolia*** Hook.)
(***C. occidentalis*** Greene) not accepted
DOUGLAS' WATER HEMLOCK
(***C. douglasii*** [DC.] J. M. Coult. & Rose)
BULBIFEROUS HEMLOCK
BULB BEARING WATER HEMLOCK
(***C. bulbifera*** L.)
NARROW LEAF HEMLOCK
MACKENZIE'S HEMLOCK
NORTHERN WATER HEMLOCK
COWBANE
(***C. mackenzieana*** Raup.) not accepted
(***C. virosa*** L.)
PARTS USED- root, seed (with care)

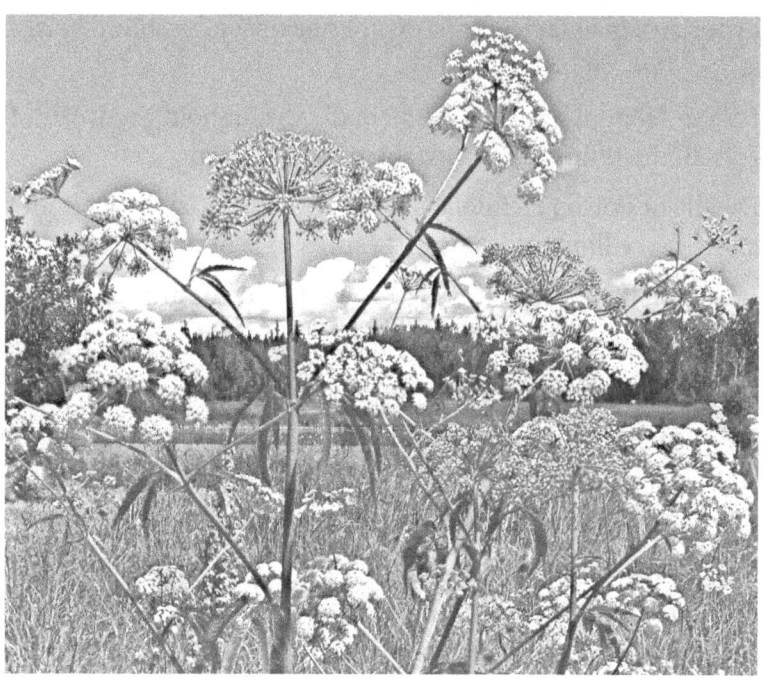

POISON HEMLOCK

We would make the men collect these roots themselves but there are several species of hemlock which are so much like the cows [Cows parsnip?] that it is difficult to discriminate them from the cows and we are afraid that they might poison themselves.
MERIWETHER LEWIS

The *Cicuta maculata* for instance. The concave umbel is so well spaced. The different umbellets like so many constellations or separate systems in the firmament. They get a sympathy with the stars.
THOREAU

For ye have turned judgment into gall, and the fruit of righteousness into Hemlock.
AMOS 6:12

" He that bites on every weed must needs light on poison."
JOHN RAY (1742)

Conium is from the Greek **KONEION**, or **KONAS**, meaning to spin or whirl as a top, referring to the giddy impact of the plant on the human body.

Maculatum is from the Latin, and means "spotted, blotched or bearing spots"; alluding to the purplish spots on the stem.

In English lore, the stems took their colour in sympathy with the mark placed on Cain's forehead after be murdered Abel.

Hemlock is from the Anglo Saxon, **HEMLIC** or **HYMELIC**. This is a combination of two words; **HEM** meaning shore, or **HOEM** or **HAELM**, meaning straw, and **LEAC**, meaning plant. Hemlock literally means hemp leek, and is similar to the ancient rune magic **LINA LAUKAR**.

In Old German, the plant was called **WUOTSCERLING** or **WODE-SCERNE** meaning Rage Hemlock. This is similar to the Norwegian **WODEN DUNK** and Anglo Saxon **WODE-HWISTLE**, or Wotan's Whistle.

Wotan or Odin is a Norse/Germanic God.

It was originally applied to any plant in the carrot family with hollow stalks, like straw, left after flowering.

Bulbifera means bulb bearing, and refers to the numerous small bulbs that fall off the top and develop into new plants.

The ancient Roman name for Poison Hemlock was Cicuta, that stuck until given to the Water Hemlock in 1541. Cicuta is named for a shepherd's pipe made from the hollow stemmed reed.

A Finnish myth of Lenninkainen relates his search for a maiden in the hostile north. He drove off all the men by force of his magic songs, except one miserable, blind herdsman who finally shot him with a shaft of cowbane (*C. virosa*).

Poison Hemlock is used medicinally throughout the world. In Italy, it is called Cleuta; in India, Kirdaman; in Iran Bikhi-i-Tafti; and in Arabian, Banj-e-rumi.

Deadly or Poison Hemlock is a common biennial throughout the prairies, usually found with wet feet in ditches, along fence lines and edge of swamps. It is quite rare in Saskatchewan, but sporadic.

It has the faint odor of mouse urine due to coniine, and is stronger when crushed.

Water Hemlock is less common, but can be plentiful in areas, as can Bulberous Hemlock, with its distinctive top.

Farmers and Ranchers are quick to eradicate these plants, as they will kill livestock. A single plant can produce up to 38,000 seeds that can be spread by water rodents and birds.

It can be recognized by its long, whitish root, purple spotted hollow stem, carrot-like leaves, and disagreeable "cat or mouse urine" odour when crushed. Although superficially like wild carrot, the latter has distinctly hairy leaves.

Poison Hemlock was used to kill Socrates in 399 BC; and it is just as poisonous today. Apparently, he was convicted of thinking. Under Jewish law, hemlock was given to criminals to drink before crucifixion or stoning, to help deaden the pain.

The ancient Baltic tribes associated the plant with the toad goddess.

Dioscorides recommended its use externally in herpes and staph infections; and applied as a mashed plant on the genitals in cases of priapism, or painful, persistent erections. If only I had known about this plant while in high school!

And it was the Arabian physician Avicenna that praised the plant as a cure for tumors of the breast.

Poison Hemlock was used by the Klallam as a love medicine, the roots rubbed on a woman's body to attract the attention of a man.

Linnaeus says that sheep will eat the leaves, but horses and goats refuse. An interesting experiment on woolly bear caterpillars involved giving them the choice of eating lupines or poison hemlock. Healthy caterpillars preferred the former, while those infected with fly larvae chose to feed on hemlock. Having parasites affected their diet choice, and this decision helped increase their odds of survival. Karban et al, *Ecology* 1997 78:2.

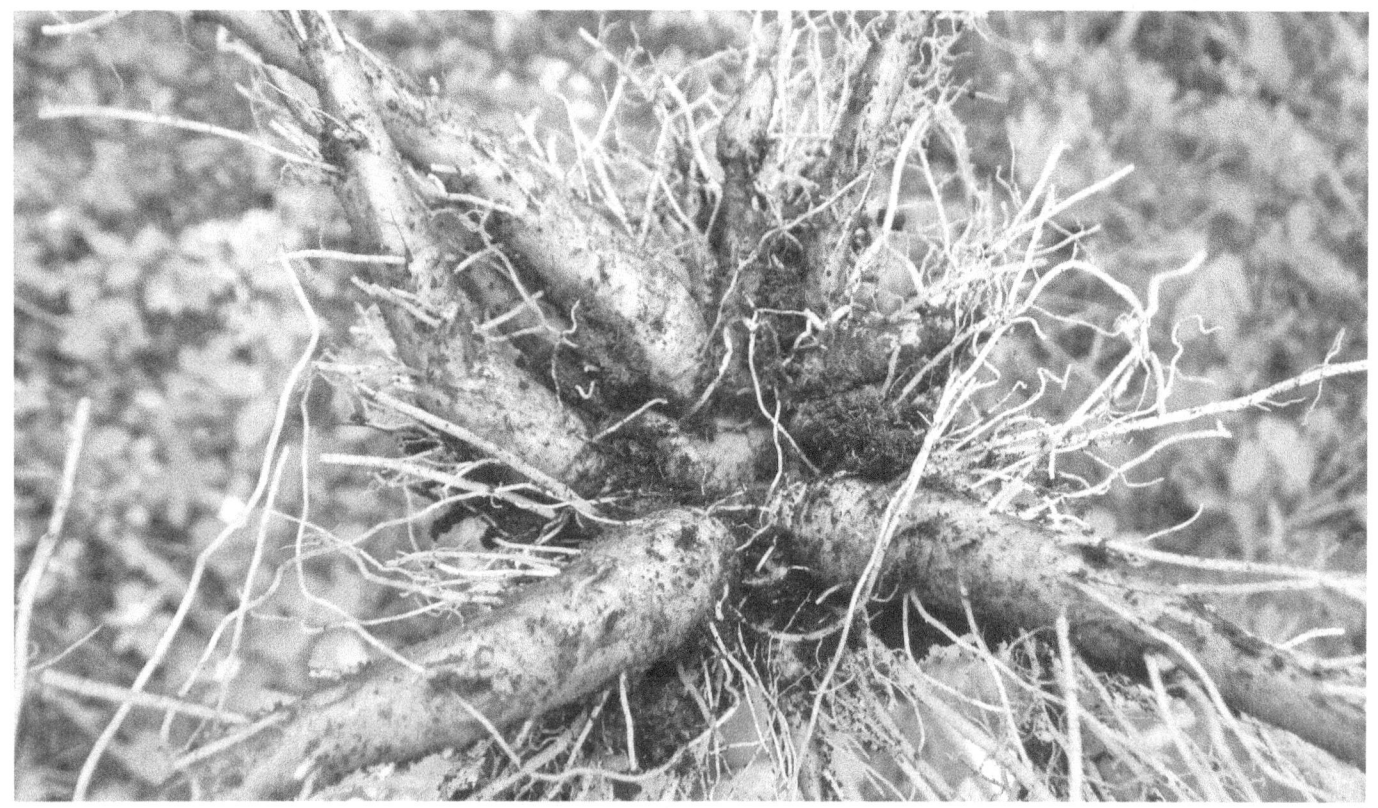

POISON HEMLOCK ROOTS

Water Hemlock has clusters of fleshy roots, cross partitions, or air chambers in the stem base, broader leaves, and wetter habitat. It doesn't have the obvious ill scent of Poison Hemlock.

Native tribes used the poison roots on their arrow tips. A Klamath tribe recipe for poison arrows was juice of western water hemlock, combined with rattlesnake venom and a decaying deer's liver.

The Blackfoot opened **TJITAATSA** root and put it directly on rattlesnake bites to draw the venom.

Western Water Hemlock (*C. douglasii*) root was mashed by the Kawaiisu, then put on a hot rock, and the sore limbs laid directly over.

A cold compounded infusion of burned and pulverized bark, was given by the Kwakiutl for diarrhea. They applied a poultice of soaked roots to the stomach as a purgative; or to draw out thorns. The Dene cut the root into small pieces and smoked it, with or without tobacco, to relieve headaches.

The Carrier heated the root and applied it to rheumatic or arthritic areas of the body. The call it **HOOGHUNAICH'O**.

The Wood Cree of Saskatchewan know Water Hemlock (*C. maculata*) as **MACI-SKATASK** meaning "bad carrot". The root was dried, powdered and made into a liniment that was applied externally.

The Cree of Alberta call it **MANITOSKATASK**, or poison carrot. Small amounts of the root are used in cancer combinations. Russell Willier, noted Cree healer, calls it God's Carrot. It is a dangerous medicine, used by some as part of a curse cure.

The Cherokee chewed the root of *C. maculata*. If dizziness occurred the person would soon die; if not, a long life could be expected.

The women of this tribe chewed the root and swallowed the juice to become sterile, generally for 4 consecutive days.

The Iroquois poultice roots for lameness, cuts, broken bones and running sores. They recognized its power, chewing roots to commit suicide.

It was used as an insecticide, with infusions of the root used to soak corn before planting.

Densmore reported that the Chippewa smoked Water Hemlock seeds, combined with their tobacco. The Ojibwa name is **WANU KONS.**

In Italy, a preparation of the crushed leaves is used as a local analgesic.

John Richardson (1832) wrote that the poisonous kinds are called **MANITOSKATASH,** and by the voyageurs "Carotte de Moreau"; or Carrot of Death, after a man in his group died from eating them.

Robin Klein, a fellow member of the American Herbalist Guild, has a catchy way to remember Water Hemlock:

"Leaf vein to the tip, all is hip.

Leaf Vein to the cut, pain in the gut".

Coniine has been proven an effective insecticide against aphids and blowflies. Gamma coniceine is a powerful anti-feedant for slugs.

MEDICINAL

CONSTITUENTS- *C. maculatum-* alkaloids including coniine (a color-less, volatile, alkaline oil) 1-2%; conhydrine, gamma-coniceine, N-methylconiine, conhydrin, conmaculatin, and pseudoconhydrin; lupeol, sitosterol, various coumarin derivatives such as umbelliferone, isopimpinellin, xanthotoxin, bergapten, and sphondin; feruloyl & sinapoly-3-0-xylosyl-glucosylgalactosides. When the plants are grown in hot, dry regions, the higher concentrations are in the fruit and seeds.
The piperidine alkaloids (coniine) are volatile and likely to be present in toxicologically harmful quantities only in the freshly harvested plant, particularly the fruit and ripe seed, 0.7-3.5%.
leaf- 0.095% alkaloids, mainly gamma coniceine.
C. maculata- cicutoxin, cicutine, cicutol, coniine (as a resinoid)
seeds- coniine, N-methyl coniine, and gamma-coniceine.
C. virosa- polynes including cicutoxic, isocicutoxin, cicudiol, cicutol, falcarindol, falcarinol; furanocoumarins similar to C. maculatum; and alkyl phthalides.

The primary action of poison hemlock is on the central nervous system. The activity is similar to nicotine poisoning, as conium alkaloids are structurally related to nicotine.

The classic symptoms of poisoning are nervousness, trembling, dilation of pupils, slow, weak pulse, rapid respiration, convulsions, paralysis, and death.

A writer of the 16th century, Banckes recorded "this herb is called humlock or herb Bennet. The virtue of this herb is thus. The joyce of this herb kepth maidens teets small."

Gerard responded saying "a very rash part to lay the leaves of Hemlocke to the stones of yong boyes, or virgins brests, by that means to keep those parts from growing great; for it doth not only easily cause those members to pine away, but also hurteth the heart and liver, being outwardly applied."

Poison Hemlock is a traditional remedy for cancer, especially of the breast and lymphatic. Ralph Moss, in his excellent book *Herbs Against Cancer*, dedicates a chapter to discussing this plant's potential.

The herb induces apoptosis in cervix (HeLa) carcinoma cell lines. Mondal J et al, *Pharmacogn Mag* 2014 10(suppl 3): S524-33.

The diluted remedy exerted cytotoxic effect against two human breast adenocarcinoma cell lines, MCF-7 and MDA-MB-23. Frenkel M et al, *Int J Oncol* 2010 36(2): 395-403.

Falcarindiol induces cell death in breast cancer cells, by induction of endoplasmic reticulum stress. It also has a synergistic effect with 5-FU and Bortezomib in killing breast cancer cells. Lu T et al, *PLoS One* 2017 12(4): e0176348. This compound is present in other members of Umbellifereae family, including carrot, angelica, devil's club, etc.

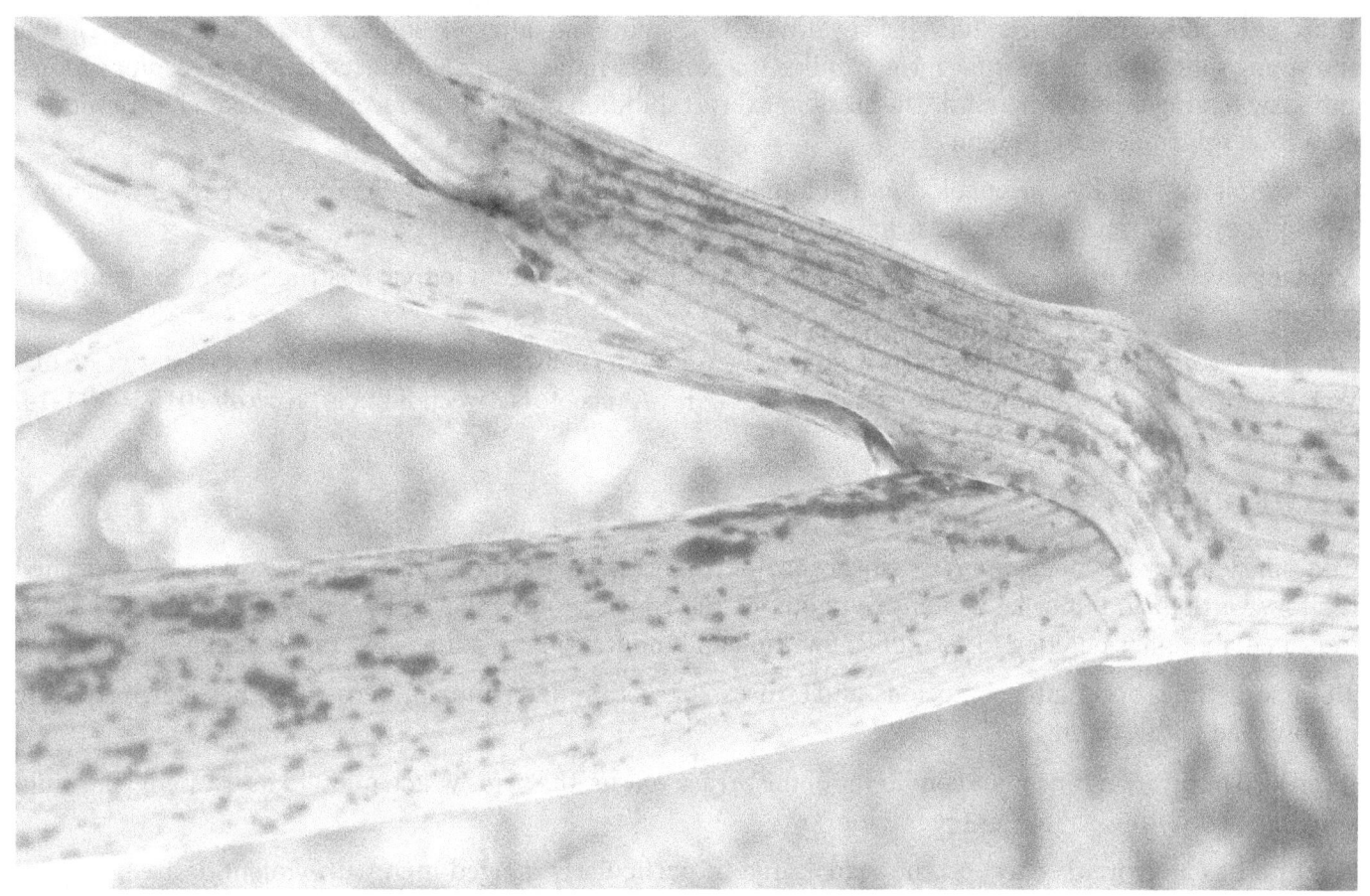

PURPLE SPOTTING ON STEMS

Falcarinol modulates GABA-A receptors, and is a reversible agonist of cannabinoid receptors. Czyzewska MM et al, *J Nat Prod* 2014 77(12): 2671-7.

Conium extracts, and tinctures have for a long time remained official drug preparations in the *US Pharmacopoeia*.

Poison Hemlock, in small, exact dosage, may help in Landry's Paralysis, or Guillain-Barré syndrome. The inexperienced should consider using a 3X homeopathic preparation.

It is very useful as a poultice or ointment for malignant glands. Continued use has a shrinking effect on reducing the gland from stony hardness.

The same ointment can be used with care in itching anus and piles.

The leaves show activity against Gram positive bacteria.

And whereas, Poison Hemlock death is more speedy and non-violent regarding paralysis; Water Hemlock is even more poisonous, with 30% of poisonings proving fatal.

The powerful nerve toxin begins 15 minutes after ingestion with excruciating cramps, pains and convulsions that people have bitten through their tongue and broken teeth.

The therapeutic and toxic dosage are so similar, that the plant medicines should be in homeopathic form (see below). It was Paracelsus, a 16th century herbalist, that said "all substances are poisons; there is none which is not a poison. The right dose differentiates a poison from a remedy."

Religious sects of the 15th and 16th centuries used roasted poison hemlock root externally to relieve the pain of gout, not only on the foot, but on their hands and wrists. In the 1700s, it was recommended for cancerous ulcers.

The juice of poison hemlock is still valued by druggists. Coniine and other alkaloids are extracted from the leaves and young shoots, just as the fruits form. Coniine is a paralysis-inducing nicotinic acetylcholine receptor agonist, and toxic teratogenetic compound. The alkaloid exerts inhibition on nicotinic receptor-mediated nitrergic and noradrenergic transmitter response.

Cicutoxin is a potent K+ current blocker that inhibits K+ channel dependent proliferation of naive and memory T lymphocytes. Strauss U et al, *Biochem Biophys Res Commun* 1996 219(2): 332-6.

A patent was issued in Germany in 1971 on medicinal extracts of Conium to treat obstructions of the lymphatic system.

Douglas' Water Hemlock water extracts were widely used, externally, by indigenous healers of western Canada. Water extracts are a non-competitive antagonist of GABA A receptors. Green BT et al, *Toxicon* 2015 108:11-14. Caution is advised.

HOMEOPATHY

Conium Hemlock (*C. maculatum*) is associated with paralysis that ascends from below upwards, with associated rotatory vertigo; and unusually intensive photophobia, which is only relieved by dark and pressure. It is also indicated, in higher potency, for glandular swelling and induration, prickling, stinging, rock hard to touch.

These sometimes occur after contusions, and bruises, such as a sudden lump in the breast. These can be quickly re-absorbed with Conium.

It can also be given in cancerous conditions of the breast, uterus; the pains which point to its use being burning, stinging or shooting, as in Apis (bee venom).

Conium has a favorable effect on the sexual organs, particularly in aged men with violent desire, amorous thoughts, and incapacity to perform. This may be accompanied with poor urine flow, which also occurs in Clematis, such as benign hypertrophic prostatitis.

It is for people whose sex drive is suppressed when they are forced into celibacy and have not chosen that path. They may close down emotionally and feel flat and depressed.

Sweating which occurs as soon as the patient falls asleep, night or day. Weakness of memory, reduced mental ability, tremors, tinnitus and sleeplessness are related to Conium.

In the mucosa, there is dryness and irritation, with a violent, tickling cough, particularly at night when lying down. This cough may be the result of a tumor of the lung, acute chill, or tuberculosis.

Other irritative states, such as ulcerative glottitis, tongue fissures, stomach pain with vomiting, thirst and craving for sour things, such as is often found in cancer of the stomach are relieved.

Aggravation is from cold, rest and night.

I made great use of the homeopathic preparation Vertigoheel during clinical practice. Conium inhibits phosphodiesterase 5, in the synergistic formulation. It works wonderfully well as a tune up of the brainstem, associated with what some practitioners call slow brainstem syndrome.

DOSE- Best in higher potencies, given infrequently, especially for growths, etc. Otherwise, 6th and 30th potency. The mother tincture is made from the whole, fresh plant in flower or unripe seed. *The French Pharmacopeia* suggests fresh flower heads only.

Eli Jones recommended 2X potency for breast cancer, five drops every two hours. Try the 3X potency for those suffering Guillain-Barré syndrome. Dr. Bastyr recommended Conium for Landry's paralysis, a particularly virulent form of Guillain-Barr. Dr. Sarkar suggested 200X for bicycle rider's prostatitis.

See *Plants* Volume One by Vermeulen and Johnston pages 288-94 for case studies of this remedy.

Water Hemlock (*Cicuta virosa*) is a European species. It is specific for creeping sensation in the limbs, by burning, pressing and tearing sensations in various parts of the body, with stiffness, cold and numbness of the arms and hands with distended veins.

This remedy is also suggested by abnormal food cravings, or lack of appetite accompanied by violent thirst.

Cicuta is indicated for a wide variety of psychoses and conditions of the brain and spinal cord, with cramps, including teething cramps in small children, especially if caused by worms.

There may be stomach cramps with bleeding, paralysis of the bladder, and skin diseases with simultaneous disturbances of the peripheral nervous system. Hard, lemon yellow crusts on the skin, chronic impetigo, and eczema with no itching may be relieved.

It is worthy of a trial in syringomyelia.

DOSE- Third to 200th potency. The mother tincture is made from the fresh rootstock with attached roots, while coming into flower. The local *C. maculata* is interchangeable, the most prominent symptoms being: falls unconscious in tetanic or clonic convulsions. The body is covered in sweat. May be useful in epilepsy or tetanus. Given in the tincture and lower potencies for these purposes.

A 3X remedy may work on Landry's paralysis, a virulent form of Guillain-Barre syndrome.

MATERIA POETICA

Where did life go?
Where once was supple
Is now crust
Hard and indurated
Glands, breasts, testes
Bruises old and deep
Life itself a tumor
Flatness of the heart
Flatness of the brain
Letting life go in increments
Until finally, like a cancer
Which spreads slowly,
Taking over its host
Your mind crumples
Leaving an imbecilic shell
Sitting in the chair.

SYLVIA CHATROUX MD

ESSENTIAL OIL

Both the leaves and roots of *C. virosa* yield 0.2% essential oil, while the seeds contain up to 5.6% oil. Thirty-one compounds have been identified.

The essential oil of the seeds of *C. virosa* var. *latisecta* contains more than 45 compounds, with gamma terpinene 40%, p-cymene 28% and cumin aldehyde 21% largest representatives. It shows anti-fungal activity that may have potent preservative benefit.

The fresh leaf of *C. maculatum* yields about 0.04% of an oil containing 23 compounds the highest 27% germacrene D, followed by E beta ocimene at 22.3% and (Z)-beta ocimene at 7.1%.

The flower yield is 0.06% with 57 compounds, the highest being germacrene D at 41%, followed by (Z)-beta ocimene at 14.3%, beta mycrene 9.3%, E beta ocimene 7.7% and (E) nerolidol 7.1%.

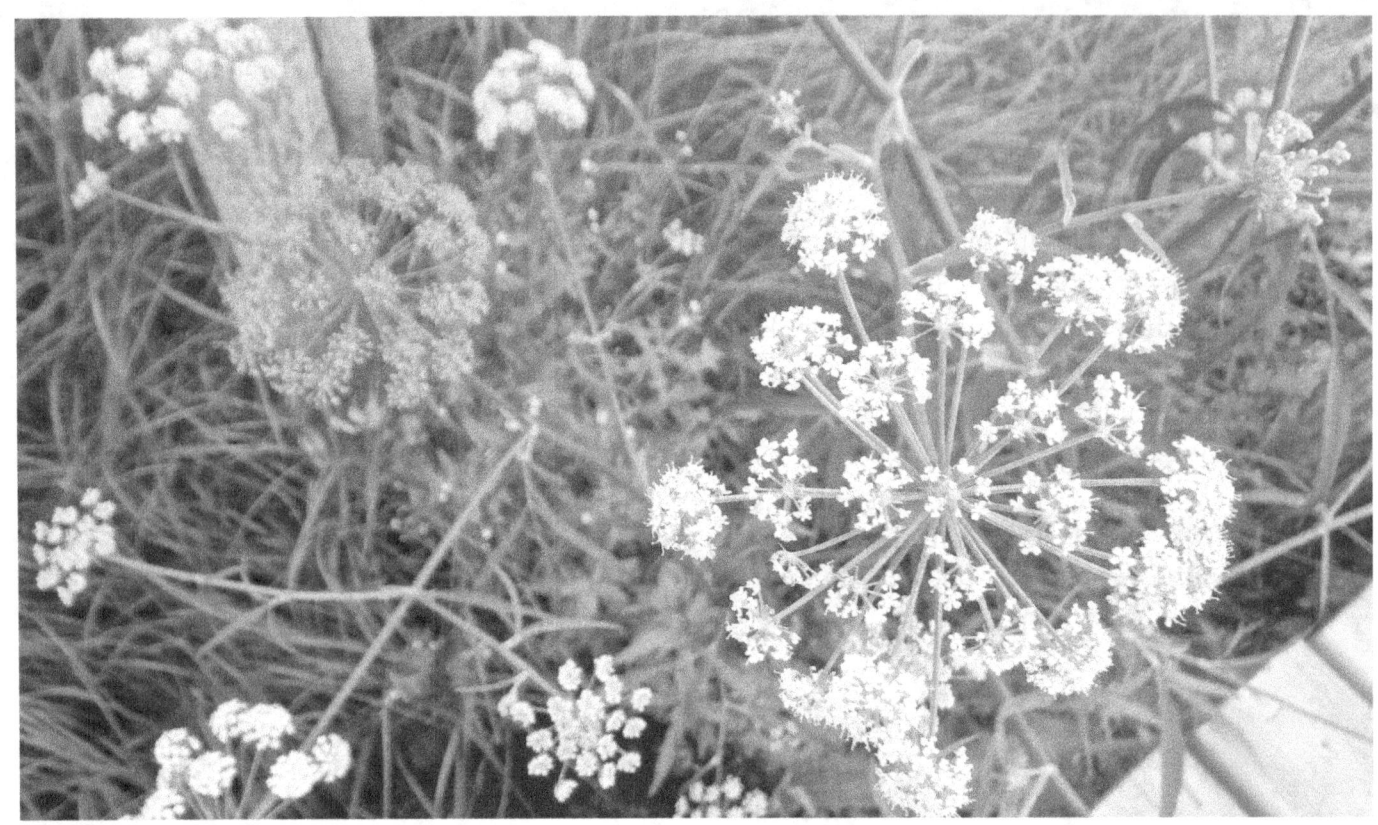

POISON HEMLOCK FLOWERS

LEAF AND SEED OIL

Poison Hemlock leaves are gathered in early summer and the seed soon after to making into oils. Use a ratio of 1part leaf/seed to four parts of canola or olive oil, and sun infuse in a safe spot for 7-10 days. The oil is used for making ointments or by itself for wheals, indolent ulcers that refuse to heal, creeping or cancerous ulcers, swollen lymph nodes throughout the body, and joint pain associated with gout.

The oil can also be used for mastitis, anal fissures and hemorrhoids. Do not use as suppository, but simply applied externally as needed.

SEED OIL

The seed oil is nearly 5% palmitic acid, 74% oleic and petroselenic acids, 20% linoleic acid, and 0.7% arachidic acid.

HYDROSOL

Hemlock (*C. virosa*) water distilled from the whole herb is, according to Brunschwig, used for reducing holy fire, or when the face is too warm. It is used for quantery fevers, paralysis, dropsy and to prevent the breasts from becoming too large. All of these uses are external only in the form of washes or wraps.

FLOWER ESSENCES

Water Hemlock (*Cicuta mackenzieana*) flower essence is for realigning one's vibration to that of one's Celestial family. It is the essence for bringing infinite nurturing and guidance to understanding one's path, the joy and a peace to follow it. **CANADIAN FOREST**

Poison Hemlock (*C. maculatum*) flower essence dissolves the emotional, mental and physical paralysis, which can arise in periods of transition and major change.

It is especially effective if we somehow believe that the change is being initiated from outside ourselves, and therefore something over which we have no control.

It is effective for stalled labour in the birthing process.

Emotionally, it helps us to release rigid feelings and to convert the energy of fear into excitement so that we can use it to move forward. Mentally, Poison Hemlock flower essence allows us to release ingrained thought patterns- repetitive and often quite unconscious thoughts which do not serve use in the moment. **PACIFIC**

PERSONALITY TRAITS

The Conium personality is weak, exhausted and early aging. They are single people who are upset because of prolonged illness or sexual repression; generally slim and pale, apathetic, inactive and desire to be alone.

They are not affectionate, owing to depression, and feel estranged from the world.

They seek comfort in sexual activity, and consider intercourse something material like eating or sleeping. Without daily intercourse with partner, and its outlet, they are subject to fits of hysteria. They are inflexible and cannot adapt to time change. The personality is overly materialistic and concerned with loss. **BIANCHI**

A sudden impact requires reaction, but Conium meets it with slow conservatism, trying to hold onto what existed before any impact. New ideas are met with the rigid, fixed ideas of resistance. Physical injuries or impacts are met with the hardening of tumour formation and the rigidity of function as in its well-known ascending paralysis. Faced with contact, Conium retreats. **VERMUELEN**

Conium's conservative nature, their retreat and their expression of the family themes including the desire to stick to the familiar rather than venturing out to the new and unexpected, is represented, surprisingly, by the interesting little rubric 'Delusion he is a goose', which has Conium as the only listing. Any animal associated with a remedy either through dreams, delusions, fears or aversion, says something important about that remedy. In this case it is a goose that represents the features of Conium. Geese are monogamous, living in permanent pairs throughout the years. Geese in pairs keep to themselves and their family group. They do not venture out to mix with other geese. **VERMUELEN**

Cicuta personality is childlike and childish and cannot explain their state. They can be a bit imbecilic. **P. CHAPPELL**

One key feature [of Conium] is slow, insidious, progressive, ascending paralysis or hardening or both, of mind and body. This is what happened to Socrates when he was poisoned with hemlock.

The other key feature is the lack of opportunity or the suppression of the sexual urges. The classic example of this I have seen is a nun with ascending paralysis.

In the common life, not dedicated to God in every moment, it's found in people who focus on esoteric and mystical writings and who suppress or neglect their natural instincts. They slowly develop an emotional flatness or hardness, leading to indifference and depression. Mentally they limit themselves within narrow, fixed ideas and become superstitious and slowly senile, so slowly they don't notice.

There is also the image of the proud old man who insists on wearing his best clothing on Sunday. They can be both dictatorial and meticulous. And there is the idea of sacrifice that *I cannot leave my husband. I have to care for him; I cannot leave because it's my duty.* It's also the older man or woman who fusses over trifles, having no sexual outlet. The image is also of the old peasant woman, dressed always in black, as her husband has died, sent went with it, and hardening up is happening. The upper lip is withered, with little vertical lines just above the lip line, indicating the womb is in trouble.

The other option is unrestrained sexual activity, resembling the cock, a belligerent and contentious individual constantly running after others for sex. This might be the teenager who abandons studies for sex, or an older male "cock".
PETER CHAPPELL

MYTHS AND LEGENDS

Haddingus, who was raised by the giants but later became a favorite of Odin, was once visited at the hearth in the evening by an apparition of a woman who wore hemlock in her garb. This woman, interpreted as a shamanic helping spirit, placed her cloak around Haddingus and led him across a bridge, into the underworld, and to the realm of the dead.
LICHTENBERGER

RECIPES

TINCTURE- One drop! In Britain, the maximum concentration for external use is 7%. The fresh root tincture is prepared at 1:10 and 60% alcohol.

EXTRACT- 0.12-0.4 grams

POWDERED LEAF- 0.12-0.5 grams

OINTMENT- Add one part of Poison Hemlock powder to ten parts of glaxol cream. This has no toxic effects if used on limited areas. Use for inflamed lymph glands, mastitis, and barber's itch (sycosis barbae).

WARNING- Do not ingest the fresh or dried plant. In the case of poison hemlock, and water hemlock use morphine and thiobarbiturates to control convulsions. When seizures have occurred, do not attempt gastric lavage without an anesthesiologist present. Prolonged mental problems and irregular ECGs have been reported. It is the antidote for strychnine poisoning, as its activity is directly antagonistic. If really isolated in the woods, try strong tannin rich teas. A 30 year-old male presented to emergency with brief cardiac arrest after injecting poison hemlock. Brtalik D et al, *J Med Toxicol* 2017 Feb 6.

EASTERN POISON IVY
(***Rhus radicans var. vulgaris*** [Michx.] DC.) not accepted
(***R. radicans ssp. rybergii*** [Small ex Rydb.] Greene) not accepted
(***Toxicodendron radicans ssp. radicans*** [L.] Kuntze.)
WESTERN POISON IVY
(***T. radicans var. rydbergii*** [Small ex Rydb.] Erskine) not accepted
(***T. rybergii***[Small ex Rydb.]Greene)
ATLANTIC POISON OAK
(***T. pubescens*** Mill.)
(***R. toxicodendron*** L.) not accepted
PACIFIC POISON IVY
(***T. diversilobum*** [Torr. & A. Gray] Greene)
PARTS USED- leaves, flowers.

Rhus is an old name for Sumac meaning either "faith" from the Greek or "red" from the Celtic. I prefer the former. ***TOXIKOS*** is from the Greek meaning poison, and radicans from the Latin ***RADICIS*** meaning "with rooting stems". Dendron is from the Greek for tree. Pubescens means hairy or downy.

Poison ivy is common in the coulees, riverbeds and open woods of the southern prairies. Strangely, it belongs to the same genus as cashew, mango and other tropical delights. The small yellow white flowers give way to green turning white berries.

The irritant sap is present all year round, but is most powerful during the night and during June and July, when the sun does not shine. It seems that dampness and lack of sunlight favour the release of the leaf toxins.

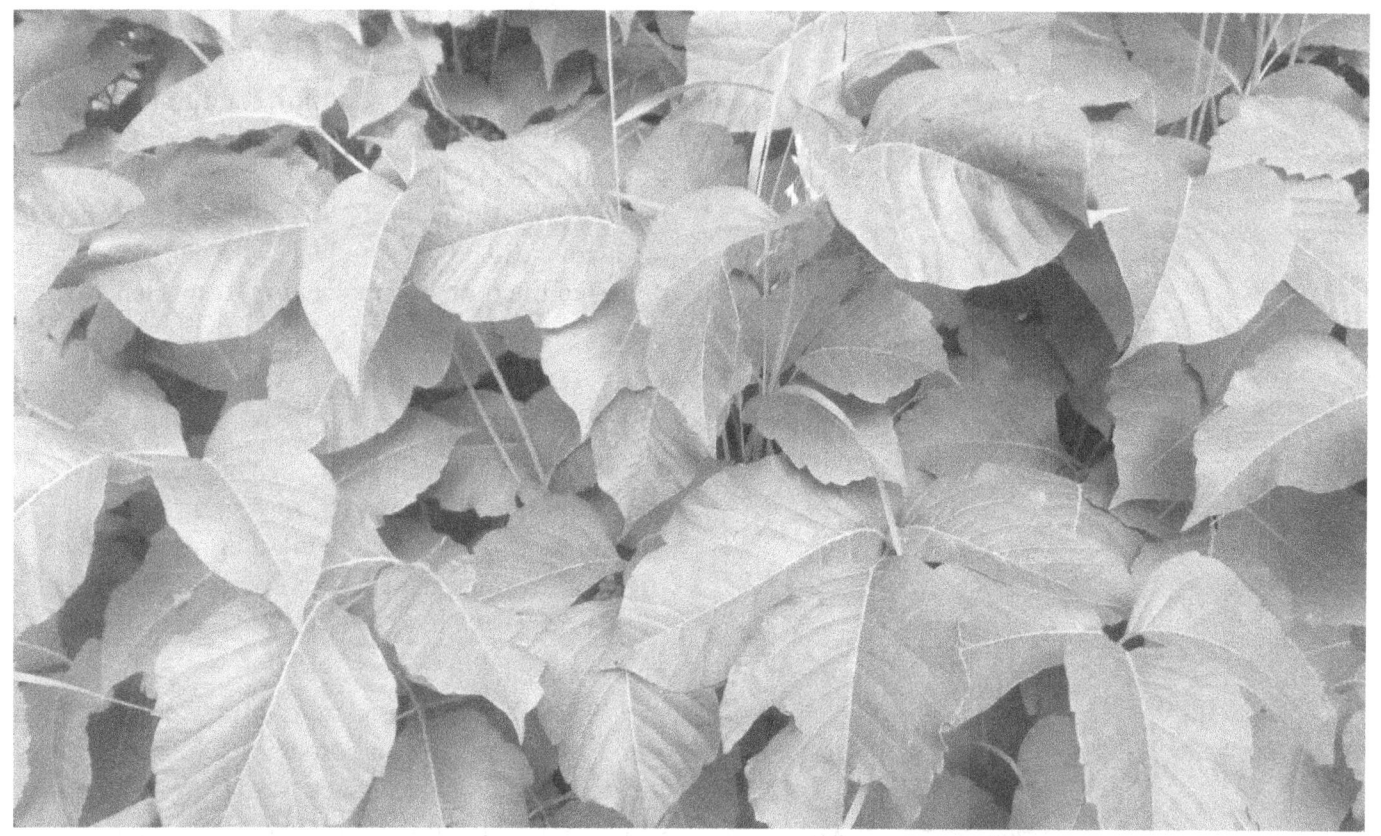

WESTERN POISON IVY

Vapors collected by simply holding over the plant can cause blisters and inflammation of the skin. According to Gillis, herbarium specimens several centuries old have induced dermatitis in sensitive people who handle them. Sap diluted five million times can create irritation! It has been estimated that 7 ml of urushiol, the active oleoresin, has the potential to affect everyone on the planet. When poison ivy molecules come in contact with skin, they instantly bind with skin protein; and cannot easily be dissolved away. Urushiol is neutralized by water and if washed off within 5-10 minutes after contact, a reaction may be avoided. Lane et al, *Austin American Statesman* 1995 June 16.

Organoclay, an ingredient in anti-perspirants, has the ability to bind with urushiol. It is known as quaternium-18 bentonite. Ivyblock is one lotion containing this compound at 5%.

One the other hand, nearly 70% of people are immune from their first exposure, and only develop allergic reaction on later contact.

Recent research at the University of Mississippi has developed an experimental vaccine that seems to prevent an allergic reaction.

This would be a welcome addition for those especially sensitive to the plant.

At one time, it was believed that swallowing a whole leaf gave a person immunity. I fear that this foolhardy act could cause serious blistering and swelling of the mouth and throat.

All that being said, it would be fairer to classify poison ivy as an allergic irritant, as some people seem quite immune, while those with sun sensitivity and light skin, are highly sensitive.

Some fresh plant leaves with antidotal relief that grow nearby include gum weed, jewelweed, mugwort and other Artemisia species, plantain, and bearberry.

Contrary to popular belief, the blister fluid does not contain urushiol, and cannot spread infection by fluid contact.

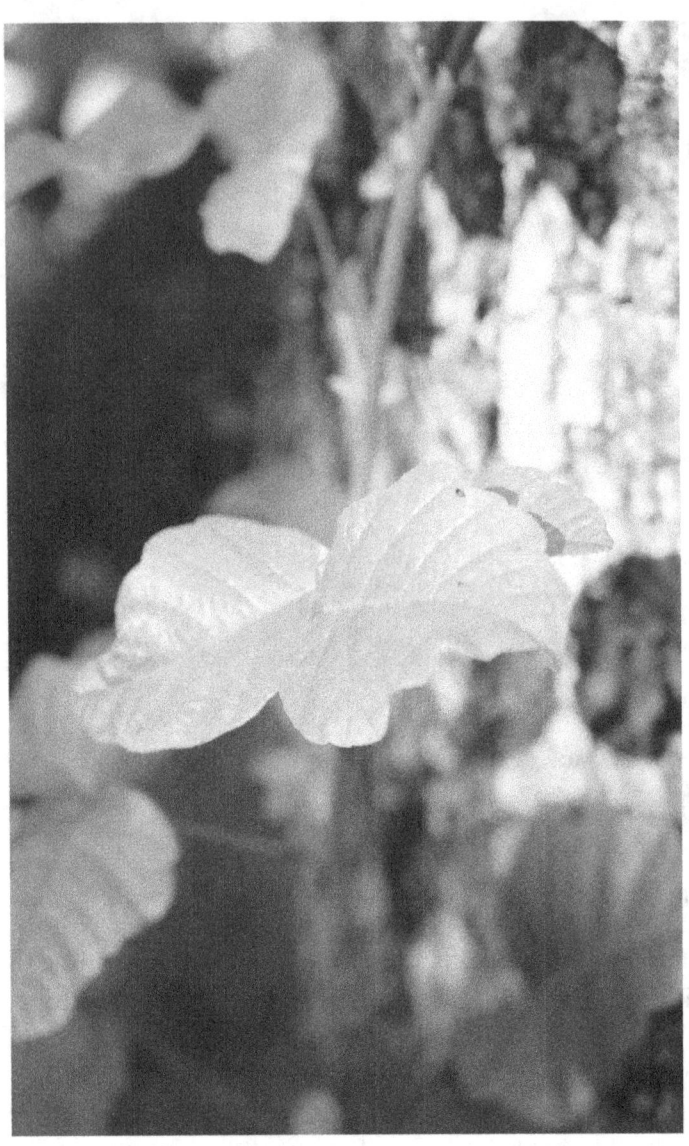

POISON OAK

There are indications that various Native tribes used the plant for medicine. The Mohegans roasted and then crushed the root for various skin conditions. Tribes of Southwestern California made poultices of the fresh leaf and applied it to warts and ringworm. The Navaho used it and other plants in a poison combination for arrowheads. Both the Delaware and Fox people pounded the roots for application to swollen glands.

The Cree of Alberta know the plant as **KA PISCIPOMAKAHKWAW NEPEYA**, or **PICIPOSKAKIS**.

The sap is initially milky, and then becomes black and sticky upon exposure to air. At one time, this was a valuable source of indelible ink that becomes darker the more it was washed. The Pomo tribe made use of this rich black dye, a colour otherwise difficult to obtain from nature.

In 1798, a French physician examined a young man who had suffered from a herpes infection on the wrist for years. After an exposure to poison ivy, the rash disappeared. Further inquiry led to the preparation of various extracts for Streptococcus and shingle (herpes zoster) inflammation. This led to the safer and very successful use in Homeopathy below.

Secondary compounds in the leaves have been used to treat bacterial infections such as gonorrhea, dysentery and gangrene. Laboratory studies appear to confirm these antimicrobial properties.

It is my belief, shared with other botanists, that *R. radicans* and *R toxicodendron* are merely varieties of the same species. It is suggested that *T. rydbergii* is a non-climbing shrub, while *T. radicans* can be a bush or vine. Work by Gillis has identified nine subspecies of *T. radicans* for those who need to know. My classifications at top of chapter are most recent, as of 2017.

An interesting study conducted in Japan involved a poison ivy-like plant. Children allergic to this plant had a leaf rubbed on one forearm. A non-poisonous leaf was rubbed on the other as a control. As expected almost all the children developed a rash on the one arm. What they did not know is that the leaves were deliberately mislabeled. The negative thought of being touched by the toxic leaf led to the rash. And the majority of arms rubbed with the toxic leaf did not develop a rash. Ikema & Nakagawa, *Kyoshu J Med Sci* 1962 13.

MEDICINAL

CONSTITUENTS- *R. toxicodendron or R. radicans*-an oil resin called urushiol, made up mainly of phenolic substances like 3-n-pentadecylcatechol; from toxicodendrol. Urushiol is from the Japanese meaning sap.
Also contains ureshenol (up to 3.3% in leaves). Tannins compose up to 40% of the leaf. The seed oil has been investigated and yields 22%, composed of 62% saturated fatty acids, 10% oleic and linoleic (24%) acids. The dry fruits contain 10.6% protein and 22.4% fat; and neicosandicarbonic acid.

Eleven endophytic bacteria have been identified from vine tissue, with five belonging to Pseudomonas genus.

In small doses, Poison ivy is a sympathetic stimulant, affecting the vasomotor and glandular fibres. In large doses, it depresses the central and sympathetic nervous system. At the turn of the century, many practitioners found poison ivy an effective remedy for teething children and the delirium around high fevered states.

Work by Patil et al, *Homeopathy* 2009 98:3 found mother tinctures to 1000 C dilutions all stimulate the immune system, with lower doses more potent.

It is useful for individuals that are keyed up, inwardly excited with a reddish complexion. It has been found useful in the past in restored nerve function in some cases. It has proven useful in sciatic and facial neuritis. For opthalmic herpes, it has brought relief to a very painful disease. The irritation and light sensitivity are improved, and corneal ulcerations are less deforming, and in many cases, free of nebula formation.

Urushiols stimulate the immune system in a non-specific manner, and inhibit cyclooxygenase and lipoxygenase, *in vitro*.

Urushiols are haptens that have to bind with skin proteins to form complete antigens.

HOMEOPATHY

Rhus toxicodendron (Rhus tox), or *T. pubescens* as it is now known, is specific to the relief of joint pain with movement. The joints, ligaments, tendons and connective tissue are achy, sore, stiff and swollen, leading to the nickname "rusty gate".

Generally, the Rhus tox patient is restless, anxious and cannot get comfortable without moving. They toss and turn, making sleep difficult. The evening, or a lack of sun, makes the symptoms worse, and they can become depressed and weep easily.

They feel chilly, and are aggravated by cold and damp weather. Symptoms are improved by dry, warm weather, warm applications and stretching.

Eruptions caused by poison ivy are red, inflamed and itchy. The blisters fill with a clear liquid that oozes. This makes Rhus Tox the perfect antidote for chicken pox, impetigo, herpes and even contact from the plant itself. In urticaria, follow with puffball.

Itchiness is present in the genital organs of both sexes.

They may be superstitious and exhibit patterns such as not stepping on sidewalk cracks or compulsively checking that all electrical appliances are turned off.

One peculiar symptom, sometimes present and helpful in diagnosis, is a triangulated area on the tip of the tongue.

DOSE- Mother tincture must have adequate amounts of quercitrin and rutin for optimal benefit. Sixth to 30th potency. Mice studies suggest 30X increases COX-2 expression, and decreases nitric oxide generation, thus modulating inflammation.

At dilutions of 1M, 10M and CM, the remedy reduced serum levels of C-reactive protein and improved pain threshold in rats. Patel DR et al, *Homeopathy* 2012 101(3): 165-70.

It is worthy of a trial for fibromyalgia at 30C potency. Take 2-4 doses daily, the last one at bedtime. Try 6X potency as a preventative measure against dermatitis. Signore RJ presents two open studies and anecdotal experience with homeopathic poison ivy in prevention of acute allergic contact dermatitis. *Dermatol Online J* 2017 23(1).

A 9CH remedy may decrease joint pain and stiffness in breast cancer patients treated with aromatase inhibitors. Karp JC et al, *Homepathy* 2016 105(4): 299-308.

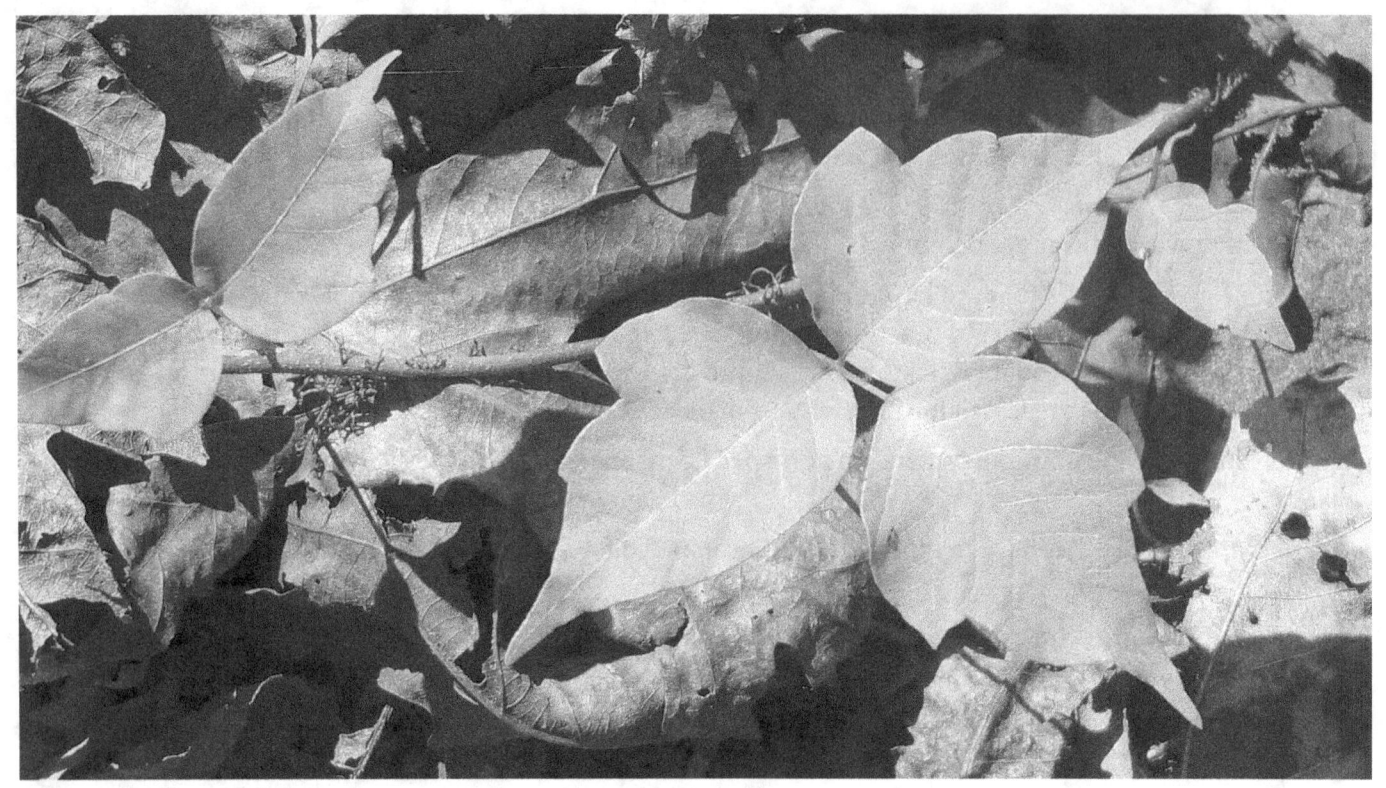

YOUNG POISON IVY

Rhus radicans, is almost identical in action, with one addition. The symptoms abate after an electrical storm has set in. And there is better relief from headaches in the occiput and nape of the neck than from Rhus tox. There is also a yearly aggravation of a symptom, pointing the way to its use.

DOSE- Sixth to 30th potency. The 200th will antidote poisoning from the plant or tincture. In cases where the patient jumps out of their sleep, try third potency at bedtime.

The mother tincture is made from the fresh leaves, before it flowers, during the night or in cloudy weather to increase potency. The mother tincture of *Rhus radicans* is prepared from the fresh root.

I don't recommend amateurs make their own mother tincture. It is extremely volatile and is best prepared in a vacuum setting.

Self experiments by Joslin with *R. radicans* at 3x, 6x, 30x, and 50x in 1846 gives some further interesting insights.

Nightmares, with inability to move and sensation of pressure on the right upper portion of chest. There is superstitious fear connected with the supposed presence and agency of some invisible, sly and malicious being. There is a disposition to criticize, find fault and utter reproaches.

Cutting pains in bladder or rectum with urination.

In the 1780s, Dufresnoy observed paralysis on lower part of body, or hot things feel cold and vice-versa.

Melancholy turns merry and disposed to work after infusion of *R. radicans*.

Vermeulen and Johnston present several good case studies in Plants Volume One pages 207-15.

Western poison oak (*Rhus diversiloba*)

It is similar to *R. radicans*, but greater intensity of heat. Restlessness is a way of distracting the person from physical symptoms, while in *R. radicans* the restlessness appears to be an amelioration of physical symptoms.

Less thirst, but helped by cold drinks, cold showers and more swelling and edema.

MATERIA POETICA

Rhus toxicodendron
Lively jester, you seemed fine
Until I looked into your mind
Behind your nervous overwear
I see a fellow bathed in fear
You didn't want the world to see
Your underlying energy
Quite a hyperactive sort
Now you snap out some retort
Stiffened up as if from rust
You need oil to warm you up
Once you move, then pace you must
Joints inflamed and craving heat
Drink cold milk and something sweet
You won't like a stormy day
So much worse when skies are gray
Skin eruptions drive you mad
Better in a real hot bath
In your sleep you toss the night
And morning is no better sight
First we begged you to sit still
Now you're stiff and cannot move
Rhus Tox, I was fooled by you!
Discontent and weeping too
Fighting back your enemy
These strange ideas won't set you free
And when all else cannot succeed
You try jokes and even greed
You think of jumping in a lake
Don't make this terrible mistake
One high dose could help you through
Cure your joints, your skin and you!

SYLVIA CHATROUX MD

ESSENTIAL OIL

Essential oil from poison ivy contains the irritant urushiol, and has great inhibitory effect on prostaglandin synthesis, similar to Labrador tea oil.

FLOWER ESSENCE

The plant signature of poison ivy is that it irritates the skin. Use of the flower essence is indicated for those with anxiety and irritability. The Etheric body is strengthened so that the individual is not so easily affected by negativity.   **PEGASUS**

Poison ivy flower essence is for impatience. The person is irritable and restless, and yet they are reluctant to move on. In the negative state, these are a passive and yielding disposition. They are unsure of their irritation, and yet very likely to stay hidden in their room. Like the plant, their symptoms are exaggerated during cloudy and rainy nights of summer.

On the positive side, the flower essence helps the person feel like exploring the true source of their irritation. This can lead to necessary changes in lifestyle or belief systems that have exacerbated the irritation.

PRAIRIE DEVA

SPIRITUAL PROPERTIES

Western re-incarnationists generally do not believe in plant transmigration, but certain Hindu sects embrace this concept. The cactus and poison ivy are thought to be the re-embodiment of criminals or those who lived a life of vice.

BOLTON

PERSONALITY TRAITS

This remedy does not have a personality, except they tell jokes and pass the time of day. Restless types, always changing position. Hard workers, gravediggers, road menders, gardeners, builders. Dream of hard work. You spot them as they get out of a chair.

P. CHAPPELL

Poison ivy, whose impact has been immortalized in a Lieber and Stoller ditty, one of a small group of rock songs to be titled after a weed….In the lyrics, poison ivy is likened to a scheming woman, who'll 'get under your skin', whereupon—and it's one of the great rhyming couplets of pop music—'You're gonna need an ocean/ Of calamine lotion'.

RICHARD MABEY

RECIPES

RHUS TOX MOTHER TINCTURE- Use with extreme caution. For the inexperienced, it would be best to purchase the homeopathic dilutions. The standard single dose is 0.03 grams.

Even these dilutions must be used with caution. Over dose of homeopathic preparations can lead to severe mucous membrane irritation, queasiness, vomiting, intestinal colic, diarrhea and symptoms of resorption, including kidney damage.

PURPLE LOOSESTRIFE
(***Lythrum salicaria*** L.)
PARTS USED- flowering tops

I love the river's sedgy bank,
Where purple loose-strife bends,
Near fleur-de-lis, and meadow sweet,
All those dear ancient friends.

TWAMLEY

Lythrum is from the Greek **LYTHRON** meaning gore or blood. This may be due to its hemostatic action or the bright red of the related Red Loosestrife flower.

Salicaria is from the similarity of leaves on plants of the willow (*Salix* genus).

Loosestrife may come from the relaxing effect of the herb on nervous disorders.

Purple Loosestrife is a naturalized noxious weed that is aggressively choking out native vegetation in the wetlands of both Canada and the United States. Since its introduction from Europe in the 1800s it has taken advantage of no natural enemy to spread at an alarming rate.

It is an extremely aggressive seed producer- up to 2.7 million seeds per plant! Germination rate is over 90%, and from 10-20 thousand seedlings can sprout on one square metre of land.

The only truly effective eradication is by pulling the complete root, with a mature root weighing more than two pounds. Work is proceeding on the introduction, from its native Europe, insects that feed upon the plant.

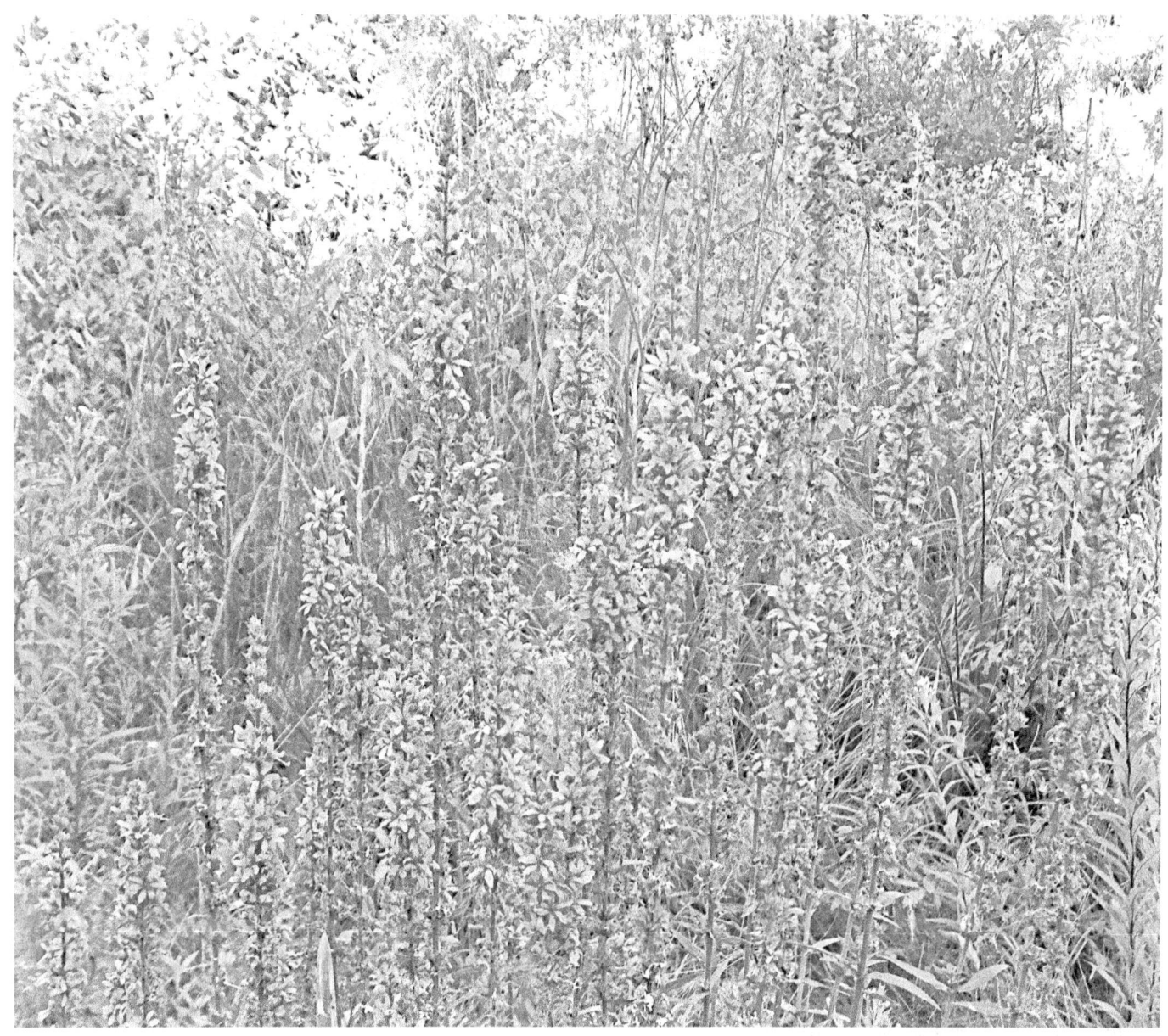

PURPLE LOOSESTRIFE

One of two leaf-eating beetle larvae, *Galerucella calmariensis*, is being used in trials for bio-control, as well as a weevil, *Nanophyes marmoratus*, which eats the flowers.

The astringent properties of the leaves and flowers have been appreciated since antiquity, even used for tanning leather.

Traditionally, it was dried and then burnt to drive away biting insects; like fleabane. In a garden, it attracts butterflies.

Dioscorides wrote about the plant. "The herb is tart and strong in taste, with an astringent and refrigerant nature, good for staunching both outward and inward bleeding. Sap extracted from the leaves and drunk stops blood-spitting and dysentery, and sour wine in which the leaves have been boiled when taken internally will have the same effect."

In Celtic mythology, purple loosestrife was said to be home to elves. In magical lore, the herb has to ability to encourage development of psychic powers and restore memory of past lives.

Turner, the famous English herbalist, coined the common plant name in 1548.

Its use for dysentery was described by Camardon (1883), with infusions and macerations being most effective. This work in France led to two preparations in the 1920s, Salicairine and Salitol, recommended for acute and chronic dysentery, and diarrhea.

Maud Grieve suggests the plant is "superior to Eyebright for preserving the sight and curing sore eyes…even in blindness if the crystalline humour is not destroyed".

Its Gaelic name translates as Wound Herb, with use in Ireland restricted to astringency in diarrhea and dysentery.

The plant is a complexion restorative, helping soothe wrinkles and tighten skin; and has been used traditionally as a hair dye, for those wishing a blond tinge; and leaving the hair glossy and silky. The root sap provides a red dye.

It fell out of use for several centuries, and was re-discovered in the nineteenth century for its "electrical" effect on cholera and dysentery.

Today, in Switzerland and France, it is still used in a number of over the counter products; including syrup for infant diarrhea related to allergy during breastfeeding.

Traditionally, the plant was used for diarrhea, hemorrhoids, eczema, varicose veins and insufficiency. Recent research shows it effective against the amoeba that cause dysentery as well as typhus bacillus.

The blossoms are trimorphous, meaning there are three distinct forms of flowers, with differing lengths of stamen and styles. This helps ensure that self- fertilization is impossible. The plant requires 13 hours of daylight to begin flowering.

Recent studies have shown that ornamental cultivars, once believed sterile, do produce viable seed. It produces six different yellow and green pollens with two sets of stamens and three different length stigmas.

Honey, produced from Purple Loosestrife flowers, is a specialty product that has a distinctive squash-like flavor, but considered by some of marginal quality.

The tender young leaves are edible when gathered in spring, either raw or steamed. Mears and Hillman, in *Wild Foods*, write "our experience suggests that they should not be eaten raw later in the year, partly because they become bitter, and more importantly because, in many people, they induce curious (and somewhat disturbing) neurological effects." I should give it a try!

It is interesting to note, that after its introduction, the Iroquois began using Purple Loosestrife in decoctions for fever and sickness caused by the dead.

Purple Loosestrife helps bio-remediate Flumequine, an animal antibiotic used extensively in aquaculture. The drug has a half-life of 150 days and may be destructive to the environment. Migliore et al, *Chemosphere* 2000:40.

Diet supplementation with the ground leaves or Cunirel®, a commercial herb mixture containing the herb, showed favorable parameters on rabbit nutrition. No adverse effects were noted, but an increase in total white blood cells, total volatile fatty acids and acetic acid concentration, and decrease in ammonia levels were noted. Kovitvadhi A et al, *Animal* 2016 10(1): 10-18.

The plant concentrates lead up to 2000 mg/litre, suggesting a use in bioremediation.

Early work by Uveges et al, *Envir Poll* 2002:120 requires further study.

Two beetles, *Neogalerucella calmariensis* and *G. pusilla*, mentioned above, have been introduced into North America as bio-control agents. Although they cause severe leaf defoliation throughout the larval and adult leaf feeding, the plants do not stress enough to die; but it helps somewhat to prevent flower and seed formation.

Recent study suggests the plant is responding to the introduced herbivores by evolving higher resistance. Stastny M & Sargent RD, *J Evol Biol* 2017 30(5): 1042-52.

MEDICINAL

CONSTITUENTS-leaf and stem-contains various glycosides including vitexin, orientin, isovitexin, isoorientin, and salicarin, up to 10% C-glucosidic ellagitannins such as lythrines A-D, castalagin, vescalagin, pedunculagin and dimeric salicarinins A-C; galloylglucose derivatives; phenolics and triterpenes including ellagic, oleanolic, ursolic, cholorogenic, isochlorogenic, p-coumaric, ferulic, vanillic, gallic, syringic betulinic, ursolic and caffeic acid; daucosterol; essential oil, narcissin; isomeric luteolin C-glucosides including orientin, isoorientin, vitexin and isovitexin, pectin, vanoleic acid dilactone, loliolide, resin, mucilage; and a variety of C-glucosidic flavonoids including rutin, hyperoside, catechin, quercitin, myricetin, kaempferol, leucodelphinidin, luteolin, apigenin and leucocyanidin. Also contains various phthalides including di-isobutyl-, butyl-, isobutyl-di-butylphthalides, di-n-butyl phthalate; plant sterols; phytol, dodecanoic acid, oleanolic acid, corosolic acid, peucedanin, buntansin, erythrodiol; coumarins including umbelliferone-6-carboxylic acid, bunstansin and peucedanin. Alkaloids include lythranine, lythranidine, lythramine, lythracine I-VII, and lythrancepine I-III.

flowers- various anthocyanins including orientin, vitexin, flavone glucosides, and gallotannins; as well as two dominating dyes, malvidin 3,5-di-O-glucoside and cyanidine 3-O-glucoside.

Traditionally, the herb was used for hemorrhoids, dysentery, chronic intestinal catarrh, eczema, varicose veins, periodontosis and gingivitis.

Purple Loosestrife is today, used for its anti-bacterial effect; very valued in treating amebic dysentery. It can be a very effective douche for persistent vaginal irritation caused by *Trichomonas* amoebae.

The herb industry today still manufactures an anti-diarrhea product called extract of salicaria. In Europe, it is known as Red Sally, and is available as a 1:2 extract by several commercial companies.

A study by Spyropoulos et al, *J Physiol Pathol Gen* 1930(28): 69-71 began the investigation into glucose metabolism. Healthy children were given salicairine (two times 20 drops p.o.) before and after subcutaneous injection of phlorizin, and was shown to prevent induced glycosuria.

Work conducted at *US Dept of Agriculture* by Richard Anderson and James Duke found a wide variety of herbs and spices may help control diabetes.

They tested 24 and found nine medicinal plants that boosted insulin activity in test tube experiment. This follows early work by Cadavid and Calleja, *J Nat Prod* 1980 43:5.

Work on rabbits and rats found the plant may provoke the liberation of insulin, with later work finding ether extracts of the stems, the most effective hypoglycemic agent.

Reduced triglycerides and an 80% increase in free fatty acids were noted.

A follow-up study by Lamela, Cadavid et al, *J Ethnopharm* 1985 14 found the hypoglycemia effect peaked at 30 minutes after glucose loading, and that the extract significantly reduced the hyperglycemic effect of epinephrine.

Other studies have found elevated blood sugar levels partially reduced in alloxan diabetic rats, and in another animals receiving the extract "showed significant enzyme variations relative to diabetic controls."

Hops, birch, bearberry and dandelion all showed some effect on blood sugar. But Loosestrife showed an astounding 450% increase in insulin activity. It certainly fits into the philosophical mood of the author, in that plants that are needed for today's health issue are all around us. Diabetes is rampant; and so is Purple Loosestrife!

Lamela et al, *Journal of Ethnopharmacology* 1985 14:1 showed that extracts of the stems and flowers at a dose equivalent to 10 g/kg of crude plant material caused significant reduction in blood glucose four hours after administration. This effect was associated with an increase in circulating insulin.

Puri et al, *Journal of the Nepal Medical Association* 1997 36:123 found Purple Loosestrife used for lowering serum cholesterol, glucose and triglyceride levels, and exhibiting anti-atherosclerotic activity.

Its antioxidant activity is similar to vitamin E, probably due to phenolic compounds. The strongest anti-oxidant activity was observed from water extracts, while the strongest anti-inflammatory and anti-nociceptive activity was noted, *in vivo*, at 50% alcohol.

Isoorientin and isovitexin are believed most responsible.

The herb lowers blood glucose levels and inhibits *Helicobacter pylori* bacterium associated with gastric and duodenal ulcers. Manayi A et al, *DARU* 2013 21(1): 61.

Gryzbek et al, looked at the bioactivity of various Polish plants, and found water extracts of this herb displayed moderate inhibitory activity against the HIV-1 reverse transcriptase.

Purple Loosestrife shows indications of protecting liver cells from carbon tetrachloride poisoning. A Romanian study also conducted in 1985 cites therapeutic efficacy of plant extracts on liver damage.

Internally, it combines astringency and stimulation. This is a useful combination, similar to sweet gale, in that it is a diaphoretic stimulant, and a bitter, cold, drying astringent.

This is due to both the unique tannins, and the glycoside salcarin, which has special anti-microbial effect in the intestinal tract. This makes it of special value in the treatment of irritable bowel syndrome, combining well with Fleabane.

The ellagitannins may be a source of bioavailable gut microbiota metabolites such as urolithins, that reduce inflammation of mucosal tissue. Piwowarski JP et al, *J Ethnopharm* 2014 155(1): 801-9. Urolithins and ellagic acid inhibit colon cancer stem cells. Nunez-Sanchez MA et al, *Food Chem Toxicol* 2016 92:8-16.

The ellagitannins, particularly water extracts of the dimeric salicarinins demonstrate potent activity on stimulating neutrophils, causing changes in skin and mucosa tissue. Inhibition of hyaluronidase was noted in the study. Piwowarski JP & Kiss AK, *J Nat Med* 2015 69(1): 100-110.

Corosolic acid suppresses octanoylated ghrelin levels in human gastric carcinoma cells. Ghrelin is an appetite-stimulating peptide hormone, suggesting possible benefit in some cases of obesity.

Corosolic acid inhibits osteosarcoma by inducing apoptosis. Jia Y et al, *Oncol Lett* 2016 12(5): 4187-94.

It may combine well with actinomycin D in the treatment of liver cancer. Xu Y et al, *Cell Signal* 2017 29: 209-17.

It may also protect from diabetic nephropathy associated with diabetes, by inhibiting proliferation of glomerular mesangial cells and preventing renal damage. Li XQ et al, *Sci Rep* 2016 6:26854.

Corsolic acid is also found in the tropical herb banaba. It is reported to decrease blood sugar levels within one hour in humans. Both corsolic acid and ellagitannins are believed responsible for hypoglycemic and anti-hyperlipidemic effect.

Water extracts of the flowers have a moderate muscarinic receptor agonist effect on ileum tissue. The relaxing of smooth muscle involves prostanoids and purinoceptor mechanisms to some extent. Bencsik T et al, *Nat Prod Commun* 2013 8(9): 1247-50.

Laboratory tests reveal plant extracts exhibit activity against gram-negative bacteria. Work by Becker et al, in *Fitoterapia* found oleanolic and ursolic acid active against *Cladosporium cucumerinum*, and vescabagin active against *Micrococcus luteus*.

Extracts of the flowering spikes, seeds and leaves show activity against *Staphylococcus aureus*, *E. coli*, *Candida albicans* and *Pseudomonas aeruginosa*. Borchardt et al, *J Med Plants Res* 2008 2:5.

It contains enough mucilage that it prevents the drying out of tissue, particularly the mucous membranes, so that it reduces inflammation in those individuals with constitutional dryness.

Felter and Lloyd suggested the demulcent and astringent decoction for diarrhea, and dysentery over a century ago.

This unique combination is also useful for respiratory complaints including bronchitis and asthma. The herb influences smooth muscle reactivity of airways more favorably than salbutamol, a commercial bronchodilator. Antitussive effects were noted in work by Sutovska M et al, *Int J Biol Macromol* 2012 51(5): 794-9.

Early work by Vincent and Segonzac in 1954 found activity against both *Staphylococcus* and dysenteric *Bacillus*.

Water extracts inhibit hyaluronidase activity, in a manner stronger than heparin. It is also a strong inhibitor of elastase release from neutrophils. Piwowarski et al, *J Ethnopharmacology* 2011 137: 937-41.

Topical ointments appear beneficial for second-degree burn wounds. Vafi F et al, *Wounds* 2016 Sept 29. Activity against *S. aureus* and *C. albicans* was noted.

Growth against *E. coli, Pseudomonas aeruginosa, Shigella species, typhoid, paratyphoid bacteria, Bacillus cereus, Mycobacterium smegnatis, Proteus mirabilis* and *Micrococcus luteus* has been noted in various studies from 1949 to present day.

Activity against some Listeria, including *L. monocytogenes* and *L. innocua* has been noted, but not against all species.

Recent work found activity against 30 *Acinetobacter baumannii* and 27 *P. aeruginosa* multi-drug resistant pathogens. Guclu E et al, *Annu Res Rev Biol* 2014(4): 1099-1105.

As a stimulant, it reduces the symptoms associated sore throat, fever, flu and upper respiratory infections. This is especially true of the spring and fall colds and flu more present in those with internal stagnation and toxemia.

It makes a good substitute for eyebright, in the treatment of allergies and sinusitis, as well as sore eyes. In Europe, the herb is used for eye soreness and conjunctivitis. I don't think I'd recommend that, but in Europe, the cooled, well-filtered infusion in eyecups is used in the treatment of ophthalmic ulcers. Taken internally, the tea is used for blurred vision, and poor night vision.

David Winston suggests simply chewing on the stems for bleeding gums resulting from pyorrhea and gingivitis. He suggests trying the herb in cases of leaky gut syndrome and irritable bowel.

It combines very well with Marsh Cudweed (*Gnaphalium uliginosum*) as a gargle for sore throats; and with white pond lily root and Bur marigold (*B. tripartita*) for leucorrhea, hemorrhage of passive bleeding of the vagina or uterus.

At the same time, the plant has dual anti-platelet activity with erythrodiol inhibiting ADP induced platelet activation and oleanolic acid inhibited TRAP-induced platelet activation. Kontogianni VG et al, *J Agric Food Chem* 2016 64(22): 4511-21.

The plant is used to treat excessive vaginal discharge and vaginal itching. Cystitis with blood in the urine may also indicate using this herb.

This probably has more to do with its cleansing action on the kidneys, through stimulation, as well as regular bowel movement due to its gentle cholagogue effect on bile. The flowering tops are useful for relieving symptoms of venous insufficiency and hemorrhoids.

Some herbalists use it to arrest diarrhea in breastfeeding babies.

Externally, the plant extracts can be used in enemas, gargles, washes and prepared into salves from a sun infused oil.

A number of compounds, including daucosterol, corosolic acid, beta-sitosterol and erythrodiol are active against HT-29 colon carcinoma cells, with the latter compound 6.4 times more selective than methotrexate. Daucosterol is highly active against K-562 leukemia cell lines with selectivity 13.3 times that of methotrexate. Manayi A et al, *Z Naturforsch C* 2013 68(9-10): 367-75.

Various extracts show weak cytotoxicity against colon carcinoma HT-29, leukemia K562, and breast ductal carcinoma T47D cell lines. Khanavi M et al, *Res J Biol Sci* 2011(6): 55-7.

Oleanolic acid and erythrodiol restricted the development of features associated with multiple sclerosis, in an animal model. They switched cytokine production towards a Th2 regulatory profile with lower levels of Th1 and Th17 cytokines, and higher expression of Th2 in both serum and spinal cord. They also affected humoral response causing inhibition of auto-antibody production. Martin R et al, *Br J Pharmacol* 2012 166(5): 1708-23.

Erythrodiol and oleanolic acid are cytotoxic to human breast cancer cells (MCF-7). The former inhibits growth through apoptosis, and the latter through cell cycle arrest. Allouche Y et al, *J Agric Food Chem* 2011 59(11): 121-30.

Peucedanin was used at one time for *alopecia areata* and *alopecia totalis*. Zheltakov MM et al, *Sov Med* 1965 28(8): 126-9.

Muscle tone and weakness of ligaments, tendons and joints, will benefit from Loosestrife.

Work by Ranha, *International Journal of Food Microbiology* 2000 56:1 found Purple Loosestrife the most active, of forty some plant extracts tested against *Candida albicans*.

Coban et al, *Pharm Biol* 2003 41:8 showed the plant to possess anti-oxidant activity, but activity lower than *Plantago major* or *Juglans regia*.

The seed, however, is a very powerful anti-oxidant with a TE/100 grams of 261,384. This compares with blueberries at 3300 TE/100 grams. Borchardt et al, 2008 above.

Tunalier et al, *J Ethnopharm* 2007 110: 539-47 found anti-oxidant, anti-inflammatory and pain-relieving properties in the herb.

Iso-orientin has been found to relieve the last two conditions. Kupeli et al, *Z Naturforsch* 59. It shares some properties with Creeping Jenny, a close relative.

The closely related *L. anceps* contains Oenothein B, a macrocyclic tannin that reduces prostate inflammation, and is of possible value in prostatic adenoma.

An excellent review of the herb is written by Piwowarski JP et al, *Journal of Ethnopharmacology* 2015 170:226-250.

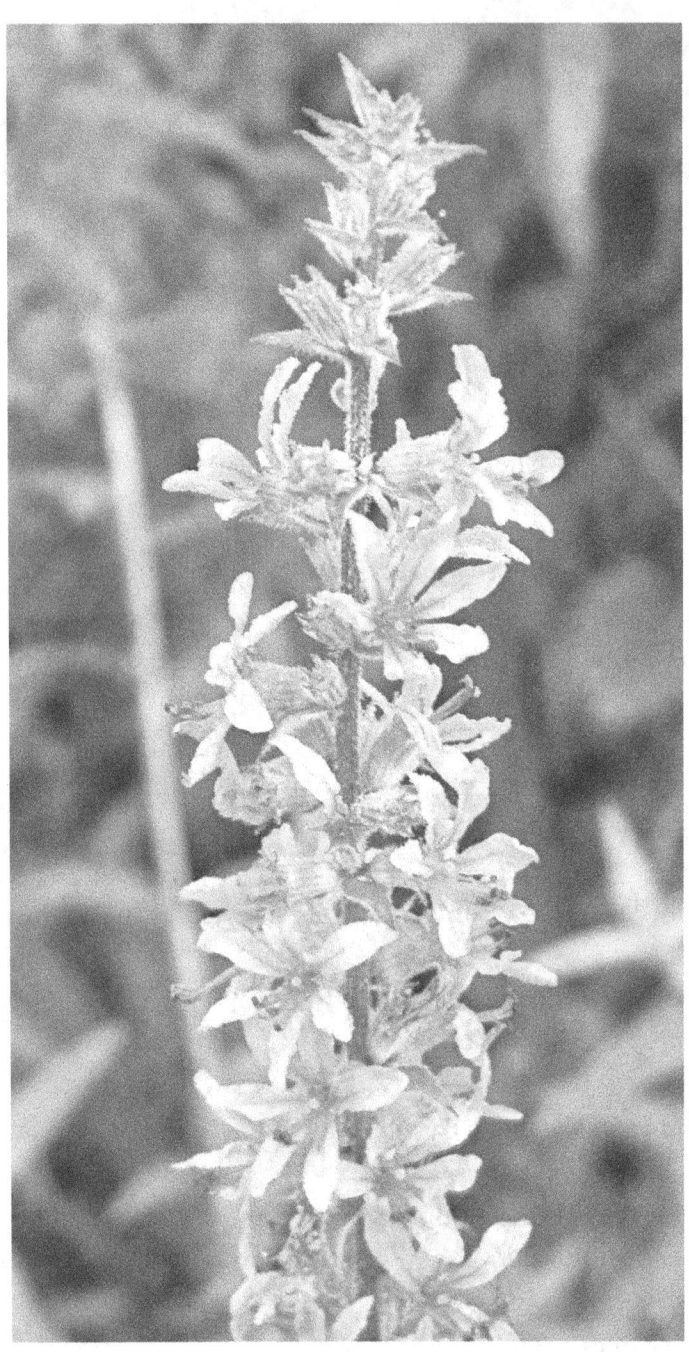

PURPLE LOOSESTRIFE

ESSENTIAL OIL

The flowering aerial parts were steam distilled and 43 constituents were found in the essential oil. Manayi et al, *Res J Pharmacogn* 2014 (1): 33-38.

HYDROSOL

Distilled waters were applied to bruised or sore eyes, as well as gargled for sore throats.

Culpepper wrote, "the distilled waster is a present remedy for hurts and blows on the eyes, and for blindness... it also cleareth the eyes of dust or any other thing gotten into them, and preserveth the sight".

FLOWER ESSENCES

Purple Loosestrife is a superior essence for New Agers. It is an enhancer for individuals who want to bring the three lower chakras into proper alignment so that they can apply spiritually inspired information, which is often received through the crown chakra.

The heart chakra is frequently open with these people because they generally have a giving nature. And usually this essence works best with people whose crown chakra is already active, so they can receive higher inspiration.

When mercury is in transition from retrograde to direct and back again, or Mercury is stationary, consider using this essence.

GURUDAS

Purple Loosestrife (*L. salicaria*) flower essence is for helping release strife. It helps one keep events in perspective. It is also for knowing that as opportunities close, new ones open.

RUNNING FOX

Purple Loosestrife essence promotes a centered, peaceful, non-attached state of being. It reduces ego consciousness and helps one to be a clear channel through which spiritual energies may flow at all times.

LIGHT MOUNTAIN

Purple Loosestrife essence helps one see change as opportunity.

MIRIANA

SPIRITUAL PROPERTIES

Loosestrife is associated with the spiritual lessons of water. Water has the ability to cut through stone, but also is able to fill a container. There are individuals who struggle with such lessons. People are often required to be flexible but also to have great power. This often occurs in management type positions.

Greater understanding is imparted concerning the ability to be fully flexible yet remain strong and focused as to what one can and cannot do. One learns to trust the way they work and, at the appropriate time, to share with others in a way that blends personal experiences with that which one has newly learned.

In healing, the energy of pure softness develops. This is very important for many healers who are working with people who have hard muscles, a rigid disposition, or who are struggling with concepts that are binding or chafing.

In Lemuria, the plant was understood for its ability to transform water. It actually raised its frequency so that individuals near the plant understood the water more directly- where it had been and the things it had worked with. As a result, a deep cleansing of the aura took place.

Through attuning to Loosestrife, aspects of water can be transferred to humanity. Today, a massage application can be made with Loosestrife for athletes, especially runners, to ease tired muscles.

The chakras in the knees, calves, thighs and the first three chakras are energized. The kidney meridian is less stressed; the radiation miasm is eased. There is a clear connection with the sign of Cancer.

There can be benefit when there is difficulty from plants being watered too much. Root and stem rot can result. A tincture at the rate of two drops to ten gallons of water may be sufficient to impart the vibration into the water.

GURUDAS

The over-lighting spirit of the Purple Loosestrife flower tells you to find another perspective, maybe a more detached approach, moving away from the minutiae and out into the bigger picture. It takes you on a journey and asks you to see yourself moving through a dark tunnel or corridor with no light and a feeling of claustrophobia.

ECLARE

RECIPES

DECOCTION- One tbsp of dried leaves or root to one pint of water. Slow simmer for twenty minutes. For diarrhea use a decoction of the aerial parts rather than infusion.

The decoction can also be cooled for douche, or external washes for eczema, skin sores, or ulcers, as it is quite mucilaginous.

INFUSION- hot infusions are more astringent, while cold infusion are more demulcent (slimy).

TINCTURE- 20-30 drops as needed. Make it from the dried flowering tops at 1:5 and 30% alcohol, or 1:2 fresh, aerial plant at 50% alcohol.

Flavonoid content is highest during main blooming in August. Polyphenol and tannin content is higher in flowering branch tips in August, and higher in leaves and shoots in July. Leaves contain highest flavonoid content, flowering branches highest polyphenols and tannins. I pick it when I have the opportunity, usually in flower.

CAUTION- Work by Latinen et al, *Pharm Res* 2004 21:10 found extracts decreased in-vitro absorption of Verpamil (calcium channel blocker), Metroprolol (beta blocker), due to tannins and phenolic acids. The same extract increased absorption of Ketoprofen (NSAID), Furosemide (loop diuretic), and Paracetamol (acetaminophen).

Do not use for extended periods of time due to high levels of tannins and calcium oxalate.

Studies on anti-coagulant or pro-coagulant activity are mixed and confusing.

WILD PURSLANE
(***Portulaca oleracea*** L.)
(***P. neglecta***) not accepted
(***P. retusa***) not accepted
GARDEN PURSLANE
(***P. oleracea*** L. **var.** *sativa*)
PARTS USED- root, seeds, leaves

The worts, the purslane and the mess of watercress.   **HERRICK**

"I have made a satisfactory dinner...simply off a dish of purslane... boiled and salted."   **HENRY THOREAU**

Portulaca is the diminutive from the Latin **PORTULA** or little gate. Linnaeus noted the lid of the seed capsule opened like a gate.

It may derive from the Latin **PORCILACA** which means, both "fleshy herb" and "cowrie shell". From the Old French **PORCELAINE** to the Old English **PURCELAN** to **PURSLANE** is another root of its common name. Porcelain, the white clay pottery, is derived from its appearance like the shiny white surface of the cowrie shell.

Portulaca may also derive from the Latin **PORTO** meaning, "to carry"; and **LAC** meaning milk; in reference to the milky sap of the injured tissue. Doubtful.

Purslane means "herb of the womb", and may derive from **PORCELLA** a sow, or vulva. Oleracea refers to its use as a garden vegetable from the Latin **OLUS** meaning vegetable.

Purslane was once thought an introduced and naturalized plant, until 1974, when archeologists discovered *portulaca* seeds in the Salt Caves in Kentucky, dated back to the first millenium BC. This means it is indigenous or was introduced in very early times.

The Iroquois made use of the nutritious plant. The Onondaga called the plant **NONIAGAI'I'I' UHIAGWI'IA'** meaning "partridge toes", and the neighboring Cayuga **DAKSAI'DASUSI"DA'**, "chicken feet".

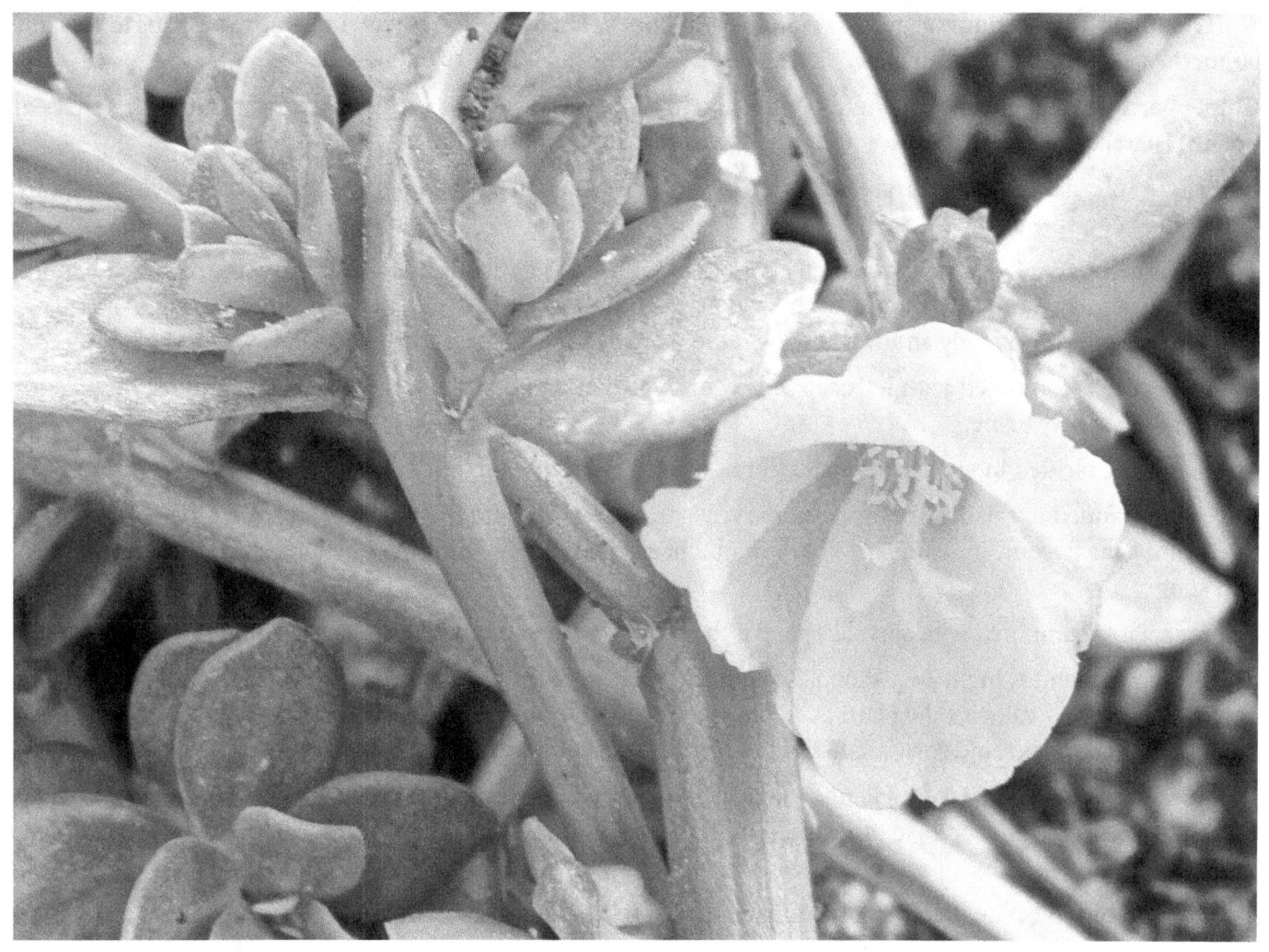

PURSLANE IN FLOWER

Purslane is an annual in our extreme climate often found near pineapple weed or plantain, where humans have trod, but especially liking the fertile soil of our garden beds. It tolerates both dry and salty soil, or areas that have been long irrigated. It increases the water holding capacity of soil and counteracts erosion and dehydration.

Garden Purslane has been developed from the wild, and has thicker stems and more succulent leaves. Otherwise, it is identical. On a trip to Santa Cruz in the summer of 2008, I was delighted to see organic purslane offered at the local market.

It makes an excellent living mulch, which reduce the need for herbicides, and tillage, increases soil surface humidity and conserves soil moisture. In studies conducted by Dr. Ellis et al, at the Storrs Agricultural Research Station at the U of Connecticut, purslane as a living mulch for broccoli, proved more economical than mechanical weeding, chemical control, or black plastic mulch. It is ranked the 8th most common plant in the world.

The Arabs, in the Middle Ages, called the plant **BAQLA HAMQA'**, which means a mad or crazy vegetable because of the way it spreads with no control. Today, in the Middle East, the plant is added to sauces and salads, especially **FATTOUSH**.

Dioscorides wrote Portulaca, "doth assuage the stupidity of the teeth, and the burning of the stomach and entrails, and the flux, and doth help the eroded kidneys and the bladder, and doth dissolve the hot desire to conjunctions."

The Old English Herbarium suggested wild purslane "for excessive flow of semen", a reference perhaps to extreme gonorrhea, or seminal incontinence.

Culpepper suggested juice of the herb be mixed with honey and sugar, to relieve dry coughs and shortness of breath. He recommended the juice be applied with rose oil to ruptured navels in infants.

In Europe, all parts are used for greens, as a potherb like asparagus. It has a mild, nutty flavour, with a texture like mung bean sprouts.

The seeds can be cooked for a type of mush or bread; or used as a substitute for poppy seeds. For this purpose, gather the plants before they mature and dry on a baking sheet for a week or so. The seed capsules ripen, and can be obtained by crushing and winnowing. One plant can produce up to 50,000 seeds.

Purslane seeds, combined with lettuce seeds, were powdered and combined with sugar in older herbals for burning and scanty urine.

The stems are pickled in vinegar, or stale beer as a condiment in Holland.

I like it best added to salads with fig-balsamic vinegar; or steamed and then used in stir fries where it imparts a sweet and sour flavour. It is similar to okra in mucilaginous content and this can be used for thickening stews and soups.

In France, it is combined with sorrel as part of the soup *Bonne Femme* or various pea soups.

The protein content is high, averaging 27-44% of dry matter in the mature growth stage. The root, predictably, declines in protein value as the plant ages, but the iron content increases. Manganese in soluble organic form is highest in the leaves and roots. Ashes of the plant make a good salt substitute.

In Greece, the plant is fed to chickens to increase the levels of omega 3 fatty acids in eggs. One study of free-range chicken eggs with access to purslane, found one yolk contained 300 mg of omega 3, the same as a standard fish oil capsule.

The content of GLA may find purslane utilized in cosmetic skin products.

The seeds can survive up to forty years awaiting their chance to sprout.

Ingested, they may encourage delayed menstruation, and were used traditionally as a vermifuge after crushing and heating in oil.

Purslane has a magical history of guarding against evil spirits, strewn around a person's bed to dispel nightmares.

In China, the leaves are used medicinally for dysentery, diarrhea, hemorrhoids, and internal bleeding, and the seeds to provoke menstruation. Its earliest recorded use in China dates to 500 AD in *Ben Cao Jing Ji Zhu*, and was called **MA CHI XIAN**, meaning Horse Tooth Amaranth. It is also known as **FEI-CHU NAN**, meaning Hog Fattening Cedar; Nine Headed Lion Grass, Five Lines Grass, Mouse's Ear and Live Forever Plant.

Another interesting name is **WU FANG CAO**, or Five Directions Herb, due to the plant colours and correspondence to compass points. The leaves are green for east, stems red for south, roots white for west, seeds black for north, and flowers yellow for centre. It is known as the Five Phases Vegetable, or Vegetable for Long Life.

An older text cites, "its leaves are unusually thick, as is its stalk; on the hottest day it does not easily dry up. It is readily seen that its nature is pure yin cold, and thus it excels at resolving swollen sores and heat toxin; it can also be applied externally…the leaves of this plant, likewise are green on the face but purplish red on the back, and its stalk is also purple, thus it enters the blood level and breaks up stasis and stagnant blood disorders."

Another name, *Vegetable Mercury*, stems from *The Illustrated Pharmacopoeia*, by Su Sung, who claimed to have acquired 8-10 ounces of mercury from 10 catties' weight of dried purslane. If purslane has the ability to absorb mercury, it may be of use in bioremediation of contaminated soil.

In the West Indies, purslane seed is often combined with other herbs for de-worming children. Confirmed bioactive compounds for treating intestinal worms are based on ethno-physiology studies in Dominica. Quinlan et al, *J Ethnopharmacology* 2002 80:1.

The seeds are taken orally to bring on menstruation.

In Brazil, the herb, known as **BELDROEGA** is applied as a fresh poultice to wounds building up keloid scar tissue.

In Indonesia, the whole plant is used for cardiac weakness, and the seeds for breathing difficulties.

In the Canary Islands, a favorite vacation spot of mine, a hot water extract of the dried leaves is used as a diuretic, dissolve sand and gravel, and treat migraines.

In West Africa, purslane leaves are used for muscle spasticity resulting from spinal injury. The fresh juice and water extracts relieve earache, toothache, swelling, boils and topical abscesses; and is taken internally as a fresh juice for asthma.

Infusions of the plants are used as an anthelminthic for children, to expel roundworms. It is a cooling drink with mild diuretic effect.

The Mawali name translates as "buttocks of the wife of the chief" in reference to the plant's succulent, round leaves and juicy stem.

The plant is a children's good luck charm in West Africa, and a symbol of goodwill.

The Mayan of Central America revere it as a food to protect, build and strengthen bones, and is known as **VERDALAGA**, or **XUCUL**.

Several North American natives used the fresh juice for earaches in an identical manner, applied to skin wounds and burns.

In 1885, C.P. Traill wrote a book on the plant life of Canada, and suggested purslane be applied to inflammatory tumours, and used as a source of blue dye.

Purslane is rich in Vitamins A, C and E, and the fresh blended plant makes a great facial mask for preventing wrinkles and restoring the skin. Simply apply and wash off 15 minutes later.

Water extracts are anti-aging, and prevent cancer due to primary targeting of p21 and p53 pathways. Hao et al, *Phytother Res* 2009 April 15.

Ancient Iranian medical texts suggest the herb for broncho-dilating effect in asthma and related conditions. It combines well with mullein leaf.

A Chinese patent for purslane was granted in 1990 as anti-fungal composition for plants and animals. It is prepared by stirring purslane extract (39-70%) with urea (29-60%) at 40 degrees Celsius. The preparations are non-toxic and do not cause environmental pollution. The ash of burnt plant has been used as a salt substitute in various countries.

And of course, the fresh juice is poured on anthills, as an insecticide.

It is used for diarrhea and immune enhancement when added to animal feed. It has been used for treating hookworm and amoebic dysentery.

Chickens fed extracts showed lowered levels of *E. coli* from ceca. Zhao XH et al, *Poult Sci* 2013 92(5): 1343-7. When fed to laying hens, it increased omega-3 fatty acid content of yolk. Aydin R et al, *J Sci Food Agric* 2010 90(10): 1759-63.

For those wishing to grow purslane commercially, studies have shown seed stored at room temperature for five months, germinated significantly faster and with a higher percentage than freshly harvested seed.

MEDICINAL

CONSTITUENTS- alicyclic hydrocarbons, portulosides A-B, alpha-linolenic acid, oxalic acid, isoprenoids, l-noradrenaline, noradrenalin (0.25% fresh), dopamine (0.20%), L-dopa, melatonin, alanine, sylvite, aspartic, ferulic, glutamic, citric and malic acid, oleracin I and II, olercein E and various phenolics such as scopoletin, bergapten, isopimpinellin, lonchocarpic acid, robustin. Triterpenes include beta amyrin, lupeol, stigmast-4-en-3-one, butyrospermol, parkeol, 24-methylene-24-dihydroparkeol, cyclo-artenol, beta sitosterol, stigmasterol and campesterol; flavonoids (11.8mg/g) including quercitin, kaempferol, myricetin, agpigenin genistein, genistin and luteolin; and nicotinic acid. Aurantiamide and aurantiamide acetate are also present, as well as portulacanones B-D. Only kaempferol and apigenin are present in ethanol extracts of leaf and stems.

Monoterpenes include portulosides A and B, diterpenes like portulene and beta amyrin type triterpenoids.

Also contains alkaloids such as cyclo-dopa, di-ketopiperacine, (3R)-3,5-bis(3-methoxy-4-hydroxyphenyl0-2,3-dihydro-2(1H)-pyridinone; oleracone, 1,5-dimethyl-6-phenyl-1,2-dihydro-1,2,4-triazin-3(2H)-one; (7'R)-N-feruloyl normetanephrine, N-trans-feruloyl tyramine; oleraciamide A-B, thymine, uracil, trollisine, aurantimide and scopoletin.

The plant contains abundant minerals, including lithium, phosphorus, calcium, magnesium, iron (4419 ppm), potassium salts (7.5%), manganese, boron (29 ppm), tin, molybdenum zinc (265 ppm) and copper. The plant hyperaccumulates selenium. Protein is 18.6% and 13.8% soluble.

The stems and leaves contain one of the richest green plant sources of omega 3 -alpha linolenic fatty acids (300-400 mg/100g). It is very rich in vitamin C (700 mg per 100 grams of fresh plant), vitamin A (1.9 mg) and E (alpha-tocopherol)- 0.3-0.4% (12.2mg/100 grams) of fresh leaf; as well as B complex vitamins such as niacin, pyridoxine and riboflavin.

In a study comparing spinach and purslane, the latter contained 10 times higher amounts of alpha linolenic acid, ascorbic acid, alpha tocopherol (7 times more vitamin E), and glutathione (14.8 mg/100 grams) an anti-oxidant. In fact, it contains the highest amounts of all three important anti-oxidant vitamins of any plant material. Sea Buckthorn fruit is a close second.

The short chain fatty acids (C4-C6) isobutyric, butyric, isovaleric, valeric, and caproic acids are also present.

flower buds- betalmic acid

The herb is cold in nature and sour in taste, and was used traditionally to cool the blood, staunch bleeding, clear heat and resolve toxins.

The dried aerial parts have been used for fever, dysentery, diarrhea, carbuncles, eczema

Work on experimental diabetic rats suggests that purslane possesses only moderate anti-diabetic activity, but does possess potent antioxidant potential in diabetic conditions. Sharma et al, *J Compl Integr Med* 2009 6:1.

Portusana, an extract manufactured by Frutarom, normalizes blood glucose in three ways. Modulation of cell sensitivity to insulin, increased glucose uptake from the blood stream into cells, and reduced glucose absorption from intestines into blood stream.

The herb increases beta cell growth and improves glucose metabolism. Ramadan BK et al, *BMC Complement Altern Med* 2017 17(1): 37. Increases in C peptide and insulin were significant over control group.

A study on type two diabetic women taking purslane seeds (2.5grams twice daily) and aerobic exercise for sixteen weeks found significant improvement in all parameters, including atherosclerosis plaque biomarkers. Dehghan F et al, *Sci Rep* 2016 6: 37819.

A double-blind, placebo-controlled clinical trial of 63 type two diabetic patients involved three capsules of purslane powder daily or placebo for 3 months. Both HbA1c and systolic blood pressure was significantly reduced in purslane group. Wainstein J et al, *J Med Food* 2016 19(2): 133-40.

Induction of GLUT4 translocation in the absence of insulin helps decrease blood glucose in diabetics. Purslane does this, via the P13K pathway. Stadlbauer V et al, *PLoS One* 2016 11(1).

Water extracts prevent diabetic vascular inflammation, hyperglycemia and diabetic endothelial dysfunction in diabetic mice. Lee AS et al, *Evid Based Complement and Altern Medicine* 2012 Article ID 741824, nine pages.

The herb increases insulin sensitivity, and ameliorates impaired glucose tolerance and lipid metabolism in diabetic rat study. Shen L & FE Lee, *Chin Journal of Integrative Medicine* 2003 9(4): 289-92.

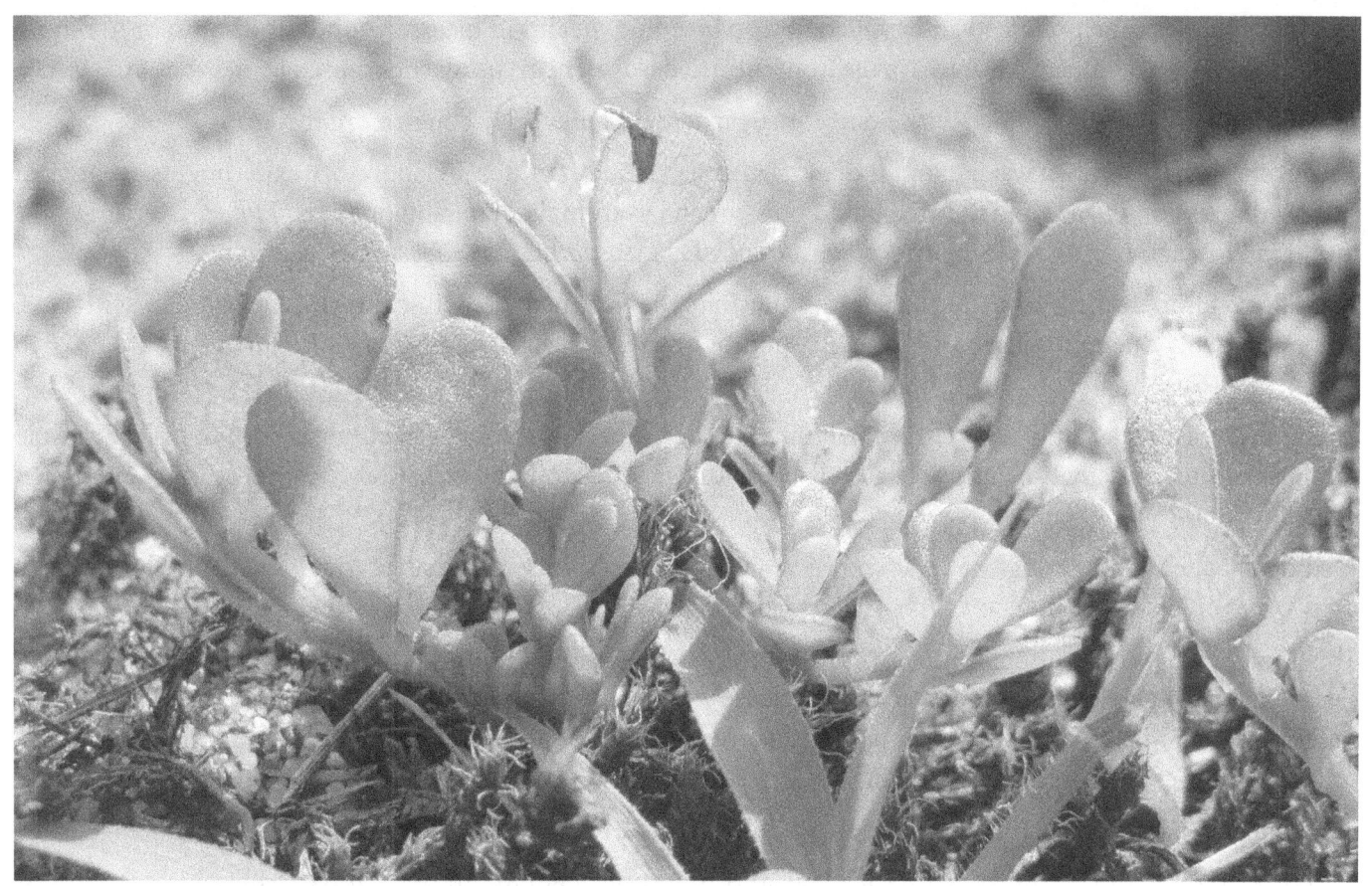

YOUNG PURSLANE LEAVES

Both fresh and dried herb possess anti-diabetic activity, but the fresh herb is stronger. Gu JF et al, *J Ethnopharm* 2015 161: 214-23.

Crude polysaccharide extracts lower blood glucose and modulate the metabolism of lipids and glucose in induced diabetic mice. Gong F et al, *Int J Mol Sci* 2009 10(3): 880-888.

It helps ameliorate diabetic nephropathy through suppression of renal fibrosis and inflammation. Lee AS et al, *Am J Chin Med* 2012 40(3): 495-510.

The seeds were studied in a diabetic study of thirty subjects. Five grams of seeds were taken by one group of fifteen, while the others received 1500 mg of metformin. Results were similar in both, suggesting an adjunctive or alternative therapy. El-Sayed M. I. K. et al, *J Ethnopharm* 2011 137(1): 643-51.

A triple-blinded, randomized, placebo-controlled study on obese adolescents, given 500 mg capsules twice daily for one month, showed improved lipid levels. Sabzghabaee AM et al, *Med Arch* 2014 68(3): 195-9.

Water extracts inhibit vascular inflammation such as atherosclerosis probably due to suppression of tumor necrosis factor alpha. Lee AS et al, *Int J Mol Sci* 2012 13(5): 5628-44.

A water extract showed significant anti-anxiety effects, improved spatial cognitive improvement, and reduction of stress in diabetic, ovariectomized rats. Fatemi SR et al, *Iran J Pharm Res* 2016 15(2): 561-71.

The leaves and stems are cool, moistening and nourishing as they cleanse the blood and act as a mild diuretic with emollient and soothing effect on the bladder and urinary tract. For severe pain in the urethra with a strong desire to pass water, take 2-3 teaspoons of the fresh juice.

The fresh plant can be poulticed and applied to stop bleeding, heal skin ulcers, wounds and sores; or to relieve headaches caused by sunstroke. A tea, made from the dried leaves, helps headaches caused by nervous excitability.

The fresh juice can be combined with honey or sugar to help relieve dry cough, sore throat.

Recent studies have shown water extracts of purslane relax smooth muscle in laboratory experiments. It induced cardiac depression *in vitro* and reduced blood pressure in lab animals. Hanuantappa et al, *J Pharm Res* 2011 4:10 found *in vitro* activity against *Staphylococcus aureus, Bacillus subtilis* and *Klebsiella pneumoniae.*

Two fatty acids in the herb combine with erythromycin in the treatment of methicillin-resistant *S. aureus* (MRSA). This is probably due to inhibition of the efflux pumps of the bacteria. Chan BC et al, *J Pharm Pharmacol* 2015 67(1): 107-16.

The leaf juice is weakly anti-tuberculin and stimulates beta-adrenoceptors of tracheal smooth muscle. Purslane exhibits anti-tussive activity comparable to codeine, at least in guinea pig research. Boroushaki et al, *Iran J Pharm Res* 2004 3:3.

A study of 54 whooping cough patients showed a satisfactory response to purslane cough syrup given four times daily over three days. Shanghai *J Chin Med & Herb* 1959 3:40.

This may be due to the inhibition of trans-membrane calcium influx; interference with the calcium-induced release process; and/or the inhibition of the release of intracellular calcium from stores in the sarcoplasmic reticulum. Nobody really knows at this point. However, purslane contains calcium and magnesium in a 1:1 ratio, best suited for cardiovascular protection.

It also may be useful in treatment of osteoclast bone disease. Kim JY et al, *Biol Pharm Bull* 2015 38(1): 66-74.

Tinctures reduce initial transvascular leakage and pulmonary edema under hypbaric hypoxia conditions. Yue T et al, *High Alt Med Biol* 2015 16(1): 43-51.

Studies from Glasgow, Scotland in 1993 confirm that the neuromuscular activity of purslane is due to the high potassium content. Foods containing potassium and magnesium show anti-depressant activity. It is rich in folic acid and lithium. James Duke, in his book *The Green Pharmacy*, notes purslane "contains up to a whopping 16% anti-depressant compounds, figured on a dry-weight basis."

Other studies found purslane extracts inhibit twitch and tetanus tension induced in animal muscle.

The plant exhibits anti-fatigue benefit, increased fat utilization and delayed accumulation of lactic acid and ammonia. Lu et al, *J Med Plants Res* 2009 3:7.

The same year, a study by Wang et al, *Phytomed* Oct 30 found betacyanins ameliorate cognition deficits induced in mice, suggesting brain protection.

An animal study found phenolic extracts enhanced cognitive function in senile mice, in a manner similar to piracetam. Wang P et al, *J Ethnopharmacology* 2017 203:252-9.

Purslane tinctures improve memory deficits in lipopolysaccharide treated rats, possibly via inhibition of TNFalpha and anti-inflammatory activity. Noorbakhshnia M et al, *Physiol Behav* 2017 169: 69-73.

Oleracein E, a tetrahydroisoquinolone with anti-oxidant activity, was studied for neuro-protection. Protection of dopaminergic neurons against rotenone toxicity, and protection on Parkinson's disease models were similar to selegiline hydrochloride. Sun H et al, *ACS Chem Neurosci* 2017 8(1): 155-164.

Dopamine and norephinephrine in purslane may be useful to inhibit acetylcholinesterase associated with Alzheimer's disease (AD). Chen YX et al, *Mol Med Rep* 2016 14(1): 446-52.

Various alkaloids inhibit acetylcholinesterase activity, suggesting benefit in AD. Yang Z et al, *Medicinal Chemistry Research* 2012 21(6): 734-8.

The herb may be useful as a neuroprotectant in Parkinson's disease. Moneim AE Abdel. *CNS & Neurological Disorders—Drug Targets* 2013 12(6): 830-841.

Animal studies suggest tinctures may protect against methyl mercury-induced neurotoxicity. Sumathi T & Christinal J, *Biol Trace Elem Res* 2016 172(1): 155-65.

A plant tincture also promotes ThI/Th2 and Treg/Th2 balance in lymphocytes suggested the benefit of purslane in inflammatory disease with decreased balance, such as asthma and cancers. Askari VR et al, *J Ethnopharmacology* 2016 194: 1112-21.

Human studies into the muscle relaxant action of purslane fomentations confirmed the plants effectiveness in 1988 studies by Dr. Parry et al, conducted in Nigeria. The plants ability to paralyze skeletal muscles is similar to dantrolene.

Purslane water extracts exhibit muscle relaxation, including external application to human subjects. Okwvasaba et al, *J Ethnopharm* 17:2 139-160 and 21:1 99-106.

Several years ago, a biochemist with multiple sclerosis wrote a letter to the *Lancet*, saying that magnesium supplementation helped him more than any other vitamin or mineral supplement. Purslane is nearly 2% magnesium on dry weight basis, giving 50 milligrams per fresh ounce of plant.

Both alcohol and water extracts appear useful for gastrointestinal conditions. Karimi G et al, *Phytotherapy Research* 2004 18(6): 484-7.

Purslane is an effective anti-fungal, antibiotic and anti-parasitic plant, combining well with pineapple weed for de-worming children, and with uva ursi or pipsissewa for bladder complaints.

Hookworm infestation in 41 patients treated with herb decoctions showed an 88% rate of complete recovery. The herb decoction was filtered and white vinegar and white sugar added, with one dose before bedtime. *New J Med Herb* 1973 8:30.

It is active against *Trichophyton rubrum*, associated with athlete's foot. For foot or nail fungus, combine with scarlet gilia, western mugwort and Oregon grape root in tincture form. Oh-Ki Bong et al, *Phytotherapy Research* 2000.

The herb is highly effective for *Shigella, Salmonella,* and *Staphylococcus* infections, but most potent, in the form of a tincture.

In Traditional Chinese Medicine the plant is know as *Ma Chi Xian* in Mandarin and *Ma Ji Yin* in Cantonese. It is considered very useful for damp heat and fire toxin conditions like dysentery with pus and blood in the stool, as well as all manner of skin, mouth, throat and gum inflammations.

Lichen planus, of the mouth, improved in 83% of 37 biopsied patients, far superior to control group. Agha-Hosseini et al, *Phytother Res* 2010 24:2. Korean research by Park et al in 1986, showed lipid fractions of purslane exhibited anti-fungal activity, and inhibited not only mycelial growth but fungal spore germination, as well.

It appears to be a novel adjunct therapy for treatment of plaque psoriasis, combining well with calcipotriol, and decreasing adverse effects, in a small study of eleven patients. Zhao H et al, *Exp Ther Med* 2015 9(2): 303-310.

In one study by Chinese researchers, purslane was found to be 90% effective in acute cases and 60% effective in recurrent cases of bacillary dysentery. A recent study identified four compounds with activity against enteropathogenic bacteria. Lei X et al, *Molecules* 2015 20(9): 6372-87.

A 70% tincture shows anti-bacterial activity against the usual suspect as well as Neisseria gonorrhea. Elkhayat ES et al, *J Asian Nat Prod Res* 2008 10(11-12): 1039-43.

Purslane is used for uro-genital infections with discharge and combined with dandelion root extract for treating appendicitis when the picture profile fits. The same combination may be used in puerperal fevers.

For urethritis, simmer ten parts purslane and one part licorice root over low heat. For swollen and itching hemorrhoids combine with *Oxalis* in equal parts, and wash affected area.

The fresh juice can be applied to shingles or herpes zoster, to both resolve and reduce the nerve pain.

Work by Dong et al, *Chem Pharm Bull* 2010 58:4 isolated a pectic polysaccharide with anti-herpes virus simplex 2 activity, suggesting fresh poultices or fomentation washes for genital herpes.

Alcohol extracts inhibit hepatitis C virus NS3 serine protease by 70%, suggesting benefit in the treatment, alone, or with interferon, of chronic HCV. Noreen S et al, *Viral Immunol* 2015 28(5): 282-9. It also appears to attenuate acetaminophen-induced liver injury. Liu XF et al, *Am J Transl Res* 2015 7(2): 309-18.

Portulacerebroside A suppresses the invasion and metastasis of human liver cancer cells (HCCLM3), by modulation of mRNA and protein expression. Ji Q et al, *Pharm Biol* 2015 53(5): 773-80.

Purslane and parsley seed extracts are cytotoxic to human liver (HepG2) cancer cells. Farshori NN et al, *Asian Pac J Cancer Prev* 2014 15(16): 6633-8.

One study found the plant polysaccharides modulate immune function in rats with ovarian cancer. Chen YG et al, *Int J Biol Macromolecules* 2009 45(5): 448-52.

The sulfation of water-soluble polysaccharides increases suppressive effect on HeLa and HepG2 cancer cell lines. Chen T et al, *Glucoconjugate Journal* 2010 27(6): 635-42.

Portulacerebroside A stimulates human liver cancer cells to commit apoptosis. Zheng GY et al, *Phytochemistry Letters* 2014 7(1): 77-84.

Various homoisoflavonoids from the herb show activity against SGC-7901 cancer cells lines as effectively as mitomycin C. Yan J et al, *Phytochemistry* 2012 80: 37-41.

One clinical trial found purslane juice effective in treating hookworms while other studies indicate use in bacillary dysentery. Taken orally, purslane juice has mild soothing activity on uterine contractions.

Two case studies in the *Australian Journal of Medical Herbalism* in 1996, examined purslane's healing qualities. In one case, fresh purslane juice successfully treated a 52 year-old woman with cystitis; and in another, a 43 year-old man used purslane for relief of gastric ulcers.

Purslane and dandelion leaf juice are used in China for intestinal abscess.

Dioscorides and other have mentioned its anaphrodisiac properties. Purslane, along with chicory, endive, and lettuce, were considered the "four cold seeds", in the 1837 *Codex of the Spanish Pharmacopoeia*. This anaphrodisiac effect is due perhaps to the presence of norepinephrine, a precursor of adrenalin, which causes a reduction in the blood flow through constriction of the main arteries. The content of l-noradrenaline in the fresh plant (2.5 mg/g) is likely to be greater than that extracted from suprarenal glands of mammals.

Noradrenaline is a hormone with vasopressor and anti-hypotensive effect that reduces hemorrhage and bleeding at the tissue level. Purslane was often used traditionally to stop postpartum bleeding; science has now confirmed it.

An ethanol extract of the seeds have a uterine stimulant and anti-spermatogenic effect in animal studies. Human application is unknown.

The roasted seed is used in Unani medicine for diuretic and anti-dysenteric properties.

A study in Iran on ten pre-menopausal women, with abnormal menstrual bleeding, and candidates for hysterectomy, was conducted by Shobeiri et al, *Phytother Res* Mar 9 2009.

Five grams of purslane seed powder was taken every four hours for two days after the onset of menses. Eight of ten women reported reduction of bleeding and volume reduced and significant improvement three months later.

Choi-ByungDon et al, *Korean Journal of Pharmacology* 2000 31:1 found purslane, *in vivo*, possesses potential anti-tumour activity.

Water extracts show inhibition or suppression of gastric tumor cell growth both *in vitro* and *in vivo*.

It shows activity against human gastric carcinoma and colon adenoma cell lines. The plant shows cytotoxicity against breast cancer cells and inhibition of xanthine oxidase associated with gout. Nile SH et al, *3 Biotech* 2017 7(1): 76.

A polysaccharide down regulates TLR4 downstream signaling pathway and induces cell apoptosis in HeLa cancer cells. Zhao R et al, *Nutr Cancer* 2017 69(1): 131-139.

Anti-oxidant and gastric anti-cancer activity of purslane polysaccharides was noted by Li Y et al, *Int J Biol Macromol* 2014 April 23.

The herb polysaccharides enhance immunity, in part by maturation of bone marrow derived dendritic cells. The herb and medicinal mushrooms may be a good combination for improving dendritic cell maturation and improved immune modulation. Zhao R et al, *Nutr Cancer* 2015 67(6): 987-93.

A mice study found ethanol extracts ameloriate induced ulcerative colitis. Yang X et al, *Am J Transl Res* 2016 8(5): 2138-48.

Ethanol extracts also attenuated aging alteration in female mice and their reproductive system, including alteration in hormone levels. Ahangarpour A et al, *Int J Reprod Biomed* (Yazd) 2016 14(3): 205-12.

A decoction of seven parts purslane and one part licorice root has been found successful in treating 212 patients with cervical erosion. A success rate, after 20 days, of 97% was noted from internal ingestion. *Tianjing Med Herb* 1973 2:5.

The plant and especially oleracein E exhibit anti-oxidant activity similar to caffeic acid. Yang et al, *Phytother Res* Jan 12 2009.

Chan, *Journal of Ethnopharmacology* 2000 73:3 showed significant analgesic and anti-inflammatory activity with a 10% alcohol extract of the dried herb. The active control, diclofenac sodium, and purslane were comparable in results.

The same team reported the next summer that opiate receptors appear be involved.

Water extracts increase SOD and decrease malondialdehyde levels, up-regulate telomere length and activity, and down-regulate p21 without changing expression of p53. Hongxing et al, *Chem Biol Interact* 2007 170:3. More research is needed.

A rare sub-class of homo-isoflavonoids show activity against four human cancer cell lines. Yan J et al, *Phytochemistry* 2012 Aug 80: 37-41.

Tian JL et al, *J Asian Nat Prod Res* 2014 16:3 259-64 found two new alkaloids with activity against lung and breast cancer cell lines.

Polysaccharides inhibit cervical cancer cell growth, *in vivo* and *in vitro*. Zhao R et al, *Carbohydrate Polym* 2013 96(2): 376-83.

Portulacerebroside A induces apoptosis on human leukemia HL60 cells, suggesting an adjunct therapy for acute myeloid leukemia. Ye Q et al, *Int J Clin Exp Pathol* 2015 8(11): 13968-77).

One unusual study found water extracts of purslane combined with fish oil, gave protection to radiation damage to liver and kidneys, in rats. Abd El-Azime AS et al, *Int J Radiat Biol* 2014 90(12): 1184-90.

Purslane tincture inhibits pancreatic lipase activity. Not sure if this is good idea or not. Conforti F et al, *Phytother Res* 2012 26(4): 600-4.

Selenium rich purslane may be useful for preventing occurrence of Keshan and Kaskin-Beck diseases. Prabha D et al, *Toxicol Indust Health* 2013.

A good review, up to 2015, of purslane was written by Zhou YX et al, *Biomed Research Int* 2015 Article ID 925631.

PLANT OIL

Purslane contains various fatty acids including palmitic, stearic, oleic, linoleic and alpha linolenic acid (omega 3).

The omega 3 fatty acid content of purslane is one of the highest in the world for plants. As these fatty acids are useful in lowering cholesterol and triglyceride levels, as well as decreasing platelet aggregation, the plant deserves consideration for green drinks and further investigation is warranted. Like flax, however, the ALA requires conversion via the liver into omega-3 found in seafood and algae.

One hundred grams of fresh leaves yield an average of 300-400 mg of omega 3 fatty acids (alpha linolenic acid), as well as around 100 mg of linoleic acid. This gives as a 3-4:1 ratio of Omega 3 to Omega 6.

Most modern day Western diets have typical ratios of 1:20-30; while health experts suggest the importance of a 1:2 ratio or better.

Palaniswamy et al, *Journal of Agric Food Chemistry* 2001 49 looked at the omega three content of purslane at different true leaf stages.

They found at the fourteen-leaf stage, oil yields were not only highest, but had an optimal Omega 3-Omega 6 ratio of 5.2:1.

Yields of 124.7 mg of alpha linolenic acid per 100 grams were found at this stage. At the six leaf stage, it was even higher, at 132.8, but linolenic acid was also higher, resulting in a 3.9:1 ratio, which is still very good.

I have been promoting purslane as a nutritional green food for a number of years, and feel it is still one of the optimal crops for the current trend of phyto-oriented functional foods.

SEED OIL

Seed oil is nutritious and has a desirable fatty acid composition. Up to 72% oil can be extracted from the seeds. The cold pressed oil has low oxidative stability and highest sensitivity to temperature changes.

The seeds contain 18.9% fatty acids composed of 39% linoleic, 28.7% oleic, 10.9% palmitic, 9.9% linolenic, 3.7% stearic, and 1.3% behenic acid.

The oil inhibits cervical cancer HeLa, esophageal cancer Eca-109, and breast cancer MCF-7 cell lines. The oil may also be useful as a substitute for synthetic antioxidants in food preservation or cosmetics. The seed oil may be useful for the prevention or mitigation of hypertensive symptoms. Guo G et al, *J Hypertens* (Los Angel) 2016 5(2).

The seed oil is cytotoxic on human liver cancer (HepG2) and lung cancer (A-549) cell lines. Al-Sheddi ES et al, *Asian Pac J Cancer Prev* 2015 16(8): 3383-7.

ESSENTIAL OIL

Purslane has been steam distilled and the volatile oil analyzed. Liu et al, *Ziran Kexueban* 1994 14:3.

The oil is composed mainly of linalool and 3,7,11,15-tetramethyl-2hexadecen-1-ol. It may be useful as a natural preservative. Sharafati CR et al, Jundishapur *J Microbiol* 2015 8(3): e20128.

HYDROSOL

The distilled water of purslane can be drunk to quench and cool all internal and external heats brought on by fever, and afflictions of the liver, stomach, and other internal organs. It also checks bloody flux and other fluxes of the stomach, cools inflamed kidneys, and eases burning urine. It stills immoderate bleedings of the hemorrhoids and so forth, and controls blood spitting. When children cannot sleep on account of a high temperature, or if they have worms, they should be given several tablespoons of this water.   **SAUER**

Purslain water cools the blood and liver, quenches thirst, helps such as spit blood, have hot coughs, or pestilences. Camerarius saith, the distilled water used by some, took away the pain of their teeth, when all other remedies failed.   **CULPEPPER**

Portulaca water from the stalks and herb is good for hot and dry cough, spitting blood, children with worms, petulance and pain in bladder.   **BRUNSCHWIG**

FLOWER ESSENCE

Purslane flower essence is for those suffering from fear of darkness. This is not only the darkness of night, which results in the need for children to have a night light in their room; but for those sensitive individuals affected by the darkness of humanity.

Carl Jung was one of the first psychologists to encourage in therapy the owning of an individual's dark side. In the owning and possibility, comes the balance many are looking for in life. Purslane flower essence assists those with muscular tightness, created by an overly controlling personality, to loosen up, relax, and find balance in their bodies and mind.   **PRAIRIE DEVA**

SPIRITUAL PROPERTIES

Purslane is an herbe for those who fear the darkness of the night. It will protect you from all bad dreams, and from any strange spirits that roam the darkness. It is most frequently used for this purpose by being made into a dream pillow.

Purslane made be taken as a daily tonic, for it attracts positive energy, and will bring a more wholesome outlook to the mentality and emotion. Purslane is said to be most effective when undergoing difficult or dangerous transits.   **BEYERL**

Opportunity comes from the Latin **PORTA**, which is an "entrance" or "passage through". For the Romans, a Porta Fenestella was a special opening that allowed Fortune to enter. The Greek root is **POROS**, which is a passageway for ships but also any passageway, including one through the skin, that is, a pore.

Poroi are all the passages that allow fluids to flow in and out of the body.

A pore, a portal, a doorway, a nick of time, a gap in the screen, a looseness in the weave- these are all opportunities in the ancient sense. Each being in the world must find the set of opportunities fitted to its nature. The giant's pathway is often blocked, but bacterial landscapes are almost pure Poroi.   **HYDE**

RECIPES

DECOCTION- 6-14 grams

TINCTURE- 2-5 ml. A fresh aerial plant tincture is made at 1:3 and 60% alcohol.

CAPSULES- 500 mg up to six daily in divided dose. The optimal drying method is vacuum dehydration, which retains the bioactive molecules.

JUICE- after juicing fresh purslane, pour into ice cube trays, freeze, pop out, bag and label. Then put the frozen cube into warm water, smoothies etc.

PICKLED PURSLANE- Take washed purslane stems only and place upright in clean jars. Pour a hot vinegar and water (equal parts) that contains garlic, salt, peppercorns, some mustard and celery seeds; or wild bergamot and dill weed. Store in sealed jars in fridge. The cultivated vegetable is far superior to the common, weedy forms.

CAUTION- Purslane should be avoided by those prone to kidney stone formation as it may increase kidney filtration, urine production and cause a stone to move. Do not take in large quantities during pregnancy due to mild uterine stimulation. Do not use purslane in cold deficient conditions.

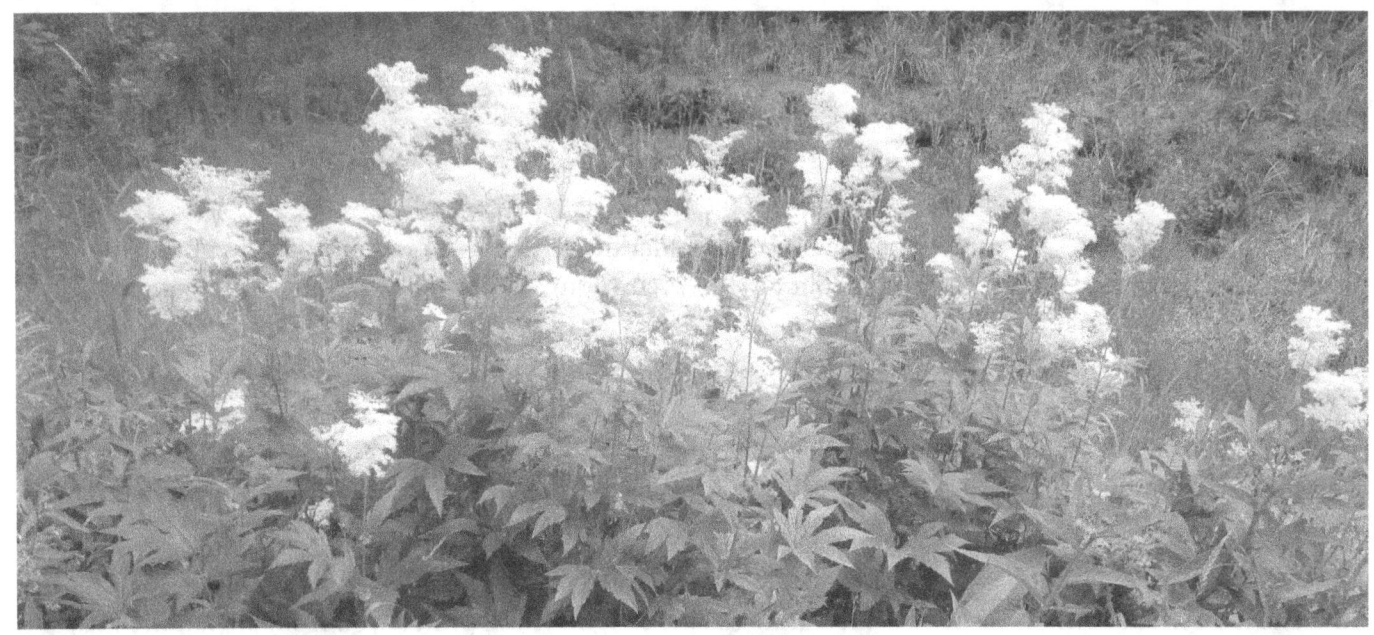

QUEEN OF THE MEADOW

QUEEN OF THE MEADOW
MEADOWSWEET
(*Filipendula ulmaria* [L.] Maxim.)
(*Spiraea ulmaria* L.) not accepted
QUEEN OF THE PRAIRIE
(*F. rubra* [Hill] B. L. Rob.)
SHINING MEADOWSWEET
WHITE MEADOWSWEET
(*S. betulifolia* Pall.)
(*S. lucida* Douglas ex Greene) not accepted
PINK SPIREA
HARDHACK
WILD LILAC
(*S. douglasii* Hook.)
(*S. douglasii ssp. menziesii*) not accepted
PARTRIDGE FOOT
CREEPING SPIRAEA
(*S. pectinata* [Pursh] Torr. & A. Gray) not accepted
(*Luetkea pectinata* [Pursh] Kuntze)

NARROW-LEAVED MEADOWSWEET
(*S. alba* Du Roi)
PINK MEADOWSWEET
ROSE MEADOWSWEET
(*S. splendens* Baumann ex K. Koch)
(*S. densiflora* Nutt ex Green nom illeg.) not accepted
DROPWORT
(*S. filipendula* L.) not accepted
(*F. vulgaris* Moench.)
(*Ulmaria filipendula* [L.] Hill) not accepted
THREE LOBED SPIRAEA
(*S. trilobata* L.)
JAPANESE SPIRAEA
(*S. japonica* L.f.)
(*Astilbe japonica*) not accepted
DWARF BUMALDA SPIRAEA
(*S. x bumalda* Burven)
CHINESE SPIRAEA
(*A. chinensis* Maxim.)
PARTS USED- leaves, flowers

Where peep the gaping speckled cuckoo-flowers
The Meadow-sweet flaunts high its showy wreath
And sweet the quaking grasses hide beneath.

CLARE

There, once upon a time, the heavy king,
Trod out its perfume from the Meadowsweet,
Strewn like a woman's love beneath his feet,
In stately dance or jovial banqueting. **WM.**

ALLINGHAM

To nod from banks, from whence depend
Rich cymes of fragrant Meadow-sweet;
Alas! those creamy clusters lend
A charm where death and ardour meet.

T. CAMPBELL

Spiraea is from the Greek **SPEIRAIRA**, a plant used for garlands; that comes from **SPEIROS**, meaning twisted, wreathed or spiral. Filipendula is from the Latin **FILUM** meaning thread, and **PENDULUS**, for hanging. This refers to the tubers being attached to long thread like roots some distance from the plant base.

Meadowsweet was originally Meadsweet, or Meadwort, referring to mead, or honey wine that it was used to flavour. It was one of the sacred herbs of the Druid.

Ulmaria is from the elm-like leaves. Luetkea is named after Count F.P. Lütke, a Russian sea captain and explorer of the 1800s. Pectinata refers to the leaves that resemble the teeth of a comb.

Dropwort, introduced from Europe, was named, according to Culpepper "because it helps such as piss by drops".

Dwarf Bumalda Spirea is a chance hybrid of *S. japonica* (pink flowers) and *S. albiflora* (white flowers) that occurred in Switzerland.

Queen of the Meadow, or Meadowsweet is common in perennial flower gardens. Its majestic, fluffy flower heads in early summer are a showy, stately sight. Their greenish-white flowers, and leaves fill the air with a honey/almond scent reminiscent of hot summer days.

Meadowsweet was one of the Druid's sacred plants, along with verbena and water mint. Queen Elizabeth I used to scatter the fragrant flowers over the floors of her private apartment, and was said to rub the plant oil on her body before lovemaking.

Another name, Courtship and Matrimony refers to the two distinct scents of the plant. The fragrant, heady flowers represent courting, while the sharper scent of dried leaves symbolized the reality of marriage.

Gerard, the English herbalist wrote, "the smell thereof maketh the heart merrie and delighteth the senses". It was one of the fifty plants in the drink called "Save", as told by the Knight in Chaucer's *Canterbury Tales*.

Culpepper mentions it for helping break fevers and colds, and when boiled in red wine, stays the flux of the belly.

The Gaelic name means Cuchullain's Belt, for in myth, the hero, ill with fierce fevers, was cured when bathed with the herb.

In the late 17th century, a woman in Bedfordshire was credited with its use in fevers and agues, combining the herb with green wheat. Various other uses include burns, itching eyes, diarrhea, stomach pain, sunburn and nervousness.

If gathered on Midsummer, it was said to give information about thieves. When placed on water, if it sinks, the thief is male, if it floats a female.

The root has been used traditionally alone or in combination for Bright's disease and dropsy.

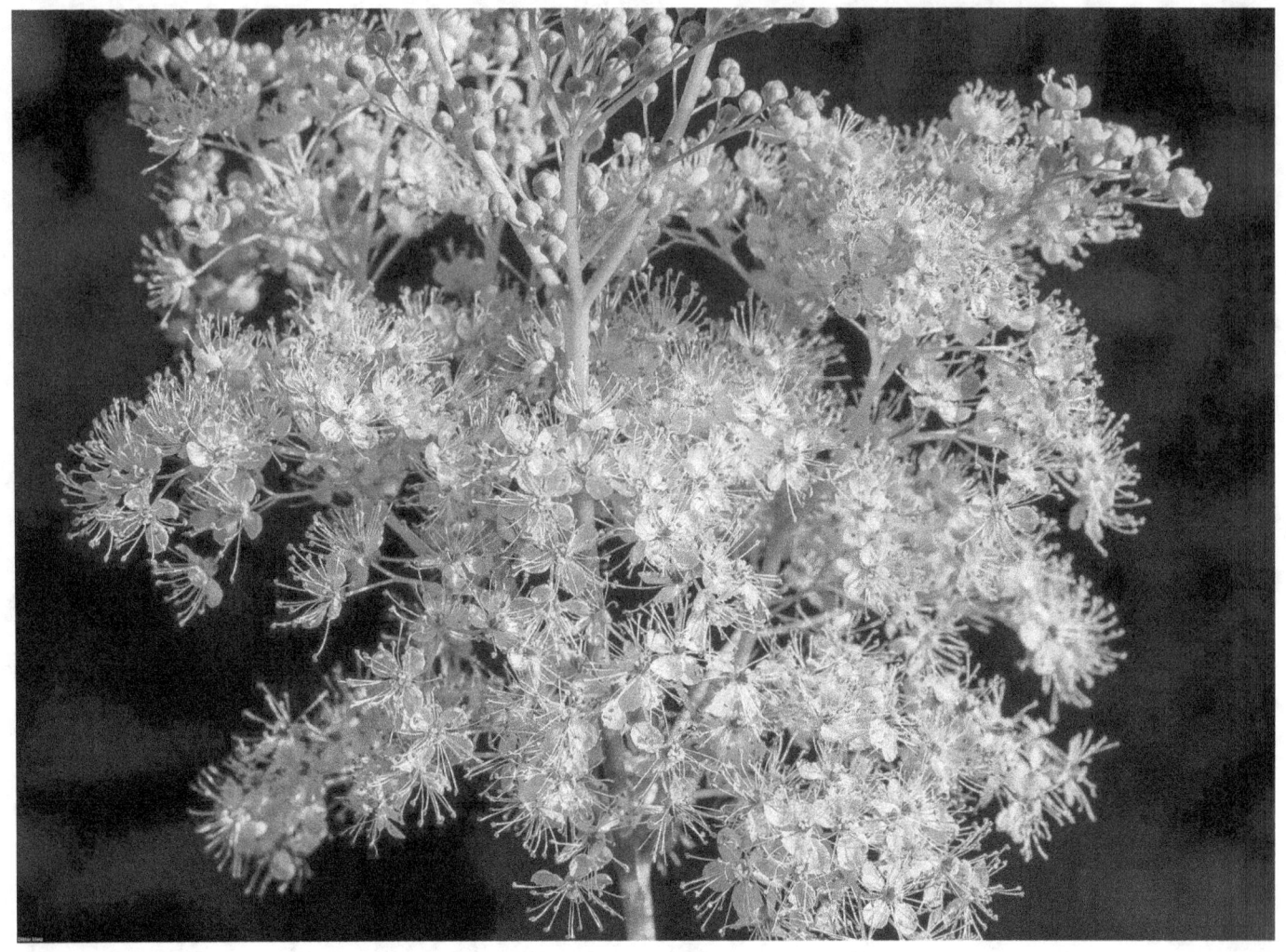

QUEEN OF THE PRAIRIE

Its cousin, Queen of the Prairie, is slightly smaller, up to 3-4 feet, with sweet scented white to pink frothy flowers. The plants do well in wet soil, even boggy and acidic.

Both the Shining and Narrow-leaved meadowsweet are native to the prairies; the former preferring thin woods and open hills, and the latter, smaller shrub more at home in wet meadows and riverbanks.

Shining Spiraea is known as "little red plant", and "venereal disease/maggot plant", by the Thompson/Nlaka'pamux. This is due to its use in treating venereal disease with decoctions of the leaves and branches internally, as well as baths.

Narrow-leaved Meadowsweet (*S. alba*) was used by the Fox to stop bloody flux; the immature seed heads being specific as a cool infusion.

The Iroquois used the mashed and powdered dried root as part of a compound decoction with yarrow for side pain, and nausea. The Mahuna boiled the roots for coughs and colds. The Ojibway used the root as trap bait, and know it as **DEMA'GENE-MINS**.

To many natives, the dried leaves of narrow-leaved meadowsweet made the best tasting wilderness tea.

Shining Meadowsweet roots and leaves were decocted by the Shuswap to treat diarrhea and upset stomach.

Some tribes used an eagle bone to help insert root infusions as an enema in various bowel complaints, including bloody stools.

Hardhack, or Pink Spiraea, seeds were infused by the Lummi for diarrhea.

The dried leaves of meadowsweet contain coumarin, and have been used to give a vanilla like scent to port, claret, and mead. In fact, the common name is believed derived from Meadsweet, rather than a description of locale.

In Europe, the herb is used as natural food flavouring.

The root of red-flowered Queen of the Prairie was gathered by indigenous healers for heart trouble. It was used, as a love medicine, which makes perfect sense.

Its high tannin content gives it astringent action, and combined with natural salicylates, was used to treat arthritis, flu and fever, as well as diarrhea and intestinal bleeding.

Cosmetic companies utilize the plant's ability to protect against UV exposure. In one trial of five subjects, 50% protection was shown. A fibroblast study also showed significant protection from sun exposure. Another study showed an 88% increase in cell proliferation when treated with 0.01% extracts. Skin respiration was measured using the Warburg Assay, and a Gilson IG-14 differential respirometer, with 10% extracts increasing cellular respiration by 55%.

Meadowsweet extracts are used in several Revlon personal care lotions, tonics and creams.

Pink Spirea is a handsome shrub up to six feet tall, with pink to rose-colored flowers. It loves wet feet and grows aggressively in the right setting.

The Nuu-chah-nulth utilized the wiry twigs to make broom like-implements to gather tubular dentalium shells on the west coast of Vancouver Island. These shells were called Wampum, and used as a form of currency throughout northwest North America.

The Nuxalk used Hardhack branches to make hooks for drying and smoking fish.

The Salish made blades, halibut hooks, and cambium scrapers from the fire- hardened wood.

On a veterinary note, studies conducted by Flouvier et al, *Phytochemistry* 1986 indicate that meadowsweet alters the composition and function of bacteria in the colon of animals such that less ammonia is released into the atmosphere and feed conversion is improved.

Adding meadowsweet, 20-30 grams daily in the food of horses, helps reduce inflammation and digestive irritability.

Partridge Foot is a short shrub found in the foothills, north of the North Saskatchewan and Athabasca River in western Alberta.

The Thompson, or Nlaka'pamux used the fresh plant as a poultice on sores. Plant decoctions were given for abdominal pain, and for women suffering from long or excessive menstruation. Its name roughly translates as "sharp leaf".

Three-lobed Spirea (*S. trilobata*) is an introduced native of Asia that grows up to a metre with a multitude of flowers in early summer.

Japanese Spiraeas (*S. japonica, S. thunbergii* and *S. prunifolia*) are introduced and hardy in gardens and hedges throughout the prairies.

Both the introduced Dropwort (*S. vulgaris*) and Siberian Meadowsweet (*F. palmata*) are hardy to -40° C.

Dropwort was considered by Culpepper, a good kidney remedy, the root combined with white wine with a little honey. The doctrine of signatures plays a role here, as the small drop-like tubers represent small piss drops.

"It is also very effectual for all diseases of the lungs, as shortness of breath, wheezing, hoarseness of the throat; and to expectorate tough phlegm".

On the Isle of Man, the juice is used as rennet for making cheese, and for binjeen. In Sweden, the slightly bitter roots are dried and baked into bread.

In fall, the tubers are dug up and have a pleasant odor, reminiscent of neroli, and a sweet taste similar to hazelnuts but with slight bitterness. In spring they are very bitter.

If made into a fresh fall root tincture, it gives a dark red tincture with starch deposit.

The look-alike False Spiraea (*Sorbaria sorbifolia*) is very hardy to the region, but is not related.

Pink Meadowsweet is restricted to the extreme southwest corner of Alberta.

MEDICINAL

CONSTITUENTS-*F. ulmaria* flowers- spiraein (salicylaldehyde) primveroside (3.47%), monotropitin, gaultherin, methyl salicylate, salicin, salicylic acid, spirein, isosalicin, anthocyanin and heparin.
flowering tops- spiraeoside (0.71%) and hyperoside (0.58%) are the main flavonoids; as well as rutoside, avicularoside, quercitin 4'-0-beta-D-glucopyranoside, and kaempferol-4-'-0-beta-D-gluco-pyranoside. Small amounts of chalcone, phenylcarboxylic acid, coumarin, citric and ascorbic acid, as well as volatile oils. Tannins, mainly hydrolysable, compose about 10-20%, mainly rugosins A, B, D and E, gallic and hexahydroxydiphenic esters of glucose. Various trace minerals include iron, sulphur, calcium and silica. Leaves also contain catechols.
The chief components salicylaldehyde and methyl salicylate are derived after dehydration. The main phenolic glycoside is spiraein, which is the primeveroside of salicylaldehyde. Polyphenol content of flowers is 165 mg/g.
Also includes hexa-hydroxydiphenic acid esters of glucose.
leaves and stems- coumarin and other flavanoids; as well as monotropitin (methyl salicylate primveroside).
roots- tannins, mainly rugosin-D. A new comprehensive study of 119 plant compounds was published by Bijttebier S et al, *Planta Med* 2016 82(6): 559-72.
S. douglasii- various salicylates including salicin, gaultherin and spiraein, tannins mucilage, flavonoids, gallic acid, and essential oils.
S. japonica root- spiramines A, B, P, T, Q, W and U, spiridine F.
S. japonica var. *acuminata*- two atisine-type diterpene alkaloids, two atisane-type diterpenes, spiramine C2.

Queen of the Meadow is well known in herbal literature. Its cool, dry properties have been used traditionally for analgesic and diuretic purpose.

It is rich in organic silica, like horsetail, and is therefore of use in all kinds of connective tissue weakness, and inflammation; including cellulitis.

Queen of the Meadow is analgesic, due in part, to its content of salicylate compounds.

In fact the name aspirin is derived from the plant, and was first discovered in Spiraea, the plant's former botanical name. It was first isolated from the flower buds in 1838, by an Italian professor Raphael Piria; and then synthesized by the German Felix Hoffman for Bayer fifty years later.

Unfortunately, salicylic acid caused so much gastric discomfort and nausea, that the drug acetylsalicylic acid was developed, "a" for acetyl, and "spirin" from Spiraea.

Methyl salicylate is found in the flowers and stems, but not in the leaves, as monotropitin, a primeveroside of methyl salicylate.

It is probable that spiraein and monotropitin are converted into salicin in the stomach or small intestine, and then into saligenin and then oxidized to salicylic acid in the blood and liver, but this has not been totally proven. The mechanism for salicin from Poplar and Willow is similar.

Meadowsweet shows anti-ulcer effects against aspirin and ethanol, but not histamine induced ulcers; suggesting the phenolic glycosides and volatile oil are not exerting exactly the same effects as other salicylates. Work by Yanutsh et al, *Farmatsevtychnyi Zhurnal* 1982 37 studied the anti-ulcerative action in some detail.

Meadowsweet extracts inhibit complement activation and T cell proliferation, as well as modulatory activity towards parts of the cellular immune system. Beside salicylates, the plant contains flavonoids which have much more significant anti-inflammatory effects. The diethyl ether root extracts were the most potent at inhibiting lymphocyte proliferation. Halkes et al, *Phytotherapy Research* 1997 11:7.

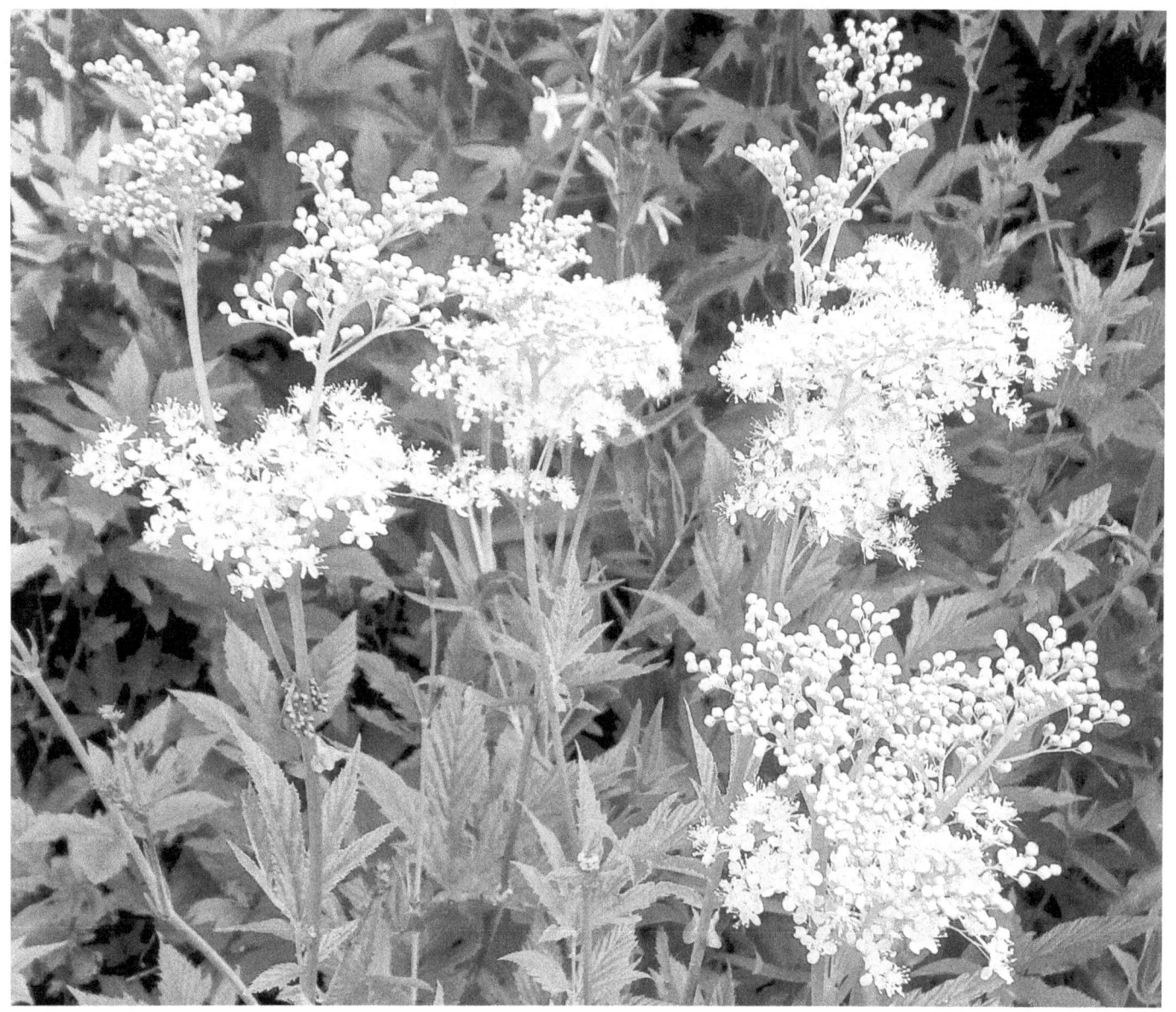

QUEEN OF THE MEADOW

Calliste et al, *J Agric Food Chemistry* 2001 49 showed that meadowsweet possesses high anti-oxidant activity, using grape seed as a reference. It showed anti-proliferative effect on B16 melanoma cells. Follow up work by Kähkönen et al, *J Agric Food Chem* 2003 47:10 confirmed the anti-oxidant effect attributed, in part, to phenolic content.

Quercitin from this herb inhibits protein kinase the best of 81 plants tested. Galkin et al, *Nat Prod Commun* 2009 4:1.

It is therefore good in fevers and inflammations causing pain such as acute and chronic rheumatism, articular rheumatism, tendinitis, gouty arthritis; and in conditions of water retention. Scientific evidence shows that the plant's active principles help promote excretion of uric acid.

The plant is a balancer of stomach acidity, reducing when necessary and increasing when deficient.

It is often combined with other gentle stomachic herbs for this purpose, such as peppermint or pineapple weed. At least one study has shown salicin to reduce blood sugar levels.

For individuals taking antacids, combine the herb with mallow, and gold thread.

Thomas Garran, in his excellent book, puts this herb into proper perspective with regards to stomach problems.

"Chronic (and, to a lesser extent, acute) inflammation of the gastric mucosa damages the tissue, which can lead to a variety of problems.

In the stomach, the first sign is a reddening and edema of the tissue with adherent mucus and potentially, erosions and bleeding. As the condition becomes chronic, there is atrophy of the glandular epithelium with loss of the parietal and chief cells, leading to decreased production of HCL, pepsin and intrinsic factor.

In such cases, meadowsweet's anti-inflammatory and astringent properties cool the tissue while gently toning with a mild astringent action. Toning the tissue and reducing inflammation results in proper blood and lymphatic flow, thus encouraging healing and correct functioning of the organ". Well put!

The flower extracts have been shown to fight bacterial infections of the urinary tract, such as *Staphylococcus aureus* and *E. coli*, according to studies by Catanicin-Hintz, *Clujul-Medica* 1983. It works well for frequent, painful and small voiding of urine associated with damp heat of the bladder, the perfect condition for microbial growth.

Recent work found anti-microbial effect against *E. coli* and *E. faecalis*. Katanic J et al, *Food Funct* 2015 6(4): 1164-75.

Meadowsweet flower extracts have been found to inhibit *Staphylococcus epidermis*, *Proteus vulgaris*, *Shigella*, *Bacillus subtilis*, *Corynebacterium diphtheriae*, *Diplococcus pneumoniae* and *Pseudomonas aeruginosa*.

Rauha et al, *Int J Food Microbiol* 2000 56:1 found meadowsweet, fireweed, cloudberry and raspberry herbs had the greatest effect on inhibiting bacteria.

Meadowsweet tea is useful in cases of red, sandy deposits in the urine, with an oily film on the surface, as well as uric acid removal.

Meadowsweet is a safe gentle and quick acting remedy for childhood diarrhea, due to its cool and bitter nature.

Adults with abdominal pain, anal burning or itching, desire for cold beverages and blood tinged urine will also benefit.

Meadowsweet is a useful cardiotonic, with help in hypertension and arteriosclerosis, and other signs of heat from the heart such as blotching and redness of the face.

Work by Bespalov et al in 1992, and Paresun'ko et al, in the following year, indicates that meadowsweet administered to rats can suppress certain kinds of tumors, including brain and spinal cord. It also helps to inhibit cervical and vaginal cancers in mice and humans. Women systemically treated with an ointment for cervical dysplasia showed benefit. Rugosin, for example, shows anti-tumor activity against sarcoma 180.

Peresun'ko et al, *Vopr Onkol* 1993 39 found flower preparations useful for treating precancerous changes and prevention of uterine and cervical cancers. A 67% drop in dysplasia occurred and no recurrence was found in 10 subjects after one year.

Recent work by Mazzio EA and Soliman KF, *Cancer Genomics Proteomics* 2017 14(1): 17-33 may explain this benefit.

Histone deacetylases (HDACs) are a major epigenetic regulator of transcriptional repression, which are highly overexpressed in advanced malignancy. Queen of the Meadow is one of 1600 plants that elicit inhibition. Other herbs of note are great burnet root (*Sanguisorba officinalis*), grapeseed extract, coffee, uva ursi, green tea, sassafras, turkey rhubarb and gossypol from cotton.

The herb also may be useful for prevention and amelioration of cisplatin chemotherapy side effects, including liver and kidney toxicity. Katanic J et al, *Food Chem Toxicol* 2017 99: 86-102. It also inhibits radiation-induced carcinogenesis. Bespalov VG et al, *Int J Radiat Biol* 2017 93(4): 394-401.

In France, the herb is used as a diuretic and diaphoretic (depending on temperature), as well as headaches and toothache pain. In Belgium, meadowsweet is used for painful articular conditions.

The leaves help soothe the sympathetic nervous system; while the flowers have also been shown to exhibit anti-ulcer, diuretic and sedative properties.

Topical administration of the flowers has been shown to decrease squamous cell carcinoma of the cervix and vagina. Application of an ointment was shown to increase regression of cervical dysplasia in 32 of 48 patients. Peresun'ko et al, *Voprosy Onkologii* 1993:39.

Heparin, from the flowers, shows some similarity to heparin of animal origin. Kudriashov et al, *Izv Akad Nauk SSSR Biology* 1991:6. Both the flowers and seeds show anti-coagulant and fibrinolytic activity *in vivo* and *in vitro*. Liapina et al, *Izv Akad Nauk Ser Biol* 1993 4.

Work by Halkes et al, *Pharm Pharmacol Lett* 1997 7:2-3 found strong complement inhibition from the flowers, suggesting immune regulating activity.

Recent work also found immune modulating benefit from the polysaccharides, as well as inhibition of amylase, alpha glucosidase and AGE formation, suggesting benefit in type 2 diabetes. Olennikov DN et al, *Molecules* 22(1). doi: 10.3390.

The flowers treat histamine-mediated symptoms such as allergies and stomach ulceration. Nitta Y et al, *Food Chem* 2013 138:2-3 1551-6.

The aerial parts are nearly 50% more effective as the root for reducing inflammation. Katanic J et al, *J Ethnopharm* 2016 193: 627-36.

The root has some effect on treating fevers; and due to the high levels of tannins is good for treating diarrhea, including infectious diarrhea like *Shigella* helping stop bleeding.

It is gentle enough for children, and yet is deep acting. Use it for intestinal infections in children where there is pain and general toxicity.

Like Water Avens, it contains elastase-inhibiting activity.

The fresh rootstock and the rubbed leaves are quite different. The "scent" is like a dental clinic, and the flavor of cheap chewing gum.

Meadowsweet extracts have been shown to lower vascular permeability, relax muscles, increase bronchial tone in cats, decrease bronchial spasm induced by histamine in guinea pigs, increase tone in vitro of guinea pig intestine and rabbit uterus, and potentiate narcotic action. Barnaulov et al, *Pharmakil Toxicol* (Moscow) 1980 43.

The same author found the anti-ulcer activity associated with the flower extracts also prolonged life expectancy in mice in study.

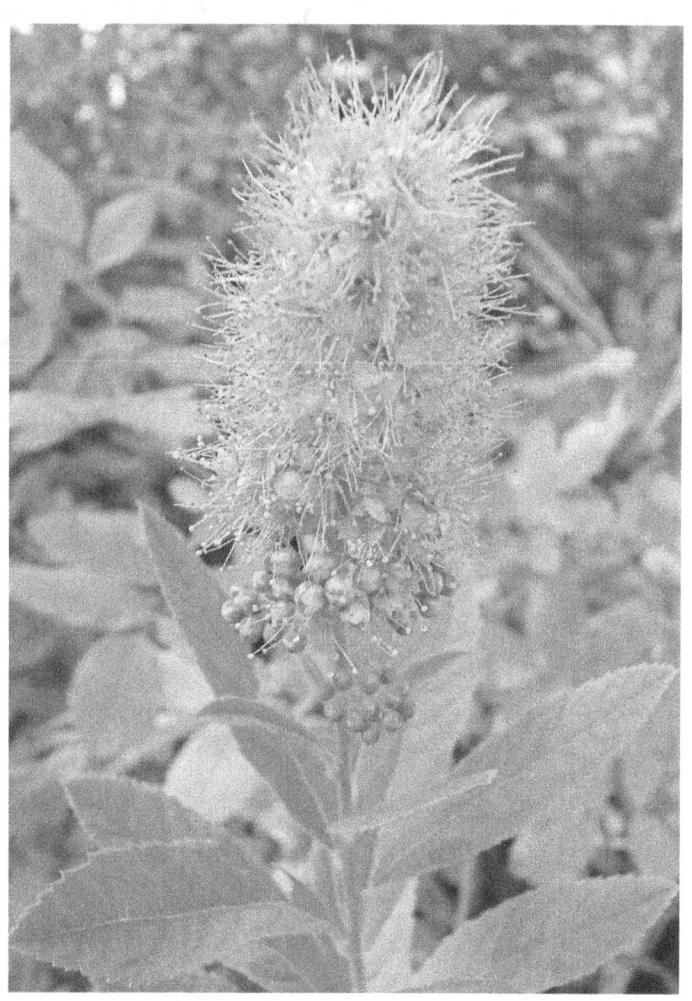

HARDHACK (PINK SPIRAEA)

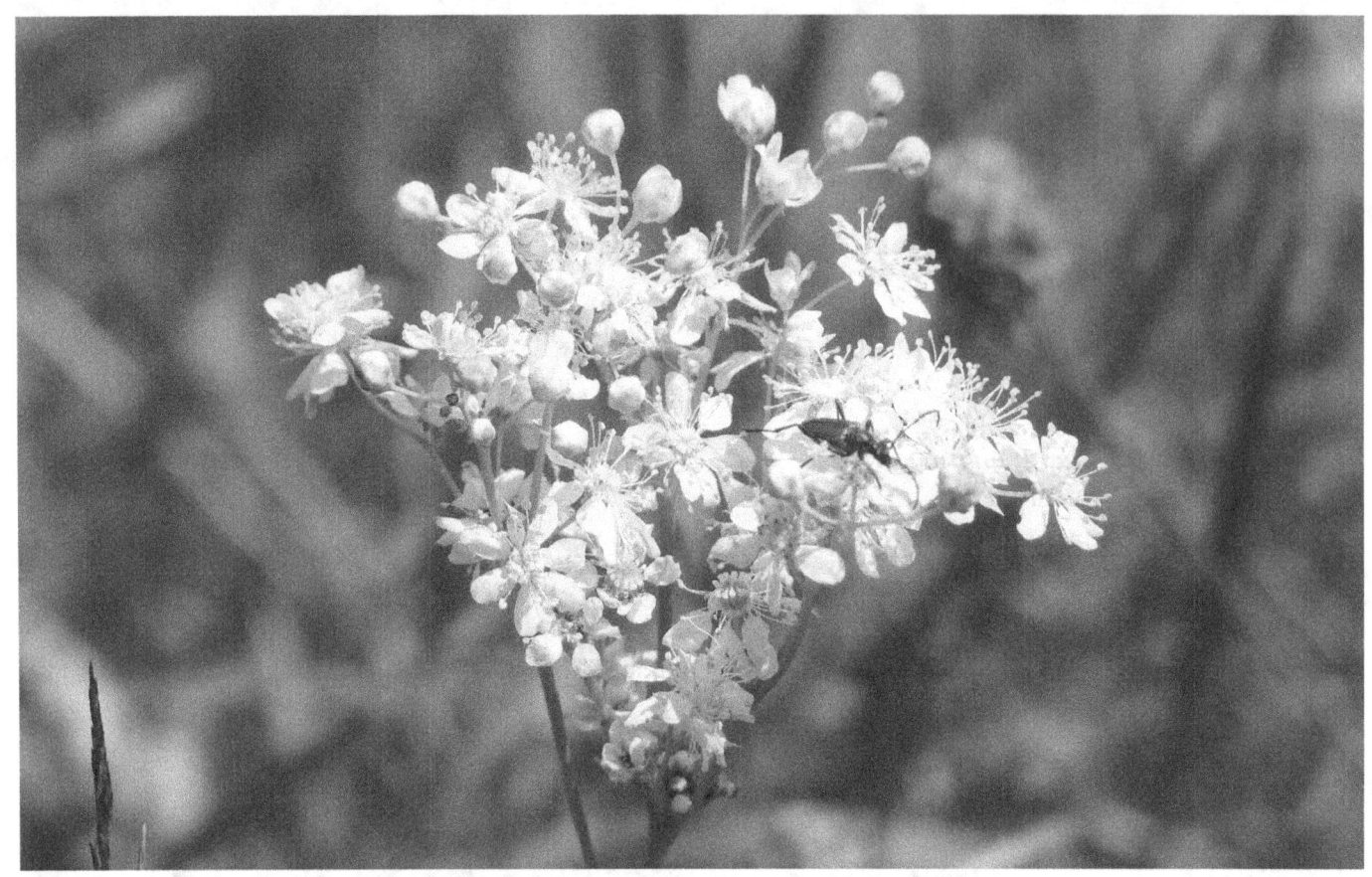

DROPWORT

The herb inhibits bacterial histidine decarboxylase and may be effective for preventing histamine production. Nitta Y et al, *J Food Prot* 2016 79(3): 463-7.

A blend of this herb with *Echinacea purpurea* and Devil's Claw (*Harpagophytum procumbens*) promotes anti-angiogenic activity and may be useful in diseases associated with excessive blood vessel formation, such as sarcoidosis. Radomska-Lesniewska DM et al, *Cent Eur J Immunol* 2016 41(1): 25-34.

The leaves of *F. rubra* and flowers, leaves and stems of *S. alba*, show activity against *Staphylococcus aureus*. Borchardt et al, *J Med Plants Res* 2008 2:5.

Hardhack fresh flower tincture is useful for treating headaches and mild to moderate muscle pain.

An infusion of dried leaves will relieve diarrhea as well as menstrual pain and heavy bleeding. It may also relieve morning sickness in some cases.

The dried bark and flowers can be ground into powder and put in "00" capsules to strengthen the kidneys and decrease incontinence.

The dried root is decocted to reduce fevers and as a digestive aid.

Dropwort water extracts reduce anxiety, far exceeding a valerian extract, in a mouse study by Venerovskii AI et al, *Eksp Klin Farmakol* 2011 74(9): 3-6.

It was also superior to valerian in improvement of mitochondrial energy product in brain of rats during experimental posthypoxic encephalopathy. Vengerovsky AI et al, *Bull Exp Biol Med* 2011 151(4): 421-4.

The herb was similar to piracetam on brain memory and behavior after hypoxic injury, in an animal study. Modulation of hippocampal activity is speculated. Shilova IV & Suslov NI, *Bull Exp Biol Med* 2015 158(5): 659-63.

Synergy between the herb and ciprofloxacin increased inhibition of *E. coli* by four times.

Fireweed and tansy also showed similar benefit. Smirnova G et al, *J Appl Microbiol* 2012 113(1): 192-9.

Japanese Spiraea shows activity against both gram positive and negative bacteria. Water and ethanol extracts of *S. thunbergii* shows activity against both bacteria as well as mycobacterium.

Li et al, *Planta Medica* 2001 67:2 found spiramine T from *S. japonica* root has neuro-protective qualities.

Spiramine Q was examined the previous year, in the same journal (66:3). This diterpene was found to possess potent anti-platelet and anti-thrombotic activity.

The herb exhibits anti-platelet aggregation.

Water extracts of *S. prunifolia* were studied, by So-HunTaeg et al, at the Wonkwang University School of Medicine in Korea.

Their work, reported in *Immunopharmacology and Immunotoxicology* 1999 21:2 found extracts exert a direct anti-malarial effect via direct cytotoxicity of nitric oxide, as well as NO mediated modulation of immune functions. Our own species have not been tested.

Compounds from *S. japonica* var. *acuminata* exhibit anti-tobacco virus activity, stronger than ningnanmycin. Ma Y et al, *Fitoterapia* 2016 109: 8-13.

False Spiraea (*Sorbaria sorbifolia*) contains a glycoside, flavosorbin that is of some interest.

HOMEOPATHY

Spiraea ulmaria (Hardhack) is for burning and pressure in the esophagus, as it feels contracted but not made worse from swallowing.

It relieves irritation of the urinary tract, and favourably influences the prostate gland; checking gleet and prostatorrhea. It has also been used for eclampsia, epilepsy and hydrophobia.

Hardhack relieves rheumatism that moves from one part of the body to another. It is used for local infiltration in cases of epicondyllitis.

Cramps in flexor muscles of forearm when lifting heavy things.It soothes heat and profuse sweating in various parts. It helps relieve the mind of the morbidly conscientious.

Nocturnal feelings of remorse from a slight fault committed long ago. Problems with sexuality, difficulty integrating with the lower part of body. Immaturity, or undeveloped sexuality. Aversion to smoking tobacco. Hot and burning pains in whole body.

DOSE- Tincture and low potencies. The mother tincture is made from the fresh root of *F. ulmaria*. Bojanus self experimented with tincture of rhizome in 1862. Proving by Schier with five provers with tincture, 2x and 3x in 1896. Clinical observations by Mangialavori.

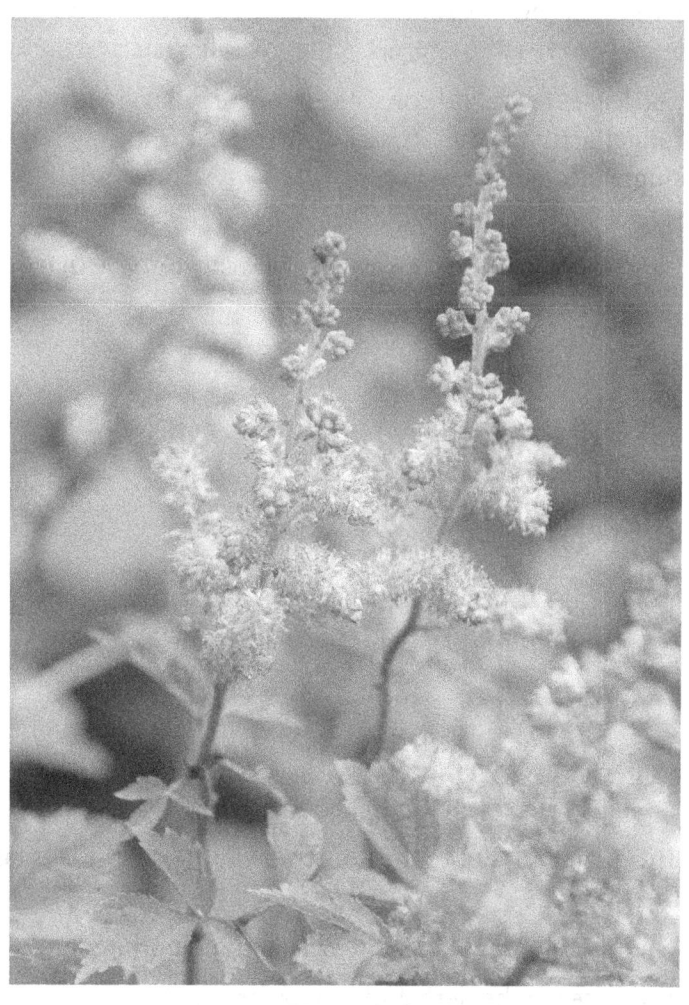

FALSE SPIRAEA

ESSENTIAL OIL

CONSTITUENTS- flowers-salicylic aldehyde (36%), methyl salicylate (19%), linalool (2.7%), trans-anethole (2.2%), heliotropin (piperonal), vanillin and beta-ionone (1.8%); over ninety individual constituents in all.
Analysis by Lindeman et al, *Wiss Technol* 1982 15 of steam distilled flowers yielded 75% salicylaldehyde, 3% phenylethyl alcohol, 2% benzyl alcohol, 2% anisaldehyde and 1.3% methyl salicylate. Other analyses show 36% salicylaldehyde and 19% methyl salicylate.
Upon distillation, the flowers of meadowsweet yield 0.2% essential oil heavier than water.
Spiraea oil congeals completely at -18°C.
roots- gaultherin, which is acted upon by gaultherase, and yields methyl salicylate. herb- salicylic aldehyde.

The flowers themselves contain no salicylic aldehyde. This is produced by the action of fermentation on an unknown substance during distillation.

Headspace analysis of the living flowers reveals a very different composition, with methyl salicylate completely absent, and only 1% salicylate aldehyde. The main component, methyl benzoate, does not occur in steam-distilled oils.

Benzonitrile, with its almond note, and anisaldehyde, with a sweet floral and vanilla like note, are both important parts of meadowsweet flower odour.

The leaf has a somewhat different composition. It consists mainly of salicylaldehyde (68%), as well as minor amounts of alpha asarone 6%, (E)-2-hexenal 4.2%, (E)-3-Hexen-1-ol 6% as well as traces of linalool, nerol, beta ionone, and benzaldehyde.

Dropwort aerial parts yield 0.1% yellow oil containing 17.9% tricosane, 13.7% salicylaldehyde, 11.9% n-nonanal, 6.8% benzyl salicylate, 6.7% methyl salicylate and 5.2% linalool.

The leaf essential oil consists mainly of salicyaldehyde (68.6%), and shows remarkable anti-microbial and anti-fungal activity. The activity is attributed to the synergistic interaction of all compounds in oil, rather than a single inhibitory agent.

Radulovic N et al, *Fitoterapia* 2007 78:7-8 found the leaf oil showed activity against a variety of bacteria and fungi. A synergy of constituents was more active than any isolated compound, with zones of inhibition similar to neomycin, gentamicin and nystatin.

WAX

The seed oil contains 17% of a wax with an extremely high melting point (240-260 degrees Celsius), and saponification number of 100.

SEED OIL

Seeds from Meadowsweet (*F. ulmaria*) contain 17% of a drying oil, resembling linseed oil composed of 47% linolenic acid, 16% linoleic, 29% oleic, and less than 8% stearic and palmitic acids. Further study would be useful.

HYDROSOL

CONSTITUENTS- *F. ulmaria-* dimethyl sulphide 70%, ethanol 6%, camphor 7%, eucalyptol 3.2% and minor amounts of bornyl formate, isobutanol, and methyl butanols.

The distilled water of the floures dropped into the eies taketh away the burning and itching thereof and cleareth the sight.   **GERARD**

The water thereof helps the heat and inflammation of the eyes.   **CULPEPPER**

The water of the herb and root is for pestilence.   **BRUNSCHWIG**

FLOWER ESSENCES

White Meadowsweet (*S. betulifolia*) flower essence is for emotional reactivity, and bringing stability to contemplate a situation, and gain broader perspective. Then, wise choices can be made.   **CANADIAN FOREST**

Meadowsweet essence brings confidence back when too much concern over material possessions.
MIRIANA

SPIRITUAL PROPERTIES

Energy that flows through the body is enhanced by Meadowsweet. This is particularly important on spiritual levels, when energy towards a project is dwindling.

This plant has a certain degree of inner or innate intelligence, so it should often be recommended for various herbal blends. At the same time, its angular stems impart the signature of the ability to change direction, to utilize various possibilities in different ways and yet maintain an alignment with the original purpose.

The herb is useful for individuals involved with groups, especially when there is a common energy towards a given project. This is particularly true when it is of a spiritual nature. There is increased ability to be flexible and change direction.

This greatly enhances the intuitive process. Many individuals need only to be exposed to other points of view to know that taking new directions is possible.

The gonorrhea miasm is eased. There is some strengthening of the impact of Uranus, particularly as it progresses through the natal chart. When it is negatively aspected, and one is involved in a project of some importance, this herb should be used.   **GURUDAS**

Meadowsweet (*S. lucida*) is a nurturer like a loving mother. It encourages and is helpful for any kind of nervous condition.

It is useful as a companion herb. It will deepen and broaden the capacity of any herb or substance it is put with.
MULDERS

In bud the big hanging creamy bundles are just bundles of loose-hung granules like farina before it is cooked. They are green and hard swelling slowly to creamy whiteness, each granule bursts and fluffs till the bush looks as if were gobbed all over with generous helps of farina pudding. No sooner has Spiraea fluffed than the sun begins to scorch it and the flowers are burnt and crisped to dark brown.   **EMILY CARR**

ASTROLOGY

In the meadowsweet, the inflorescence in the vicinity of the center shoot is a reflection of Jupiter, similar to the inflorescences of the umbellifers.   **KRANICH**

MYTHS AND LEGENDS

Russian herbalists often tell the story of a brave knight named Kudryash, the strongest man in the village. One morning he woke up filled with fear of his impending death. He was so fearful that he carefully avoided any confrontations that could lead to a fight. During this time a band of marauding thieves were planning to raid the village. The local people looked to Kudryash for leadership.

Ashamed of his fear and feeling powerless against the band of thieves, Kudryash could not sleep nights. One morning he went to the river to drown himself but came upon a beautiful girl instead. In her hand was a garland made of meadowsweet flowers. She told him to wear it for protection. Later that day he fearlessly lead the villagers into battle and they soundly defeated the invaders. Kudryash was declared the saviour of the village and was celebrated for his courage and leadership by the populace.   **ZEVIN**

RECIPES

INFUSION- leaves and/or flowers- Heaping tablespoon (4-6 g) of dried flowers to one pint of water. Steep twenty minutes. The flowers are nearly twice the potency of the leaves. For myalgia and arthralgia take 2-4 ounces twice daily.

DECOCTION- one cup 2-3 x times daily for diarrhea.

TINCTURE- 2-4 ml three times daily. Fresh flowering herb tincture is prepared at 1:2, the dried at 1:5 and 45% alcohol. For rheumatic pain, take 120 drops 3 times daily.

POWDER- One half teaspoon 3x daily in small amount of water.

BEER- Boil two ounces each of dried meadowsweet, agrimony and dandelion in six gallons of water for one half hour. Strain and add two pounds of sugar and half a pint of barm or yeast. Leave stand for twelve hours in warm place. Bottle when nearly finished working.

HARVEST- The first cutting of Meadowsweet is in flower, but includes leaves with white undersides and stems. A second and even third harvest, depending upon the year, is entirely of leaves that are green underneath and no flowers. When making tinctures, make each batch from fresh material and later combine for optimal product.

CAUTION- Do not use if sensitive to salicylates. The German authorities approve of meadowsweet for the common cold.

Do not give meadowsweet to children under sixteen for flu or chicken pox symptoms, due to the rare but serious Reye's syndrome associated with aspirin.

Maybe, this is just theoretical. If you have asthma, use meadowsweet with caution, due to its ability to stimulate bronchial spasms in some people.

COMMON RABBITBRUSH
(*Chrysothamnus nauseosus* [Pall. ex Pursh] Britton) not accepted
(*Ericameria nauseosa* var. *nauseosa* [Pall. ex Pursh] G. L. Nesom & Baird)
GREEN RABBITBRUSH
YELLOW RABBITBRUSH
DOUGLAS RABBITBRUSH
(*C. viscidiflorus* [Hook.] Nutt.)
PARTS USED- flowering tops

Chrysothamnus means, "gold shrub" with **CHRYSOS** from the Greek meaning Gold, and **THAMNOS** meaning, a shrub. Nauseosa is obvious. Ericameria is derived from the Greek, **EREIKE** meaning heath or heather and **MEROS** for part, in reference to the leaf shape. Visidiflorus is derived from Latin **VISCUM**, or bird lime, meaning sticky or clammy, like Viscum (mistletoe) berries. And florus, means flower, hence sticky flower.

The species name refers to the smell of the plant that is sweet and tenacious, but hardly nauseating. It combines visible beauty with invisible digestive upset to cattle, and so the name fits in both respects. Rabbits hide amongst the odorous branches to disguise their scent.

Rabbitbrush was used, by indigenous tribes, for ceremonial and practical purpose. As a tea, it was given to new mothers to relieve after-birth cramping.

Rabbitbrush is called Hairy Plant, **ME?ESHKAATSEH?ESTSE**, or **O'IV IS SE' EYO**, meaning "scabby medicine", by the Cheyenne.

They treated eruptions or sores on the body by washing with infusions from the leaves and stems. If this didn't help, they would next rub it on hard, and in severe cases, the infusion was drunk at the same time.

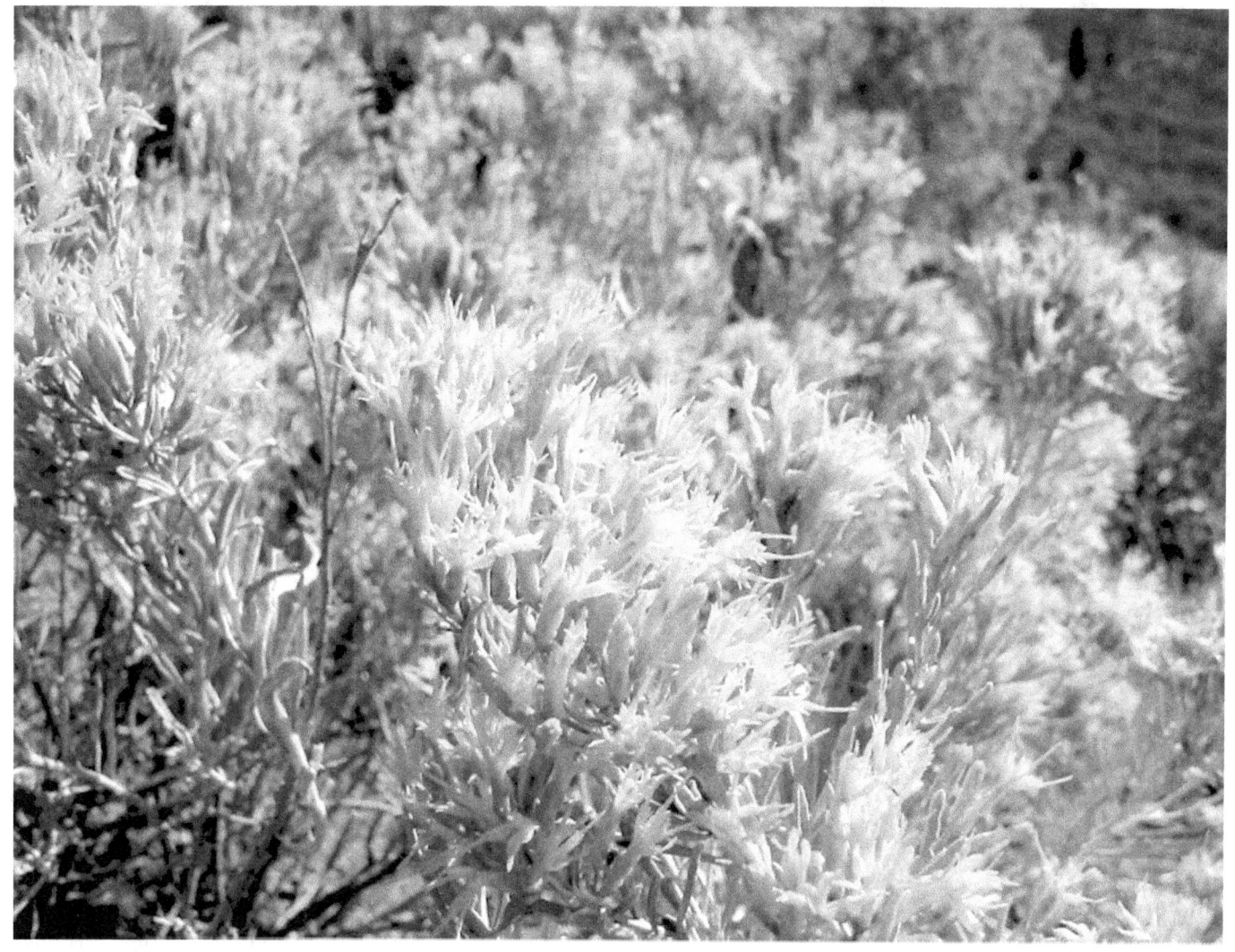

RABBITBRUSH

It was used for smallpox, coughs, colds and tuberculosis, by combining it with one of the many *Artemisia* species.

The cold leaf tea was sometimes applied externally to relieve headaches, and hot internally for constipation, to reduce fevers, colds and stomach pain.

For toothaches, the leaves were crushed, packed into the decayed area, and bitten down on.

The Blackfoot call it Blue Stick Grass. They considered the plant useful for fall and winter forage of their horses. Salves were made of the branches and leaves to help keep flies off horses in the summer.

The women of the Okanagan tribe used the leaves in the manner of sanitary napkins after childbirth. Other tribes, including the Northern Secwepemc drank the tea from the leaves to ease menstrual cramping. The St'at'imc made a leaf infusion and gargled for sore throat.

Other indigenous tribes boiled root decoctions for treating coughs, fevers, colds and menstrual cramps.

Rabbitbrush was used for nightmares; the leaves and branches burnt on coals made from Manitoba Maple. This smoke was believed to drive away the spirits that cause nightmares.

The green branches were burned slowly to smoke hides, and where plentiful for the floors and coverings of sweats.

The milky latex contains rubber compounds that were used by various native tribes as chewing gum.

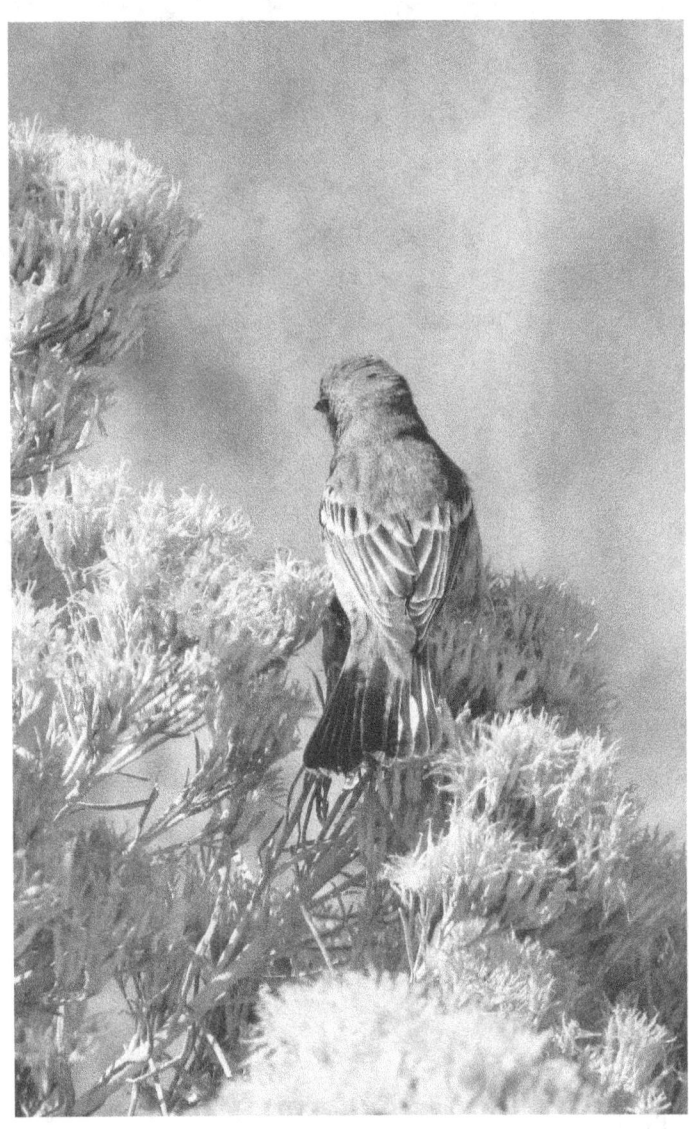
RABBITBRUSH

The Paiute call the plant **SIGUPI**. They dug up the roots in summer and peeled off the bark. If there is a green color, then gum is present.

The outer skin is peeled off and the green part is chewed into fine pieces. The bark is spit out and the gum remains in rubber-like balls.

This is chewed, making a delightful noise that is greatly appreciated for both sexes. This is chewed day after day, lasting a long time, with an entertaining sound. The gum is called **SIGUSANANKA'A**.

The Paiute colored the gum with Tiger lily (*Lilium lanciflorum*) petals.

The leaves were steeped for colds and stomach problems.

The Kawaiisu threaded pine nuts onto sharpened twigs to improve the nuts' flavor.

A tea from *C. viscidiflorus* was used for coughs and colds and leaves a poultice for rheumatism.

The pitch was used on water jugs, and the branches were used for roofing of brush lodges. Today, elders use the flowers for funeral wreaths.

During World War I, the American government considered Rabbitbrush as a potential source of rubber.

Rabbitbrush may be a valuable plant for re-vegetation, wildlife and livestock forage, as well as production of natural rubber, resins for polymer plastics, biomass hydrocarbons for fuel and a source of natural chemical compounds.

Seeds germinate readily, even on saline soils, and the plant can tolerate freezing temperatures as well as hot arid conditions. Several species contain up to 7% rubber, with an average molecular weight of 585,000. Resins are up to 35% in some species with application as plastic extender. These resins contain a wide range of terpenoid compounds including monoterpenes and pregnanes. The latter is chemically related to animal hormones, while the terpenes have known insect inhibiting properties.

The mature flowers and buds were boiled overnight, and baskets are set into the liquid for a few hours to produce a bright yellow dye. In parts of the American Southwest the yellow flowers are boiled with Rocky Mountain Bee Plant for a yellow paint.

Green Rabbitbrush is similar, with brittle twigs that are only slightly hairy.

It is found on dry, open sites on the plains or foothills of southern British Columbia all the way down to New Mexico.

The Paiute infused the leaves for colds, and decocted them for more severe coughs. They also used the branches as beds in sweats for relieving rheumatism. The Shoshone poulticed the crushed stems and leaves on affected rheumatic joints or muscles, and drank decoctions internally for the flu.

Finely mashed leaves were inserted into toothache cavities, for temporary relief.

Bears consume ants, and their damaged nests allow for the spread of Green Rabbitbrush. Grinath JB et al, *Ecol Lett* 2015 18(2): 164-73.

Both species show anthelmintic activity against Barber Pole worm, *Haemonchus contortus*, a gastro-intestinal nematode that affects sheep, goats and range animals. They are rarely an issue for humans, but females can produce up to ten thousand eggs a day. Acharya J et al, *Vet Parasitol* 2014 201(1-2): 75-81.

MEDICINAL

CONSTITUENTS- *C. viscidiflorus*- aerial parts- chrysothol, sesquiterpenes, cinnamic derivatives, ketoalcohol derivatives, and coumarin glucoside.

Both rabbitbrush species change their chemical composition of leaves from summer to winter. This may influence the dietary changes of mule deer and other browsers.

Several compounds in Yellow Rabbitbrush, including chrysothol show anti-cancer activity against human breast cancer cells. Ahmed AA et al, *Phytochemistry* 2006 67(4): 1547-53.

Chrysothol inhibits LPS induced nitric oxide production in RAW264.7 cells, suggesting anti-inflammatory activity. This compound is also found in Water Plantain (*Alisma* sp.). Li HM et al, *Chem Pharm Bull* (Tokyo) 2017 65(4): 403-7.

ESSENTIAL OIL

Rabbitbrush has been steam distilled and found to contain an essential oil with 22.8% beta phellandrene and 19.8% beta pinene. Complete analysis found at Tabanca et al, *J Ag Food Chem* 2007 55:21.

FLOWER ESSENCES

Rabbitbrush (*C. nauseosus*) flower essence is for individuals who are easily overwhelmed by details, and are unable to cope with simultaneous events or demanding situations. The essence helps create an active and lively consciousness, with an alert, flexible and mobile state of mind.   **FLOWER ESSENCE SOCIETY**

Rabbitbrush is about the power and wisdom of stillness. It's very good for people who have a hard time doing that at all, like those who are compensating for their wounding by being overly active and busy.
HIGH SIERRA

PERSONALITY TRAITS

Psychologically, Rabbitbrush functions at a much different level because it touches the instinctual/little kid self with innocence and a sense of wonder, like when you see a wild animal and it looks you in the eye…It helps one use stillness as part of being a whole medicine person, teaching the necessity of stillness to fully understand anything at all.

A beautiful comparison is the silence that happens when snow falls, almost like one can become so still that even intense activity takes on a gentle, calming, soothing quality.   **HIGH SIERRA**

MYTHS AND LEGENDS

The rabbit is, in most mythologies, a trickster, culture hero or symbol of fertility. Brer Rabbit, for example, came from the Trickster Hare of West Africa and slaves introduced to America.

The Japanese story of White Rabbit, who tricked crocodiles into making a bridge for him, is an example. As he approached the last jump, and began boasting, the angry croc caught him and skinned him alive.

In Greece and Rome, the rabbit was linked with fertility and Aphrodite, the goddess of love and sexuality. The German goddess Eostra (Easter) owned a hare in the moon that laid eggs, symbolizing renewed life.

The Aztec deities known as the Centzon Totochtin, means Four Hundred Rabbits, and represented both sexuality and trickery.   **VARIOUS SOURCES**

Hares and Rabbits have strong lunar symbolism possibly because the moon's patches resembled leaping hares to the ancients. As a result, they were linked with menstruation and with fertility in African, Native American, Celtic, Buddhist, Chinese, Egyptian, Greek, Hindu and Teutonic tradition. The hare was an attribute of lunar and hunter goddesses in the classical and Celtic worlds, and also of the Greek gods Eros (as passion) and Hermes (as speedy messenger)…Folklore attributes harmless guile to rabbits, and in North American myths the lunar hare plays a creative role in shaping nature to human advantage.   **JACK TRESIDDER**

GARDEN RADISH
(*Raphanus sativus* L.)
(*R. raphanistrum* ssp. *sativus* [L.] Domin)
BLACK RADISH
(*R. sativus* L. var. *nigra* [Mill.] S.K.)
(*Raphanus nigrum* Mill.)
WILD RADISH
JOINTED CHARLOCK
(*R. raphanistrum* L.)
(*Raphanistrum arvense* Wallr.) not accepted
DAIKON RADISH
(*R. sativa* var. *longpinnatus* L H Bailey)
(*R. sativa* L. var. *hortensis* Baker.)
(*R. sativa* var. *macropodus* [H. Levi] Makino)

MOUGRI RADISH
RAT TAIL RADISH
CAUDATUS
(*R. mougri* H. W. J. Helm) not accepted
(*R. sativa* L. var. *caudatus*)
FODDER or OIL RADISH
(*R. oleifera*)
(*R. sativus* L. var. *oleifera* Stokes)
PART USED- root, seeds, leaves

"Radishes are eaten with salt alone, as carrying their pepper in them".
What do I know of man's destiny? I could tell you more about radishes.   **SAMUEL BECKETT**

If you eat more radish in winter, and more ginger in summer, you needn't see the doctor.
                                                                                                CHINESE SAYING

Radish is from the Latin **RADIX** meaning root, and hence the Old English **RAEDIC**. Raphanus is a corruption of the Greek **RA** quickly; and **PHAINO** to appear, attesting to the rapid easy germination and growth of the plant. The French call radish a poetic, Roses d'hiver, or Roses of Winter.

The wild radish was introduced from Europe and is considered a widespread weed throughout the eastern prairies.

The seedpods when immature are fleshy, juicy and quite delicious, and a good addition to a spring salad.

The radish was grown in ancient Egypt over four thousand years ago and distributed to the thousands of slaves who built the pyramids to protect them from disease. It then made its way to China about 500 BC, and later to Japan about 700 AD. Radishes were so valued in ancient Greece that offerings to the God Apollo were small replicas of radishes formed from gold. Beets rated silver, and the lowly turnip lead.

Most consumers are familiar with the white fleshed, red-coated variety found in supermarkets. But there are several species with culinary and medicinal value.

A new red dye, derived from red radish, is now available from RFI ingredients, for use in functional foods, beverages, dairy products, salad dressings, etc.

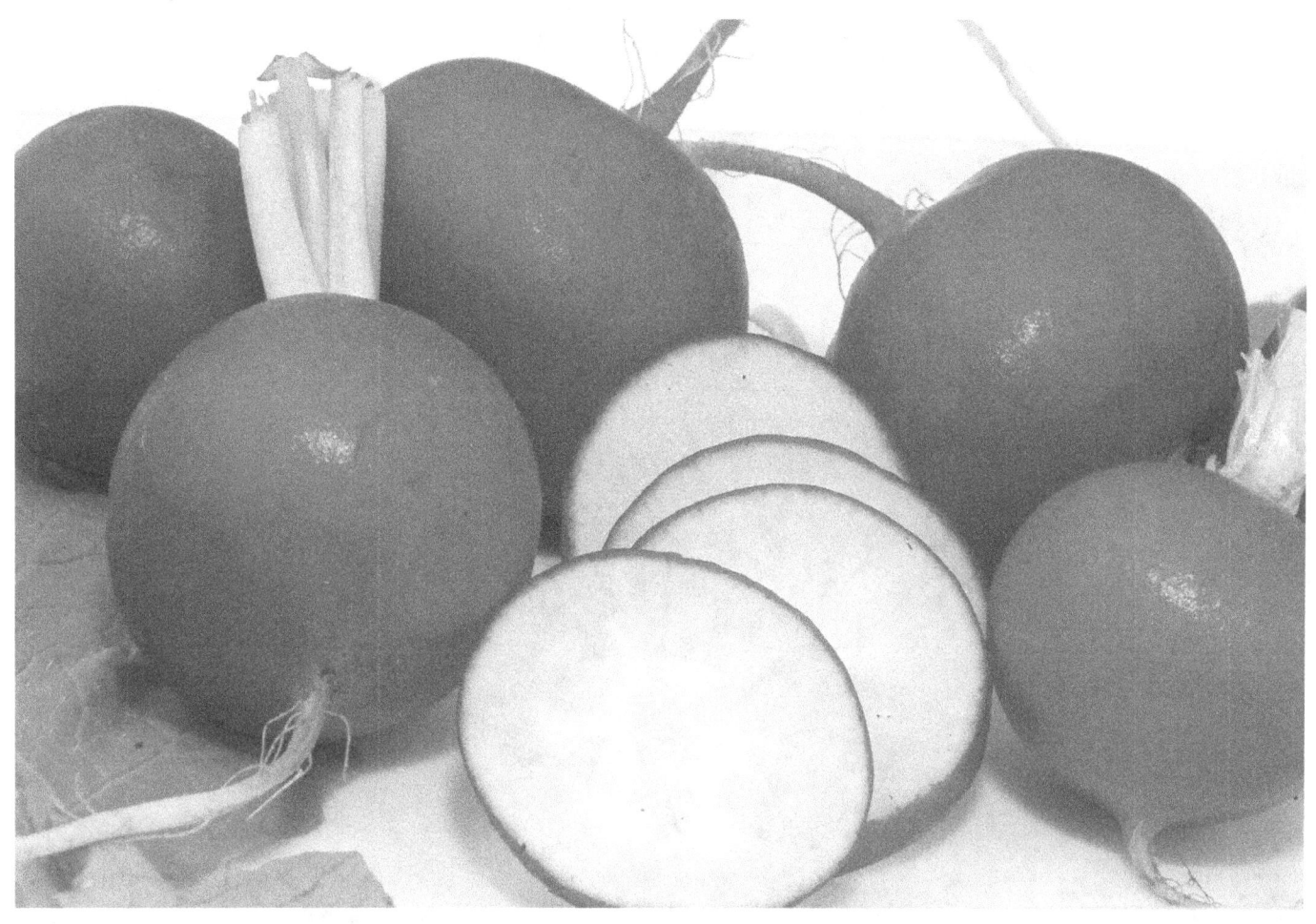

GARDEN RADISH

The Radish was originally introduced to Europe as a long white-rooted variety in the 16ᵗʰ century. In Bavaria, the white radish is eaten as an accompaniment with beer and is called Bier Radi.

The Black or Spanish Radish originated in the Mediterranean region.

One of my favorites is the Violet de Gourney Radish, from a cross between the red and black over many years of selection in France. The Gourney is a cold hardy variety that can take a hard frost without splitting; and both its intense violet colour and flavour add zest to salads, or when steamed like a turnip.

In Mexico, the wild radish leaves are harvested for cattle feed, and eaten during food shortages by humans.

Artists carve the long, white radishes grown near Oaxaca into sculptures to celebrate the annual Night of the Radishes. Prizes are given for best carvings.

In a study by Patil et al, *Adv in Agric Research in India* 1997 8 it was found that tomatoes inter-cropped with radish were significantly less infected with tomato fruit borer. Radish growth is helped by Redroot Pigweed, that helps loosen the soil, and by Nasturtiums. Never plant radish and hyssop together, as they dislike each other.

Radish Feast, first held in 1280, was a common, peculiar annual custom in England.

Today, radish sprouts can be found in most supermarkets, alongside alfalfa, broccoli, buckwheat, and others. The unripe fruit are delicious raw, and in Asia are made into a green sauce from the extracted juice.

The flowers themselves make a spicy and decorative touch to salads. The flower buds and tender tips can also be steamed like the broccoli they resemble. When fresh and tender, the leaves may be cooked like spinach, or added to soups. They can also be dried for later use as tea infusions.

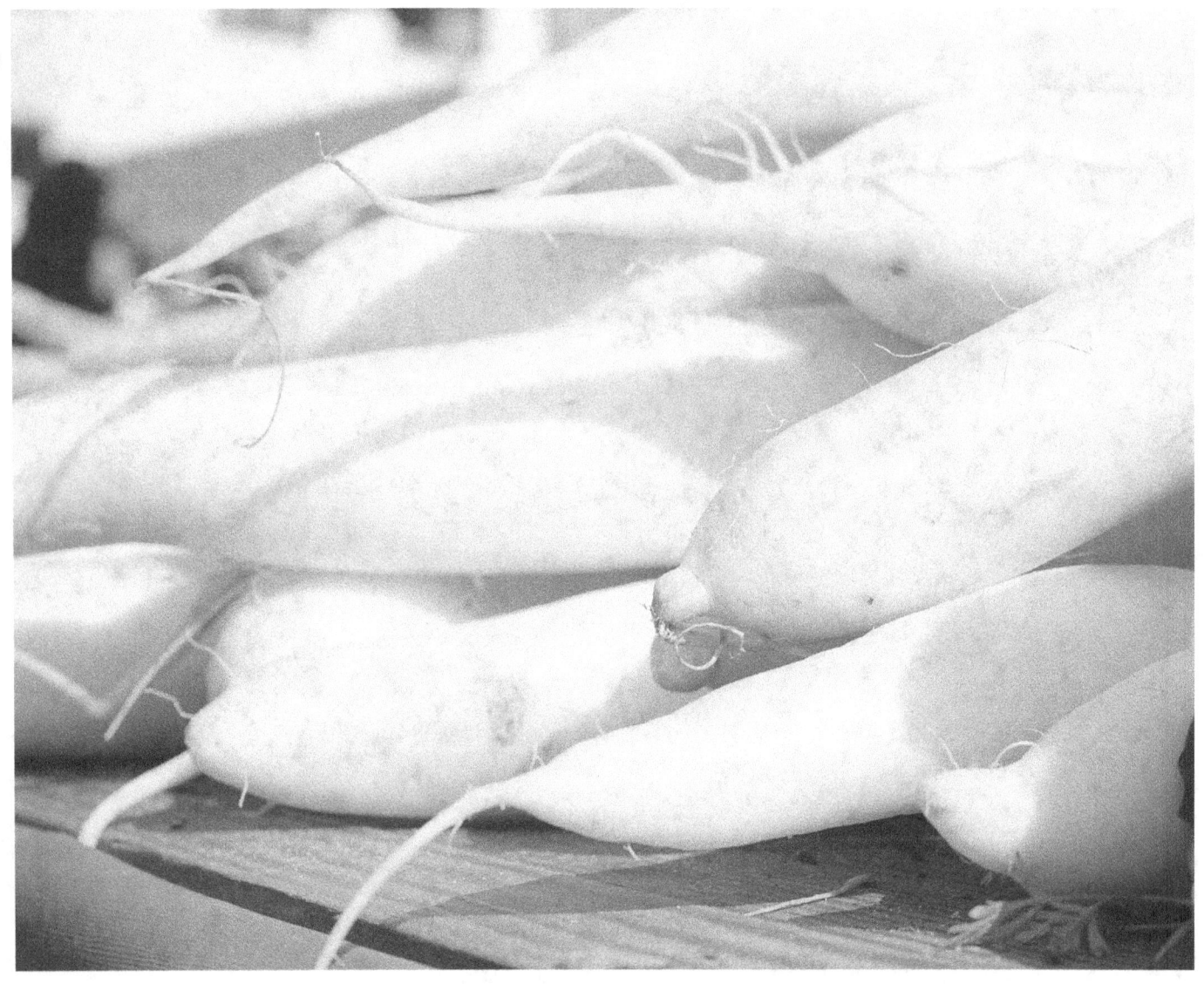

DAIKON RADISH

A new type of cuisine, sweeping North America, involves infant vegetables, including radish, beets, carrots, leeks, etc. The immature plants are the hottest trend in what Lee Jones from Ohio, calls the "first stages of a vegetable revolution. We can affect the nutrient and sugar level in our plants by 300%, just by improving the soil. We actually measure the brix (sugar content) in our lettuce. The rest of the world is rushing forward, but we're going back."

Jones has identified six stages of growth, each with its own flavour spectrum: cotyledon, micro, petite, ultra, young, flowering and seed stage. "At every stage of life, a plant offers something to the plate", he says.

Not all experiments with breeding radish have been a success. In 1924, the Soviet geneticist Alexi Karpenchinko crossed a radish and cabbage. He named this Rabage, expecting a plump cabbage head on an edible round root. Instead what developed was a head of scraggly radish leaves and thin, useless roots of a cabbage.

Peroxidase from radish is a good substitute for that extracted from horseradish to degrade phenols and various other aromatic, toxic chemicals. Ziai et al, *J Med Plants* 5.

Methyl marcapten, present in both the root and seed, has anti-fungal and pesticide properties. As a chemical, it is a jet fuel additive.

Daikon Radish, a long, white rooted vegetable familiar as a sushi condiment, can weight up to 20 kilograms each. One variety can grow up to 100 pounds!

The two Japanese characters making up the word Daikon mean, "Great Root". The name is connected in myth with Daikoku, a famous hero and Buddhist guardian of good harvests. A ritual marriage of a radish and Daikoku is still performed around the winter solstice to placate the gods and the return of spring and growth.

It has only 20 calories per cup, and yet supplies 36% of our recommended, daily amount of vitamin C.

As well, it has a well-earned reputation for aiding the digestion of fatty foods. It is the most important cruciferous vegetable in Japan. The pickled or simply shredded radish is often served with Japanese or Korean meals as a digestive aid. The technique of shaving Katsura Muki into a massive strip is difficult to master, even for sushi chefs.

The Chinese grate the root to make **LO BAAK GOR** a heavy radish and rice flour pudding that is steamed, then sliced and fried. It is commonly served at good Dim Sum restaurants.

Laboratory analysis shows the juice of raw daikon is abundant in digestive enzymes similar to those found in the human digestive tract-diastase, amylase, and esterase.

It is a great aid to those with weak digestive systems. But it must be used immediately, as 50% of the enzymes are destroyed only thirty minutes after grating.

In traditional Indonesian herbal healing, or Jamu, the daikon is known as **LOBAK**, and used to relieve edema.

In China, the dried daikon radish leaf *LUO BO YE* is used to relieve diarrhea and dysentery. It also relieves appetite and helps regulate the flow of vital energy in the body.

Decoctions of the fresh root *LUO BO* are given for digestive distress, hoarseness, thirst, migraine, nosebleed and blood in the sputum.

The fresh juice helps lower blood pressure when taken in small amounts for week or two.

Decoctions of the dried, shrunken root, *DI GU LUO* are a soothing diuretic, used in urinary irritation and water retention.

The seeds contain fats and oils, and help keep the Chi from becoming overactive, and help in the treatment of asthma, indigestion and excessive phlegm.

Radishes over 100 pounds have been grown; Sukarijma being the largest cultivar.

Mougri (Mouli) or Rat-tailed Radish is cultivated in India and Southeast Asia for its edible leaves and seedpods, which grow up to three feet in length. The long white radish is valued for its liver regenerative properties and constipation.

Korean Radish, known as **MU**, usually refers to Joseon radish to distinguish it from **WAE** the Japanese variety, which is longer, thinner and moister. Korean radish is shorter, more sturdy, and pale green halfway down root.

The soft greens, known as **MUCHEONG** are used as a vegetable.

Oilseed Radish is being grown for its foliage as animal fodder more frequently in Canada. It is a cross between Fodder Radish, Fodder rape and Rapeseed.

The annual grows very fast, becoming two to three feet tall in four to six weeks, and can yield up to 10 tons of green matter in 45 days, or 1.5 tons of dry matter in 60 days.

It is a good cover crop for weed control, and a natural nematode when disked under. It contains 22-24% protein.

If grown for seed, swath when the seeds start to turn brown, and leave to mature for week on ground.

Ozawa et al, have reported the isolation and identification of a novel yellow beta barboline pigment in salted garden radish roots.

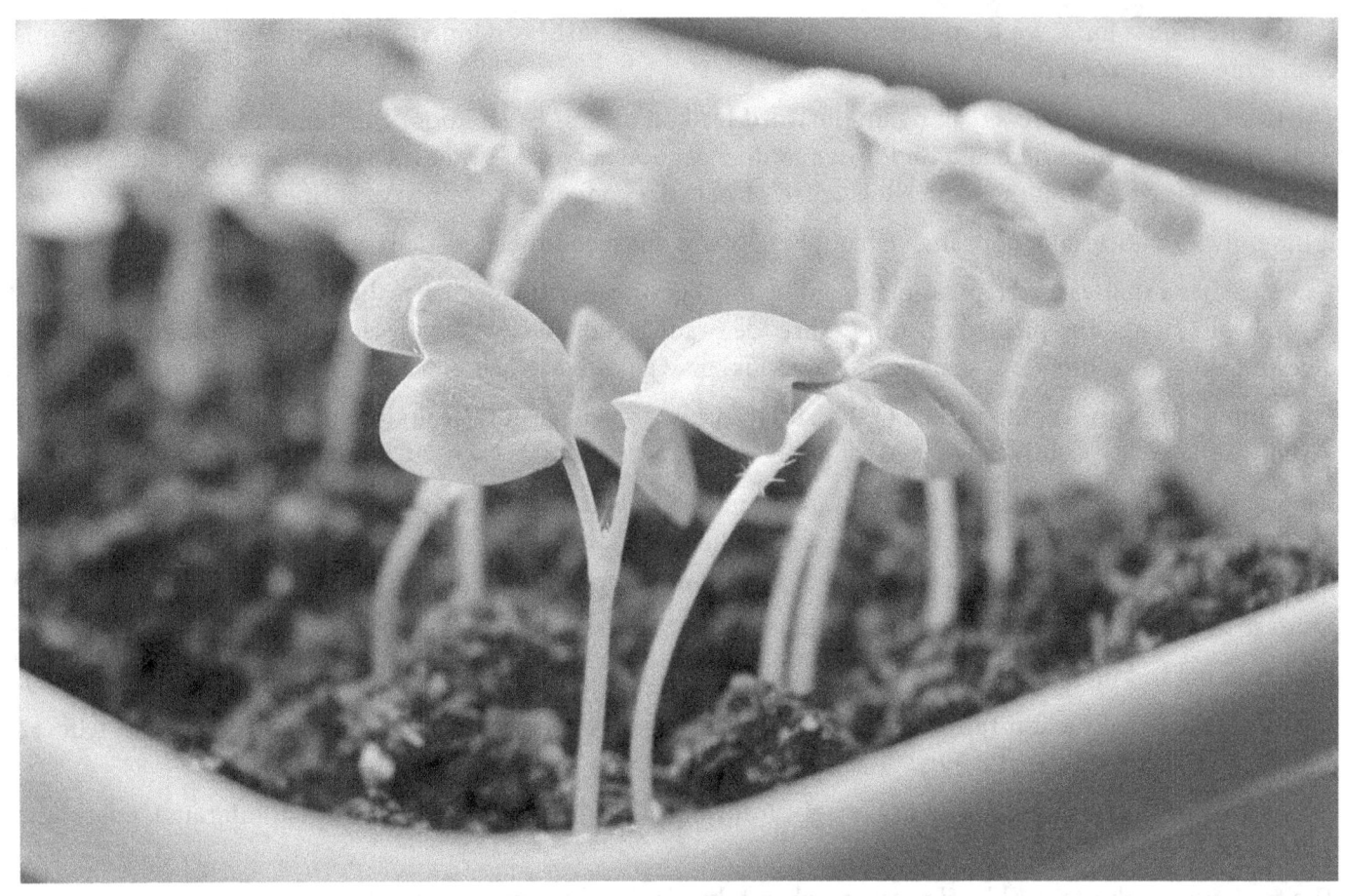

RADISH SPROUTS

MEDICINAL

CONSTITUENTS- *R. sativus* fresh root- glucosinolates, pentosane, adeneine, arginine, histidine, choline, trigonelline, diastaste, oxydase, phospholipase D, catalase, Vit A, B and C, allyl isothiocyanate, sulfuraphene, and oxalic acid. The root also contains trans-4-(methylthio)-3-butenyl glucosinolate, methanethiol, rasatiol, protease inhibitors, defensin, and dithiolthiones. The pink radish contains anthocyanic pigments such as cyanin and pelargonin; while the black lacks this, but has glucoraphene, a sulphurated heteroside with antibiotic properties. The pigment in the purplish coloured edible part is malvin chloride. Roots contain trace minerals such as aluminum, barium, lithium, manganese, silicon, titanium, fluorine and iodine (18 mcg/100 grams). Six day old seedling roots contain alpha-L-fucosyltransferase.
Cotyledons- olomucine.
leaves- essential oil, vit A and C
seed- 30-40% fatty oil with erucic acid, linoleic and linolenic acid, glycerol sinapate, sinapic acid, raphanin and methyl mercaptan; eight phenylpropanoid sucrosides, including raphasativuside A-B; seven 4-methyl thiobutanyl derivatives.
Also contains Rs-AFP2, a 51 amino acid cysteine rich peptide, sulphoraphene, and galactan/arabinogalactans in 16:83 ratio.
R. raphanistrum- fresh plant- glucoputranjivine, that yields isopropyl mustard oil as the cells are destroyed; senevol, glucoraphenine, zinc, nickel, cobalt and sulphur.
R. sativa var. hortensis root- brassitin, N-methoxyspirobrassinol methyl ether, and N-methoxyspirobrassinol.
sprout- sinapinic acid esters, flavonoids

The common garden radish has many medicinal uses for those willing to look.

The leaves are diuretic, laxative, and able to break or crush kidney and gall stones. The fresh leaf juice is useful for slow or painful urine flow with calculi or gravel in small frequent doses with lots of water. Decoctions of the leaf are used in China for application to the temples in headaches, chest congestion, hiccups, indigestion and sore throats. The leaves are also used for breast swelling, or shortage of milk secretion.

The dry radish leaves are also boiled in water with some salt, and used to bath irritated or itchy genital areas in women.

Korean Radish leaves shows anti-inflammatory activity, suppressing COX-2 and iNOS expression. Park HJ & Song M, *Prev Nutr Food* 2017 22(1): 50-55.

The flowers possess cholagogue properties.

The root is useful for urinary complaints or hemorrhoids. The root can be made into syrup for hoarseness, whooping cough, and other bronchial or chest complaints. The dried root powder will work just as well. The fresh root is a good digestive.

Radish root juice is one-third potassium and one-third sodium, helping to both build muscle tissue and prevent accumulation of acidic deposits in the blood stream. Refrigerate for several hours before using to moderate the acrid taste.

It also contains iodine and chlorine, having good influence on thyroid health.

If the fresh leaf and root are juiced, combine one part with seven of celery juice. Do not take when the stomach is inflamed.

Radish contains raphanin, a sulphur compound with the ability to both suppress and balance thyroid problems. Radish is used extensively in Russia specifically for hyperthyroidism, Grave's disease; as well as low thyroid. Raphanin helps keep calcitonin levels normalized in the blood stream, something of interest to those suffering osteoporosis.

Radishes contain isothiocyanates and protease inhibitors that suppress and prevent cancer and viral growth. Conoway et al, *Curr Drug Metab* 2002:3.

Methanethiol, present in both red and white varieties, suppresses abnormal cell growth.

Sulphoraphene is anti-bacterial against *Streptococcus, Pyococcus, Pneumococcus and E. coli*. Raphinin shows inhibition of *Staphylococcus aureus, Bacillus dysenteriae, Salmonella typhi* and *E. coli*.

Radishes are rather good accumulators of vanadium, a catalytic of enzymes and insulin production.

Radish root juice impregnated in a cotton ball has been found effective against *Trichomonas vaginalis*. In one study 62 out of 68 human cases were cured.

Fresh radish juice is anti-fungal and anti-bacterial, and useful in chronic bronchial conditions such as silicosis, or tuberculosis of the lungs. Slice radish and cover with honey overnight for a superior cough syrup.

Defensin, or AFP2, also found in fruit flies, is an active anti-fungal of radish root. Work by Aerts et al, *FEBS* 583:15 found the anti-fungal protein induces apoptosis and triggers activation of caspases against *Candida albicans*.

In enemas, it is diluted, and useful for treating allergic colitis, diarrhea and chronic ulcerative colitis.

Radish root is a potent protector against hepatoxicity induced by chemicals. Chaturvedi et al, *Int J Vit Nutr Res* 77:1.

Radish root juice shows anti-diabetic activity. Shukla et al, *Pharm Biol* 2010 August 5. Radish extracts lower blood sugar, and contain a SOD-like protein. Habib et al, *Biochimie* 2012 94:5.

The roots contain sulforaphene, also present in broccoli, cabbage and related Brassica species. When combined with the chemotherapy drug carboplatin, enhanced apoptosis and anti-proliferation of A549, non-small cell lung carcinoma was noted. Chatterjee S et al, *J Med Food* 2016 19(9): 860-9.

The root contains rasatiol, which stimulates fibrous components of extracellular matrix produced by dermal fibroblasts, suggesting application for maintenance of connective tissue integrity. Roh SS et al, *Ann Dermatol* 2013 25(3): 315-20.

The waste peel of radish root shows activity against various bacteria. Ethanol extracts show high MIC against *Salmonella typhi* and *Klebsiella pneumoniae*; and very high zones of inhibition against *Micrococcus luteus, Pseudomonas aeruginosa, Bordetella bronchiseptica* and *Enterobacter aerogenes*. Janjua S et al, *Adv in Med Plant Research* 2012 1:1.

Radish, fermented in brine, undergoes a series of bacterial population, but Lactibacillus brevis is present in final product, along with lactic acid, acetic acid and ethanol.

Garden Radish leaf and stem tea has been shown to improve sperm motility and numbers as well as alleviate prostatitis. A US patent 5736144 for this purpose has been granted, based on submission of several case studies.

The Garden Radish is known in Ayurvedic medicine as **MULAKA**. The root is considered heavy, wind forming and sharp. Alone it aggravates all doshas but when prepared with fat, alleviates all three. The seed alleviates kapha and pitta; while the flower alleviates kapha and vata imbalance.

The seeds are easy to harvest and make excellent hot, spicy sprouts. They take 5-6 days to mature, with the shells falling off easily. A white fur is common in early growth and easily rinsed away. This is indicative of inadequate watering pressure, frequency or volume. China Rose Radish is the best sprout.

Radish sprouts have 29 times more vitamin C, and four times more vitamin A than milk, ten times more calcium than a potato and more vitamin C than pineapple. Takaya et al, *J Ag Food Chem* 2003:51 found radish sprouts exhibit free radical scavenging nearly double that of L-ascorbic acid.

Medicinally, they can be taken for their laxative, diuretic and expectorant properties like above. They can be infused for soothing and carminative action on the stomach.

Radish sprout juice decreased diet-induced obesity in an animal study, lowering total cholesterol levels, body and liver weight. Vivarelli F et al, *PLoS One* 2016 11(3).

Raphanin is an active anti-bacterial present in seeds.

Water extractions of the seeds show activity against gram-positive, gram-negative bacteria and mycobacterium.

Activity against *S. aureus, E. coli, Salmonella typhi-H, S. typhi-O, S. paratyphi B, Pseudomonas pyocyanea, Bacillus anthracis, B. subtilis* and *Chromobact prodigiosum* was noted in work by Ivanovics and Horvath in 1947. Recent work found ethanol extracts inhibit *Streptococcus pyogenes* and *E. coli*. Jadoun J et al, *Evid Based Complement Altern Med* 2016;2016:9271285.

Work by Shishu et al, *Planta Medica* 2003 69:2 found sulphurophanes inhibit various cooked food mutagens (heterocylic amines).

Arabinogalactan polysaccharides in radish seed are immune stimulating and modulating.

In Traditional Chinese Medicine, the dried ripe radish seed is known in Mandarin as **LAI FU ZI**. In Cantonese, the seed is called **LAAI FUK JI**, and in Japanese Kampo Herbal Medicine, it is known as **RAIFUKUSHI.**

The seed tea relieves coughs and resolves phlegm, removing copious expectoration. In asthma, with a tight chest, it acts as a bronchodilator.

When stir-fried until yellow, the seed tea is more useful for food stagnation, distention of the abdomen, and vomiting of undigested food, combining well with stir fried Hawthorn fruits.

Studies conducted in India in 1986, showed seed extracts possessed human anti-fungal activity, including *Candida albicans.*

Additional work by Alves et al, in Belgium 1994 showed that radish seed isolates exhibited potent anti-fungal activity. One compound, machrolysin, is a specific against *Mycobacterium tuberculosis.*

The seeds contain both essential and fatty oils, and can be considered a digestive stimulant that removes stagnant food, dysbiosis and toxicosis of the gut. They are relaxing, and as such are both laxative and useful in simple and infectious diarrhea. The seeds exhibit both anti-viral and anti-bacterial activity. Raphanin from water extracts of the seeds exhibit activity against both gram positive and gram-negative bacteria.

Radish seed water extract may be useful in ameliorating intestinal oxidative and inflammatory damage in ulcerative colitis animal models. Choi KC et al, *J Ethnopharm* 2016 179:55-65.

Phenylpropanoids, derived from radish seeds are cytotoxic against A549, SK-OV-3, SK-MEL-2 and HCT-15. Kim KH et al, *Bioorg Med Chem Lett* 2015 25(1): 96-9.

Derivatives of 4-methyl thiobutanyl in seeds showed anti-proliferative activity against HCT-15 cancer cell lines. Kim KH et al, *J Ethnopharm* 2014 151(1): 503-8.

Sprouted radish seeds, or **KAIWARE**, make a hot, peppery addition to salads and garnish.

During sprouting of Daikon radish seeds, the levels of glucoraphasatin increase 25 fold in ten days. The compound shows significant antioxidant activity in work by Barillari et al, *J Ag Food Chem* 2005 53. Work by Taniguchi et al, *Phytother Res* 20:4 found radish sprouts prevent and treat elevated blood sugar levels.

Papi et al, *J Ag Food Chem* 2008 56:3 found daikon radish sprouts active against three colon carcinoma cell lines.

Water-soluble extracts have been found to lower glucose levels without increasing insulin secretion in diabetic rats. Lower levels of glucoalbumin and fructosamine were found.

Radish sprout powder may be effective for habitual constipation. In one study of 32 elderly patients given the dry powder in water, 20 had a bowel movement within 12 hours, nine within 24 hours and 3 still had none. Chongching *Med Herb* 1986 6:46.

The sprout powder was also tested on 467 patients with hypertension with a reduction noted in 92% and significant lowering of blood pressure in 49.8%. Effect was attributed to either dilation of blood vessels or sedation of CNS. *Report of Medical Studies* 1986 6:46.

In one study in China, tablets were prepared of the dried seeds (5 gram each) and given to 70 essential hypertensive patients (4-6 tablets twice daily). Marked improvement was noted in 31 cases and some improvement in 29 others. The systolic pressure was decreased by 25 mmHg and diastolic by 13 mmHg after two to five weeks.

The cotyledons of red radish contain olomucine. This compound has been used as a template for development of drug roscovtine, also known as seliciclib or CYC202. It is currently in phase two clinical trials for treatment of non-small cell lung cancer, and may be useful for leukemia, AIDS and cystic fibrosis. Meijer et al, *Accounts of Chem Res* 2003 36.

Daikon radish contains isothiocyanate that possesses both anti-cancer and anti-inflammatory properties. The compound degrades in water, but is best picked up and absorbed with fats and oils. Ippoushi K et al, *Food Chem* 2014 161: 176-80.

Dr. Fohr, a German physician, re-discovered the therapeutic properties of Black Radish. In some parts of Germany, gallstones were very rare, and studying the eating habits, he noted they always began their meals with a black radish salad. He experimented and noted the radish provoked progressive contractions of the gallbladder, insuring its continual drainage.

Black Radish is noted for medicinal benefit from the root, acting initially in the intestine, increasing peristaltic action.

It is not a true cholagogue that promotes bile formation but increases secretion of bile by stimulating gall bladder contraction, and allowing a freer flow. This choleretic combination makes it useful for biliary tract congestion, gas and heartburn; combining well with dandelion root juice for added benefit.

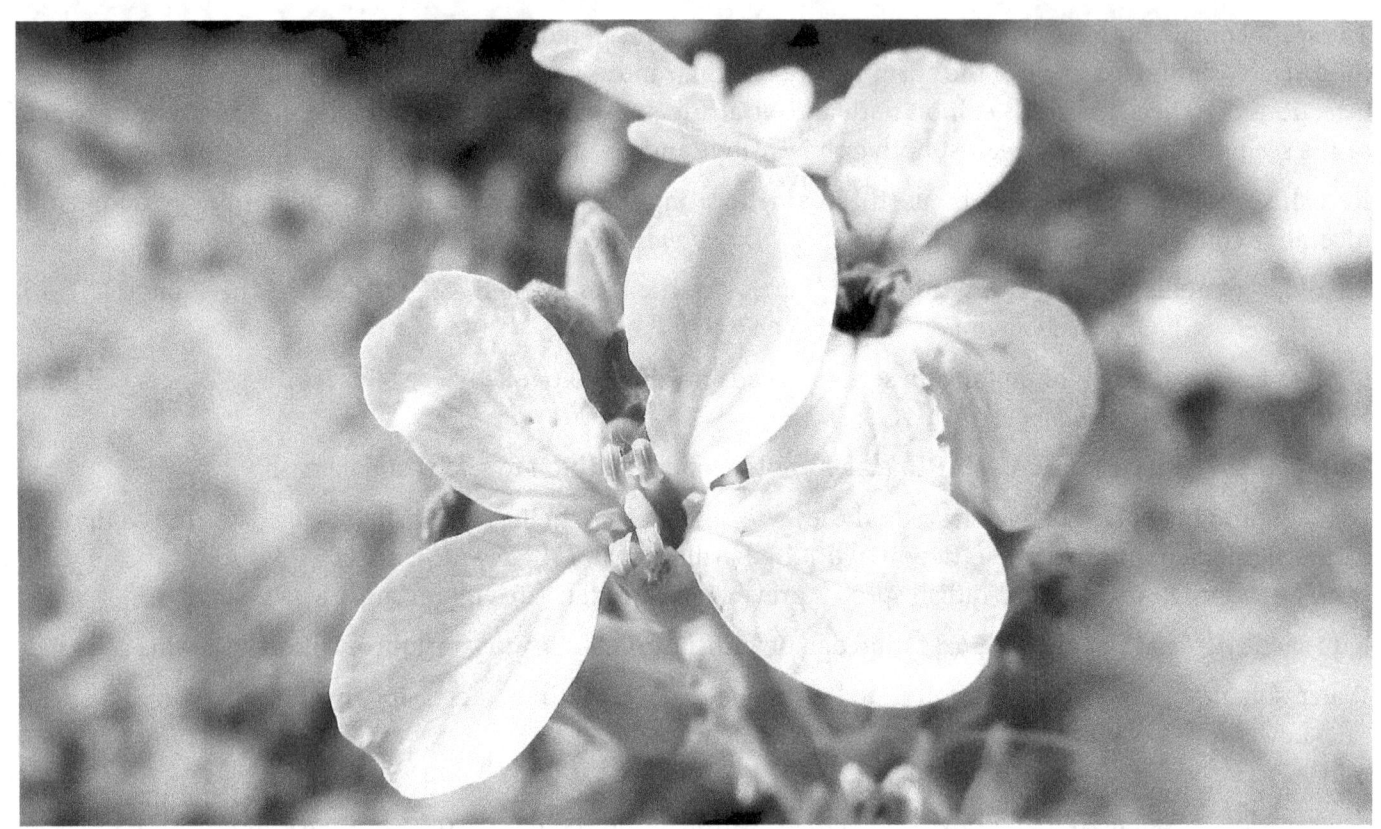

WILD RADISH FLOWER

Black radish contains compounds that prevent formation of cholesterol gallstones, including glucosinolates. Castro-Torres IG et al, *Phytother Res* 2014 28(2): 167-71.

Work by Kumar et al, *Nepal Med Coll J* 2004:6 showed a diet containing radish increased excretion of calcium oxalate in both genders.

The stem bark, decocted as a water extract, reduces the size of kidney stones. Vargas et al, *J Ag Food Chem* 68:1-3.

Lugasi et al, *Phytother Res* 19:7 found black radish juice decreases hyperlipidemia. Water extracts have been found to induce detoxification enzymes in HepG2 cell lines. Hanlon et al, *J Ag Food Chem* 55:16.

Radish is a potent liver protectant, helping reduce zearalenone related liver damage. This is a common toxin in corn products. Salah-Abbes et al, *J Pharm Pharmacol* 2009 61:11.

The healing benefits of black radish are believed due, at least in part, to raphanol, a sulphuric etheric oil, and glycoside.

The root is used for bronchitis, as well as inflammation of the urinary tract. In fact, it can be a powerful sedative for coughs and is used for treating asthma in certain constitutions.

Black radish can also act as an anti-allergic against urticaria.

For whooping cough, or chronic bronchitis, take a whole fresh root and cut the top off and make a hole. Fill this with honey, and allow to stand a day or two. Take a teaspoon 2-3 times daily.

Tinctures of black radish root can prevent the aggravation of pulmonary fibrosis via decreasing transforming growth factor-beta1 levels, associated with this ailment. Asghari MH et al, *Res Pharm Sci* 2015 10(5): 429-35.

Research conducted by Prahoveanu et al in Romania found that water extracts of black radish administered nasally before introduction of the influenza virus, ensured some protection.

Hanna Kroger uses Black Radish in one of her formulas for strep throat.

It should be avoided in cases of acute gastritis, or liver inflammation due to its stimulating properties. It should also be used with caution in thyroid conditions, as glycosinolates can have goitergenic effect.

The anti-oxidant and free radical scavenging properties of fresh black radish juice have been confirmed in a study by Lugasi, *Phytotherapy Research* 1998 12:7.

Wild Radish herb is used as a ground leaf or alcohol extraction in Germany for various skin conditions and stomach disorders. Extracts of the plant indicate both gram positive and negative bacteria killing activity.

At flowering, the plant contains up to 50% glucosinolates. It is often planted and plowed under at this point for weed suppression. Malik et al, *Phytochem* 2010 58:6.

Slight cardiotoxicity has been noted in frogs, so be careful not to feed your amphibian friends too many radishes.

In Traditional Chinese Medicine, Daikon Radish, or **LAI FU TZU**, is used for resolving phlegm and curing intestinal parasites. It is most often used for indigestion, abdominal distention, hiccups, excessive sputum, asthma, abdominal pain and diarrhea. Take 5-10 grams of raw root in decoction.

Researchers at Tokyo's College of Pharmacy have discovered that daikon juice actually inhibits the formation of dangerous chemicals in the body.

Nitrosamines which form in the stomach, from natural and processed foods, are neutralized by the phenolic compounds in daikon juice.

Daikon is an effective diuretic, increasing urination in cases of edema. The enzymes also help to dissolve mucous and phlegm in the respiratory system, and assist removal from the body. The root is a good source of calcium.

Daikon radish sprout extracts exhibit 1.8 times the anti-oxidant potency of vitamin C. Takaya et al, *J Ag Food Chem* 2003 51.

Rat Tail Radish ethanol extracts demonstrated notable anti-depressant activity in a mice study. Younus I et al, *Afr J Tradit Complement Altern Med* 2017 14(3): 142-6.

HOMEOPATHY

Raphanus (Black Garden Radish) is for burning and vomiting from the stomach, with attendant loss of appetite. The stomach and intestine are hard, and yet gas will not pass upward nor down.

The mind may be sad, with headaches where the brain is sore and tender. There may be edema of the lower eyelids.

In the female, there may be nervous irritation of the genitals, with profuse and long lasting menses. There may be nymphomania or sexual insomnia; with aversion to her own sex, and children.

Extreme anxiety, thinks she will die. Feeling of aversion towards women but attracted to all men. Fears she will be burden to everyone. Anger alternating with depression. Dreams of killing own children.

The urine is copious, thick and cloudy like milk.

Chest pains with coldness in the centre, and the sensation of a heavy lump.

DOSE- Third to thirtieth potency. The mother tincture is prepared from the fresh root. Proving by Nusser with tincture and second dilution in 1830s. Proving by Curie with one female with tincture, 15th and 30th dilutions around 1854 plus clinical observations of Hering and Mangialavori.

Raphanistrum arvense is for a kind of appetite without hunger, at 4 am in bed. Talking during sleep, light sleep with painful dreams of death, sleep better toward morning.

Frequent shivering descending along back, perspiration in morning.

Heat at root of tongue, frequent burning in forepart of tongue. Heat in lower abdomen, especially left side. Pain in left tonsil. Many left sided indications including tearing in skin of left thigh, coldness of left foot in bed at night, tearing on top of left shoulder.

DOSE- Third to 30th potency. Nusser observed symptoms in the 1830s fater eating large quantity of wild radish. In materia medica of Allen.

SEED OIL

The yield of seed oil from wild radish varies from 26.5-29.3%. It is composed of fatty acids such as rapic (60%), linoleic (8-10%), linolenic (5-7%), arachidonic (1.5-2%). There are also assorted sterols as well as glucoraphenin, glucoalyssin and assored quercitin flavanoids.

The cultivated radish seed yields about 40% of 10% saturated fats, 60% oleic, 4.5% linoleic, 3.7% linolenic, and 22% erucic acid. The iodine value varies from 93-112 with about 1% unsaponifiables. It has a saponification value of 180-82.

It is a wonderful secret which till now has been described by no one; take a liter each of carrot oil and radish oil, a quarter-liter of mustard oil, mix all together and add a half-liter of live, saffron-yellow ants to this. Place the oil for 4-7 days in the sun.

Then may it be used. Massage the penis with this for two hours before intercourse. Wash it then with warm water, and you will have an erection even after ejaculation.   **OVID**

ESSENTIAL OILS

Upon distillation with water, the root of R. *sativus* yields a colour-less oil containing sulphur that is heavier than water. It possesses the taste but not the odour of radish. Yield of the root essential oil is from 0.032- 0.035%.

The white root oil consists mainly of butyl-crotonyl isothiocyanate sulfide, and a thiocyanate, a substance with a salve like consistency. Methyl mercaptan is the unpleasant component in the oil.

Black or Spanish Radish was distilled with water vapour, and an unpleasant odour was obtained. It smelled of the unpleasant odour of cabbage, and contained traces of sulphur, but was free of mustard oil. Yield is 0.04%.

When grated black radish is extracted with ether, a brownish oil is obtained with the characteristic odour and taste. After standing for awhile, crystals containing raphanol appeared. This melts at 62° C; and is only 0.0025%.

This substance has also been found in common garden radish, white and common turnips, and watercress.

The green leaves can be steam distilled and yield a leaf aldehyde 2-hexen-1-al; a leaf alcohol, 3-hexen-1-ol; and small quantities of n- and isobutyraldehyde and isovaleraldehyde.

The seeds, when distilled, yield an isolated sulforaphene, a mustard oil containing a sulfoxide group. It occurs in the seeds as a glucoside.

A small amount of 4-methylsulfoxide-3-butenyl cyanide is also present.

Black radish seeds, upon distillation, yield ten different variations of isothiocyanates.

HYDROSOLS

The water of red and white radish is good for breaking the stone in the bladder, increasing urination, dropsy, stoppage of the entrails, and improving digestion. It provokes the menses, and is good for them that have eaten evil mushrooms, according to Brunschwig, Book of Distillation.

Radish root water is produced with the Sun in Leo and Moon in Aries. It is used to wash tuberculin wounds of the legs, for tertiary and quaternary fevers, purging the stomach, urinating and passing stone and blood, gout in gut, liver abscesses and opening of liver bile, itching sores that do not open, canker sores, and brown blains.
                                                                                    CULPEPPER

FLOWER ESSENCES

Radish flower essence is a psychologically strengthening essence for anyone suffering from bereavement or sense of being unable to cope.

It specifically strengthens and re-orders the mind, affording mental objectivity, well-being and comfort, in the difficult time immediately following the death of someone close. It integrates the mind after the shock and trauma of bereavement.   **ADITI HIMALAYA**

Radish flower essence is a catalyst that can be added to combinations to amplify the other essences, to give them a "kick".   **GREEN HOPE FARM**

Radish flower essence stabilizes the subconscious and dream state. It increases the life force, yang energy, and opens the lower two chakras.   **PEGASUS**

SPIRITUAL PROPERTIES

The primary property of radish is its ability to extend energy at certain levels of spiritual development in the 7th and 12th chakras. As the crown chakra awakens, there is a gradual change in which people have more energy to work with their own potential.

Certain states of ecstasy and a greater sense of purpose develops, and potential psychic abilities are activated.

In Lemuria, the radish was not primarily used as food. It was grown to understand mankind's destiny of the heavens. The glowing in radish is quite clear; and they absorbed some of that energy directly in themselves to unite the highest spiritual aspects with that of pure Earth existence.

The karmic purpose of radish is to provide all these patterns as symbolic representations of what is possible for all humans.

There is extra energy in the gall bladder meridian, and the nadis in the head are stimulated. The soul body is energized, the psora miasm is eased slightly, and the 10th, 11th, and 12th rays are activated.   **GURUDAS**

MYTHS AND LEGENDS

In the view of Charles M. Skinner [1911], the mountain gnome Rubezahl in the old German fairy tale of the same name represents the soul of the radish, 'a harsh, peppery, odious creature.' Rubezahl steals a princess and shuts her in his castle, so she cannot avoid listening to his protestations of love. She begs him to solace her loneliness with other company so he touches a number of radishes, which instantly take on human form, but which can keep it only so long as a radish can keep its leaves.

When these companions fade, she begs others; so to show his power, Rubezahl changes another radish to a bee and the princess, whispering her plight into its ear, sends it off to seek her human lover in the great world. The bee does not return. Another radish becomes a cricket and that also is pushed out of the window with a message to her lover. It never returns.

Still pestered by the attentions of Rubezahl, the princess beseeches him to count the radishes he has left with her and he begins to do so, whereupon the girl, seizing his wand, changes one of the radishes into a horse and gallops off on it to meet her lover.   **VERMEULEN**

Rapunzel is another fairy tale concerning a Maiden in the Tower. In some interpretations of the tale the name Rapunzel is taken as a variation of the name Radish, for while pregnant with her, Rapunzel's mother had cravings for the vegetable. The pregnant woman sends her husband to take some radish from the garden of a witch. He get caught and has to promise to give the witch the baby. As soon as the child, a girl, is born, the witch appears, takes it with her, promising to care for it like a mother. When the girl is twelve years old, the witch locks her up in a tower with a single window at the top.

The witch is cast as an overprotective parent, for worse or for better, depending on the tale's interpretation. She pays the girl a visit now and then by climbing up by the girl's long golden hair. To make a long story short, a prince appears, the girl gets pregnant and the witch angry, cutting off Rapunzel's hair and leaving her in a waste and deserted place. The prince, after wandering several years in misery in search of her, finds her and takes her to his kingdom, where they live happily every after.

Trichobezoar, an extremely rare intestinal condition resulting from the eating of one's own hair has been named after her, being called the Rapunzel Syndrome. The syndrome occurs in about 1% of cases engaging in hair-eating, trichophagia, as part of a disorder termed trichotillomania, the compulsive pulling of one's own hair.

In the cases of a young girl with the syndrome, one author conceptualized it "as physically holding on to her past life by literally ingesting it and holding it within". According to both Mangialavori and Karl-Josef Muller, it mirrors perhaps a social background that is not uncommon for Brassicales remedies, symbolized by an undigested ball, lump, hard object or foreign body.   **VERMEULEN**

RECIPES

FRESH ROOT JUICE- One to two tablespoons before meals as needed. Radish contains salicylate, similar to willow, and may cause sensitivity or allergic reaction in those sensitive.

SEED POWDER- 5-9 grams. Use the seed decoction or tincture with caution in cases of Qi deficiency conditions where the patient is weak and tired. When used for coughs, it is usually roasted first. Raphanine, the potent antibiotic from the seeds, kills mice when injected intravenously at a dose of 7-10 mg. Now you know.

LEAF JUICE- 3-5ml.

LEAF TEA- Take 50 grams of radish leaves to 500 ml of boiling water. Let infuse ten minutes. Let cool, and take one cup after meals for removing toxins associated with water retention.

ROOT DECOCTION- 1-2 oz. as needed.

ROOT POWDER- one to two grams

BLACK RADISH CAPSULES- For cleansing regimes, begin with one capsule daily for three days, then one twice daily for three more, etc up to 2 capsules three times daily and discontinue. Drinks lots of water!

Black radish is rarely available as a fresh vegetable. Peel off black exterior for eating as part of a salad.

It is sometimes available as a fresh plant juice, in health food stores. Salus and Schoenenberger are two good German organic products.

RADISH-HONEY JUICE- Take the grating of one radish or more and mix with honey. Allow to stand for 10 hours, and take a spoonful as needed, for whooping cough. The seed can be substituted when needed. Commercial products are also available.

PERENNIAL RAGWEED	**GREAT RAGWEED**
WESTERN RAGWEED	**TALL AMBROSIA**
BURSAGE	(*A. trifida* L.)
(*Ambrosia psilostachya* DC.)	**BURR RAGWEED**
(*A. coronopifolia* Torr. & A. Gray)	**BURSAGE RAGWEED**
COMMON RAGWEED	**FALSE RAGWEED**
ROMAN WORMWOOD	(*A. acanthicarpa* Hook.)
BASTARD WORMWOOD	(*Franseria acanthicarpa* [Hook.] Coville) not accepted
(*A. artemisiifolia* L.)	(*Gaertneria acanthicarpa* [Hook.] Britton)
(*A. elatior* L.) not accepted	not accepted
	PARTS USED- leaves, roots, stems

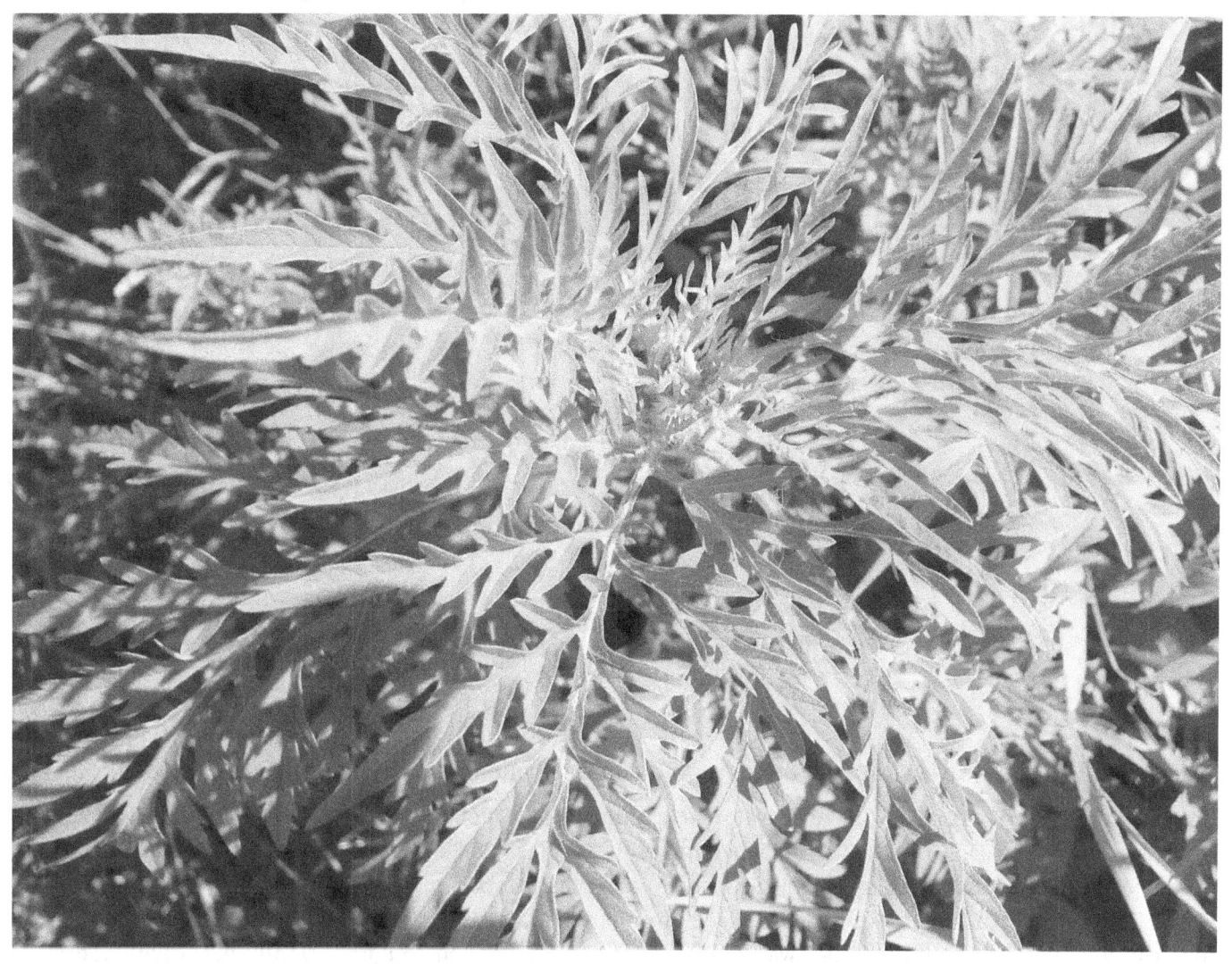

COMMON RAGWEED

And did you hear wild music blow
All down the boreen, long and low,
The tramp of ragweed horses' feet,
And Una's laughter wild and sweet.

N. HOPPER

Ambrosia means Immortal, related to the Food of the Gods that imparted immortality. This ambrosia was said to be fragrant. A plant known as sea ambrosia, native to Europe and Asia was named *Ambrosia maritima,* by Linnaeus.

As well as a food, nine times sweeter than honey, according to the 6th century BC Greek poet, ambrosia was also a perfume of the Gods.

In Hinduism, the counterpart is amrita, meaning "not to die". Soma, the mystical food or beverage may be the precursor to the Greek nectar.

Buddhists believe an ambrosia tree made of gemstones, originated at the center of the universe, also known as the Cloud Tree, or Tree of Wisdom.

A Norse myth involves the goddess Idun, who kept a basket of golden apples that were fed to gods and goddesses when they began to age.

A new apple variety from British Columbia is named Ambrosia. It is ok, but I prefer Honey Crisp if given the choice.

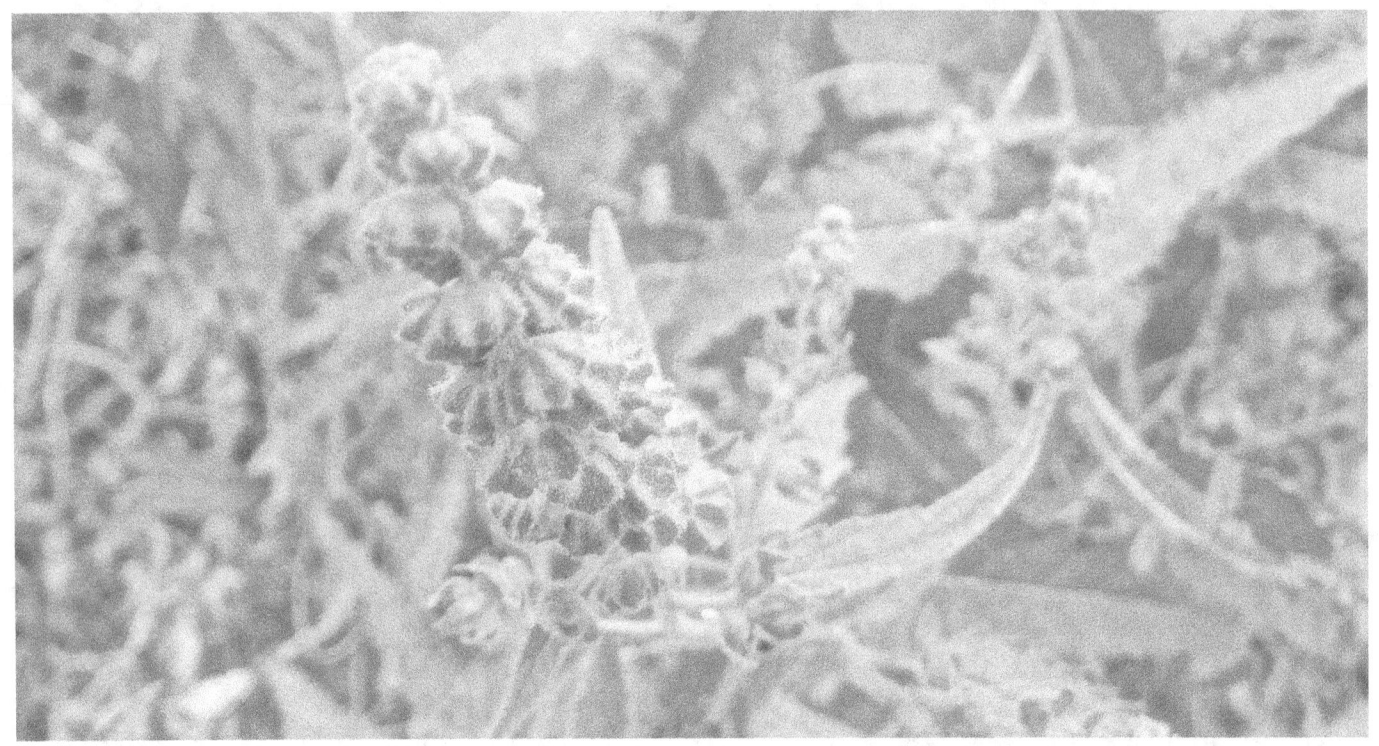

GREAT RAGWEED

Artemisiifolia means leaves similar to those from Artemisia. Trifida means three-cleft and refers to the leaves.

Ragweed pollen is one of our worst aggravators of asthma and hay fever. Wind pollinated ragweed will change sex according to the ease or difficulty of dispersing pollen. It has been estimated that a quarter of a billion tons of ragweed pollen is dispersed into American skies each season. Each plant is capable of producing up to one billion grains that can travel several miles. Each grain is so small that 100 grains measure the distance across the head of a pin. Or to put it another way, one gram of ragweed pollen contains 90 million individual grains.

When surrounded by taller weeds, it is a female. Those taller than surrounding plants are probably male.

The seeds of Great Ragweed have been found in prehistoric sites, and were 4-5 times larger than those of the present plant, seeming to indicate culture by selection.

Work by Peter Wayne, at Harvard found that ragweed grown in an atmosphere with double the normal carbon dioxide are taller, and produce 61% more pollen. Global warming will make this worse. The tallest Ragweed ever recorded was 18 feet 4 inches.

The Cheyenne ground the leaves and stems, and about a pinch of the powder was used to make a tea for bowel cramps, and to stop bloody stools, and colds. Ironically, leaf infusions were also used as a laxative in constipation.

It is known as **MO OHTAA VANO** or Black Sage, by the Cheyenne.

The Costanoan made poultices of the heated leaves and applied them to aching joints. The Gosiute poulticed the steeped leaves for sore eyes.

The Kiowa decocted the whole plant to wash sores on humans and horses, the latter probably related to botflies or another parasitic condition.

The roots of Great Ragweed (*A. trifida*), were chewed by various indigenous peoples, for nerves and bad dreams. Simply chew the root before going to bed to drive nightmares and fear from your sleep. The Cree call it **MASKIHKEWAHTIK**.

The Cherokee used Great or Common ragweed as an ingredient in the Green Corn medicine. The leaves were crushed and rubbed on insect bites or infused and the water rubbed on hives. Internally, the infusion was given for pneumonia or fevers.

A juice of the wilted leaves was applied to infected toes.

The crushed heads yield a red colour used for dye.

The Kiowa name means bloody weed, and although children liked watching the "bloody" juice excrete from the stems, it was held in fear by most of the tribe.

The Lakota name is either **CANHLO'GANWAS' TE'MNA** meaning "bulky weed", or **YAMNMU' MNUGA IYE'CECA** that translates, "it is like making noise crunching with teeth".

The seeds may or may not have been a cultivated food. It ranked second to the cultivated Marsh Elder (*Iva annua*) in residue at the Koster archaeological site along the Illinois River.

According to Dr. King, farmers used the herb for "slabbers" in horses, affecting a cure in a few hours.

King also mentioned the plant for its slightly stimulant, astringent, hemostatic and antiseptic properties.

Decoctions are cooled and injected vaginally to treat leucorrhea, prolapsed uterus, chronic gonorrhea, and gleet. He recommended it as a gargle for sore mouth, and as a wash for ulcers, including gangrene.

Internally, decoctions are useful for fevers, attendant with diarrhea and dysentery.

Rafinesque said that various natives used the stems of Giant Ragweed to make a sort of rope.

The Iroquois used Common or Great Ragweed as part of a compound decoction for diarrhea with bleeding. The Nanticoke of Virginia decocted the roots to treat constipation.

An infusion of the Common Ragweed roots was used for stroke victims, while a decoction of the whole plant was taken for cramps from picking berries.

Common Ragweed root was used, by the Houma to treat menstrual problems.

John Lame Deer, a Lakota healer, says "**CAN HLOGAN WASTEMNA**- a ragweed- helps a woman during a bad child-bearing".

Folk healers of the Ozarks prepare cold infusions of the fresh leaf for diarrhea. Ragweed and Tansy soaked in whiskey is said good for hiccoughs.

Common Ragweed was formerly recognized in the *Mexican Pharmacopoeia* for its emmenagogue, febrifuge and anthelmintic activity.

In Brazil, the herb is known as **ARTEMIJO VERDADEIRO**, and recommended by traditional healers for stomach diseases.

Dr. King felt common ragweed was best as a fomentation in recent inflammation from wounds and injury. As a salve, it can be very useful for hemorrhoid tumours and some forms of ulcers.

Dr. William Cook wrote "the leaves are stimulating and astringing, bitter and permanent in action.

An infusion is useful in diarrhea and dysentery of passive character; in uterine, gastric and pulmonic hemorrhages; and in degenerate leucorrhea as an injection and drink…A strong decoction influences the kidneys considerably, sustains the tone of the stomach, and slowly elevates the circulation; and these actions render it useful in the treatment of chronic dropsies, especially when combined with hepatics and stimulating diaphoretics."

The flower heads can be dried and feed to caged birds. Hay made with harvested common ragweed before blooming, and cured with a little salt, was shown in 1940 studies to be preferred by cattle over alfalfa. Sheep and pigs love the fresh plant.

The compound isabelin may be useful as a bioherbicide, due to its ability to inhibit various plants ability to germinate.

Burr Ragweed is so named due to its clinging burrs. It is fairly uncommon, but if found will be growing around prairie sand dunes.

The Zuni tribe infused the whole plant and used it as a wash for obstructed menstruation. The plant is probably abortifacient, and should be used with caution, especially internally.

They took the ground root and applied it to hollow teeth and toothaches.

The related *A. chamissonis*, in a study by McCutcheon, showed activity against methicillin-resistant *Staphylococcus aureus*. The root and to lesser extent, the leaves, contain thiarubrine compounds.

Perennial Ragweed leaves are often burned in various sweat lodges throughout North America.

The presence of Ragweed, often times, indicates soil deficient in potassium.

An insect, *Ophreaell communa*, has been trialed in attempts to control ragweed distribution, with limited success.

MEDICINAL

CONSTITUENTS- *A. artemisiifolia*- artemisiifolin, ambrosic acid, ambrosin, peruvin, isabelin, psilostachyins A-C, coronopilin (1600 ppm), 6a-hydroxy-eudesm-4(15)-ene-9b-0-anisate, 1-hydroxyeudesm-4, 11(13)-dien-12-oic acid, damsinic acid, 1b,6a-dihydroxyeudesm-4(15)-ene, cholest-7-en-3-ol, 4a,14-dimethyl-9,19-cyclo-cholestan-3b,24xi-diol & -3b,24xi, 25-triol, lophenol, lophenone, paulitin, isopaulitin, dumosin, reynosin, cumanin, 1,2-dihydroparthenin.
seed- agmatin
pollen- isorhamnetin-glucoside
A. psilostachya- ambrosiol, coronopolin, psilostachyin, and parthenin.

All species of Ragweed have some use in head colds, allergies and moderate histamine reactions. In some ways, the herb makes a suitable replacement for Eyebright or Ground Ivy.

It is a very efficient astringent whenever there are copious respiratory secretions with inflammation. Itchy eyes, and nose along with discharge, as well as asthma associated with cat allergies show great relief.

For pollen allergies begin dose drops two weeks before season. Or simply chew a leaf a day during the season to reduce the allergic response.

For allergic rhinitis use drop doses of flowering tops.

Two large epidemiological studies indicate a link between pollen allergies and depression. In one study of 700 children, those with hay fever at age 5 or 6 were twice as likely to develop a major depression episode over next 17 years compared to those without hay fever.

A recent study suggests more mental and motivational fatigue than physical.

Sixty nine percent of participants reported increased irritability, 63% more fatigue, 41% difficulty staying awake, and 31% feeling sad. The researchers concluded that ragweed allergy releases pro-inflammatory cytokines that directly affect the central nervous system. This suggests that hypothetically, the reaction is similar to psychological stressors and that there is a common genetic aetiology rather than environmental aetiology for allergy and depression. Marshall et al, *Psychosomatic Medicine* 2002 July-August.

The leaf is mildly bitter, pungent and slightly astringent, according to Matthew Wood. I would add slightly drying as well.

Common Ragweed (*A. artemisiifolia*) leaves, roots, stems and seeds have all been tested as alcohol and water extracts, and found active against both gram negative and positive bacteria, as well as mycobacterium.

The fluid extract has been, in past years, used to stop bleeding, or as a bitter tonic for dyspepsia.

Early work by Sanders et al, *J Bact* 1945 49 found strong inhibition of *Bacillus subtilis* and *E. coli*.

The flowers show activity against *S. aureus*. Borchardt et al, *J Med Plants Res* 2008 2:5.

Kim et al, *Korean Journal of Weed Science* 1993 showed broad anti-bacterial properties and inhibition against *Phytophthora capsici*.

Paulitin, a sesquiterpene lactone, has been found cytotoxic. David et al, *Pharm Biology* 1999 37:2. It exhibits significant inhibition against HeLa, MCF-7 and A431 cancer cells lines. This compound is present in yarrow flowers. Csupor-Loffler B et al, *Phytother Res* 2009 23(5): 672-6.

Both paulitin and isopaulitin exhibit activity against chloroquine-sensitive and resistant *Plasmodium falciparum* (malaria).

Ambrosin exhibits cytotoxic and anti-tumour activity, especially towards sensitive and multidrug-resistant cancer cells. Saeed ME et al, *J Ethnopharm* 2015 174: 644-58.

Ambrosin induces apoptosis in Jurket leukemia T cells, in work by Dirsch VM et al, *Planta Medica* 2001 67(6): 557-9. The compound is, however, poorly water-soluble.

Psilostachyins A and C exhibit modulation of the G2 checkpoint, blocked cells in mitosis and caused formation of aberrant microtubule spindles. Sturgeon CM et al, *Planta Medica* 2005 71(10): 938-43.

An alcohol extract of Common Ragweed leaves has been found to possess significant anti-inflammatory activity, in a study conducted by Perez, *Phytomedicine* 1996 3:2. The results four different experimental models of inflammation, found the extract comparable to phenylbutazone and betamethasone; two standard anti-The fresh leaf poultice is used like plantain for insect bites, stings, hives, poison ivy rash, etc. This may be due, in part, to the content of lophenol, also found in *Aloe vera*. This sterol simulates collagen and hyaluronic acid production in human dermal fibroblasts. Tanaka M et al, *Clin Cosmet Investig Dermatol* 2015 8:95-104.

Lophenol is an anti-diabetic phytosterol that may have benefit in metabolic disorders, including diabetes and obesity. Misawa E et al, *J Agric Food Chem* 2012 60(11): 2799-806.

Jung followed up this work in Korea, and found reynosin, a sesquiterpene lactone exhibited a dose dependent inhibition of CINC-1 (cytokine induced neutrophil chemoattractant-1) in LPS stimulated NRK-52E cells. The IC50 value is 1 microM, and suggests significant anti-inflammatory activity. *Plant Medica* 1998 64:5.

Reynosin inhibits clinical strains of *Mycobacterium tuberculosis*. Coronado-Acebes EW et al, *Pharm Biol* 2016 54(11): 2623-2628.

A 70% ethanol extract shows significant anti-oxidant activity. Maksimovic et al, *Indust Crops Prod* 28:3.

The herb combines well with eyebright or goldenrod in the treatment of acute hay fever and sinusitis.

Peruvin, a sesquiterpene lactone, and psilostachyin are cytochrome P450-linked aromatase compounds. It shows activity against *Plasmodium falciparum*, responsible for malaria.

Peruvin induced apoptosis and cell cycle arrest in work by Martino R et al, *Toxicol in Vitro* 2015 29(7): 1529-36. Psilostachyin C was also found most active.

Coronopilin has been found to arrest cancer cells in mitosis. Bosco A et al, *Molecules* 2017 22(3). Coronopilin inhibits cancer cell proliferation, DNA biosynthesis and NF-kappa B and STAT2 pathways, suggesting multiple anti-cancer effects. Villagomez R et al, *Anticancer Res* 2013 33(9): 3799-805. The sesquiterpene lactone inhibit leukemia cell growth by triggering cell type-specific responses, with normal white blood cell viability not affected. Cotugno R et al, *Cell Prolif* 2012 45(1): 53-65.

Bhagwath et al, *Journal of Biotechnology* 2000 23:8 looked at culturing the hairy roots for thiarubrine-A.

Several members of the *Ambrosia* genus contain thiarubrine-based chemicals in their foliage; a potent anti-fungal, anti-bacterial compound at low concentrations. It is also anti-viral, and has been found to reduce some solid tumors; with three patent applications for medical use.

This compound, also found in Hoary Yellow Yarrow, and Black Eyed Susan, is a potent anti-viral, anti-fungal and anti-parasitic agent. This team of scientists found they could increase the levels in hairy root culture by 8 times over 72 hours by adding vanadyl sulphate to the water medium.

Perennial Ragweed was tested as an expressed juice of the entire plant, and showed activity against Gram positive bacteria.

Great Ragweed was extracted by both ethanol and saline solutions and showed activity against both Gram positive and negative bacteria.

Ragweed has a selective action on the female reproductive system, and is used to both promote menstruation and to alleviate menstrual pain.

Cumanin possesses anti-protozoa activity, and in model of *Trypanosoma cruzi* infection, was 8-fold more active during acute phase of infection than benznidazole. It did not show hepatoxicity. Sulsen VP et al, *PLoS Negl Trop Dis* 2013 7(10): e2494.

Parthenin and Parthenolide are sesquiterpene lactones found in some Ambrosia species. Our local species should be studied further, as parthenolide is the active constituent of Feverfew (*Tanacetum parthenium*) an herb used to treat migraines.

While in Peru, I noted the related *A. peruviana* was often used to treat cancer. Studies by Klinar et al, *Fitoterapia* 1995 66:4 confirmed extracts of this plant reduce tumour formation.

The related *A. maritima* contains a chemical so toxic to snails related to schistosomiasis that one part in a thousand kills all of them. This is a serious disease affecting up to 12% of the world's population, mainly in tropical and sub-tropical countries.

Two sesquiterpene lactones, neoambrosin and damsin show significant cytotoxicity against various drug-resistant tumor cell lines. Saeed M et al, *Front Pharmacol* 2015 6: 267.

The related *A. tenufolia* contains psilostachyin and peruvin, exhibiting significant activity against Chagas' disease and Leishmaniasis. Sülsen et al, *Antimicrob Agents Chemother* 2008 52:7.

The related *A. paniculata* has been used traditionally in Cuba and elsewhere for treating epilepsy. Work by Buznego et al, *Epilepsy Behav* 2004 5:6 suggests the dry plant decoctions may enhance GABAnergic neurotransmission.

Rhizosphere fungi associated with *A. ambrosoides* contains the metabolite terrequinone, which exhibits moderate activity against various cancer cell lines. He J et al, *J Nat Prod* 2004 67(12): 1985-91.

HOMEOPATHY

Ambrosia (Ragweed) is a remedy for hay-fever, lachrymation and intolerable itching of the eyelids.

It is useful in some forms of whooping coughs, and in irritation of the trachea and bronchial tubes, leading to asthmatic attacks. The nose is stuffy, with sneezing and watery discharge, sometimes with blood.

It can be useful for many forms of diarrhea, especially in the hot summer months. In Germany the mother tincture is used for worm infestations and associated problems.

DOSE- Tincture to 3rd potency. Ten drops in water during and after attack of nosebleeds. Use 30th and higher potencies in treating hay fever. The mother tincture is prepared from the green parts of *A. artemisiaefolia*. Millspaugh did clinical observations in four cases in 1870. Boericke and Blackwood also contributed clinical observations.

Work by Bowen et al, *Ann Allergy Asthma Immunol* 2004 93:5 found sublingual swallow immunotherapy safe and efficacious for ragweed rhino-conjunctivitis, even when started just before pollen season.

This randomized, double-blind, placebo-controlled study was conducted at nine Canadian allergy centers. If this study was called homeopathic instead of sublingual swallow immunotherapy, it might well have never been funded, and the peer review may have been prejudiced. Just saying!

ESSENTIAL OILS

The related *A. tenufolia*, gives a yield of 1.32% essential oil upon steam distillation. Of 32 components found to represent over 99.2% of the oil, the major component is alpha thujone (79.3%).

The essential oil of *A. elatior* (*A. artemisiifolia*) is a deep green color with a specific gravity of 0.87. It has an aromatic, not unpleasant odour.

The essential oil of *A. artemisiifolia* contains 60 compounds of which 18 have been identified including germacrene D 24%, p-cymene, alpha pinene 8%, sabinene, beta pinene, limonene 17%, 1,8-cineole, mycrene 7.4%, gamma terpinene, cis and trans-artemisia ketones.

Giant Ragweed (*A. trifida*) dried aerial parts were steam distilled and yielded about 0.12% essential oil. Thirty-five compounds were identified with 15.5% bornyl acetate, 8.5% borneol, 8.3% caryophyllene oxide, 8% alpha pinene, 6.3% germacrene D, 4.6% beta-caryophyllene, 2.9% trans-carveol, 2.6% beta-myrcene, 2.4% camphor and 3.2% limonene. Activity was noted against six bacterial strains and two fungal strains. Wang P et al, *Molecules* 2006 11(7): 549-55.

SEED OIL

Common Ragweed seed contains over 20% oil composed of 69.5% linoleic acid, 19.2% oleic acid, 7.6% palmitic acid and minor amounts of stearic acid. In 1942, Roedel and Thorton wrote a paper for the *American Journal of Oil Chemistry Society* 19 suggesting the oil be used for paints and varnish. The oil is said to be similar to soybean oil.

Giant Ragweed seeds contain over 44.1% oil, composed of 70.6% linoleic acid, 17.8% oleic acid, 3.6% stearic acid, and 8% palmitic acid.

FLOWER ESSENCE

Great Ragweed (*Ambrosia trifida*) flower essence is for those suffering restless dreams, and insomnia. It helps both children and adults who suffer from fear of the dark, and feel anguished by the onset of evening.

The essence can be especially useful to children who require a night-light, or who frequently wake and want to crawl into bed with their mother or father. **PRAIRIE DEVA**

SPIRITUAL PROPERTIES

Experiments with *Ambrosia* roots have indicated that these plants are capable of self-recognition through differentiation between self and non-self, an ability that has been considered by some as basic for self-aware beings: the root system of the *Ambrosia* plant detects and avoids other *Ambrosia* plants and plants of different species, indicating self-recognition. The mechanism that helps the plant differentiate between the roots of other plants and its own is unknown, but can be interpreted on a molecular level. Likewise, it is essential for the human immune system to differentiate between self and non-self by chemical means, without resorting to conscious processes. Further, as far as defensive tactics are concerned, there are flowers that detect the approach of pests that visit to steal their nectar, and react by closing up when these insects are nearby. **DR. EDE FRECSKA**

MYTHS AND LEGENDS

Tantalus was a wealthy king and the son of Zeus and the nymph Pluto. For numerous crimes, including stealing nectar and ambrosia from the gods, he was condemned to an eternity of hunger and thirst in the Underworld, where he was placed in a lake the waters of which receded whenever he tried to drink, while above his head were boughs of fruit always tantalizingly beyond his reach. Tantalize is a word derived from this tale.

SMALL

The gods were served ambrosia and nectar by Hebe, goddess of youth, the daughter of Zeus and Hera, and the wife of Heracles. One day she tripped and fell, and Zeus dismissed her. Zeus then took the shape of an eagle and flew to earth to seize Ganymeade, the son of the king of Troy, as a replacement servant for the Gods.

SMALL

Psyche, a princess, mysteriously became pregnant. Eros, who had in fact inseminated her while she was asleep, told her the child would be divine if she did not try to find out who the father was. When Psyche discovered that Eros was responsible, he fled from her.

The goddess Aphrodite offered to force Eros to marry Psyche, if she could complete a series of nearly impossible tasks. When she did carry out the tasks, the shotgun marriage took place, and Psyche was fed ambrosia to make her immortal.

SMALL

In the Greek myth, it [cornucopia] was one of the horns of Amalthaea, a goat which nursed the god Zeus when he was a baby. The horn produced ambrosia and nectar, the food and drink of the gods. In Roman mythology, the cornucopia was the horn of the river god, Archelous, who often took the form of a bull. Hercules broke off the horn in combat with him. Nymphs filled the horn with flowers and fruit and offered it to Copia, the goddess of plenty.

SMALL

RECIPES

TINCTURE- 1-2 drops in water as needed. The tincture is made of the whole plant of Common Ragweed fresh, and while full of pollen. Use a 1:4 ratio of 40% alcohol, or better yet 1:2 at 95% of fresh leaves before pollen.

The resulting tincture smells and has initial taste of chocolate, and then bitter and acidic.

DECOCTION- *A. trifida or A. elatior*-1-2 ounces as needed.

CAUTION: If allergic to ragweed, do not eat cantaloupe, melons, bananas, sunflower seeds, chamomile tea and honey from Asteraceae family as they contain some of the same proteins. Also, although obvious, those allergic to ragweed should not be gathering the flowering plant for tinctures. Prolfilin, also found in birch, mugwort and celery pollen may also cause cross-reactivity.

SPINY REST HARROW
(***Ononis spinosa*** L.)
SPINELESS REST HARROW
FIELD REST HARROW
(***O. arvensis*** L.)
REST HARROW
(***O. repens*** L.)
PARTS USED- roots, leaves, flowers

Ononis may be from the Greek **ONOS** meaning donkey, or an ancient jar with big handles on it that they also called Onos. However, I'm just speculating because I have found no other source. It is relished food by donkeys and goats. Spinosa means spiny, and I didn't even have to look that one up.

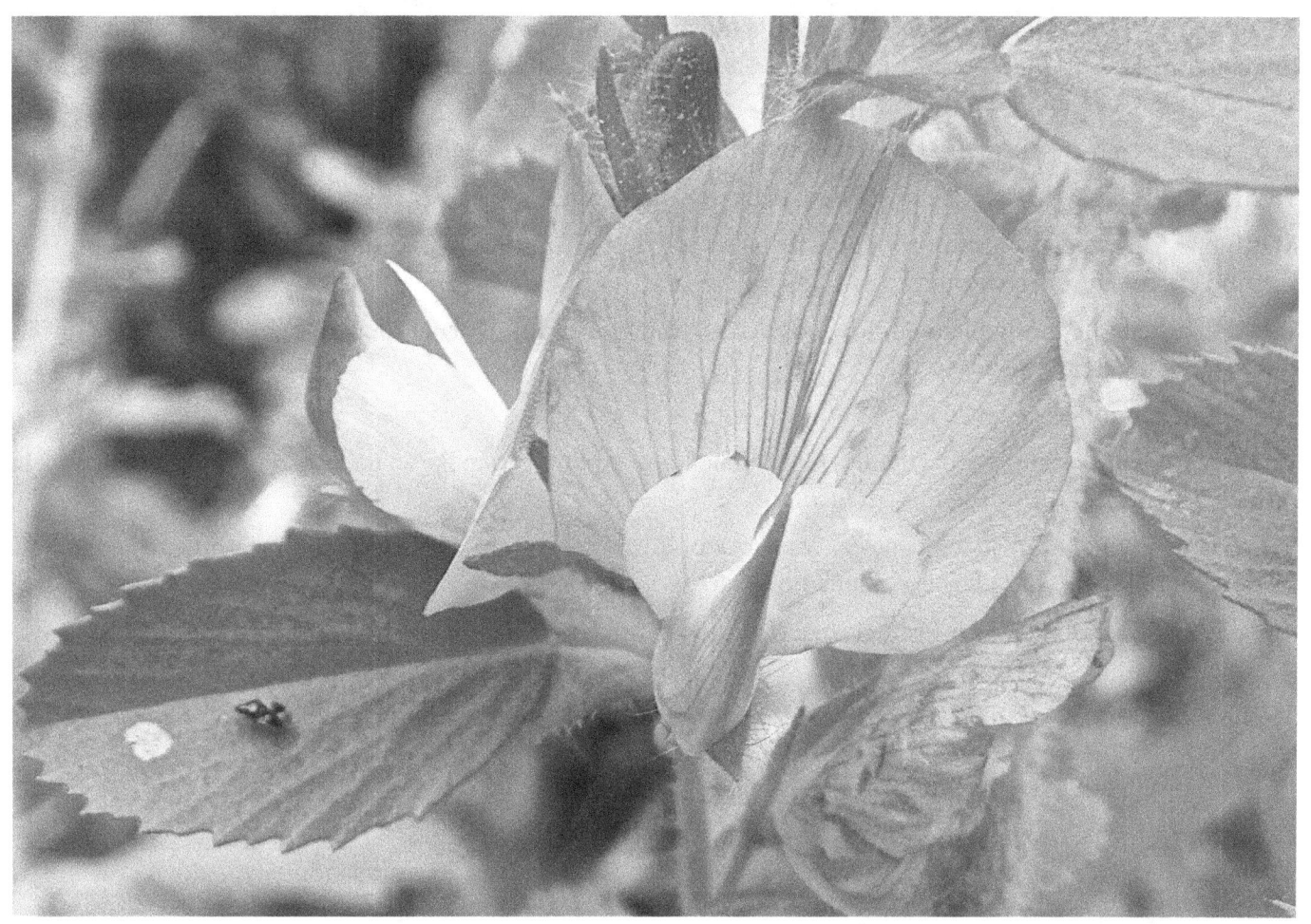

REST HARROW FLOWER AND LEAF

Rest Harrow stems from "arrest harrow", brought in from "remore ararti", literally a plough hindrance.

It is said that traditionally, this was the plant from which the crown of thorns was plaited for the crucifixion.

Another name in England was Ground Furze and in France it was known as Bugrane.

Field Rest Harrow is an introduced plant in Alberta, Oregon and parts of eastern USA. It is found occasionally in waste areas, near fence lines. It has prickly thorns and has an unusual odour that some people find unpleasant. Rest Harrow (*O. repens*) is common in Washington and Oregon.

Spiny Ononis is found in Pennsylvania and adjacent states.

Ononis is a somewhat woody perennial and a member of the legume family. It is rare and introduced, found occasionally in roadside ditches. In parts of Europe, it is cultivated in hopes to improve and stabilize the quality of the medicinal herb.

The highly variable essential oil content of *O. spinosa* is believed responsible for its somewhat unreliable action.

Parkinson wrote that "four pounds of the roots first sliced small and afterwards steeped in a gallon of Canary Wine… and put into a stone pot close stopped… and so set to boyle in a Balneo Marie for 24 hours is as daintie a medicine for tender stomachs as any of the daintiest Lady in the land can desire to take…It is recorded that in former times the young shoots and tender stalks before they become prickly were pickled up to bee eaten as a meate or sauce, wonderfully commended against a stinking breath, and to take away the smell of wine in them that had drunk too much."

Rest Harrow (*O. repens*) roots are very sweet, and when young, have the flavour of liquorice. Traditionally, in England, workmen would suck the juice out of the roots to quench their thirst in the hot sun. The young shoots are very sweet and succulent, boiled and eaten.

In parts of England, Rest harrow is called Wild Liquorice. Older roots are sweetish, but have a harsh, irritating aftertaste.

Traditionally, the herb was used to subdue delirium, and bladder stones.

Matthiolus said that Rest harrow root powder helps cure fleshy ruptures that would seem incurable by any other method except cutting or burning.

When touched, the bushy plant emits a wonderful, resinous odour. During the day there is not much, but in the evening it is very sweetly scented.

The leaf juice soothes chapped skin.

All three roots are so similar, that there is movement afoot in Europe to make all three part of the pharmacopoeia monograph of the crude drug *Radix Ononidis*.

Bacteria of the genera Rhizobium and Mesorhizobium form symbiotic interactions with *O. arvensis* and *O. spinosa*; but not with red clover, alfalfa nor bird's foot trefoil.

The related *O. rotundifolia* has been given a hardiness rating of 7.8 by the Morden Research Station; *O. spinosa* a rating of 8.7-8.9.

Methanol extracts of related *O. hirta* induce apoptosis on breast cancer cell lines. Talib et al, *Sci Pharm* 78:1.

MEDICINAL

CONSTITUENTS- *O. spinosa-* root-flavonoids like rutin, kaempferol, hyperoside, cosmosiin (apigetrin), myricetrin, apigenin, vitexin, luleolin, quercitin, faceidin, penduletin; free isoflavonoids like genistein, formononetin, biochanin A 7-glucoside and its 6"-malonate; glycosides like spinonin, ononine, ononin-6-malonylester, homoptero-carpin-7-glucoside and trifolirhizin; triterpenes including alpha onocerin; ononid, ononine, trifolirhizin, triterpenoids like onocerol, triterpenes 9,19cyclo27-lanostan-25-on, beta sitosterol, medicarpin, maachiain, tannins, resins, homopter-carpin, volatile oils (mainly trans-anethole), 18 phenolic acids, including trifolirfizin and other pterocarpans, ononetin and lectins.
aerial parts- flavonoids, sterols, and triterpenes especially onocol (alpha onocerin).
O. arvensis- isoflavones like onogenin, and phenolics like 7-0-beta-D-glucopyranoside-3,4'-methylenedioxy-pterocarpan

The whole plant of Rest Harrow is used in rheumatism, gout and various skin disorders. It is of equal value in kidney and bladder complaints, as well as gravel and small stones. One of its great advantages is diuretic action that does not irritate the kidneys.

This may be due to the fact that the volatile oil is diuretic, and the other constituents are not.

Therefore, decoctions of the root are anti-diuretic, since the oils are lost to steam.

Cold infusions are best for strictly diuretic action; especially in cases of excess fluid retention. Maria Treben suggests cold infusions overnight, slightly warmed in the morning and taken half an hour before and after breakfast for edema.

The flowers, leaves and roots can all be used for their salty/sour cooling effect.

Therefore, in cases of inflammation of the urinary tract and bladder, as well as after colic suffered from passing stones and gravel, it excels as a urinary antiseptic.

It is used to treat hypertension and renal edema in cases of kidney depletion, that result in swollen ankles.

The leaves can be used externally as a poultice on wounds and injuries.

The root extract have definite diuretic activity, and are used for this purpose in Austria, Hungary and Poland.

Spinonin has been found inactive against a number of human cancer cell lines and HIV-1 reverse transcriptase. It shows weak activity against *Pseudomonoas aeruginosa*. Ononin shows activity against beta-hemolytic *Streptococcus*.

Mahasneh et al, *J Ethnopharm* 1999 64:3 found butanol extracts *of O. spinosa* possess high moderate anti-fungal activity against *Aspergillus flavus, Fusarium moniliforme* and *Candida albicans*. Kirmizigul et al, *J Nat Products* 60:4 found the root of *O. spinosa subspecies leiosperma* is weakly active against *Pseudomonas aeruginosa* and *beta hemolytic Streptococcus*.

Both water and ethanol extracts of the root show benefit in skin disease and lesions. Altuner et al, *Mikrobiyol Bul* 2010 44:4.

In studies conducted in 1995 by Langer, Engler and Kubelka at the University of Wien, Austria, various Ononis roots were compared for similarity of action.

It has been suggested that *O. arvensis, O. repens, and O. spinosa* are similar enough to place all of them in the pharmacopoeia monographs of the crude drug *Radix Ononidis*. The plant should be further investigated for its remarkable content of isoflavones in the roots.

For example, it contains in nmol/gram of fresh weight 1020 biochanin A, as compared to 29 in red clover roots, and 6.8 in the stems. It contains 123 genistein, as compared to red clover stems of 51. And it is rich in formononetin (230), formononetin-7-O-glucoside (74), and formononetin-7-O-glucoside-6"-malonate (2947).

Formononetin is considered an isoflavone, somewhat instrumental in the effects of Black Cohosh, resulting in LH, luteinizing hormone and estrogen binding hormonal activity. Formononetin acts as a mild prostaglandin synthase inhibitor (Guengerich, 1987).

Formononetin has been found to inhibit bone loss associated with estrogen deficiency. Hyekyung Ha et al, *Arch Pharm Res* 33:4.

With biochanin A, it appears to inhibit human alcohol dehydrogenase; and by itself is abortifacient, and fungicidal. Biochanin A is heat sensitive, and loses much of its estrogenic activity upon drying.

The root is often combined with licorice root, juniper berries and used as a component of diuretic teas.

Yolmaz et al, *Phytother Res* 20:6 found the root of *O. spinosa* possesses analgesic activity equivalent to aspirin.

Cosmosiin (apigetrin) inhibits neuro-inflammation and may have potential for prevention or treatment of neurodegenerative disease and injury. Lim HS et al, *J Med Food* 2016 19(11): 1032-40.

Apigetrin, also known as apigenin-7-glucoside, binds to 17 cancer drug targets, suggesting further research. Gogoi B et al, *Mol Biosyst* 2017 13(2): 406-16.

It exhibits significant anti-proliferative activity against melanoma B16F10 cells. Nasr Bouzaiene N et al, *Life Sci* 2016 144: 80-5. The compound is present in german chamomile flowers, and dandelion root.

The root exhibits anti-inflammatory activity in work by Ergene, Oz B et al, *Biomed Pharmacother* 2017 91:1096-1105. Targeting cytosolic phospholipase A2alpha is a potential target to reduce inflammation since the enzyme is involved in heart disorders, asthma, arthritis, and neuronal disease. Spiny Restharrow shows great activity, lower than black currant, but better than stinging nettle, birch, and Petasites species. Arnold E et al, *Molecules* 2015 20(8): 15033-48.

Ononetin, a deoxybenzoin derived from *O. spinosa* root selectively inhibits transient receptor potential melastatin 3, that inhibits dorsal root and trigeminal ganglia sensory neurons. Straub I et al, *Mol Pharmacol* 2013 84(5): 736-50. This suggests a trial for trigeminal neuralgia and related conditions, perhaps combined with Cow Parsnip green seed tincture.

Tumova et al, *Herba Polonica* 1999 45:2 tested flavonoid production of *O. arvensis* callus cultures. Chitosan solution in a 1% acetic solution increased flavonoid production in the first 24 hours by 516%.

Later work by the same researcher looked at the effect of jasminic acid, with a 55% increase in flavonoids, and with 4-hydroxyanilide-6-chloro-5-terc.butyl-pyrazine-2-carboxylic acid; an increase of 976%. *Ceska Slov Farm* 2002 51:4.

HOMEOPATHY

Rest-Harrow (*Ononis spinosa*) is a remedy associated with renal function and edema, similar to juniper. It is also useful for chronic nephritis, and tendency to stone formation.

It is used for calculus nosebleeds upon washing the face.

Headaches, epistaxis, and epileptic convulsions.

DOSE- 1st to 6th potency. Mother tincture is made from the whole, fresh plant in flower.

ESSENTIAL OILS

Restharrow roots contain from 0.02-0.2% of a volatile oil containing anethole, cis-anethole, menthone, isomenthone, camphor, linalool, estragole, borneol, carvone and menthol. The related *O. viscosa* has been hydro-distilled and yields 0.24% of an essential oil composed of 10% carvacrol, 5.5% nonanal, 12.5% hexahydrofarnesyl-acetone, 8.3% lauric acid, and 4.8% dodecanal and 36 other compounds.

HYDROSOL

A distilled water in Balneo Mariae, with four pounds of the root hereof first sliced small, and afterwards steeped in a gallon of Canary wine, is singularly good to cleanse the urinary passages.

The flowers of *O. hircina* are distilled and the water used for red spots, pimples and little red blains in the face. A spoonful every time of water his nature to cure again. **BRUNSCHWIG**

RECIPES

INFUSION- Take 2-3 grams of dry root powder to one pint of hot water and steep for twenty minutes. Take 2-4 times daily as needed. (3 grams = one heaping tsp)

ROBERT'S KIDNEY INFECTION TEA- Combine one part rest harrow root, birch leaf, kidney bean pods, with two parts couch grass, corn silk and rose hips. Steep, strain and serve cool.

For kidney stones, combine rest harrow root, bearberry, valerian root and marshmallow root.

DIAPHORETIC TEA- Combine one part rest harrow, parsley seed, and juniper berries as a hot infusion. Let cool and drink up to four ounces every hour as needed.

CAUTION- Do not use for edema if caused by cardiac or kidney insufficiency.

GARDEN RHUBARB
ENGLISH RHUBARB
(***Rheum x hybridum***)
(***R x cultorum***)
(***R. rhaponticum*** L.)
(***R. rhabarbarum*** L.)
SIBERIAN RHUBARB
(***R. undulatum*** L.)
CHINESE RHUBARB
TURKEY RHUBARB
(***R. palmatum*** L.)
(***R. officinale*** Baill.)

PARTS USED- stem, root, seed.

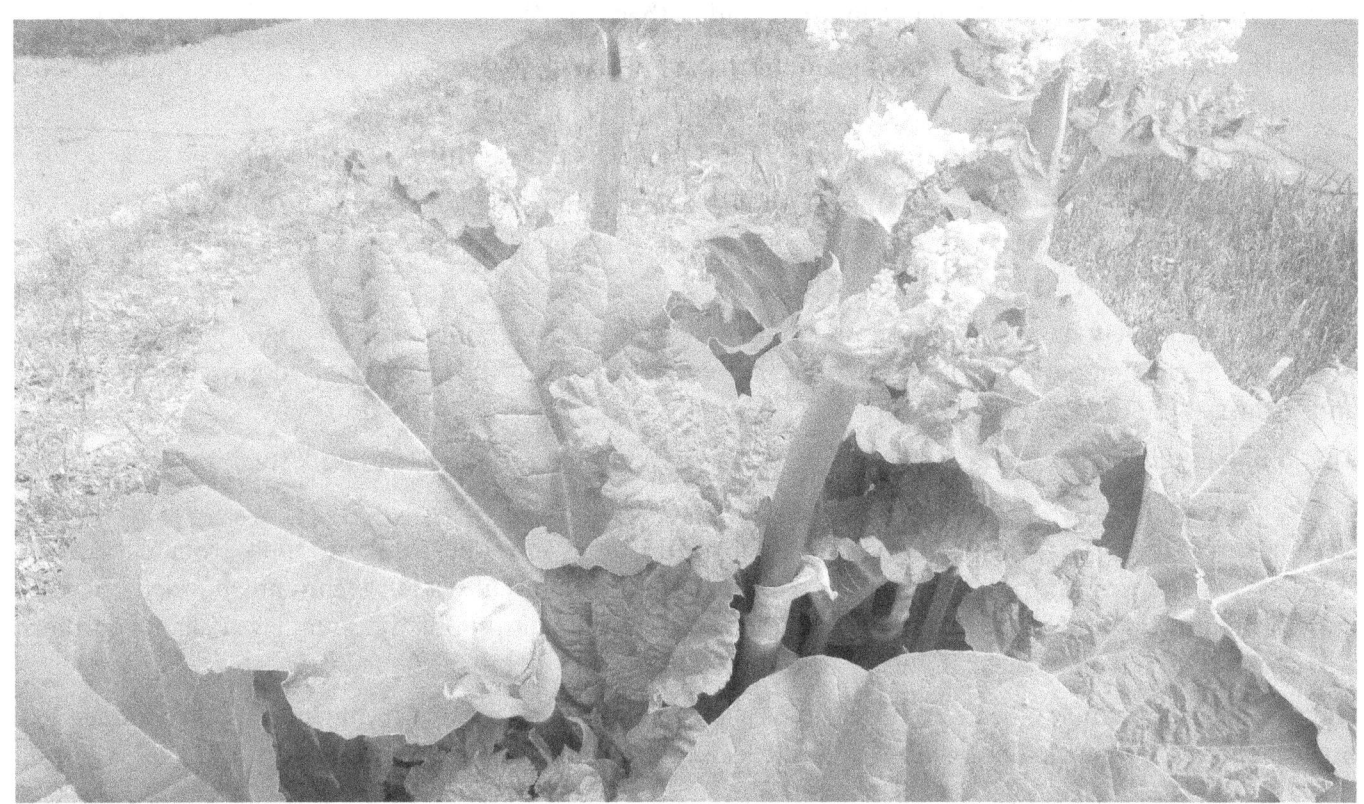

GARDEN RHUBARB

Never rub another man's rhubarb.   **THE JOKER (BATMAN)**

Now let us all praise the Rhubarb...
Its roseate stalks are a treat
Especially when stewed or otherwise brewed
In concoctions delectably sweet.   **C. FRANCISCO**

Rest, with nothing else, results in rust.
The rhubarb that no one picks go to seed.   **WILDER PENFIELD**

Rheum is from the Greek **RHEO**, meaning to flow, and thought to be related to the purgative nature of the plant. Rhubarb may be from the Middle Latin **RHA BARBARUM**, meaning "root of the barbarians". Rha is an early name for the Volga River. Rhaponticum is from the Greek, meaning rhubarb of Pontus, a province in Asia Minor near the Black Sea. Rha comes originally from the Indo European **SREU**, which means to flow, or river.

Rhaflowers are the rhubarb blossom heads that look similar to cauliflower. It was believed that if rhubarb goes to seed, someone in the family would die during the year.

In magic, it was believed that a piece of rhubarb root, worn around the neck on a string would protect against stomach pains. Symbolically, rhubarb is related to advice, and birth date of March 21st.

In Tibet, rhubarb leaves are dried and smoked with tobacco. Some authors believe the original Soma drink was fermented from rhubarb stem juice.

Rhubarb pie, one of my favorites, was traditionally served to one's mate, and said to help maintain his or her fidelity.

Rhubarb stalks are a good source of fibre, more than two grams in a half-cup serving. Other interesting products include rhubarb jerky, catsup, butter, hamburger and leather.

Edible rhubarb is believed brought to England from the Volga region of Russia in 1573 or from the mountains of Bulgaria.

Seeds were brought to England from Italy, and given to the botanist Parkinson.

It was introduced originally for the therapeutic properties of the root, but did not live up to its laxative reputation. It was not until the 1800s that the stem was prepared as a fruit or preserve. It is believed to be a cultivar or hybrid of wild *R. rhaponticum*.

The cultivated variety has 44 chromosomes, double the wild. Today, *R. rhaponticum* and *R. rhabarbarum* are often considered synonymous, although some authors may disagree. The former is used for both food (stalk) and a source of herbal medicine (root).

The *R. officinale* root has blackish veins while *R. rhaponticum* has red veins, and pink fractures. In the latter, the bark is generally not removed.

Attempts in 17th century England to produce rhubarb rhizomes and roots similar to those from China, were consistently disappointing. Whether it was the climate, the soil, or cultivation technique, puzzled botanists and horticulturists. I grew *R. palmatum* very successfully on the south shore of Lesser Slave Lake, in northern Alberta, considered only zone 2 in most garden books.

Culpepper recommended the English variety, as a suitable substitute for that from China. He recommended, however, that the roots not be collected until the leaves have turned red and are gone.

Today, in Canada, there are about ten cultivars. The most common are the German Wine, with large green-purple stalks, and McDonald with small dark red purple stalks.

Adding sweet cicely roots, or anise seed to rhubarb while cooking can significantly reduce the amount of sugar or honey needed to balance the tartness. Red currants in small amounts, and of course, strawberries, help bring out the best flavour in rhubarb desserts.

Nine million pounds of rhubarb stalk were produced in Washington in 1988; 1.25 million from hothouse production and sold fresh.

Rhubarb is an ingredient in Seraglio pastilles, an aphrodisiac lozenge available in Paris.

Elixir Rabarbaro, made from the Chinese root, is produced in Milan and is the second largest selling apertif in Italy. In Poland it is cooked as a vegetable dish with potatoes, while in Iran, it is added to stews. Of course it is a vegetable, but for trade purposes, the US Customs ruled in 1947 it a fruit.

Rhubarb juice is a natural anti-browning agent that at 20% concentration inhibited apple browning for several hours. The juice has a slight pink colour, and at 20% contains 0.07% oxalic acid. Commercial opportunities for natural substances with this property are wide spread throughout the food industry.

Scientists at Yale have found a chemical in rhubarb leaves that harmlessly breaks down Freon and other chloro-fluoro-carbons. Previously the leaves were used to tan hides, and clean chrome and other metals. The boiled leaf decoction is poured on the soil before seed sowing to prevent club root, and is a useful spray against greenfly and black spot on roses.

The leaves cannot be eaten, but their juice makes a cooling poultice when applied to stinging nettle irritated skin.

The young flowers, which look somewhat like cauliflower, can be steamed, or deep-fried.

Both Garden and Chinese Rhubarb are use commercially in flavouring. The roots bitter addition to carbonated beverages, syrups, liqueurs, candies and other food products is substantial

Rhubarb Garden root is permitted, by the FDA, as ingredient in alcoholic beverages.

Garden Rhubarb root, sliced thin and dried, can be chewed to relieve sore throats, canker sores and bleeding gums. Although tolerant of great variation in soils, Garden Rhubarb prefers pH of 6.5-7, of a rich sandy loam and is a rabid consumer of nitrogen and potassium, with corresponding higher yields.

It also needs lots of water. Composted manure is best fertilizer, applied in late fall to avoid promoting growth.

Rhubarb dislikes warm temperatures and will stop growing above 26 degrees Celsius.

Root division is the most common method of propagation, and is quite productive for at least seven years. Plants do not come true from seed, so plant them 6 cm below soil and place at least a metre apart. Spring and fall division is best when root is dormant.

Two year-old plants can be picked 6-15 times a season, with yields of 40-70t/ha typical.

Some favourite varieties are Honey Red, a non-stringy type from Saskatchewan that like Canada Red, is sweeter than some others. I grew MacDonald when I lived near Lesser Slave Lake, and it is a good producer.

Roy Beck lives near Sedgewick, and collects information and various heritage rhubarb varieties. He may be contacted at rwbeck@telusplanet.net.

The Rosy Rhubarb Festival, in Shedden, Ontario, is one example of numerous festivals held in North America, England and Australia. Intercourse, Pennsylvania has an annual festival, but you would think they could have come up with a more interesting event, given their name.

Garden rhubarb rhizome extracts possess anti-oxidant, and anti-tyrosinase activity, suggesting use in cosmetic, sunscreen and skin care products for prevention or reduction of photo damage. Silveira JP et al, *BMC Complement Altern Med* 2013 Feb 27.

Mechanical rhubarb harvesters can harvest up to one ton of large stalked cultivars in only seven man hours, compared to eighteen for hand harvest.

Rhubarb, companion planted with Columbines, helps protect against red spider mite. The leaves can be boiled to produce a spray that is effective in Cabbage family plantings, to help prevent club root, or simply put a piece of leaf or stem in planting hole.

Leaf spray helps control greenfly and black spot on roses.

MEDICINAL

CONSTITUENTS- *R. rhaponticum* root- chyrosphanic acid, and glycosides; hydroxystilbene derivatives including rhaponticin (rhapontin), rhaponiticin, rhapontigen, piceatannol, resveratrol, deoxy-rhapontigen, pterostilbene acetyl glucosides; anthracene compounds 19.8 mg/g, anthroquinones 16.6 mg/g including rhein, emodin, chrysophanol and physcion; sennasides A-F, sennidin A, phenolic glycosides like lindleyin, iso-lindleyin, cinnamic and gallic acids, volatile oils, rutin, fatty acids, oxalic acid; tannins like rhatannin, and glucogallin.
stalk- 2% soluble and 53% insoluble fibre, 96% moisture in fresh; also contains protein, minerals, flavonoids, including cyanidin 3-glucoside and rutinoside; lutein, organic acids such as oxalic (0.1-1.4%), malic (0.7-2.2%), citric and ascorbic; sugars (0.3-2.3%), pectin. The pH is 3.0-3.6. Anthranoids are lowest (0.001%) close to root and highest (0.004%) closest to leaf, but still very low and not associated with any food risk. Oxalic acid (1336 mg/100 grams) is approximately double that of spinach.
panicle (unopened flower)- various brassinosteroids including brassinolide, castasterone and 24-epicastasterone; phytosterols, campesterol, stigmasterol, sitosterol, and isofucosterol, and a pentacyclic triterpene, 1up-20-(29)-en-2alpha,3beta,28-triol and its 3,28-dipalmitoyl ester.
leaves- emodin, emodin-8beta-D-glyco-pyranoside (vitexin), rutin, citrerosein, chrysophanol, physcion (0.6% in spring),
R. palmatum/officinale root- 34mg/g anthraquinone compounds, including 32 mg/100 grams emodin; 21 mg/100 gr chrysophanol, 1.8 mg/100 grams rhein; physcion, aloe-emodin, rhabarberone, sennosides (dianthrone glycosides) stilbenes glucosides such as rhaponticin and 4-0-methyl-piceid, alizarin, cinnamic and gallic acid, galloyl esters, catechin, tannins, calcium and potassium oxalate, flavonoids (2-3%).

English Rhubarb root is both laxative and astringent in action, but considerably milder than the Chinese rhubarb (*R. officinale/ R. palmatum*). The roots bitter and cooling properties are useful in constipation, as well as liver and gall bladder problems.

It combines well with dandelion root for gastritis and constipation, with burdock for acute eczema and with figwort and Oregon grape root for acute psoriasis.

It is very useful in treating infant's stomach troubles and loose stools. In large amounts, it acts as a laxative, but nowhere near the activity of its more famous cousins.

English Rhubarb root is laxative, and will accelerate peristalsis within 6 to 8 hours, in most cases; but is dependant upon healthy bowel flora. Overuse of antibiotics, or poor diet can create poor intestinal bacteria content, which prevents anthrene compounds breaking down to emodins, which possess laxative activity.

Rhubarb root, when boiled for several hours, loses its laxative compounds, and instead exudes constipating causing tannins.

Matthew Wood considers rhubarb a badger medicine, a designation also given to yellow dock. "That is to say, it is a yellow root that moves things downward through the digestive tract."

Emodins and rheins have been shown to inhibit the growth of breast, liver and skin cancers, due in part to angiogenesis, and partly because rheins reduce the rate at which cancer cells can create proteins and use glucose as a cellular fuel. Castiglione et al, *Biochem Pharmacology* 1990 40:5.

Rhein appears to distort and disrupt the membranes of mitochondria and cells through altered actin microfilaments, which collapse into ring-like structures in the cell cytoplasm. The christae of mitochondria are disrupted which may lead to impairment of energy metabolism, variations in cellular permeability and altered receptor molecule activity. Iosi et al, *Anticancer Res* 1993 13.

Rhein appears to reduce hepatocellular carcinoma. Shi et al, *Am J Chin Med* 2008 36:4. It also gives renal protection and lowers lipids in a manner different from statin drugs. Gao et al, *Planta Med* 2009 July 28.

Rhein inhibits angiogenesis, suggesting anti-tumor and anti-inflammatory activity. He et al, *Phytomed* 2011 18:6.

A study by Cyong et al, *J Ethnopharm* 1987 19:3 looked at 178 herbs for activity against *Bacteriodes fragilis*, a major anaerobic microorganism of the human intestinal flora. Only rhein, from rhubarb root, had significant activity. This bacterium is very common in patients suffering gall bladder concerns.

Emodin is protective of cholestatic hepatitis. Work by Ding et al, *Zhong Yi Xue Za Zhi* 2009 89:10 found decreased levels of bilirubin, and other markers were lowered by emodin quicker than ursodeoxycholic acid and better effect than dexamethasone.

Emodins stimulate the production of white blood cells, which help fight cancer. In one study of 67 patients, emodin increased WBC counts by more than one thousand cells per cubic centimetre of blood. This makes emodin useful for treating white blood cell deficiency during chemotherapy.

Emodin makes breast cancer cells more sensitive to paclitaxel, suggesting rhubarb root, sheep sorrel or yellow dock combines well with hazelnut leaf or twigs for prevention. Emodin makes lung cancer cells more sensitive to cisplatin and doxorubicin.

The compound appears to cause apoptosis of esophageal cancer cells. Wang et al, *Biochem Cell Bio* 2010 88:4.

Emodin inhibits VeroE6 cells that play a role in SARS-Cov S protein and may help to reduce effects of this life threatening infection. Emodin was found in the same study by Ho et al, *Antiviral Res* 2007 74:2 to have angio-tensive benefit.

Combining rhubarb root with licorice root increases the rate at which the large intestine can absorb these compounds; as does a mild alcohol water extract.

Rhubarb root is used for treating trichomonas that causes vaginal infections, with early research indicating 1:1000 concentrations lethal to *Trichomonas hominis*, and recent research showing inhibition of *T. vaginalis*. Kajo, *Chem Abstr* 1959 47; Wang, *J Ethnopharm* 1993 40:2. His work suggests anti-oxidants increase effectiveness of this herbal therapy.

Rhaponticin is metabolized, by intestinal bacteria to rhapontigenin, which exhibits anti-allergic activity. It inhibits platelet aggregation induced by arachidonic acid or collagen. Ko et al, *Arch Pharm Res* 1999 22:4

Methanol extracts of *R. undulatum*, or its isolated rhapontigenin, show anti-allergic activity. Matsuda et al, *Bio Pharm Bull* 2000 24:3.

Rhaponiticin shows lowering of blood sugar and improvement of diabetic symptoms in mice. Chen et al, *Planta Medica* 2009 75:5.

Rhubarb is not only laxative, but a diuretic that can alkalize urine up to pH 8.4; much higher than the organisms preferred level of 5.5-5.8.

In a study conducted at the University of Alberta, researchers led by Dr. Tapan Basu and Dr. B. Ooraikul found rhubarb stalk fibre significantly reduces cholesterol, especially the harmful LDL. It also helped lower triglycerides in the blood.

Ten hyper-cholesterol men in the study consumed 27 grams of powdered rhubarb stalk daily for 30 days. Average cholesterol reduction was 9%, and triglycerides averaged an 18% decrease. *Journal Am College of Nutrition* 1997 16:6.

They found that processed dry stalk powder holds water up to 20 times its own weight.

It is theorized that because rhubarb stalk has the ability to bind eleven times more bile salts than cellulose, and 2.5 times oat, rice and wheat bran, that this must be the mechanism of action. *Nutrition Research* 1998 18:5.

Despite the presence of oxalic acid, the fibre does not interfere with calcium absorption, at least in lab animals.

Recent testing with both rhubarb juice and pulp led to their use as an acid coagulant for the production of Quark, a dairy product similar to cottage cheese. This led to significantly reduced loss of calcium to the whey. This high calcium Quark, when fed to rats, in comparison to regular lactic acid coagulated product, led to an interesting observation.

Although the rate of calcium absorption was half of the diet containing regular quark, the actual amount absorbed was about twice as much.

It may prevent cancer. Researchers at the University of Mainz in Germany tested raw rhubarb juice against cancer causing agents. They found rhubarb near the top in preventing cell mutations that lead to cancer, but only in the test tube.

More study on humans would be the next logical step.

Rhubarb contains Vitamin C, another immune booster that prevents the oxidation of LDL cholesterol.

Rhubarb contains high amounts of calcium oxalate, which can antagonize sufferers of kidney stones, if they are also low consumers of calcium.

For years, doctors have recommended patients prone to kidney stones limit their intake of calcium. However, a study in 1992, of over 45000 men, showed a higher risk of kidney stones for those with low calcium intake. Why?

Dietary calcium binds oxalates so they cannot be absorbed, and if dietary calcium levels are too low, they are free to enter the bloodstream. Curhan et al, *NEJ of Medicine* 1993 328. Maybe.

Oxalates in rhubarb, spinach, sorrel and other foods temporarily bind to calcium in teeth, feeling like sandpaper.

During World War II it was claimed that people died from eating rhubarb leaves that contained oxalates. The stalks contain as much oxalates as the leaves, and spinach 30% more. The leaves are poisonous for reasons that have nothing to do with oxalates.

In a normal healthy diet, oxalates are excreted with little absorption through intestinal walls. Plants high in oxalates are also high in calcium so the often-repeated suggestion that they block calcium absorption is suspect.

Oxalates bind to heavy metals and help remove them from the body.

There is little science to suggest that oxalates promote development of kidney stones or gallstones in healthy individuals. People who develop kidney stones have a physiological abnormality that promotes creation and deposition of oxalates in body.

In normal metabolism, excess vitamin C is converted to oxalates and other breakdown constituents that filter through kidneys. High intake of vitamin C results in much greater metabolic oxalate production than high oxalate vegetables. Oxalates in the blood do not bind with calcium in healthy people because our blood chemistry and pH will not allow it. High levels of ascorbic acid and oxalates at same time may be bad idea, unless you wish to develop kidney stones.

Oxalic acid appears to neutralize chlorofluorocarbons (CFCs) associated with destruction of the ozone layer. Sodium oxalate was found by Yale researchers in 1995 to break down these compounds in a less costly and dangerous manner.

Dr. Bibby, of the Eastman Dental Centre in Rochester, New York observed that the mineral salts in rhubarb juice appear to coat teeth with a thin, protective film against decay. Simply rub the expressed juice on the teeth every other day.

According to James Duke, rhubarb is a good source of lutein, which has benefit in prevention of macular degeneration in eyes.

The root has a mild laxative action that improves appetite and stimulates the liver. Two components of the English Garden Rhubarb root, lindleyin and iso-lindleyin, have been found as effective as aspirin and phenylbutazone regarding anti-inflammatory and analgesic properties.

The root of garden rhubarb contains trans-resveratrol and hydroxystilbenes that reduce liver damage caused by ethanol. Raal et al, *Phytother Res* 2009 23:4.

Individuals taking rhubarb root will find their urine turns red, a harmless alkaline reaction.

The rhizomes of *R. rhaponticum* were studied by Starec et al, *Acta Veterinaria Brno* 1996 65:3. A new substance, RG tannin, purified from the root has interesting neurolyptic properties that could be useful in veterinary and human medicine.

Work by Kaszkin-Bettag et al, Menopause 14:2 found an extract of *R. rhaponticum* root called ERr 731 decreases anxiety and improves general well-being in peri-menopausal women.

Wober et al, *J Steroid Biochem Mol Biol* 2007 107:3-5 found this compound to be an estrogen receptor beta agonist, suggesting use in both peri-menopause and menopause as well.

Further work by Möller et al, *Phytomed* 2007 14:11 on this compound found the Er alpha influence to be associated with bone cells, not endometrial, suggesting benefit in osteoporosis.

The extract has been in use since 1993, with no side effects in human trials. A study by Kaszkin-Bettag et al, *Food Chem Tox* 2008 46:5 found the compound exhibits extremely low toxicity.

The same authors did a six-month study of 363 menopausal women and found the Menopause Rating Scale, a subjective evaluation of various symptoms such as vaginal dryness, depression, anxiety, and hot flushes, reduced from 14.5 to 6.5. *Alter Ther Health Med* 2008 14:6.

Hasper et al, *Menopause* 2009 16:1 followed 48 perimenopausal women for a half-year, and noted improvements in many parameters, while taking ERr 731.

Papke et al, *J Steroid Biochem Mol Biol* 2009 117:4-5 found the extract safe as well.

Work by Hussain et al, *Fitoterapia* 1997 68:5 found ethanol extracts of the root active against various bacteria including *E. coli, Staphylococcus aureus, S. epidermis, Klebsiella pneumoniae, Enterobacter aerogenes,* and *Bacillus cereus.*

Superficial skin infections from *S. aureus* and *S. epidermis* may be treated with *R. rhaponticum* root extracts. Kosikowska et al, *Centr Eur J Bio* 5:6.

Alcohol extracts containing athracene and stilbene derivatives show activity against various tuberculosis mycobacterium, including *M. tuberculosis* H37Ra and *M. bovis.* Smolarz HD et al, *J AOAC Int* 2013 96:1 155-60.

Rhubarb extracts have been found to be effective against various fungi including *Trichophyton, Microsporum* and *Epidermaphyton* species.

Thomas Bartram, noted English herbalist, wrote Garden Rhubarb is a mild stimulant for the production of estrogen, and useful for menopause and estrogen deficient conditions. He does not say, however, whether he is speaking of the roots, or stalk. The former I assume.

A decoction of seeds is useful to ease stomach pain and increase appetite.

Rhubarb seeds, in the immature stage, contain the biologically active gibberellin A. This is an important class of growth regulators. Yosh Kimura, *J of Agr Food Chemistry*, Oct 2001. My herbal students have used hot water extracts of the seed as growth promoters in gardens and greenhouses with excellent results.

In Egypt, the seeds of *R. officinale* are combined with fenugreek, lupine (*L. albus*), and other seeds as an anti-diabetic preparation. Work by Nada el al, *Fitoterapia* 1997 68:3 found the mixture induced significant decrease of serum cholesterol, triglycerides, creatinine, and aspartate amino-transferase.

It induced a significant increase in hemoglobin levels and red blood cell counts, as well as a significant decrease of total white blood cell count after four weeks treatment.

Chinese Rhubarb, and its medicinal uses, can take up an entire book, so I've chosen to concentrate on the garden variety. For more information on official rhubarb, there is no better source than *Rhubarb, the Wondrous Drug*, by Clifford M. Foust.

Our Garden Rhubarb stems should be checked for content of rhuscholide, present in *R. chinensis*, as this compound showed significant anti-HIV activity in work by Gu et al, *Planta Med* 73:3.

Rhubarb leaves can be inserted under a bra to help relieve breast pain, including mastitis.

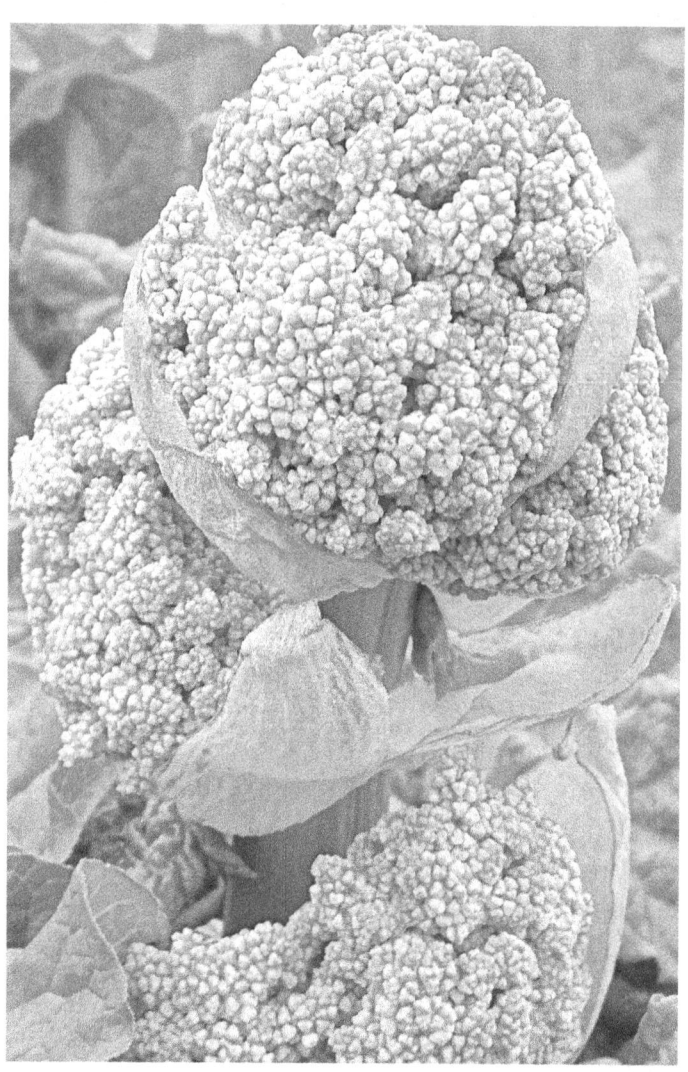

GARDEN RHUBARB SEED HEAD

HOMEOPATHY

Rhubarb (*R. officinale/palmatum*) is mainly indicated in diarrhea that is sour and full of mucus. The anus is red and sore, and there is accompanied stomach and abdominal pain. There is a constant, yet unsuccessful urge to urinate before stool.

Summer complaint in children with teething pain is a classic symptom.

There may be a sweat on the hairy scalp that is constant and profuse, with a cold sweat on the face.

Symptoms are worse from uncovering, after eating, or moving about.

Anxiety as if they had done something bad. Sulky, silent, reserved, laconic and indolent. Mental state as if half asleep.

Whimsical impatience, and dreams of deceased relatives.

DOSE- Third to sixth potency. The mother tincture is prepared from the rootstock, peeled off almost to the cambium. First proving by Hahnemann with six provers.

ESSENTIAL OILS

The root of Garden Rhubarb (*R. rhaponticum*) has been steam distilled and yields about 0.0041% oil containing chrysophanic acid.

The oil is intensely yellow, and is a concrete that melts at 25.5 ° C.

The root of *R. palmatum* has been steam distilled and yields oil containing 108 components, of which over 27% were terpenoids.

The main constituents were palmitic acid (22.5%), paeonol (16.2%), alpha-copaene (9.8%), methyl stearate (9.3%), delta-cadinene (5.7%), and methyl eugenol (5.4%).

The stalks of *R. rhabarbarum* contain methyl branched alcohols and acids including 2-methylbutanol, 4-methylhexanol, 2-methylbutanoic acid, and 4-methylhexanoic acid.

More than 65% of volatiles contain C6 skeletons. In additions to unsaturated C6 aldehydes and alcohols, substantial amounts of less common (E)-2- and (E)-3-hexanoic acid were found among the 59 components identified so far.

FLOWER ESSENCE

Rhubarb (*R. officinale*) flower essence helps create more tolerance, compassion and ability to discover the true core of others.
                                                                                                   MIRIANA

SPIRITUAL PROPERTIES

With Rhubarb, there is a strong tendency for energy in the root chakra to rise through the spine. This liberates energy stored in the other chakras.

As a result of this pattern, the energy already dealt with in life is more available. This is why rhubarb can sometimes cause difficulty in pregnancy. A great deal of changing energy, which is largely under the control and direction of the being that is newly conceived, is taking place in the root and second chakras. Rhubarb also cleanses the root chakra.

There is an enhanced ability to accept sexuality, to share in the energy of creation. The root chakra is relaxed and its energy is dispersed, while the natural movement through the bladder meridian is slightly accelerated.

When Mars is retrograde for any individual, there will be some enhanced absorption in working with rhubarb.
                                                                                                   GURUDAS

PERSONALITY TRAITS

The [Rhubarb] patient has always tended to constipation, which can vary in severity. During the acute phases, the patient has hard dry stools and some rectal bleeding. This may be accompanied by distension and discomfort of both the epigastrium and abdomen, bad breath, and a bitter taste in the mouth. The patient has recurring eczema with red lesions, and a sensation of heat in the skin.   **ROSS**

"To rhubarb" also means muffled rather than sharp declamation. As a dramatic term, it refers to a group of actors giving the impression of indistinct background conversation, made by mumbling "rhubarb" over and over again, used because the word contains no sharp or recognizable phonemes. Rhubarb can describe a heated dispute, usually over insignificant matters. Here is a word that can be both instrument and obfuscation, while the real vegetable, impertinent as it is determined, presents an audacious face to the retreating back of winter.

ARITHA van HERK, NEW TRAIL WINTER 2011

MYTHS AND LEGENDS

There was an herbalist who was called Mr. Five Yellow because he was known to have mastered five yellow herbs-yellow bark, yellow essence, greater yellow root, yellow root and yellow pearl rhizome.

One year he went to pick herbs and found that his friend Mr. Mah was living alone in a cave after his house burned down and he lost his family.

Mr. Five Yellow found his friend and asked if he wanted to work with him. Mr. Mah wanted to be an herbalist so he agreed, but Mr. Five Yellow did not want him to treat patients.

"You are not careful enough to be an herbalist", said Mr. Five Yellow.

One day, while his friend was away, Mr. Mah started to treat patients on his own, and initially was doing all right. One day, however, a woman with diarrhea came to see him, and she was very weak and pale.

He remembered his friend used yellow root, so he decocted this for the patient. But after drinking it, the patient got much worse and almost died from severe diarrhea.

Mr. Mah did not know what went wrong. When his friend returned he told him. Mr. Five Yellow knew he had used the wrong yellow root, as there was one for constipation and one for diarrhea.   **HENRY C. LU**

RECIPES

ROOT DECOCTION- 3-12 grams dry root in 500 ml of water for 20 minutes. Drink 50-100 ml as needed.

DRIED POWDER- One to four grams of dried root powder at bedtime in water. Standardized capsules contain 30-100 mg of hydroxyanthracene derivatives.

TINCTURE- 5 ml three times daily in water of 1:5 at 40% alcohol for dried root. Do not use fresh root.

DISEASE SPRAY- Take three pounds of leaves to six pints of water and boil for 30 minutes. Strain, bottle and mix with liquid soap for roses, apples, etc. For Cabbage family, simply cut a piece of stem and insert with seed in hole.

One 1973 report from Liverpool found 90% immunity from clubfoot with this method.

CAUTION- Do not use for Crohn's disease or ulcerative colitis, or acute abdominal pain of unknown origin, including appendicitis. Long-term use can lead to loss of electrolytes, and possibly hyper-aldosteronism, and enhancement of cardioactive steroids. Heart arrhythmia, nephropathy, edema and accelerated bone deterioration MAY result.

ESCOP does not recommend the herb during breastfeeding. I doubt this would be a problem at normal dosage. Cathartic constituents may cross the blood brain barrier, causing infant diarrhea or feeding problems.

Senna (*Cassia senna*) has been found safe for use during breastfeeding.

ROCK JASMINE
NORTHERN ROCK CANDELABRA
PYGMY FLOWER
(***Androsace septentrionalis*** L.)
FAIRY CANDELABRA
WESTERN ROCK JASMINE
(***A. occidentalis*** Pursh.)
ALPINE ROCK JASMINE
SWEET FLOWER ROCK JASMINE
FAIRY CANDELABRA
(***A. chamaejasme*** Wulfen ex Host)
(***A. lehmanniana*** Spreng.) not accepted
PARTS USED- whole plant

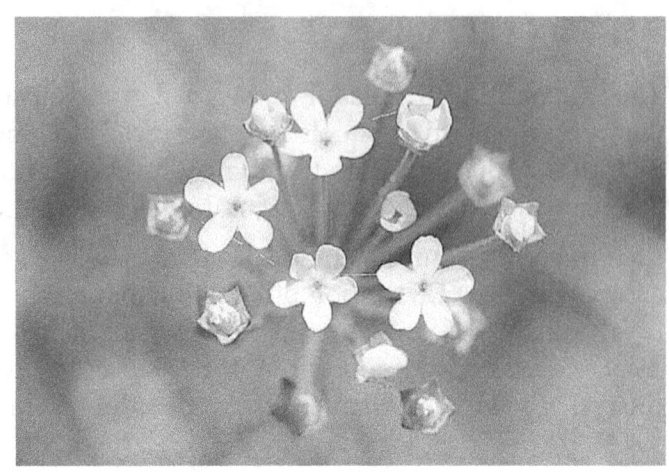

ANDROSACE SEPTENTRIONALIS

Androsace is from the Greek **ANER**, meaning a man and **SAKOS**, a shield, or buckle referring to the resemblance of the anthers to an ancient buckler. This was the name given to another plant by Dioscorides. Androsakes is the Greek name for a marine plant.

Occidentalis means from the West; and septentrionalis means Northern, from septentriones, the seven stars of the constellation *Ursa Minor*. Chamaejasme means jasmine-like, referring to the strong scented and pleasant scent of the flower.

Fairy Candelabra is a fairly common annual, on the prairies. It likes dry, open country of southeastern Alberta. The closely related Alpine Rock Jasmine is also a lover of dry soils, but is circumpolar and more widely spread, even up to alpine elevations.

Both plants have whitish-pink flowers with yellow eyes that are short lived.

Native tribes, including the Navaho-Ramah used Fairy Candelabra as part of decoctions for birth injury, or postpartum hemorrhage.

The closely related Rock Jasmine (*A. septentrionalis*) was used as a life medicine. Cold infusions were given for internal pain or the pain of "witch's arrows".

In Siberia, the plant was used in folk medicine for angina, epilepsy, gonorrhea, and as a contraceptive.

It was often made into a lotion with which one anointed themselves for protection from witches.

It was usually taken as a cold infusion of the leaves and flowers as a "life medicine" or combined with other plants in decoction and drunk before entering sweats for treating venereal disease.

The Slave of Canada's boreal forest call Rock Jasmine "Lice Medicine", or **YAH NAYDI**.

A whole plant decoction was used to wash the hair and other body parts to kill lice.

Milky Pygmy Flower is an introduced plant, not native to the Canadian prairies.

MEDICINAL

CONSTITUENTS- *A. occidentalis*-fifteen triterpene glycosides, the aglycones being oleonolic acid, primulagenin, and more than 15 phenolic compounds including quercitin, 3,4-dihydroxycinnamic (caffeic) acid, kaemferol, rutin, and coumarins. *A. septentrionalis*- androseptosides (saponins), quercitin, kaempferol, rutin, caffeic acid. Various triterpene glycosides are present including androspetosides A, B, C1, D and D1; andro-septoside F.

Rock Jasmine has been investigated for its contraceptive action. Work by Mats et al, *Farm Toksikol* 1986 49(2) 38-9 show the triterpene glycosides from Rock Jasmine change the concentrations of lutropin and follitropin in the pituitary gland and blood plasma.

In turn, this influences the ration of these hormones in the blood in the active phase of the menstrual cycle.

This leads to the change of the ovarian hormonal activity in the direction of estrogenic action, and an increase in uterine contractions.

Research conducted in Leningrad in 1984, by same author found the triterpene glycosides have contraceptive effect because of their powerful spermicidal activity.

Work by Sokolow and Surina have investigated the pharmacology of *A. septentrionalis*. The results confirm the tranquilizing and contraceptive effect with respect to influence on corpus luteum.

The related *A. strigilosa*, which can be grown in zone 3, shows strong anti-viral activity against influenza. Rajbhadari et al, *Evid Based Comp Alt Med* 2007 6:4.

The related *A. umbellata* contains saxifragifolin A-D, compounds that strong strong cytotoxicity and induce apoptosis in multi-drug resistant tumor cell lines. Park et al, *Arch Pharmacal Res* 33:8.

Saxifragifolin C induced apoptotis in breast cancer cells, with MDA-MB-231 cells more sensitive than MCF-7 cells. Kim KH et al, *Arch Pharm Res* 2016 39(4): 577-89. Earlier work by same author found saxifragifolin also induced apoptosis. *Phytomed* 2015 22(9).

The compound myricetin 3-O-beta-D-glycopyranoside from this herb was identified as one of four plants out of 88 with high inhibition of hyaluronidase, associated with snake venom. Wood Sorrel (*Oxalis corniculata*) also rated high. Liu Y et al, *Phytochemistry* 2015 119:62-9.

HOMEOPATHY

Milky Pygmy Flower (*A. lactea*) is used in cases of urinary troubles, and as a diuretic in cases of dropsy.

DOSE- 6th to 30th potency.

SEED OIL

The seeds of *A. septentrionalis* contain two unusual fatty acids. These are 11-cis-hexadecenoic acid (16:1 delta11c or 16:1n-5) and 9-cis, 12-cis-hexadecadienoic acid (16:2delta9c or 16:2n-4).

These compounds are found in members of the Asclepiadaceae and Ranunculus species.

The oil is rich in 9-cis-hexadecenoic acid (21.4%) and 18:1delta11c (3.8%).

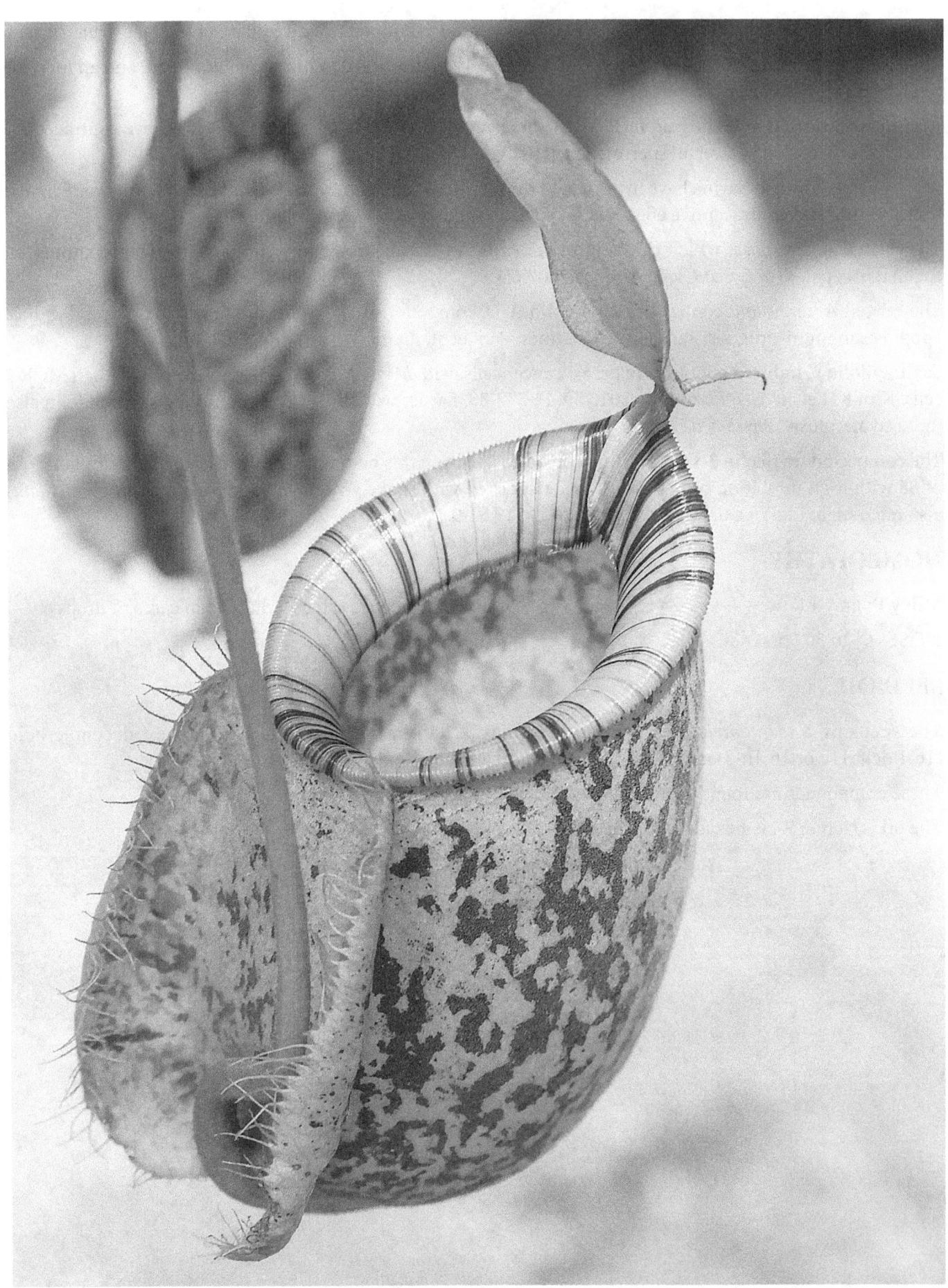

ABOUT THE AUTHOR

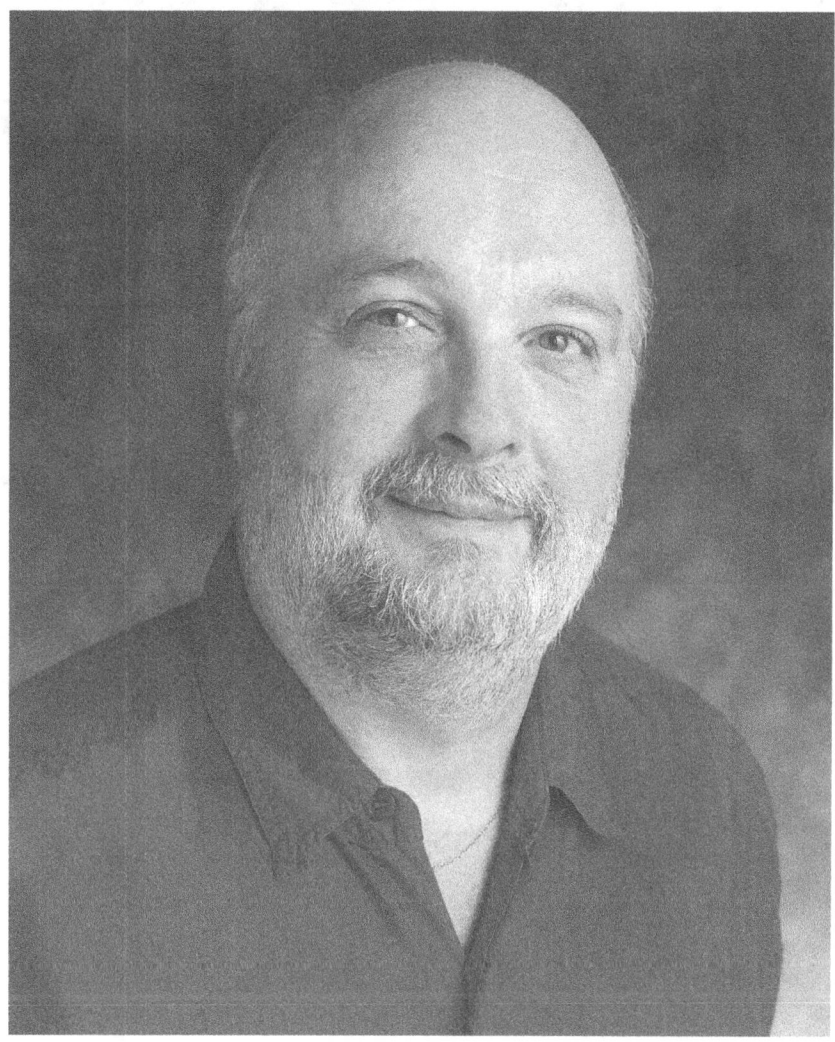

Robert Dale Rogers has been an herbalist for over forty-five years. He has a Bachelor of Science from the University of Alberta, where he is an assistant clinical professor in Family Medicine. He teaches plant medicine, including herbology and flower essences in the Earth Spirit Medicine Program at the Northern Star College of Mystical Studies in Edmonton, Alberta, Canada.

Robert is past chair of the Alberta Natural Health Agricultural Network and Community Health Council of Capital Health. He is a Fellow of the International College of Nutrition, past chair of the medicinal mushroom committee of the North American Mycological Association and on the editorial board of the International Journal of Medicinal Mushrooms. He writes occasional article for Fungi magazine.

Robert co-hosts The Alberta Herb Gathering held every second year (www.albertaherbgathering.com)

He lives on Millcreek Ravine in Edmonton with his beautiful and talented wife, Laurie Szott–Rogers and out of control cat Ceres.

You can email him at scents@telusplanet.net
or visit
www.selfhealdistributing.com

BIBLIOGRAPHY

Abbe, Elfriede, *The Fern Herbal,* Cornell University Press, Ithaca, 1981

Acorn, J. Bugs of Alberta, Lone Pine Publishing, Edmonton, AB, 2000.

Adams, J. *Les Plantes Medicinales.* Bulletin 23, Agriculture Canada. 1916

Adams, Jean. *Insect Potpourri, Adventures in Entomology.* Sandhill Crane Press, FL. 1992

Aggarwal, Bharat. Healing Spices. Sterling Pub. New York 2011.

Albert-Puleo, Michael. *Economic Botany, 32, Jan-Mar, 1978.*

Allaby, Michael. *Temperate Forests.* Facts on File. New York. 1999.

Allen, D & Hatfield, G. *Medicinal Plants in Folk Tradition.* Timber Press, Portland. 2004

Allen,E, Morrison,D, &Wallis,G. *Common Tree Diseases of B.C. Canada Forest Service,* '96

Allende, Isabel. *Aphrodite- A Memoir of the Senses.* Harper Flamingo. New York. 1998.

Alstat, Ed. *Electic Dispensatory of Botanical Therapeutics.* Ecl Med. Oregon. 1989.

Anderson, Anne, *Some Native Herbal Remedies,* Pub 8A, Devonian Botanical Gardens 1980

_____*Plants in Cree.* Duval House Pub. Edmonton AB 2000.

Anderson, C.&Tischer,T. *Poinsettias, the December Flower,* Waters Edge Press, CA, 1997

Andoh, Anthony. *The Science & Romance of Selected Herbs used in Medicine and Religious Ceremony.* North Scale Institute. San Francisco. 1986.

Andre, Alestine & Fehr, Alan. *Gwich'in Ethnobotany.* Gwich'in Social and Cultural Institute, Box 46, Tsiigehtchie, NWT, X0E 0B0, fax 1867-953-3820.

Andrews, Tamra. Nectar and Ambrosia. ABC-CLIO Box 1911 Santa Barbara CA. 2000.

Andrews, Ted. *Animal Speak- The Spiritual and Magical Powers,* Llewellyn. Minn. 1996.

_____*Animal Wise,* DragonHawk, Jackson, TN, 1999.

Antol, Marie. *The Incredible Secrets of Mustard.* Avery Pub. New York. 1999.

Aronson J K Ed. Meyler's Side Effects of Herbal Medicines. Elsevier Amsterdam. 2009.

Arrowsmith, Nancy. Essential Herbal Wisdom. Llewellyn Pub. Woodbury, Minn. 2009.

Arsdall, Anne Van. *Medieval Herbal Remedies.* Routledge, New York. 2002.

Arvigo & Balick, *Rainforest Remedies,* Lotus Press, Twin Lakes, WI. 1993

Arvigo & Epstein. *Rainforest Home Remedies,* Harper SanFrancisco, 2001.

Assiniwi, Bernard. *La Medecine des Indiens d' Amerique,* Guerin Literature, 1988

Atal C.K. & Kapur B. *Cultivation and Utilization of Medicinal Plants,* Jammu-Tawi, 1982

Attenborough, David. *The Private Life of Plants.* Princeton U Press. Princeton NJ 1995.

Ausubel, K. *Seeds of Change The Living Treasure.* HarperSanFrancisco, 1994.

Aversano, Laura. *The Divine Nature of Plants.* Swan•Raven & Co. Columbus, NC, 2002.

Ayensu, Edward,S. *Medicinal Plants of the West Indies,* Reference Publications, 1981

Baïracli Levy, Juliette *Herbal Handbook for Farm and Stable,* Faber&Faber, London, 1952

Baker, Phil. The Dedalus Book of Absinthe. Dedalus 2001.

Barl, Branka et al, *Saskatchewan Herb Database,* U. of Sask. Saskatoon, 1996.

Barlow, Max. *From the Shepherd's Purse.* 1990

Barnes J, Anderson L, &Phillipson J. *Herbal Medicines, A guide for healthcare professionals.* Pharmaceutical Press, London, 2002.

Barnett, Robert A. *Tonics,* Harper Collins, New York, N.Y. 1997

Bartram, Thomas. *Bartram's Encyl. of Herbal Medicine,* Robinson Pub. London, 1998.

Bascom, Angella. *Incorporating Herbal Medicine into Clinical Practice.* F. Davis Co. 2002

Beals, Katherine, M. *Flower Lore and Legend,* Henry Holt, 1917

Beers, Susan-Jane. *Jamu The ancient Indonesian Art of Herbal Healing,* Periplus, 2001.

Belcourt, Christi. Medicines to Help Us. Gabriel Dumont Instit. Saskatoon, SK 2007.

Béliveau, R & Gingras,D. *Foods That Fight Cancer.* McClelland & Stewart Toronto. 2006.

Belsinger S & Dille C. *Cooking with Herbs.* CBI- Van Nostrand Reinhold, N.Y. 1984.

Benjamin, D.R. *Mushrooms: Poisons and Panaceas.* WH Freeman, San Francisco, 1995.

Bennet, Doug & Tiner, Tim. *Up North.* Reed Books Canada. Markham, Ont. 1993.

_____*Up North Again.* McClelland and Stewart. Toronto, 1997.

Bennet, J & Rowley S. *Uqalurait An Oral History of Nunavut.* McGill Queens, Mont. 2004

Benyus, Janine. *Biomimicry Innovation Inspired by Nature.* William Morrow. 1997.

Berenbaum,May R. *Buzzwords, A Scientists Muses on Sex, Bugs and Rock N Roll,* Joseph Henry Press, Washington, D.C. 2000.

_____*Bugs in the System.* Helix Books, Addison-Wesley Pub. 1995.

Beresford-Kroeger, Diana. The Global Forest. Viking Penguin. 2010.

_____Arboretum Borealis. U Michigan Press. 2010.

Berliocchi,Luigi. *The Orchid in Lore and Legend.* Timber Press, Portland Oregon, 2000.

Berlund B & Bolsby C. *The Edible Wild* Pagurian Press, Toronto, Ont. 1971.

Berkowsky, Bruce. *Mount Julius Flower Remedies. Mt. Vernon Washington, 1986*

Bermejo, J & Leon,J. *Neglected Crops-1492 ...* FAO Series 26, United Nations, Rome, 1994.

Bernhardt, P. *The Rose's Kiss, A Natural History of Flowers* . Island Press, Covelo CA 1999

Bianchi, Ivo. *Geriatrics and Homotoxicology.* Aurelia-Verlag GmbH, Baden Baden, 1994.

Bianchini, F. *The Complete Book of Health Plants.* Crescent Books, New York, 1975.

Biship, Carol. *The Book of Home Remedies &Herbal Cures,* Jonathan-James, Toronto, 1979.

Bisset, Norman G. *Herbal Drugs and Phytopharmaceuticals.* 2nd Ed. CRC Press, 2001.

Blackburn, Thomas. *December's Child: A Book of Chumash Oral Narratives* , U of California Press, Berkeley, 1975.

Blanchan, Neltje. *Nature's Garden.* Doubleday, Page&Co. New York, 1900.

Bland, John. *Forests of Liliput.* Prentice Hall, Englewood Cliffs, New Jersey, 1971.

Bliss, Anne. *Rocky Mountain Dye Plants.* Juniper House, Boulder, Colorado, 1976

Blouin, Glen. *Weeds of the Woods.* Goose Lane, Fredericton, New Brunswick 1992.

_____*An Eclectic Guide to Trees, east of the Rockies.* Boston Mills, 2001.

Boas, F. *Ethnology of the Kwakiutl.* Bureau of Am. Ethnology, 35th annual report, 1921.

Boericke, Wm. *Materia Medica with Repetory.* B. Jain Publishers. 1976

Boik, John. *Natural Compunds in Cancer Therapy.* Oregon Med Press, Princeton,Minn 2001

Boland, Bridget. *Gardener's Magic &Other Old Wives' Lore.* The Bodley Head, London, 77.

Bolton, Brett L. *The Secret Powers of Plants.* Berkley Pub Co. New York. 1974.

Bolton, J.L. *Alfalfa, Botany, Cultivation &Utilization.* Interscience Pub, New York, 1962.

Bone, Kerry. *A Clinical Guide to Blending Liquid Herbs.* Churchill Livingstone. 2003

Borrel, Marie. *Healing Plants.* Cassell & Co. Wellington House, London. 2001.

Bouchardon, Patrice. *The Healing Energies of Trees.* Journey Editions, Boston, 1999.

Bossenmaier, Eugene. *Mushrooms of the Boreal Forest.* U. of Saskatchewan Press, 1997

Boulos, Loutfy. *Medicinal Plants of North Africa,* Reference Pub. Algonac, Mich. 1983

Bowles, E. Joy. *The Chemistry of Aromatherapeutic Oils.* Allen & Unwin, Crow's Nest, Australia, 2003.

Bowman, Daria. *Hydrangeas.* Friedman/Fairfax Pub. New York. 1999.

Bradley, Peter. British Herbal Compendium Vol 2 Brit Herb Med Assoc. Bournemouth 2006.

Brahmachari, Goutam Ed. Natural Products, Alpha Sci Int Ltd. Oxford UK 2009.

Brandeis, Gayle. *Fruitflesh.* Harper Collins, San Francisco. 2002.

Brennan, M. *Complete Holistic Care & Healing for Horses*. Trafalgar Sq. Pub. VT. 2001.

Bringhurst, Robert. *A Story as Sharp as a Knife*. Douglas&Mc Intyre Vancouver, 1999.

Brinker, Francis N.D. *Herb Contraindications and Drug Interactions*. Third Edition Eclectic Medical Publications, Sandy, Oregon, 2001

_____*The Toxicology of Botanical Medicines,* revised 2nd. Eclectic Med, Oregon, 1996.

_____*Eclectic Dispensatory of Botanical Therapeutics,* Vol 2, Ecl. Med . Oregon, 1995.

Brodo, Irwin & Sharnoff. *Lichens of North America*. Yale University Press, 2001.

Brown, Deni. *Encyclopedia of Herbs and Their Uses*. Reader's Digest Press, Que. 1995.

Bruneton, J *Pharmacognosy, Phtyochemistry, Medicinal Plants,* Lavoisier Pub. Paris, 1995

_____*Toxic Plants Dangerous to Humans and Animals*. Editions TEC&Doc, Paris, '99.

Brunschwig, Hieronymus. *Book of Distillation*. Johnson Reprint Co No. 79. New York, 1971.

Brynaherb Essences 29, Kells Meend Berry Hill, Gloucestershire GL16 7AD

Bubar, Carol et al. *Weeds of the Prairies*. Alberta Agriculture Pub. Edmonton, 2000.

Buchanan, Carol. *Brothers Crow, Sister Corn*. Ten Speed Press, Berkeley, 1997.

Buckle, Jane. *Clinical Aromatherapy. 2nd ed.* Churchill Livingstone, Toronto, 2003.

Buhner, Stephen H. *Sacred and Herbal Healing Beers,* Siris Books, Boulder, Co, 1998

_____*Sacred Plant Medicine*. Robert Rinehart, Boulder, Co. 1996.

_____Herbal Antibiotics. Storey Books, Vermont, 1999.

_____*The Lost Language of Plants*. Chelsea Green Pub. White River, Vt. 2002

_____Secret Teachings of Plants. Bear & Co. Rochester, Vt. 2004.

_____The Natural Testosterone Plan. Healing Arts Press, Rochester VT. 2007

Burbridge, Joan. *Wildflowers of the Southern Interior of B.C.* U. of B.C. Press, 1989.

Burger, W. Flowers- *How they changed the world. Prometheus Books.* Amherst NY 2006.

Burgess, Isla. *Weeds Heal*. Viriditas Pub Group. Cambridge NZ 1998.

Burlando, Bruno et al, Herbal Principles in Cosmetics. CRC Press Boca Raton 2010.

Caius, Rev. Fr. Jean F., *The Medicinal and Poisonous Plants of India*, Scientific Pub, 1986.

Cameron, Elizabeth. *A Floral ABC*. John Wiley and Sons. Toronto. 1980.

Carpenter D. Snr Pub. *Nursing Herbal Medicine Handbook,* Springhouse Corp. 2001.

Carpinella, Maria et al. Novel Therapeutic Agents from Plants. Sci Pub. Enfield NJ 2009.

Carr, Emily. *Wild Flowers*. Royal BC Museum, Victoria, B.C, 2006

Carroll, Roisin. *The Crane Bag Celtic Tree Ogam Oils* , Feasibility Pub. Dublin

Carter, Bernard F. *The Floral Birthday Book*. Bloomsbury Books, London. 1990.

Casselman, Bill. *Canadian Garden Words*. Little, Brown & Co. Toronto, 1997.

Castleman, Michael. *The Healing Herbs*. Bantam Books. 1995.

Castro, Miranda. *The Complete Homeopathy Handbook*. MacMillan, 1990

Catty, Suzanne. *Hydrosols the next Aromatherapy,* Healing Arts Press, Vermont, 2001.

Cavers, Paul ed, *The Biology of Canadian Weeds* 62-83,Ag Institute of Canada, Ottawa, 1995

_____84-102 Ag Inst. of Canada, Ottawa, 2000.

_____103-129 Ag Inst. of Canada, Ottawa 2005

Ceres. *Herbal Teas for Health and Healing*. Healing Arts Press, Rochester, Vermont, 1984.

Chan, K, and Cheung L. *Interactions between Chincese Herbal Medicinal Products and Orthodox Drugs*. Harwood Academic Publishers, Canada, 2000.

Chandler, F. *Herbs-Everyday Reference for Health Professionals,* Can. Pharm Assoc. 2000

Chang & But. *Pharmacology &Applications of Chinese Materia Medica,* World Scientific, 86

Chang Chao-liang et al, *Vegetables as Medicine,* Pelanduk Pub, Malaysia, 1999.

Chappell, P. Emotional Healing with Homeopathy. North Atlantic Books. Berkeley, 2003.

Charissa's Cauldron. www.charissacauldron.com

Chase, Pamela & Pawlik, J. *Newcastle Trees for Healing* , Newcastle Pub. Van Nuys,1991

Chatroux, Sylvia. *Botanica Poetica*. Poetica Press 2004 1-877-POETICA.

_____*Materica Poetica*. Poetica Press 1998.

Chen, John K & Chen, Tina T. Chinese Medical Herbology & Pharmacology. Art of Medicine Press, City of Industry, CA 2004.

Chevalllier, Andrew. *The Encyclopedia of Medicinal Plants*. Reader's Digest, 1996.

Chishti, Hakim. *The Traditional Healer*, Healing Arts Press, Vermont,1988.

Christchurch Flower Essences. www.christchurchfloweressences.com

Clark, Ella E. *Indian Legends of Canada*. McClelland & Stewart. Toronto, 1960.

Coats, Peter. *Flowers in History*. Weidenfeld and Nicolson, London. 1970.

Coffey, Timothy.*The History and Folklore of North American Wildflowers,* Houghton-Mifflin, 1993.

Cohen, Kenneth. *Honoring the Medicine*. Random House, Toronto. 2003.

Conrad, Chris, *Hemp for Health,* Healing Arts Press, Rochester, Vermont, 1997.

Cook, Wm.H. *The Physio-Medical Dispensatory.* 1869. Reprinted by Eclectic Medical Publications, Portland, Oregon, 1985.

_____A compendium of the new Materia medica together with additional descriptions of some old remedies. Wm. Cook Publisher, Chicago, 1896.

Cooper, J.C. *Dictionary of Symbolic & Mythological Animals,* Thorsons, London, 1992.

Cormack, R.G.H. *Wild Flowers of Alberta*. Hurtig Publishers, 1977

Coupland, Francois. *The Encyclopedia of Edible Plants of N. America*. Keats Pub. 1998.

Cousin, Pierre J. *Eat Well, Be Well*. Thorsons, London. 2001.

Cowan, Eliot. *Plant Spirit Medicine*. Swan Raven & Co. Box 726 Newberg, Oregon, 1995.

Cowan, Thomas. The Fourfold Path to Healing. New Trends Pub. Washington DC 2007.

Crane, Eva. *Honey- A Comprhensive Survey* , Heinemann Pub. London 1975.

Craydon D. & Bellows W. Floral Acupuncture. The Crossing Press Berkeley CA 2005.

Creekmore, H. *Daffodils are Dangerous*. Walker and Co. New York. 1966.

Crow, Tis Mal. *Native Plants, Native Healing*. Native Voices Book Pub. Box 99 Summertown, Tennessee, 2001 1-888-260-8458.

Crowell, Robert L. *The Lore & Legends of Flowers*. Thomas Crowell, New York, 1982.

Crowfoot & Baldensperger. *From Cedar to Hyssop*. Sheldon Press, London, 1932.

Cruden, Loren. Medicine Grove. Destiny Books. Inner Traditions Vermont. 1997.

Cummings, S. and Ullman, Dana. *Everyone's Guide to Homeopathic Medicines,* St. Martins

Cupp, Melanie. *Toxicology and Clinical Pharmacology of Herbal Products*. Humana P. 1999

Curtin, LSM. *Healing Herbs of the Upper Rio Grande*. SouthWest Museum, Los Angeles 1965

Cutler & Cutler Eds. Biologically Active Natural Products: Agrochemicals, CRC Press 1999.

Dai Yin-fang&Liu Cheng-jun. *Fruit As Medicine*. Rams Skull Press, Kuranda, Aust. 1987

Dalton, David. Stars of the Meadow. Lindisfarne Books. Great Barrington, Mass. 2006.

D'Amelio Sr. Frank. *Botanicals A Phytocosmetic Desk Reference* CRC Press, Boca Raton, 99

Darby,Wm et al. *Food: The Gift of Osiris,* Vol 1. Academic Press, San Francisco, 1977

Darwin, Tess. The Scots Herbal, the Plant Lore of Scotland. Birlinn Ltd, Edinburgh 2008

Davidow, Joie. *Infusions of Healing, A Treasury of Mexican-American Herbal Remedies,* Fireside Books, New York, 1999.

Davis,W. *El Gringo, New Mexico and Her People*. Harpers, New York, 1857.

Demargaux, N. *Phytotherapy*. Herbal Health Publishers Ltd. 1989

De Bairacli Levy, Juliette. *Herbal Handbook for Farm and Stable,* Faber and Faber 1952

Deer Lame, J & Erdoes, R. *Lame Deer Seeker of Visions.* Washington Sq Press, 1976.

Deer, Thea Summer. Wisdom of the Plant Devas. Bear&Company Vermont 2011.

Delta Gardens Flower Essences. www.deltagardens.com

De Smet et al. *Adverse Effects of Herbal Drugs.* Springer-Verlag, Berlin. 1997.

Der Marderosian, Ara & Liberti L. *Natural Product Medicine,* George Stickley Co, Philadel.

DeRios, Marlene D. *Hallucinogens: Cross Cultural Perspectives.* U. New Mexico Press, 1984

DeSmet, P. et al. *Adverse Effects of Herbal Drugs. vol 2* Springer-Verlag

Devi, Lila. The Essential Flower Essence Handbook. Crystal Clarity Pub. Nevada City 2007.

Dewey, Laurel. *Plant Power- revised.* Safe Goods/New Century Pub, Markham Ont, 2001.

Dewick, Paul M. *Medicinal Natural Products.*3rd Ed John Wiley and Sons, West Sussex, 2009.

Diederichsen, Axel. *Coriander.* Int. Plant Genetic Resources Institute. Rome, Italy. 1996.

Dixon, Bernard.*Power Unseen, How Microbes Rule the World.* W.H. Freeman, Oxford, 1994

Dow, Elaine. *Simples and Worts.* Historical Presentations, Topsfield, MA. 1982.

Duke, James. *Handbook of Medicinal Herbs.* CRC Press, Boca Raton, Florida, 1985

_____*Handbook of Edible Weeds.* CRC Press. 1992

_____*The Green Pharmacy,* Rodale Press, Emmaus, Pennsylvania, 1997.

_____*The Green Pharmacy Herbal Handbook,* Rodale Press, 2000.

_____*Anti-aging Prescriptions.* Rodale Press. 2001.

Dumas, Anne. Book of Plants and Symbols. English Ed. Octopus Pub. London 2004.

Dymock,Wm. *Pharmacographia Indica, Vol 2,* Kegan Paul, Trench, Trubner and Co. 1891

Earle, Liz. *Vital Oils,* Ebury Press, London, 1991.

Eason, Cassandra. Fabulous Creatures, Mythical Monsters... Greenwood Press, CT. 2008.

Eastman, John. *The Book of Swamp and Bog...* Stackpole Books, Mechanicsburg, Penn, 1995

Ebadi, M. *Pharmacodynamic Basis of Herbal Medicine,* CRC Press, Boca Raton. 2002.

Eckey, E.W. *Vegetable Fats and Oils,* Rheingold Publishing Co, New York, 1954.

Eclare, Melanie. *Flower Spirit Cards.* Quadrille Publishing, London, England, 2004.

Edwards, Lawrence. *The Vortex of Life.* Floris Books. Edinburgh 2nd Ed. 2006.

Eisner T et al. *Secret Weapons.* Belknap Press, Harvard U Press. Cambridge & London 2005.

Ellingwood F. *American Materia Medica,* Eclectic Med. Pub. Portand, Oregon, reprint, 1983

Elliot, Douglas B. *Roots .* Chatham Press, Old Greenwich Conneticut.

Ellis, Hattie. *Sweetness & Light.* Hodder and Stoughton, London, 2004.

Erdoes & Ortiz. *American Indian Myths and Legends,* Pantethon Books, New York, 1984.

Erichsen-Brown,Charlotte. *Use of Plants for the Past 500 Years,* Breezy Creeks Press, 1979

_____*Medicinal and Other Uses of North American Plants,* General Pub, 1979.

Erickson, David, Wai Kit Nip *Food uses of whole oil and protein seeds,* Amer. Oil Chemists Society, 1989.

Eskin, N. A. Michael, Tamir, S. *Dictionary of Nutraceuticals and Functional Foods.* CRC Press, 2006.

Etkin, Nina. Edible Medicines, An Ethnopharmacology of Food. U Arizona Press. 2006.

Evans, W.C. *Trease and Evans' Pharmacognosy.* WB Saunders Co. Toronto, 2000.

Fang Jing Pei, Dr. *Natural Remedies from the Chinese Cupboard.* Weatherhill, 1998.

Farmer-Knowles,Helen. *The Healing Garden.* Sterling Publishing, New York, 1998.

Fielder, Mildred. *Plant Medicne and Folklore,* Winchester Press, New York, 1975.

Felter, Harvery and Lloyd, John. *King's American Dispensatory .* 1898. Reprinted by Eclectic Medical Publications, Portland Oregon, 1983.

Ferguson, Gary. *Spirits of the Wild.* Clarkson Potter/Random New York, 1996.

Fernie, W.T. Dr. *Old Fashioned Herbal Remedies.* Coles Pub. Toronto, 1980. Reprint.

Fingerman M. et al editors. *Bioremediation of Aquatic and Terresrial Ecosytems.* Sci Pub. Enfield NH 2005.

Fischer-Rizzi, S. *Complete Aromatherapy Handbook,* Sterling Pub. New York. 1990.

_____*The Complete Incense Book,* Sterling Pub. New York. 1998.

_____*Medicine of the Earth,* Rudra Press, Portland, Oregon, 1996

Florey, H.W. et al. Antibiotics vol 1. Oxford University Press. London 1949.

Ford, Gillian. *Plant Names Explained.* Friends of the Devonian Botanic Garden, #16, 1984

Foster, Steven. *Herbal Renaissance,* Gibbs Smith Pub. Salt Lake City

_____& Yue Chongxi. *Herbal Emissaries,* Healing Arts Press, Vermont, 1992

_____& Johnson R. *Desk Reference to Nature's Medicine.* Nat Geographic. Washington, D.C.

Fox, H. M. Gardening with Herbs. Macmillan Pub. New York 1933.

Freeman, D. & Mongeau D. Nettles and More…Vol One. Self published 2nd printing 2009.

Freeman, Lyn. *Mosby's Complementary & Alternative Medicine.*3rd Ed. Mosby Elsevier 2009

Friedman, Sara Ann, *Celebrating the Wild Mushroom,* Dodd, Mead & Co. New York, 1986

Friend, Tim. The Third Domain: the Untold Story of Archaea. Joseph Henry Press. 2007.

Fugh-Berman, Adriane. *The 5-minute Herb &Dietary Supplement Consult.* Lippincott Williams &Wilkins, Philadelphia 2003.

Gaertner, Erika. *Reap without Sowing.* General Store Publishing, Burnstown, Ont. 1995

Galun, Margalith. *Handbook of Lichenology,* CRC Press, 1988

Garran, Thomas. *Western herbs according to Traditional Chinese Medicine.* Healing Arts Press. 2008.

Garrett, J.T. *The Cherokee Herbal.* Bear&Company, Rochester, Vermont. 2003.

Genders, Roy. *Floral Scents of the World .* St. Martin's Press, London, 1977

Geuter, *Herbs in Nutrition.* Bio-Dynamic Agricultural Assoc. London. 1978.

Gildemeister, E. *The Volatile Oils.* John Wiley and Sons, New York. 1916

Gifford, Jane. The Wisdom of Trees. Sterling Pub. New York 2000.

Gill S. & Sullivan I. *Dictionary of Native American Mythology.* Oxford U Press 1992.

Gilmore, M.R. Uses of Plants by Indians of the Missouri river region. 33rd Annual Report Bureau American Ethnology, 1911-12, Washington D.C. 1919.

Gladstar R & Hirsch P. *Planting the Future.* Healing Arts Press, Rochester, Vt. 2000.

Gladstar, Rosemary. *Family Herbal.* Storey Books, North Adams, Mass. 2001.

Glasby, J.S. *Dictionary of Plants Containing Secondary Metabolites,* Taylor & Francis, London 1991.

Godfrey, A & Saunders P. Principles and Practices of Naturopathic Botanical Medicine, Vol 1, CCNM Press Toronto ON 2010.

Goodrick-Clarke, Clare. Alchemical Medicine for the 21st Century. Healing Arts Press. 2010.

Gordon, David G. *The Compleat Cockroach.* Ten Speed Press, Berkeley, CA. 1996.

Gordon, Lesley. The Mystery and Magic of Trees & Flowers. Grange Books. London 1993.

Gottesfeld, Leslie M. Johnson. *Plants, Land and People, A Study of Wet'suwet'en Ethnobotany.*U of A, 1993.

Grae, Ida. *Nature's Colors, Dyes From Plants.* Macmillan Pub. New York, 1974.

Graham, Frances K. *Plant lore of an Alaskan Island.* Alaska Northwest Pub. 1985

Grandparents of the Forest flower essences. www.grandparentsoftheforest.com

Grange, Michael etal, *Handbook of Plants with Pest Control Properties,* J. Wiley& Son 1988

Gray, Bev. The Boreal Herbal. Wild Food & Medicine Plants of the North. Aroma Borealis Press 2011

Green, James. *The Male Herbal .* Crossing Press, Freedom, California, 1991.

_____*The Herbal Medicine-Maker's Handbook.* Crossing Press, Freedom CA 2000

Green, Jonathan. *Consuming Passions.* Sphere Books, London, 1985.

Grey Wolf. *Earth Signs,* Raincoast Books, Vancouver, B.C. 1998.

Grieve, M. *A Modern Herbal.* Jonathan Cape. 1931

Griffiths, Deirdre. *Elk Island National Park.* U. of Alberta Press, 1979.

Grigson, Geoffrey. *A Herbal of All Sorts*. Phoenix House, London

Grimaud, Baptiste, Paul. *TAROT DES FLEURS*, France Cartes, France 1989

Grimshaw, John. *The Gardener's Atlas*. Firefly Books, Willowdale, Ont. 2002.

Grohmann, Gerbert. *The Plant Vol 2*, Bio-Dynamic Farming & Gardening Assoc. 1989.

Gruenwald et al, Ed. PDR for Herbal Medicines. 4th Ed. Thomson Pub. 2007.

Guillet, Alma. *Make Friends of Trees and Shrubs*. Doubleday & Co. New York, 1962.

Gumbel, Dietrich. *Principles of Holistic Skin Therapy with Herb Essences*. Haug Pub. Heidelberg 1986.

Gurudas. *The Spiritual Properties of Herbs* , Cassandra Press, 1988

_____*Flower Essences and Vibrational Healing*, Cassandra Press, 1983

Hageneder, Fred. The Spirit of Trees. Continuum. NY and London. 2005.

Hale, Mason. *The Biology of Lichens*. Edward Arnold Pub. London, 1967.

Hall, Dorothy. *Creating Your Herbal Profile* , Keats, 1988

Hallworth, B & Chinnappa CC. *Plants of the Kananaskis Country* U of A Press 1997.

Hanchuk, Rena. *The Word and Wax*. Can Inst of Ukrainian Studies Press, Edmonton, 1999.

Hanson, J, & Morrison D. *Of Kinkajous, Capybaras, Horned Beetles...*Harper Collins, NY '91

Harbourne & Baxter. *The Handbook of Natural Flavonoids Vol 1&2*. John Wiley & Sons, 1999

_____*Phytochemical Dictionary*. Taylor & Francis 1993.

Harrington, Geri. *Growing Your Own Chinese Vegetables*, MacMillan, N.Y. 1978.

Harrington, H.D. *Edible Native Plants of the Rocky Mtns*. U. of New Mexico Press, 1967.

Harris, Ben C. *Eat the Weeds,* Keats Pub. New Cannan, Conneticut 1973.

_____*Make Use of Your Garden Plants*. General Pub. New York. 1978.

Harris, Marjorie. *Botanica North America*. Harper Collins, New York, 2003.

Harrison, Nora. *Flower Remedy Rhymes* , self published, England, 1990.

Hart, Jeff. *Montana Native Plants and Early Peoples*, Montana Historical Society Press. '92

_____The Ethnobotany of the Northern Cheyenne Indians of Montana. Journal of Ethnopharmacology 1981 4.

Hartung, Tammi. *Growing 101 Herbs That Heal*. Storey Books, Pownal, Vt. 2000.

Hartwell, Jonathan, *Plants Used Against Cancer*. Quarterman Pub. 1982

Hartzell, Jr. H. *The Yew Tree A Thousand Whispers*. Hulogosi, Box 1188, Eugene, OR 1991.

Harvey, C & Cochrane A. *The Healing Spirit of Plants*. Godsfield Press, Sterling Pr N.Y. 1999

Harvey Clare. The New Encyclopedia of Flower Remedies. Watkins Pub. London 2007.

Hatfield, Gabrielle. *Encyclopedia of Folk Medicine*. ABC CLIO Santa Barbara. 2004.

Haughton, Claire. *Green Immigrants*. Harcourt Brace Jovanovich. New York and London.

Hawksworth, Frank & Wiens, D. Dwarf Mistletoes, Ag Handbook 709, USDA, Wash, DC, '96

Health Canada, Native Foods and Nutrition. Medical Services Branch, 1995.

Heatherington, M. and Steck, W. *Natural Chemicals from Northern Prairie Plants,* Ag West Biotech Publishers, Saskatoon, Canada. 1997.

Heilmeyer, Marina. The Language of Flowers-Symbols & Myths. Prestel Pub. Munich 2001.

Heinerman, John. *Encyclopedia of Nuts, Berries and Seeds*, Parker Publishing, 1995.

_____*Encyclopedia of Healing Herbs & Spices*. Parker Pub. N.Y. 1996.

Heinrich, Bernd. *Winter World The Ingenuity of animal survival*. HarperCollins. NY 2003.

Heinrich, Clark. *Magic Mushrooms in Religion and Alchemy*. Park St. Press, VT. 2002.

Heiser, Charles B. Jr. *Of Plants and People*. U. of Oklahoma Press, 1985.

Hellson, John C, *Ethnobotany of the Blackfoot Indians* No. 19, National Museums of Canada, Ottawa 1974.

Henderson, Robert K. *The Neighborhood Forager*. Key Porter Books, Toronto, 2000.

Hendrickson, Robert. *Encycl of Word and Phrase Origins*. Facts on File Inc. NewYork, 1997.

Hendry, G. *Natural Food Colorants* , Blackie and Son, Glasgow Scotland, 1992.

Henry, J. David. *Canada's Boreal Forest.* Smithsonian Institute. 2002.

Hilarion. *Wildflowers, Their Occult Gifts.* Marcus Books, Queensville, Ont. 1982.

Hobbs, Christopher. *Usnea : The Herbal Antibiotic.* Botanica Press. 1986.

_____*Medicinal Mushrooms*, Botanica Press, Santa Cruz, 1995.

Hoffman, David. *The Holistic Herbal.* Findhorn Press, 1983.

_____*Welsh Herbal Medicine.* Abercastle Publications, Dyfed, 1978.

_____*Medical Herbalism.* Healing Arts Press, Rochester, VT, 2003.

Hole, Lois. *Favorite Trees and Shrubs.* Lone Pine Pub. Edmonton Alta. 1997.

_____*Perennial Favorites.* Lone Pine Pub. 1995.

Holm, LeRoy G. *World Weeds,* John Wiley and Sons, 1997.

Holmes, Peter. *The Energetics of Western Herbs, Vol 1 and 2,* Artemis Press, 1989.

_____*Jade Remedies, Vol 1 and 2,* Snow Lotus Press, Boulder 1996.

Hopman, Ellen. *A Druid's Herbal,* Destiny Books, Rochester, Vermont. 1995.

Howarth, D& Kahlee Keane. *Wild Medicines of the Prairies* Self Published, 1995.

_____*Native Medecines* Self Published , 1995

Hozeski, Bruce. *Hildegard's Healing Plants.* Beacon Press. Boston, Mass. 2001.

Hsu, Hong-Yen. *Oriental Materia Medica,* Keats Publishing,Connecticut, 1986.

Huang, Kee Chang. *The Pharmacolocy of Chinese Herbs.* 2nd Edition, CRC Press, 1999.

Hu-Nan. *A Barefoot Doctor's Manual.* Running Press, Philadelphia, 1977.

Hudson, James B. *Antiviral Compounds from Plants,* CRC Press, Florida, 1990

Hudson, Rick. *A Field Guide to Gold, Gemstone and Mineral Sites.* Orca Pub, Victoria, 1999

Hurley, Judith. *The Good Herb* Wm. Morrow and Co. New York, 1995.

Hutchens, Alma. *Indian Herbology of North America.* Merco. 1969

Ingram, Cass. *Supermarket Remedies.* Knowledge House, Buffalo Grove, Ill. 1998.

Injoynow essences.

Inkpen W & Van Eyk, R. *Guide to the Common Native Trees and Shrubs of Alberta,* Government of Alberta, Environmental Protection, 1995.

James & Keeler, *Poisonous Plants- 3rd Int. Symposium,* Iowa State U. Press, 1992.

Jason, Dan & Nancy. *Some Useful Wild Plants,* Talon Books, Vancouver, 1972.

Jiao Shu-De. *Ten Lectures on the Use of Medicinals.* Paradigm Pub. Brookline, Mass. 2003.

Johnson, Kershaw, MacKinnon & Pojar *Plants of the Western Boreal Forest and Aspen Parkland,* Lone Pine Press, Edmonton, Alberta 1995.

Johnson, L. *Tending the Earth A Gardener's Manifesto.* Penguin Books, Toronto, 2002.

Johnson, Leslie. Journal of Ethnobotany and Ethnomedicine. 2006 2:29.

_____*Health, Wholeness & the Land: Gitksan Traditional Plant Use and Healing.* U of Alberta 1997.

Jones, Alison. *Larousse Dictionary of World Folklore.* Larousse, New York, 1995.

Jones, Pamela. *Just Weed, History, Myths and Uses.* Prentice Hall Press, Toronto, 1991.

Kamm, Minnie W. *Old Time Herbs for Northern Gardens* Little Brown & Co. 1938.

Kane, Charles W. Herbal Medicine of the American Southwest. Lincoln Town Press. 2007.

_____Herbal Medicine: trends and traditions. Lincoln Town Press 2009.

Kapoor, L.D. *CRC Handbook of Ayurvedic Medicinal Plants,* CRC Press, Boca Raton, 1990.

Kari, Priscilla. *Tanaina Plantlore.* National Park Service, Alaska Region 1987.

Kaur, Sat Dharam. *The Complete Natural Medicine Guide to Breast Cancer.* Robert Rose Inc Toronto, 2003.

Kavash E, Barrie & Barr K, *American Indian Healing Arts.* Bantam Books, Toronto 1999.

_____*The Medicine Wheel Garden.* Bantam Books, N.Y. 2002.

Kay, Margarita Artschwager. *Healing with Plants in the American and Mexican West,* The University of Arizona Press, Tucson. 1996

Kays, S & Nottingham S. Biology and Chemistry of Jerusalem Artichoke. CRC Press 2008.

Keane, Kahlee & Howarth,D. *The Standing People.* Saskatoon, Saskatchewan. 2003.

Kee Chang Huang, *The Pharmacology of Chinese Herbs,* 2nd Edition, CRC Press, 1999.

Kemp, Cynthia. *Cactus and Company.* Desert Alchemy, Tucson, Arizona, 1993.

Kenner D &Requena Y. *Botanical Medicine: .*Paradigm Pub. Brookline, Mass, 1996.

Kerik, Joan. *Living with the Land:Use of Plants by the Native People of Alberta,* Alberta Culture, Circulating Exhibits Program, National Museums of Canada Fund, 1981.

Kershaw, Linda. Edible & Medicinal Plants of the Rockies, Lone Pine, Edmonton 2000.

_____*Alberta Wayside Wildflowers.* Lone Pine, Edmonton, 2003.

_____*Saskatchewan Wayside Wildflowers.* Lone Pine, Edmonton, 2003.

_____*Manitoba Wayside Wildflowers.* Lone Pine, Edmonton, 2003.

Kershaw, L. et al. *Rare Vascular Plants of Alberta.* U. of Alberta Press, Edmonton, 2001.

Kershaw, MacKinnon & Pojar. *Plants of the Rocky Mountains.* Lone Pine, Edmonton 1998.

Keys, John. D. *Chinese Herbs,* Charles E. Tuttle Co. 1976.

Kimmerer,Robin. *Gathering Moss.* Oregon State University Press, Corvallis, 2003.

Kindscher, Kelly. *Medicnal Wild Plants of the Prairies.* Univ. Press of Kansas. 1987.

King, Francis X. *Rudolf Steiner and Holistic Medicine.* Rider & Co. England, 1986.

Klein, Carol. Plant Personalities. Timber Press, Portland, Oregon. 2005.

Klein, Richard. *The Green World.* 2nd edition. Harper Collins, 1987.

Kloss, Jethro. *Back to Eden.* Woodbridge Press Pub.Co. Santa Barbara, Ca. 1975.

Knab, Sophie H. *Polish Herbs, Flowers and Folk Medicine.* Hippocrene Books, N.Y. 1999.

Knowles, Hugh. *Woody Ornamentals for the Prairies.* U. of Alberta , 1995.

Knudtson,P & Suzuki D. Wisdom of the Elders. Greystone Books. Vancouver BC 2006.

Kraft, K & Hobbs C. *Pocket Guide to Herbal Medicine.* Thieme, N.Y. 2004.

Kranich, Ernst M. Planetary Influences Upon Plants. Bio-Dynamic Lit. Wyoming RI 1984.

Krymow, V. Healing Plants of the Bible. Wild Goose Pub. Glasgow, UK 2002.

Kuhnlein, Harriet and Turner, Nancy. *Traditional Plant Foods of Canadian Indigenous Peoples.* Gordon and Breach Science Publishers. 1991.

Kuijt, Job. *The Biology of Parasitic Flowering Plants,* U. of California Press, 1969

Kunkele, U. & Lohmeyer, T. *Herbs for Healthy Living.* Parragon Pub. Bath UK 2007.

Lacey, Laurie. *Micmac Medicines Remedies and Recollections.* Nimbus Pub. Halifax, 1993.

Lahring, Heinjo. *Water and Wetland Plants of the Prairie Provinces,* Can Plains Research Center, U. of Regina, 2003

Lambert, Grant. *Falling Leaf Essences.* Healing Arts Press, Rochester Vermont, 2002.

Lamont, SM. *The Fisherman Lake Slave and their environment: a story of floral and faunal resources.* Master's thesis. U. of Saskatchewan, Saskatoon, 1977.

Langenheim, Jean. *Medicinal Plant Resins.* Timber Press Portland Oregon 2003.

Larsen,Henning. *An Old Icelandic Medical Miscellany,* Norske Akademi, Oslo, Norway '31

Lavabre, Marcel. *Aromatherapy Workbook.* Healing Arts Press, Vermont. 1990.

Lawless, Julia, *The Encyclopedia of Essential Oils* , Element Books, 1992.

LeClaire,N &Cardinal,G. *Alberta Elders' Cree Dictionary,* U of Alberta Press, 1998.

Leduc, M.A. *The Explorers Guide to Boreal Forest Plants,* Hwy Book Shop, Cobalt, Ont. 1997

Leighton, Anna L. *Wild Plant Use by the Woods Cree (NIHITHAWAK) of East-Central Saskatchewan .* Paper no. 101, National Museums of Canada, Ottawa, 1985

Lepore, Donald. *The Ultimate Healing System*. Woodland Books, Provo, Utah, 1988.

Le Strange, Richard, *A History of Herbal Plants*. Arco Pub. New York. 1977.

Leung, Albert. *Chinese Herbal Remedies*. Universe Books, New York, 1984.

Leung & Foster, *Encyclopedia of Common Natural Ingredients,* J. Wiley&Sons, N.Y. 1996.

Levey,M. *The Medical Formulary or Aqrabadhin of Al-Kindi* U of Wisconsin Press, 1966

Leyel, C.F. *Elixirs of Life,* Faber and Faber, London.1948

Li, Thomas. *Medicinal Plants, Culture, Utilization & Phytopharmacology*. Technomic Publishing, Lancaster, Pennsylvania, 2000.

Li, Thomas. *Chinese and related North American Herbs*. CRC Press, Boca Raton, 2002.

Libster, Martha. *Delmar's Integrative Herb Guide for Nurses*. Delmar, 2002.

Lininger et al. *The Natural Pharmacy*. Healthnotes, Prima Pub. Rocklin Ca, 1999.

L'Orange Darlena, *Herbal Healing Secrets of the Orient*. Prentice Hall, New Jersey, 1998.

Lock, Carolyn. *Country Colours*. Nova Scotia Museum. 1981

Lovejoy, Sharon. *Sunflower Houses*. Workman Pub Co. New York 2001.

Lu, Henry. *Using Foods to Stay Young,* Sterling Press, New York, 1996.

_____*Chinese Natural Cures*. Black Dog & Leventhal Pub. New York, 1994

Luetjohann, Sylvia. *The Healing Power of Black Cumin*. Lotus Light, Twin Lakes, WI, 1998

Lyle, Katie Letcher. *The Wild Berry Book,* NorthWord Press, Minocqua, WI, 1994.

Mabey, Richard. *Plantcraft*. Universe Books. 1978.

MacKinnon, Pojar, Coupe. *Plants of Northern British Columbia*. Lone Pine Press, 1992.

Mailhebiau, Philippe. *Portraits in Oils*. C.W. Daniel Company, Essex, England, 1995.

Malmud, René. *The Amazon Problem,* trans by M. Stein, Spring Pub. Dallas TX, 1980.

Maloof, Joan. *Teaching the Trees, Lessons from the Forest*. U Georgia Pr, Athena GA. 2005.

Manandhar, N.P. *Plants and People of Nepal*. Timber Press, Portland, Oregon, 2002.

Maple, Eric. *The Secret Lore of Plants and Flowers*. Robert Hale Ltd. London 1980.

March, Kathryn & Andrew. *The Wild Plant Companion*. Meridian Hill Pub. 1986.

Marles, Robin. *The Ethnobotany of the Chipewyan of Northern Saskatchewan,* 1984. Thesis.

_____et al. *Aboriginal Plant Use in Canada's Northwest Boreal Forest*. UBC Press, Vancouver, and Natural Resources Canada, 2000

McBride, L.R. *Practical Folk Medicine of Hawaii*. Petroglyph Press, Hilo,Hawaii, 1975.

McCune B. & Geiser L. *Macrolichens of the Pacific Northwest*. Oregon State U. Press, 1997

McFarland, Phoenix. *The Complete Book of Magical Names*. Llewellyn Pub. St Paul 1996

McGrath, Judy. *Dyes from Lichens and Plants*. Van Nostrand Rheinhold, 1977.

McGuffin, Nancy. *Spectrum: dye plants of Ontario*. Burr House Spinner, Richmond Hill '86

Mc Intyre, Anne. *The Complete Woman's Herbal,* Henry Holt, New York, 1995.

Mears, R & Hillman,G. Wild Food. Hodder and Stoughton

MELODY. *Love is in the Earth, A Kaleidoscope of Crystals*. Earth Love Pub. Col. 1995.

Mercatante, A. S. The Facts on File Encyclopedia of World Mythology. New York 1988

Merriam, C. Hart. *Dawn of the World, Weird Tales of Mewan Indians*. Arthur H. Clark, Cleveland, 1910

Meyer, George et al. *Folk Medicine and Herbal Healing,* Charles Thomas, Springfield, 1981

Meyerowitz,Steve. *Sprout It!* The Sprout House, Box 1100,Great Barrington, MA, 1993.

Meyers, Edward C. *Basic Bush Survival,* Hancock House, Surrey, B.C. 1997.

Miller, L &Murray,W. *Herbal Medicinals A Clinician's Guide*. Hawthorn Press, N.Y. 1998.

Miller, Sandra. Editor Echinacea- Medicinal and Aromatic Plants. CRC Press, 2004.

Mills S. & Bone,K. *Principles and Practice of Phytotherapy*. Churchill Livingstone, 2000.

_____*The Essential Guide to Herbal Safety*. Churchill Livingstone, 2005.

Mills, Simon. *Out of the Earth*. Viking Penquin Books, Toronto. 1991.

Millsbaugh, Charles. *American Medicinal Plants,* Dover Pub. New York, 1974

Milne, Courtney. *Visions of the Goddess*, Penguin Studio, Toronto, 1998

Minnis & Elisens. *Biodiversity and Native America*. U. Oklahoma Press, 2000.

Mitchel, Jr. Wm. *Plant Medicine in Practice*. Churchill Livingstone, St. Louis, 2003.

Moerman, Daniel, *Medicinal Plants of Native America*. U of Michigan No. 19, 1986

Mohammed, G. *Catnip & Kerosene Grass* Candlenut Books, Sault Ste. Marie, Ont, 2002.

Montgomery, Pam. *Plant Spirit Healing*. Bear and Company, Rochester, VT 2008.

Moore, Michael. *Los Remedios*. Red Crane Books, 1990

_____*Medicinal Plants of the Desert and Canyon West*. Museum of New Mexico Press 1989

_____*Medicinal Plants of the Mountain West,* Museum of New Mexico Press '79

_____Med Plants of the Mountain West. Revised, expanded. 2003

_____*Medicinal Plants of the Pacific West,* Red Crane Books, 1993

More, Daphne. *The Bee Book,* Universe Books, New York, 1976.

Morelli, I. et al. *Selected Medicinal Plants*. University of Pisa. FAO 53/1

Morton, Julia. *Major Medicinal Plants* . Charles Thomas, Springfield, Illinois 1977

_____*Atlas of Medicinal Plants of Middle America, Bahamas to Yucatan*. 1981

Moss, E.H. *Flora of Alberta*. University of Toronto Press. 1983

Mother, The. *Flowers and their Messages*. Sri Aurobindo Ashram Trust, India 1979.

Mourning Dove. Coyote Stories. Caxton Press Caldwell Idaho. 1933.

Mowrey, Daniel. *The Scientific Validation of Herbal Medicine*. Cormorant Books, 1986.

Mucz, Michael. *Baba's Kitchen Medicines*. U of Alberta Press, Edmonton, 2012.

Mulders, Evelyn. *Western Herbs for Eastern Meridian & 5 Element Theory. Self publ. 2006.*

Mulligan, G editor *The biology of Canadian Weeds,* 1-32 Pub. 1693 Ag Canada 1979

_____33-61 Pub. 1765 Ag Canada 1984

Murphy, Cristine Editor, *Practical Home Care Medicine,* Lantern Books, New York, 2001

Murray, Michael. *The Pill Book Guide to Natural Medicines*. Bantam Books, April, 2002.

_____& Pizzorno, J. The condensed Encycl of Healing Foods. Pocket Books NY 2005.

Naegele, Thomas A. *Edible and Medicinal Plants of the Great Lakes Region,* Wilderness Adventure Books, Davisburg, Michigan. 1996.

Naiman, Ingrid. *Cancer Salves, A Botanical Approach to Treatment*. N. Atlantic Books, 99.

Nesse R & Williams G. *Why We Get Sick*. Vintage Books/Random House, New York, 1996.

Neuwinger H.D. *African Traditional Medicine*. Medpharm Sci. Pub. Stuttgart 2000.

_____African Ethnobotany, Poisons and Drugs. Chapman & Hall, London 1996.

Newcombe C.F. unpub notes on Haida plants. Dept of Anthro. Am Mus Nat Hist. NY 1897

_____unpublished papers. Prov Archives B.C. Victoria. 1898-1913.

Nicander. *The Poems and Poetical Fragments*. Cambridge U. Press, New York, 1953.

Norman,Howard. *Northern Tales*. Pantheon Books, New York, 1990.

Northcote, Rosalind. *The Book of Herbs*. John Lane: The Bodley Head, London, 1912.

Null, Gary. *The Clinician's Handbook of Natural Healing*. Kensington Books, N.Y. 1997.

Olive, Barbara. *The Flower Healer*. Cico Books, London and New York. 2007.

Ollsin, Don. *Herbal Healing Journey-Playful Workbook*. Aquiline Comm, Victoria,BC 1998.

Ootoova I. et al. *Interviewing Inuit Elders, Perspectives on Traditional Health*. Vol 5, Nunavut Arctic College, Box 600, Iqaluit, Nunavut X0Z 0H0.

Page, George. *Inside the Animal Mind*. Doubleday, New York, 1999.

Pallasdowney, Rhonda. *The Complete Book of Flower Essences*. New World Library, 2002.

Pappalardo, Joe. Sunflowers (the secret history). The Overlook Press. Woodstock NY 2008.

Parish, Coupé & Lloyd. *Plants of S. Interior British Columbia*. Lone Pine Edmonton 1996

Park, Willard Z. *Ethnographic Notes on the Norhern Paiute of Western Nevada, 1933-40* compiled by Catherine Fowler, U. of Utah, Salt Lake City, 1989.

Parvati, J. *Hygieia, A Woman's Herbal*. Freestone Collective. 1978

Paturi, Felix *Nature, Mother of Invention*. Harper and Row Pub. New York. 1976.

Peirce,Andrea. *Practical Guide to Natural Medicines*. Stonesong Press. 1999.

Pelikan, W. Healing Plants. Mercury Press, Spring Valley NY 1997.

Pellowski, Anne. *Hidden Stories in Plants*. MacMillan Pub. New York. 1990.

Penoel,Daniel & Franchomme, P. *L'Aromatherapie Exactement* , Roger Jollois, France, 1990

Peneol, Daniel. *Medecine Aromatique, Medecine Planetaire*. Roger Jollois France 1991.

_____& Peneol, Rose-Marie. *Natural Home Health Care Using Essential Oils*. Osmobiose Pub. 1998.

People of 'Ksan, The. *Gathering What the Great Nature Provided*. Douglas & Mc Intyre. Vancouver, B.C. 1980.

Peters, Josephine & Ortiz B. After the First Full Moon in April. Left Coast Press. Walnut Creek CA, 2010.

Pettitt,Sabina. Energy Medicine, Healing from the Kingdoms of Nature, Pacific Essences, Box 8317, Victoria, B.C. V8W 3R9 Canada, 1999

Phaneuf, Holly. Herbs Demystified. Marlowe and Company, New York. 2005

Pielou, E.C. *The Naturalist's Guide to the Arctic*. U. of Chicago Press. 1994.

Pieroni, A & Price L. Eating and Healing, Trad Food as Medicine. Haworth Press. N.Y. 2006.

Pfeiffer E. *The Earth's Face and Human Destiny*, Rodale Press, Emmaus, Pa. 1947.

Plotkin, Mark. *Medicine Quest*. Viking Penguin Books, New York, 2000.

Pojar, J & MacKinnon, A. *Plants of Coastal British Columbia* Lone Pine Edmonton 1994.

Pollock, L. With Faith and Physic: the life of a tudor gentlewoman. Collins & Brown,1993.

Polya, Gideon. *Biochemical Targets of Plant Bioactive Comp*. CRC Press, Boca Raton 2003

Pond, Barbara, *A Sampler of Wayside Herbs*, Chatham Press, Riverside, Conn.

Pressor, Arthur, *Pharmacist's Guide to Medicinal Herbs*, Smart Pub. Petaluma, CA,2000

Price, Len & Shirley. *Understanding Hydrolats*. Churchill Livingstone, Toronto, 2004.

_____Aromatherapy for Health Professionals. Churchill Livingstone 1995.

Purvis, William. *Lichens*. Smithsonian Institution Press. Washington D.C. 2000

Quin, Frederick F. *The Flora Homoeopathica*. B. Jain Pub. New Delhi, India. 1997.

Radin, Paul. *The Winnebago Tribe*, Bur of Am Ethnology, Smithsonian Inst. 37th. 1923.

Rätsch, C. *Plants of Love, The History of Aphrodisiacs*. Ten Speed Press, Berkeley,1997.

_____The Dictionary of Sacred & Magical Plants. ABC-CLIO St Barbara 1992.

_____The Encyclopedia of Psychoactive Plants. Park St Press. 2005.

Raven Essences. www.ravenessences.com

Ravenworks flower essences. www.ravenworksministries.weebly.com

Reaume, Tom. 620 Wild Plants of North America. Nature Manitoba. Canadian Plains Research Center, U of Regina, U of Toronto Press. 2009.

Reckeweg, Hans-Heinrich, *Materia Medica, Vol 1. Aurelia-Verlag GmbH, Baden Baden* 1996.

Reich, Lee. *Uncommon Fruits Worthy of Attention*, Addison-Wesley Pub. 1991.

Reid, Daniel, *A handbook of Chinese Healing Herbs*, Shambala, Boston, 1995

Rhode, David. Native Plants of Southern Nevada. U of Utah Press. 2002.

Richards B & Kanecko A. *Japanese Plants- Know Them &Use Them*. Shufunotomo, Tokyo 1995

Richardson, David. *The Vanishing Lichens*. David and Charles, Vancouver, BC, 1975

Riddle, John M. *Eve's Herbs*. Harvard U Press. Cambridge Mass. 1997.

_____Goddesses, Elixirs and Witches. Palgrave MacMillan. England 2010.

Rister, Robert. *Healing Without Medication.* Basic Health Pub. N. Bergen, N.J. 2003.

Roberts, Jonathan. *The Origins of Fruit and Vegetables.* Universe Pub. New York. 2001.

Robicsek, F. *The Smoking God: Tobacco....*Norman: U. of Oklahoma Press, 1978.

Robinson, Peggy. *Profiles of Northwest Plants.* Far West Book Service. Portland, OR 1979

Rogers, Dilwyn. *Edible, Medicinal, Useful & Poisonous Wild Plants of the Northern Great Plains —South Dakota Region.* Buechel Memorial Lakota Museum, St. Francis,SD, 1980.

Rogers, Pattiann. *Firekeeper:New & Selected Poems.* Milkweed Editions, 1994.

Rogers, Robert Dale. *Sundew Moonwort Vols-1-7, self-published.* Edmonton 1995-present.

_____Rogers' Herbal Manual. Karamat Wilderness Ways, Edmonton, 2000.

_____& Capital Health, Herbal Drug Interactions. Mediscript Comm. 2003.

_____The Fungal Pharmacy, The Complete Guide to Medicinal Mushrooms and Lichens of North America, North Atlantic Books 2011.

Rombi, Max. *Phytotherapy.* Herbal Health Publishers. U.K. 1990.

Rosengarten,Jr. F. *The Book of Edible Nuts.* Walker and Co. New York. 1984.

Ross, Gary. *Nature's Guide to Healing.* Freedom Press, Topanga, Ca. 2000.

Ross, Ivan. *Medicinal Plants of the World.* Vol 1 Humana Press, Totowa, New Jersey. 1999.

_____ Vol 2 Humana Press, Totowa, N. J. 2002.

Rotella, Rev. Alexis. *The Essence of Flowers,* Jade Mountain Press, N.J. 1991.

Royer F. & Dickinson R. *Plants of Alberta.* Lone Pine Pub. Edmonton, AB. 2007.

Rudginsky, Marlene *The Flower Speaks.* U.S. Games Systems, Stamford, Conn. 1999.

Rupp, Rebecca. *Red Oaks and Black Birches* , Storey Comm. Garden Way Publishing. 1990

Russell, Sharman Apt. *Anatomy of a Rose.* Perseus Pub. Cambridge, Mass. 2001.

_____An Obsession with Butterflies. Perseus Publishing 2003.

Ryan, J et al, *Traditional Dene Medicine.* Lac La Martre NWT, 1993.

Ryden, Hope. *Wildflowers around the year.* Clarion Books, New York. 2001.

Ryrie, Charlie. Garden Folklore That Works. Reader's Digest. Pleasantville, NY 2001.

Sagadic O. & Ozcan M. *Food Control* 2003 14.

Salmon, Wm. *Botanologia: The English Herbal.* London: I. Dawkes, 1710.

Sandberg & Corrigan. *Natural Remedies, their origins and uses.* Taylor & Francis 2001.

Sanders, Jack. *The Secrets of Wildflowers.* The Lyons Press, Guilford, CT, 2003.

Sapolsky, Robert. *The Trouble with Testosterone.* Scribner, New York. 1997.

Sauer, Johann Christopher, Compendious Herbal-see Weaver below.

Savage, Candace. Bees, Nature's Little Wonders. Greystone Books. Vancouver 2008.

Schalkwijk-Barendsen, Helene. *Mushrooms of Western Canada* . Lone Pine Pub. 1991.

Schar, Douglas. *The Backyard Medicine Chest.* Elliott&Clark Pub. Washington, DC. 1995.

Scheffer, Mechthild, *Bach Flower Therapy, Theory and Practice,* Healing Arts Press, 1988

Schenk, George. *Moss Gardening.* Timber Press, Portland Oregon. 1997.

Schnaubelt, Kurt. *Medical Aromatherapy.* Frog Ltd. Berkeley CA. 1999.

Schneider, Anny. *Wild Medicinal Plants.* Key Porter Books, Toronto. 2002.

Schnell, Donald. *Carnivorous Plants.* 2nd Ed. Timber Press, Portland, Oregon, 2002.

Schofield, Janice. *Discovering Wild Plants.* Alaska Northwest Books. 1989.

_____*Nettles.* Keats Publishing, New Canaan, Conneticut, 1998.

Schulman, Robert. *Solve It With Supplements.* Rodale Press. New York. 2007.

Shapiro, R & Rapkins J. Awakening to the Plant Kingdom, Cassandra Press 1991.

Shauenberg, Paul and Paris. *Guide to Medicinal Plants.* Keats Publishing, 1977.

Shook, Edward Dr. *Advanced Treatise on Herbology* . Reprint Health Research.

Shosteck,Robert. *Flowers and Plants.* Quadrangle/The New York Times Book Co. 1974.

Siegfried, EV. Masters Thesis, Ethnobotany of the Northern Cree of Wabasca/Desmarais. U of Calgary, Alberta. 1994.

Silverman, Maida. *A City Herbal.* David R. Godine , 1990.

Silvertown, Jonathan. An Orchard Invisible. U of Chicago Press. 2009.

Simonot, Danielle. *Bio-Manufacturing in Saskatchewan-* Assessment of the Manufacturing Potential of Select Saskatchewan Plants, Sask. Nutraceutical Network, Saskatoon, 2000

Simpson, Brenan, M. *Flowers At My Feet,* Hancock House, Surrey, B.C. 1996.

Sionneau, P. *An Introduction to the Use of Processed Chinese Medicinals.* Blue Poppy Press, Second Printing 2003, Translated by Bob Flaws.

Smagghe, Guy Ed. Ecdysone: Structures and Functions. Springer Sci 2009.

Small, E & Catling, P. *Canadian Medicinal Crops,* NRC Research Press, Ottawa 1999.

Small, Ernest. *Culinary Herbs, Second Ed.* NRC Research Press, Ottawa, 2006.

_____*Medicinal Herbs,* NRC Research Press, Ottawa, 2000.

_____Top 100 Food Plants. NRC Press, Ottawa. 2009.

Smith, Andrew. *Strangers in the Garden, the Secret Lives of Our Favorite Flowers.*McClelland & Stewart 2004.

Smith, Annie Lorrain. *Lichens,* Cambridge at the University Press, 1921.

Smith, Harlan, *Ethnobotany of the Gitksan Indians of B.C.* Edited by B. Compton, B. Rigsby, and M.L. Tarpent, Mercury Series, Can Ethno Service, Paper 132, Can Mus of Civil. 1997.

Smith, Huron H. Manataka American Indian Council. www.manataka.org.

Snell, Alma Hogan. A Taste of Heritage. Crow Indian Recipes and Herbal Medicines. University of Nebraska Press 2006.

Soule, Deb. *The Roots of Healing, A Woman's Book of Herbs.* Citadel Press, 1995.

Spencer, Kate. *The Magic of Green Buckwheat ,*Richard Clay, England, 1987.

Spinella, Marcello. *The Psychopharmacology of Herbal Medicine.* MIT Press, 2001.

Steedman, E.V. *The Ethnobotany of the Thompson Indians of British Columbia.* 1930.

Stein, Sara. *My Weeds, A Gardener's Botany.* Harper and Row, 1988.

Stern, Gai. *Australian Weeds.* Harper and Row, Australia 1986

Stern Wm. *Stern's Dictionary of Plant Names for Gardeners.* Cassell Pub, London, 1972

Stewart, Hilary. *CEDAR.* Douglas & Mc Intyre. Vancouver/Toronto, 1984.

Storl, Wolf D. Healing Lyme Disease Naturally. NorthAtlantic Books, Berkeley, CA 2010.

Strehlow,W & Hertzka,G. *Hildegard of Bingen's Medicine* Bear & Co. Santa Fe 1988

Stuart, David. *Dangerous Garden.* Harvard University Press, Cambridge, Mass. 2004

Sturdivant L.&Blakley,T. *Medicinal Herbs in the Garden, Field and Marketplace* Bootstrap Guide, San Juan Naturals, Friday Harbor,WA, 1999.

Sumner, Judith. *The Natural History of Medicinal Plants.* Timber Press, Oregon, 2000.

Sun Bear & Wabun, *The Medicine Wheel* Prentice Hall, NJ 1980.

Swanton, J.R. *Haida Texts and Myths.* Bureau Am Ethnol, Bull #29. Smithsonian Inst. Washington, D.C. 1905.

_____*Bureau of Am Ethno 26th Ann Report.* Smithsonian Inst. Washington, 1908.

Szczeklik, Andrzej. Kore: On Sickness, the Sick and the Search for the Soul of Medicine. Counterpoint Berkeley 2012.

Tainter, D& Grenis A, *Spices and Seasonings ,* VCH Pubishers, New York, 1993.

Talalaj,S.& Czechowicz,A S. *Herbal Remedies,* Hill of Content Press, Melbourne, 1989

Taylor, Wm &Farnsworth,N. The Vinca Alkaloids, Marcel Dekker, New York, 1973.

Teeguarden, Ron. *The Ancient Wisdom of the Chinese Tonic Herbs.* Warner Bros. 1998.

Telesco, Patricia. *The Victorian Flower Oracle,* Llewellyn Pub. St. Paul 1994

Temple, Robert. *The Genius of China.* Simon and Schuster. New York. 1986.

Thompson, Gerry, *Astral Sex to Zen Teabags.* Findhorn Press, 1994.

Thoreau, Henry David. *Wild Fruits.* W. W. Norton & Co. New York, 2000.

Throop, Priscilla. *Hildegard von Bingen's Physica.* Healing Arts Press, Vt. 1998.

Tick, Edward. *The Practice of Dream Healing.* Quest Books Wheaton, Illinois, 2001.

Tierra, Michael. *The Way of Herbs- revised Pocket Rooks,* New York, 1998.

Tigner, Daniel. *Canadian Forest Tree Essences,* self published,1998. ISBN 0968365809

Tilford, Gregory. *Edible and Medicinal Plants of the West.* Mountain Press, Missoula 1997.

Timbrook, Jan. Chumash Ethnobotany. St. Barbara Mus, Heyday Books, Berkeley Ca 2007.

Traill, E.C. *Studies of Plant Life in Canada.* A. S. Woodburn, Ottawa, 1885.

Traill, C. P. *The Backwoods of Canada.* McClelland and Stewart. Toronto. 1846.

Tobyn, G., Denham, A., Whitelegg, M. The Western Herbal Tradition. 2000 years of medicinal herbal knowledge. Churchill Livingstone Toronto 2011.

Toop, Edgar W & Williams, Sara. *Perennials for the Prairies.* U of A&Saskatchewan. 1991.

Treben, Maria. *Health Through God's Pharmacy.* Wilhelm Ennsthaler. 1982.

Tresidder, Jack. Symbols and Their Meaning. Friedman/Fairfax Pub. 2007.

Tucker A. & DeBaggio,T. *The Big Book of Herbs.* Interweave Press. Loveland CO. 2000.

_____The Encylcopedia of Herbs. Timber Press, Portland. 2009.

Turkington, Carol. *The Home Health Guide to Poisons and Antidotes,* Facts on File 1994

Turner, Nancy J. *Food Plants of Interior First Peoples.* UBC Press, Vancouver, 1997.

_____*Food Plants of Coastal First Peoples.* UBC Press, Vancouver, 1995.

_____*Plant Technology of First Peoples in B.C.* UBC Press, Vancouver, 1998.

_____et al. *Thompson Ethnobotany.* Memoir #3, Royal B.C. Museum, 1996.

_____*Plants of Haida Gwaii.* Sononis Press, Winlaw, B.C. 2004.

_____The Earth's Blanket. Douglas & Mc Intyre. Vancouver. 2005.

Turner, N & von Aderkas, P. Common Poisonous Plants and Mushrooms. Timber Press 2009

Turner, W.B. *Fungal Metabolites,* Academic Press, London and New York, 1971.

Twitchell, Paul. *Herbs The Magic Healers.* Eckankar, Box 3100 Menlo Park, CA, 1986.

Vermeulen, Nico. *Encyclopedia of Herbs.* Whitecap Books, Vancouver B.C. 1998.

Viereck, Eleanor, G. *Alaska's Wilderness Medicines.* Alaska Northwest Pub. 1987

Vitt, Marsh and Bovey, *Mosses, Lichens, and Ferns,* Lone Pine Press, 1988.

Vogel, A. *Swiss Nature Doctor.* A. Vogel, Switzerland. 1952

_____*Nature-Your Guide to Healthy Living.* Verlag A. Vogel, Teufen, Switzerland 1986.

Vogel, Virgil. *American Indian Medicine,* U. of Oklahoma Press, Norman, 1970

Vortex Essences (Mt. Shasta Essences) www.vortexessences.com

Walker, Barbara. *The Woman's Dictionary of Symbols&Sacred Objects.* Csstle Books, 1988.

Walker, Marilyn. Wild Plants of Eastern Canada. Nimbus Pub. Halifax NS. 2008.

Ward, Bobby J. The Plant Hunter's Garden. Timber Press, Portland. 2004.

Ward-Harris, Joan.*More Than Meets the Eye, The Life and Lore of Western Wildflowers* Oxford University Press, Toronto, 1983

Watanabe & Shibuya. *Pharmacological Research on Traditional Herbal Medicines.* Harwood Academic Publishers, 1999.

Watt, John, and Breyer-Brandwijk, Maria *The Medicinal and Poisonous Plants of Southern and Eastern Africa* . E and S. Livingstone. Edinburgh and London. 1962.

Watts, Donald. Elsevier's Dictionary of Plant Lore. Elsevier. 2007.

Waugh, F.W. *Iroquois Foods and Food Preparation* #12 Anthropological Series, Ottawa. 1916. Reprinted by Iroqrafts, RR #2, Ohsweken, Ontario N0A 1M0, 1991.

Weaver, Wm. *100 Vegetables & Where They Came From*. Workman Pub. New York, 2000.

_____*Sauer's Herbal Cures America's First Book of Botanic Healing 1762-1778*, Routledge, New York, 2001.

Weed, Susan. *Menopausal Years, The Wise Woman Way*. Ash Tree Pub. Woodstock NY, 1992

Weigle, Marta. *Spiders and Spinsters*. U. of New Mexico Press, Albuquerque, 1982.

Weiner, M. *The People's Herbal, A family guide*. Putnam Publishing, New York, 1984.

Weiss, Rudolf. *Herbal Medicine*. Beaconsfield Publishers, 1988.

_____*Herbal Medicine* 2nd Edition. Thieme, Stuttgart, New York, 2000.

Wells, Diana.*100 Flowers and How They Got Their Names*, Algonquin Books, Chapel Hill,97

Westcott, Frank. *The Beaver Nature's Master Builder*. Hounslow Press, Willowdale, ON '89.

Westrich, LoLo, *California Herbal Remedies*, Gulf Pub Co. Houston, TX, 1989.

Wetzel, Suzanne et al. Bioproducts from Canada's Forests. Springer Netherlands 2006.

WHO monographs on selected medicinal plants, vol 1, 1999; vol 2, 2002.

White, Ian. *Australian Bush Flower Essences*. Bantam Books, 1991

White, Florence. *Flowers as Food* . Jonathan Cape. 1934

Whitmont, Edward. *Psyche and Substance*. North Atlantic Books. 1980

Wilkinson, Kathleen. *Trees and Shrubs of Alberta*. Lone Pine Books, Edmonton 1990.

_____*Wildflowers of Alberta*. U of A/Lone Pine Books, Edmonton 1999.

Williams, Jude. *Nature's Gentle Cures*. Sterling Publishing. New York. 1997.

Williamson, Darcy. 130 Medicinal Plant Monographs of the NW. self pub. E-book. 2011.

Williamson, E. *Major Herbs of Ayurveda*. Churchill Livingstone, Elsevier Science, 2002.

FLOWER ESSENCE RESOURCES

Aditi Himalaya Flower Essences, 15,Jaybharat Society, 3rd Road, Khar (W), Bombay 400 052, India.

Alaskan Flower Essence Project, P.O. Box. 1369, Homer, Alaska USA 99603-1369. www.alaskanessences.com.

Australian Bush Flower Essences. Australia. www.ausflowers.com.au.

Bach- Healing Herbs English Flower Essences- in Canada by Self Heal Distributing, Box 95008, Whyte Postal Outlet, Edmonton, AB T6E 0E5, 1800-593-5956 or www.selfhealdistributing.com Also www.healingherbs.co.uk or www.fesflowers.com

Bailey Flower Essences, 8 Neslon Road, Ilkley, West Yorkshire England, LS298HN. www.flowervr.com

Bloesem Remedies. Netherlands. www.bloesem-remedies.com

BrynaHerb Essences. www.brynaherbessences.uk

Canadian Forest Essences, PO Box 29128,1996 W. Broadway, Vancouver, BC V6J 1Z0

Canadian Forest Tree Essences. Ottawa. www.essences.ca. 613-725-9764.

Choming Flower Essences. www.mkprojects.com

Clear Path Essences. www.clearpathessences.com

Dancing Light Orchid Essences. Fairbanks, Alaska. www.orchidessences.com

Desert Alchemy, PO Box 44189, Tucson, Arizona, USA 85733. www.desert-alchemy.com.

Deva Flower Essences BP3 38880, Autrans, France. www.lab-deva.com

Eastern Flower Herbal Essences. julied@hfx.eastlink.ca.

Falling Leaf Essences. Box 78, Kallista, Victoria 3791, Australia. www.advancedalchemy.com.au.

Findhorn Flower Essences, Morayshire, Scotland IV36 0TY. www.findhornessences.com

Florais des Minas, Rua Albita, 194-Sala 408, Cruziero, CEP 30310-160,BH, MG, BRAZIL

FlorAlive®, Brent Davis. Contact info@floralive.com

FES Flower Essence Society, PO Box 1769, Nevada City, California, USA, 95959. www.fesflowers.com Canadian Distributor- Self Heal Distributing, Box 95008, Whyte Postal Outlet, Edmonton, AB T6E 0E5 – www.selfhealdistributing.com

Green Hope Farm Flower Essences, PO Box 125, Meriden, New Hampshire USA 03770

Green Man Tree Essences. www.greenmantrees.demon.co.uk.

Habundia Flower Essences. c/o Peter Aziz. PO Box 90, Totnes, Devon, England TQ11 0YG.

Harebell Remedies. Scotland. ellie@harebellremedies.co.uk.

Hawaiian Gaia Flower Essences. www.gaiaessences.com

High Sierra Flower Essences. PO. Box 4275 Truclee, CA 96160. holly.hsb@highoctavehealing.com

Horus Flower Essences- horus@floweressences.de.

Hummingbird Remedies, PO Box 50161, Eugene, Oregon, USA 97405

Icelandic Flower Essences. www.kristbjorb.is.

Jade Mountain Flower Essences, Box 125, Mountain Lakes, New Jersey USA 07046-0125

Korte Phi. www.PHIessences.com

Light Heart Essences. England. www.lightheartessences.co.uk.

Light Mountain Flower Essences, Michael A. Vertolli, 1-800-667-HERB.

Living Essences of Australia, Box 355, Scarborough, 6019, Perth, Australia. www.livingessences.com.au

Living Flower Essences, www.livingfloweressences.com . Rhonda Pallasdowney.

Master's Flower Essences, 14618 Tyler Foote Rd Nevada City, California, USA, 95959. www.masteressences.com

Miriana fortem Flower Essences. www.mirianaflowers.com and info@miraflowers.com.

NaturaSacredplay, PO Box 32, Buckhorn, New Mexico, 88025, (505-535-2255).

New Millenium Flower Essences of New Zealand. info@nmessences.com.

New Zealand New Perception Flower Essences, PO Box 60-127,Titirangi, Auckland 7, NZ

Pacific Essences, Box 8317, Victoria, B.C. V8W 3R9. www.pacificessences.com.

Pegasus Products, PO Box 228, Boulder, Colorado, USA 80306-0228. 1-800- 527-6104.

Perelandra, Box 3603, Warrenton, VA. 22186. www.perelandra-ltd.com

Petite Fleur Essence, 8524 Whispering Creek Trail, Fort Worth, Texas, USA 76134. www.aromahealthtexas.com

Prairie Deva Flower Essences, Box 95008, Whyte Postal Outlet, Edmonton, AB T6E 0E5 1-(780) 433-7882. www.selfhealdistributing.com

Ravenworks- joni@ravenworksministries.org

Running Fox Farm PO Box 381,Worthington, Maryland USA 01098

Star Peruvian Flower Essences. Santa Barbara. www.starfloweressences.com

Stars of the Meadow, David Dalton, Lindisfarne Books, Mass. 2006.

Sun Essences. Norfolk, England. www.sunessence.co.uk

Sweetwater Sanctuary Essences. www.plantspirithealing.com

Tree Frog Farm Flower Essences. www.treefrogfarm.com

Whole Energy Essences, PO Box 285, Concord, Mass. 01742

Wild Rose Essences. www.wildrose.com

Woodland Essence, PO Box 206, Cold Brook, New York, USA 13324.

www.ingramcontent.com/pod-product-compliance
Lightning Source LLC
Chambersburg PA
CBHW081108170526
45165CB00008B/2370